Head, Neck, and Neuroanatomy

THIEME Atlas of Anatomy
Third Edition

Latin Nomenclature

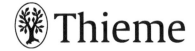

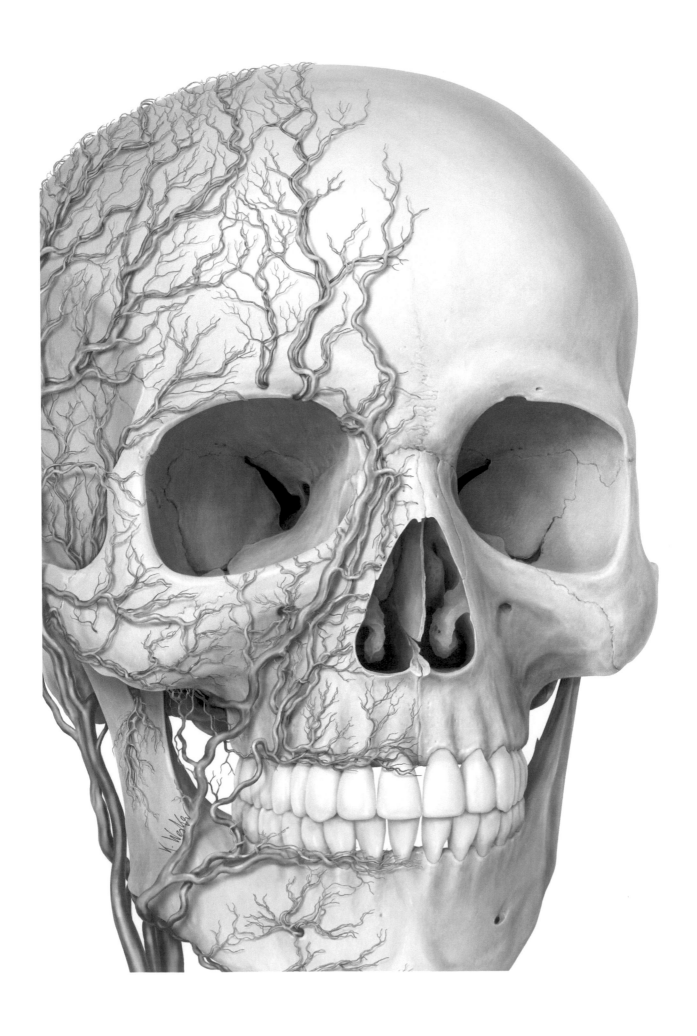

Head, Neck, and Neuroanatomy

THIEME Atlas of Anatomy
Third Edition

Latin Nomenclature

Authors

Michael Schuenke, MD, PhD
Institute of Anatomy
Christian Albrechts University, Kiel

Erik Schulte, MD
Institute of Functional and
Clinical Anatomy
Johannes Gutenberg University, Mainz

Udo Schumacher, MD
FRCPath, CBiol, FIBiol, DSc
Institute of Anatomy and Experimental
Morphology
University Medical Center,
Hamburg-Eppendorf

Illustrations by
Markus Voll
Karl Wesker

Consulting Editor
Cristian Stefan, MD
Department of Basic Science and
Craniofacial Biology
New York University College of Dentistry

Consulting Editor, Latin Nomenclature
Hugo Zeberg, MD
Department of Neuroscience
Karolinska Institute, Stockholm

Thieme
New York • Stuttgart • Delhi • Rio de Janeiro

Translators: Terry Telger, John Grossman, and Judith Tomat

Illustrators: Markus Voll and Karl Wesker

Compositor: DiTech Process Solutions

Library of Congress Cataloging-in-Publication Data is available from the publisher

Thieme Medical Publishers, Inc.
333 Seventh Avenue, 18th Floor
New York, NY 10001, USA
www.thieme.com
+1 800 782 3488, customerservice@thieme.com

Printed in Germany by Beltz Grafische Betriebe   5 4 3 2

ISBN 978-1-68420-086-3

Also available as an e-book:
eISBN 978-1-68420-087-0

Important note: Medicine is an ever-changing science undergoing continual development. Research and clinical experience are continually expanding our knowledge, in particular our knowledge of proper treatment and drug therapy. Insofar as this book mentions any dosage or application, readers may rest assured that the authors, editors, and publishers have made every effort to ensure that such references are in accordance with **the state of knowledge at the time of production of the book**.

Nevertheless, this does not involve, imply, or express any guarantee or responsibility on the part of the publishers in respect to any dosage instructions and forms of applications stated in the book. **Every user is requested to examine carefully** the manufacturer's leaflets accompanying each drug and to check, if necessary in consultation with a physician or specialist, whether the dosage schedules mentioned therein or the contraindications stated by the manufacturers differ from the statements made in the present book. Such examination is particularly important with drugs that are either rarely used or have been newly released on the market. Every dosage schedule or every form of application used is entirely at the user's own risk and responsibility. The authors and publishers request every user to report to the publishers any discrepancies or inaccuracies noticed. If errors in this work are found after publication, errata will be posted at www.thieme.com on the product description page.

Some of the product names, patents, and registered designs referred to in this book are in fact registered trademarks or proprietary names even though specific reference to this fact is not always made in the text. Therefore, the appearance of a name without designation as proprietary is not to be construed as a representation by the publisher that it is in the public domain.

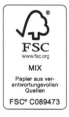

Foreword

Each of the authors of the single-volume *Thieme Atlas of Anatomy* was impressed with the extraordinary detail, accuracy, and beauty of the illustrations that were created for the Thieme three-volume series of anatomy atlases. We felt these images were one of the most significant additions to anatomic education in the past 50 years. The effective pedagogical approach of this series, with two-page learning units that combined the outstanding illustrations and captions that emphasized the functional and clinical significance of structures, coupled with the numerous tables summarizing key information, was unique. We also felt that the overall organization of each region, with structures presented first systemically—musculoskeletal, vascular, and nervous—and then topographically, supported classroom learning and active dissection in the laboratory.

This series combines the best of a clinically oriented text and an atlas. Its detail and pedagogical presentation make it a complete support for class and laboratory instruction and a reference for life in all the medical, dental, and allied health fields. Each of the volumes—*General Anatomy and Musculoskeletal System*, *Internal Organs*, and *Head, Neck, and Neuroanatomy*— can also be used as a stand-alone text/atlas for an in-depth study of systems often involved in the allied health/medical specialty fields.

We were delighted when Thieme asked us to work with them to create a single-volume atlas from this groundbreaking series, and we owe a great debt to the authors and illustrators of this series inasmuch as their materials and vision formed the general framework for the single-volume *Thieme Atlas of Anatomy.*

We thank the authors and illustrators for this very special contribution to the teaching of anatomy and recommend it for thorough mastery of anatomy and its clinically functional importance in all fields of health care-related specialties.

Lawrence M. Ross, Brian R. MacPherson, and *Anne M. Gilroy*

A Note on the Use of Latin Terminology

To introduce the Latin nomenclature into an English-language text-book is a delicate task, particularly because many Latin loanwords have passed into general use. Some loanwords are so common that fluency of the text would be disturbed if they were to be translated back into Latin. These Latin loanwords have typically undergone several adaptations before becoming part of the English language. A term such as *sympathetic trunk* (lat. *truncus sympaticus*) has undergone morphological adaptation (through the loss of masculine suffix -us), orthographical adaptation (through the substitution of a "Germanic" k for a Latin c), and phonological adaptation (th and e instead of t and i). In addition, the word order has been reversed. The Latin term *sympaticus* is in fact borrowed from the late Greek word *sympathetikos* (from sympathes "having a fellow feeling, affected by like feelings"), thereby illustrating that words move between languages when cultures meet. Other anatomical terms are so colloquial (e.g. *hand*), that a Latin word (e.g. *manus*) would be inappropriate to use at all occasions. Clearly, the text would become unreadable if a strict translation of all English terms into Latin were imposed.

As a result, Latin has been used as long as it does not disrupt the flow of the text and whenever possible in figures and tables. In some cases, dual terminology has been used, with either the English or Latin word in parentheses. As much as possible, the terminology of *Terminolgia Anatomica* (1998) has been followed.

Hugo Zeberg

Preface of the Authors and Illustrators

When Thieme started planning the first edition of this atlas, they sought the opinions of students and instructors alike in both the United States and Europe on what constituted an "ideal" atlas of anatomy — ideal to learn from, to master extensive amounts of information while on a busy class schedule, and, in the process, to acquire sound, up-to-date knowledge. The result of our work in response to what Thieme had learned is this atlas. The *Thieme Atlas of Anatomy*, unlike most other atlases, is a comprehensive educational tool that combines illustrations with explanatory text and summary tables, introducing clinical applications throughout, and presenting anatomic concepts in a step-by-step sequence that includes system-by-system and topographical views.

For the first edition we had hoped that our *Atlas of Anatomy* would help the medical student to understand the anatomical basis of clinical medicine. This indeed was accepted by the students all over the world and soon a second edition had to come on the market in Germany, which was extensively extended and revised. More and more information had been added, including spreads on important foundational information on the common imaging planes for plain film, MRI, and CT scans, the structure of skeletal muscle fibers, the structure and chemical composition of hyaline cartilage, and the regeneration of peripheral nerves, bone marrow, and paraganglia, as well as new graphical summaries in neuroanatomy. Hence the fifth German edition looks ever more distinctly different from the first one. Of course, we have also checked, corrected, and updated all of the information in this atlas.

We are grateful to the American branch of Thieme that they have made this third English edition possible. We hope that this updated version will serve the medical students and practitioners of medicine alike in helping them to understand human morphology which is indispensable for diagnosis and therapy.

Michael Schünke, Erik Schulte, Udo Schumacher,
Markus Voll, and Karl Wesker

Acknowledgments

First we wish to thank our families. This atlas is dedicated to them.

Since the publication of the first volume of the *Thieme Atlas of Anatomy* in 2006, we have received numerous suggestions for refinements and additions. We would like to take this opportunity to express our sincere thanks to all those who through the years have helped us to improve the *Thieme Atlas of Anatomy* in one way or another. Specifically, this includes Kirsten Hattermann, Ph.D.; Runhild Lucius, D.D.S.; Prof. Renate Lüllmann-Rauch, M.D.; Prof. Jobst Sievers, M.D.; Ali Therany, D.D.S.; Prof. Thilo Wedel, M.D. (all at the Anatomic Institute of Christian Albrecht University of Kiel); as well as Christian Friedrichs, D.D.S. (Practice for Tooth Preservation and Endodontics, Kiel); Prof. Reinhart Gossrau, M.D. (Charité Berlin, Institute of Anatomy); Prof. Paul Peter Lunkenheimer, M.D. (Westphalian Wilhelm University Münster); Thomas Müller, M.D., associate professor (Institute of Functional and Clinical Anatomy of the Johannes Gutenberg University of Mainz); Kai-Hinrich Olms, M.D., Foot Surgery, Bad Schwartau; Daniel Paech, M.S. physics, medical student (Department of Neuroradiology of the University Medical Center, Heidelberg); Thilo Schwalenberg, M.D., supervising physician (Urologic Clinic of the University Medical Center, Leipzig); Prof. emeritus Katharina Spanel-Borowski, M.D. (University of Leipzig); Prof. Christoph Viebahn, M.D. (Georg August University of Göttingen). For their extensive proofreading we thank Gabriele Schünke, M.S. biology; Jakob Fay, M.D.; as well as medical students Claudia Dücker, Simin Rassouli, Heike Teichmann, Susanne Tippmann, and dental student Sylvia Zilles; also, Julia Jörns-Kuhnke, M.D., especially for her assistance with the figure labels.

We extend special thanks to Stephanie Gay and Bert Sender, who prepared the layouts. Their ability to arrange the text and illustrations on facing pages for maximum clarity has contributed greatly to the quality of the atlas.

We particularly acknowledge the efforts of those who handled this project on the publishing side:

Jürgen Lüthje, M.D., Ph.D., executive editor at Thieme Medical Publishers, has "made the impossible possible." He not only reconciled the wishes of the authors and artists with the demands of reality but also managed to keep a team of five people working together for years on a project whose goal was known to us from the beginning but whose full dimensions we only came to appreciate over time. He is deserving of our most sincere and heartfelt thanks once more this year, in which Jürgen Lüthje, M.D., Ph.D., is retiring. We welcome his successor Dr. Jochen Neuberger, who has shown great initiative in taking over the *Thieme Atlas of Anatomy* and will continue to lead and develop the existing team.

Sabine Bartl, developmental editor, became a touchstone for the authors in the best sense of the word. She was able to determine whether a beginning student, and thus one who is not (yet) a professional, could clearly appreciate the logic of the presentation. The authors are indebted to her.

We are grateful to Antje Bühl, who was there from the beginning as project assistant, working "behind the scenes" on numerous tasks such as repeated proofreading and helping to arrange the figure labels.

We owe a great debt of thanks to Martin Spencker, managing director of Educational Publications at Thieme, especially to his ability to make quick and unconventional decisions when dealing with problems and uncertainties. His openness to all the concerns of the authors and artists established conditions for a cooperative partnership.

We are also indebted to Yvonne Strassburg, Michael Zepf, and Laura Diemand who saw to it that the *Thieme Atlas of Anatomy* was printed and bound on schedule, and that the project benefited from the best practical expertise throughout the entire process of publication. We also thank Susanne Tochtermann-Wenzel and Anja Jahn for their assistance with technical issues involving every aspect of the illustrations; Julia Fersch who ensured that the *Thieme Atlas of Anatomy* is also accessible via eRef; Almut Leopold for the exceptional index; Marie-Luise Kürschner and Nina Jentschke for the appealing cover design; as well as Dr. Thomas Krimmer, Liesa Arendt, Birgit Carlsen, Stephanie Eilmann, and Anne Döbler, representing all those now and previously involved in the marketing, sale, and promotion of the *Thieme Atlas of Anatomy*.

The authors, October 2019

As consulting editor I was asked to review, for accuracy and appropriateness, the English translation of the *Thieme Atlas of Anatomy: Head, Neck, and Neuroanatomy, Third Edition*. My work involved a review and edit of the translation, conversion of nomenclature to terms in common usage in English, and some small changes in presentation to reflect accepted approaches to certain anatomic structures in North American anatomy programs. This task was eased greatly by the clear organization of the original text. In all of this, I have tried diligently to remain faithful to the intentions and insights of the authors and illustrators, whom I wish to thank for this outstanding revision.

In remembrance of Ancuta (Anca) M. Stefan, M.D.

Cristian Stefan

It has been a great honor to act as a consulting editor, with responsibility for the Latin nomenclature, for *Thieme Atlas of Anatomy: Head, Neck, and Neuroanatomy, Third Edition*. There were several people from whom I received a great deal of assistance and guidance, and must express my gratitude towards. Regarding the discussion of nomenclature, I would wish to thank my mentor Prof. Peter Århem, Ph.D., my father Lennart Zeberg, M.D., and Prof. Jonas Broman, Ph.D. In addition, I would also like to express my gratitude to Prof. Björn Meister, M.D., Ph.D., for putting forward my name for this task.

Moreover, I am deeply grateful to the staff at Thieme Medical Publishers that I have been in close contact with, in particular, the editorial director Anne Sydor, Ph.D., managing editor Judith Tomat, editorial assistant Huvie Weinreich, and marketing agent David Towle.

I would also like to acknowledge the Federative International Programme for Anatomical Terminology (FIPAT) for their work towards a standard nomenclature in the field of anatomy.

In addition, I would like to express my gratitude to my talented assistant teachers — C. Stening-Soppola, D.F. Åström, A. Javanmardi, E.N. Sögutlu, A. Sotoodeh, N. Aziz, A.-M. Al-Khabbaz, K. Ma, and T. Engström — for performing an initial review of the Latin nomenclature.

Hugo Zeberg

The people behind the *Thieme Atlas of Anatomy*

A work such as the *Thieme Atlas of Anatomy* can only arise when the people involved in the project work hand in hand. The integrated educational and artistic work you now hold in your hands is the product of an intensive discourse between anatomy professors Michael Schünke, Erik Schulte, and Udo Schumacher and anatomic illustrators Markus Voll and Karl Wesker.

Creating learning units that comprehensively treat a topic on a two-page spread is a challenge in itself. The authors must carefully select the content, assemble it, and add explanatory legends. Yet how this content is presented in the atlas, how appealing and memorable it is, depends largely on the illustrations. And the *Thieme Atlas of Anatomy* now includes a good 5000 of them. In creating them, Markus Voll and

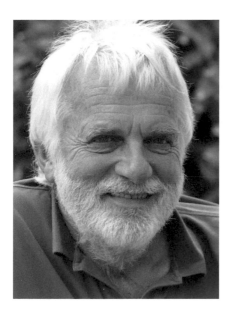 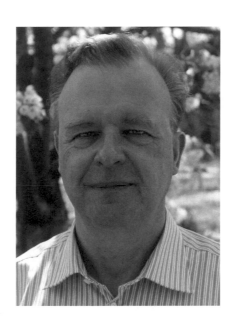 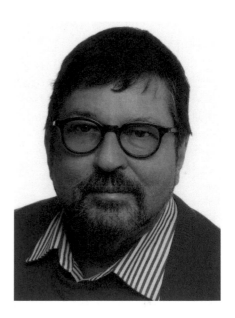

Michael Schünke, MD, PhD, professor

Institute of Anatomy of the University of Kiel, studied biology and medicine in Tübingen and Kiel, extensive teaching of medical students and physical therapists, author and translator of other textbooks.

Erik Schulte, MD, professor

Institute of Functional and Clinical Anatomy of the Johannes Gutenberg University of Mainz, studied medicine in Freiburg, extensive teaching of medical students, award for excellence in teaching in Mainz.

Udo Schumacher, MD, professor

Institute of Anatomy of the University of Hamburg; studied medicine in Kiel with one year of study at the Wistar Institute of Anatomy and Biology in Philadelphia; extensive teaching of medical students, physical therapists, and residents (FRCS). Spent several years in Southampton and gained experience in integrated interdisciplinary instruction.

Karl Wesker drew on many years of experience in anatomic illustration, visited anatomic collections, studied specimens, and immersed themselves in old and new works of anatomy. This was the foundation on which the *Thieme Atlas of Anatomy* arose.

It guides the reader through anatomy step by step, revealing what a crucial role anatomy will later play in medical practice. This was a particularly important consideration for the authors. Whether performing bowel surgery for a tumor, puncturing the tympanic membrane in a middle ear infection, or examining a pregnant patient, no physician lacking knowledge of anatomy is a good physician. Even the *Thieme Atlas of Anatomy* cannot spare you the effort of learning, yet the authors and illustrators can assure you that it will make it a lot more pleasant.

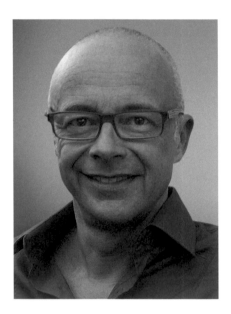 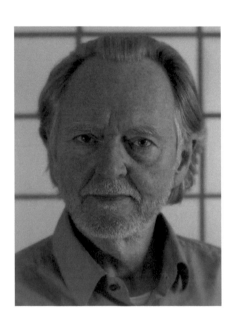

Markus Voll

Freelance illustrator and graphic artist in Munich, trained as an artist at the Blocherer School of Design in Munich, studied medicine at the University of Munich. He has worked as a scientific illustrator on numerous book projects for 25 years.

Karl Wesker

Freelance painter and graphic artist in Berlin. Apprenticeship as a plate etcher and lithographer, studied visual communication at the University of Applied Sciences in Münster and at the Berlin University of the Arts and art science at the Technical University of Berlin. For over 30 years he has been active as a freelance painter and graphic artist, including book projects in anatomy.

Contents

A Head and Neck

1 Overview

2 Bones, Ligaments, and Joints

3 Classification of the Muscles

4 Classification of the Neurovascular Structures

B Neuroanatomy

Table of Contents

C CNS:
Glossary and Synopsis

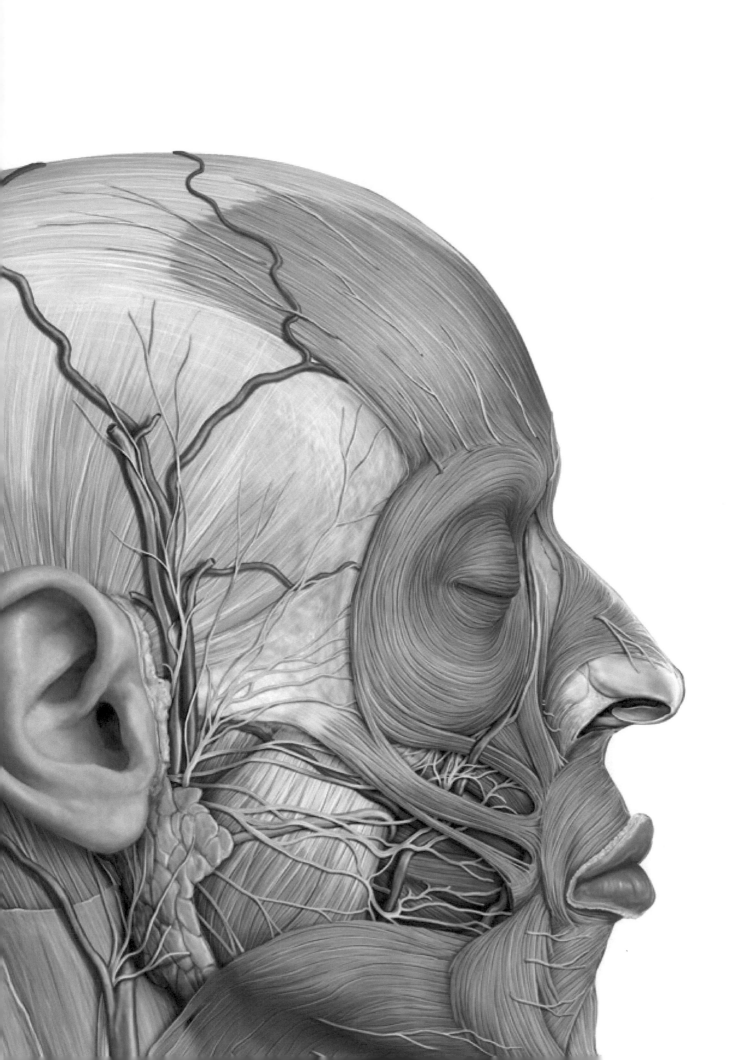

Head and Neck

1.1   Regions and Palpable Bony Landmarks

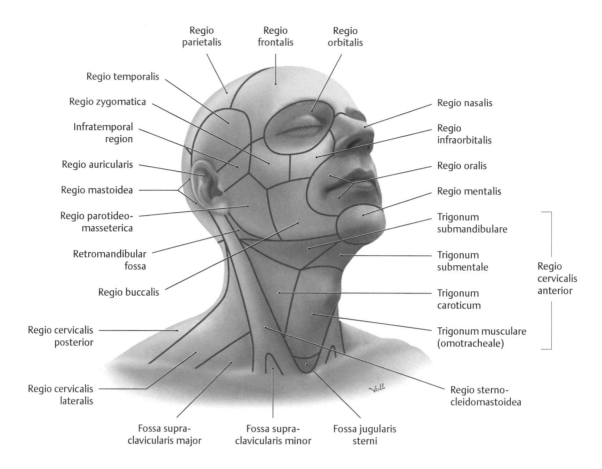

A Head and neck regions
Right anterior view.

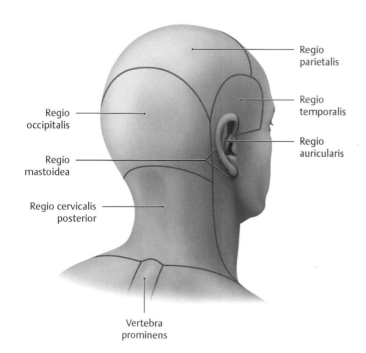

B Head and neck regions
Right posterior view.

C Head and neck regions

Head regions	Neck regions
• Regio frontalis	• Regio cervicalis anterior
• Regio parietalis	– Trigonum submandibulare
• Regio occipitalis	– Trigonum caroticum
• Regio temporalis	– Trigonum musculare
• Regio auricularis	(omotracheale)
• Regio mastoidea	– Trigonum submentale
• Regio facialis	
– Regio orbitalis	• Regio sternocleidomastoidea
– Regio infraorbitalis	– Fossa supraclavicularis minor
– Regio buccalis	
– Regio parotideomasseterica	• Regio cervicalis lateralis
– Regio zygomatica	– Trigonum omoclaviculare
– Regio nasalis	(fossa supraclavicularis
– Regio oralis	major)
– Regio mentalis	
	• Regio cervicalis posterior

The regions of the head and neck are clinically important since they can exhibit many skin lesions, the location of which must be precisely described. This is particularly important for skin cancer given that the tissue fluid, through which the tumor cells spread, drains into different groups of lymph nodes named for their location.

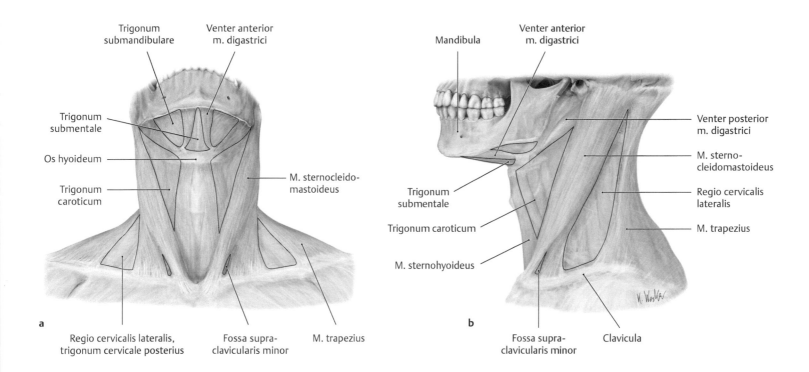

Trigonum submandibulare

Venter anterior m. digastrici

Trigonum submentale

Os hyoideum

Trigonum caroticum

M. sternocleido-mastoideus

a

Regio cervicalis lateralis, trigonum cervicale posterius

Fossa supra-clavicularis minor

M. trapezius

Mandibula

Venter anterior m. digastrici

Venter posterior m. digastrici

M. sterno-cleidomastoideus

Trigonum submentale

Regio cervicalis lateralis

Trigonum caroticum

M. trapezius

M. sternohyoideus

b

Fossa supra-clavicularis minor

Clavicula

D Regions of the neck (cervical regions)
a Right lateral view; **b** Left posterior oblique view.

These neck muscles are easily visible and palpable, making them suitable as landmarks for a topographical classification of the neck.

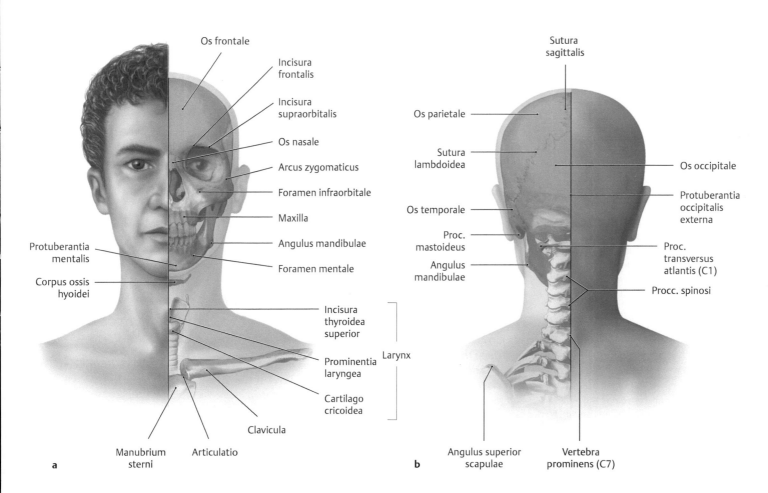

Os frontale

Incisura frontalis

Incisura supraorbitalis

Os nasale

Arcus zygomaticus

Foramen infraorbitale

Maxilla

Angulus mandibulae

Foramen mentale

Protuberantia mentalis

Corpus ossis hyoidei

Incisura thyroidea superior

Prominentia laryngea

Larynx

Cartilago cricoidea

Clavicula

a

Manubrium sterni

Articulatio

Sutura sagittalis

Os parietale

Sutura lambdoidea

Os temporale

Proc. mastoideus

Angulus mandibulae

Os occipitale

Protuberantia occipitalis externa

Proc. transversus atlantis (C1)

Procc. spinosi

b

Angulus superior scapulae

Vertebra prominens (C7)

E Palpable bony landmarks at the head and neck
a Frontal view; **b** Dorsal view.

3

1.2 Head and Neck and Cervical Fasciae

The head and neck form an anatomical and functional unit with the neck connecting the head and the trunk. The neck contains many pathways to which the cervical viscera are indirectly attached. In the head however, there is only visceral fascia around the glandula parotidea but no general fasciae. Multiple fascial layers subdivide the neck into compartments which will be referred to when describing the location of structures within the neck.

A Sequence of topics in this chapter about the head and neck

Overview	• Regions and palpable bony landmarks • Head and neck with cervical fasciae • Clinical anatomy of the head and neck • Embryology of the face • Embryology of the neck
Bones	• Cranial bones • Teeth • Cervical spine • Ligaments • Joints
Muscles	• Muscles of facial expression • Mm. masticatorii • Neck muscles
Classification of pathways	• Arteries • Veins • Lymphatics • Nerves
Organs and their pathways	• Ear • Eye • Nose • Cavitas oris • Pharynx • Gl. parotidea • Larynx • Gl. thyoridea and gl. parathyoridea
Topographical anatomy	• Anterior facial region • Neck, anterior view, superficial layers • Neck, anterior view, deep layers • Lateral head: superficial layer • Lateral head: middle and deeper layer • Fossa infratemporalis • Fossa pterygopalatina • Regio cervicalis lateralis • Apertura thoracis superior, trigonum caroticum, and trigonum omoclaviculare • Regio cervicalis posterior and regio occipitalis • Cross-section of the head and neck

B Fascia cervicalis
Deep to the skin is the superficial cervical fascia (subcutaneous tissue) which contains the platysma muscle anterolaterally. Deep to the superficial are the following layers of fascia cervicalis:

1. Lamina superficialis: envelops the entire neck, and splits to enclose the m. sternocleidomastoideus and m. trapezius.
2. Lamina pretrachealis: the muscular portion encloses the mm. infrahyoidei, while the visceral portion surrounds the gl. thyoridea, larynx, trachea, pharynx, and oesophagus.
3. Lamina prevertebralis: surrounds the cervical columna vertebralis, and the muscles associated with it.
4. Vagina carotica: encloses the a. carotis communis, v. jugularis interna, and n. vagus.
5. Visceral fascia: encloses the larynx, trachea, pharynx, oesophagus, and gl. thyoridea.

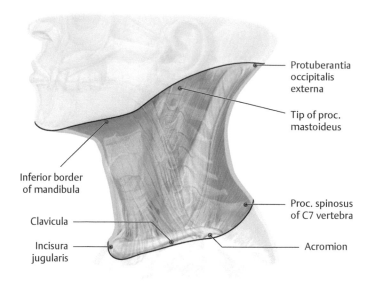

C Superficial and inferior boundaries of the neck
Left lateral view. The following palpable structures define the superior and inferior boundaries of the neck:

• Superior boundaries: inferior border of the mandibula, tip of the proc. mastoideus, and protuberantia occipitalis externa
• Inferior boundaries: incisura jugularis, clavicula, acromion, and proc. spinosus of the C 7 vertebra.

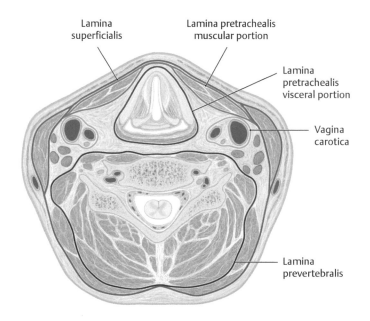

D Relationships of the fascia cervicalis in the neck. Transverse section at the level of the C 5 vertebra
The full extent of the fascia cervicalis is best appreciated in a transverse section of the neck:

• The *muscle fascia* splits into three layers:
  – Lamina superficialis (orange),
  – Lamina pretrachealis (green), and
  – Lamina prevertebralis (violet).
• There is also a neurovascular fascia, called the *vagina carotica* (light blue), and
• a *visceral fascia* (dark blue).

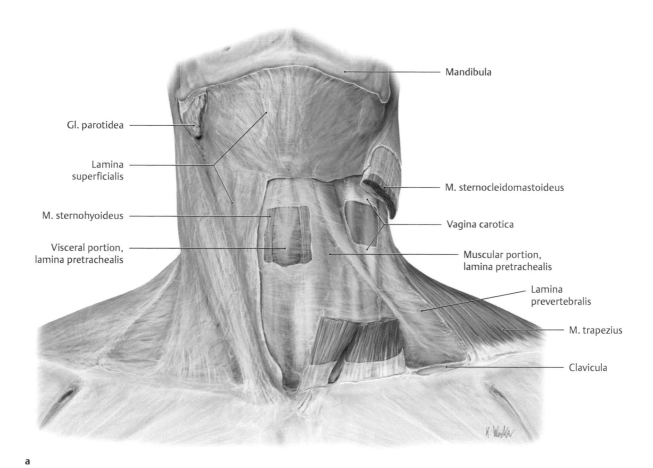

Mandibula

Gl. parotidea

Lamina superficialis

M. sternocleidomastoideus

M. sternohyoideus

Vagina carotica

Visceral portion, lamina pretrachealis

Muscular portion, lamina pretrachealis

Lamina prevertebralis

M. trapezius

Clavicula

a

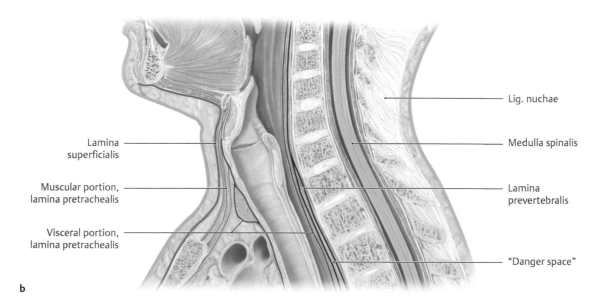

Lig. nuchae

Lamina superficialis

Medulla spinalis

Muscular portion, lamina pretrachealis

Lamina prevertebralis

Visceral portion, lamina pretrachealis

"Danger space"

b

E Fascial relationships in the neck

a Anterior view. The cutaneous muscle of the neck, the platysma, is highly variable in its development and is subcutaneous in location, overlying the superficial cervical fascia. In the dissection shown, the platysma has been removed at the level of the inferior mandibular border on each side. The cervical fasciae form a fibrous sheet that encloses the muscles, neurovascular structures, and cervical viscera (see **B** for further details). These fasciae subdivide the neck into spaces, some of which are open superiorly and inferiorly for the passage of neurovascular structures. The *lamina superficialis* of the fascia superficialis has been removed at left center in this dissection. Just deep to the lamina superficialis is the *muscular portion of the lamina pretrachealis*, part of which has been removed to display the *visceral portion of the lamina pretrachealis*. The neurovascular structures are surrounded by a condensation of the fascia cervicalis called

the *vagina carotica*. The deepest layer of the fascia cervicalis, called the *lamina prevertebralis*, is visible posteriorly on the left side. These fascia-bounded connective-tissue spaces in the neck are important clinically because they provide routes for the spread of inflammatory processes, although the inflammation may (at least initially) remain confined to the affected compartment.

b Left lateral view. This midsagittal section shows that the deepest layer of the fascia cervicalis, the lamina prevertebralis, directly overlies the columna vertebralis in the median plane and is split into two parts. With tuberculous osteomyelitis of the cervical spine, for example, a gravitation abscess may develop in the "danger space" along the lamina prevertebralis (retropharyngeal abscess). This fascia encloses muscles laterally and posteriorly (see **D**). The vagina carotica is located farther laterally and does not appear in the midsagittal section.

5

1.3 Clinical Anatomy

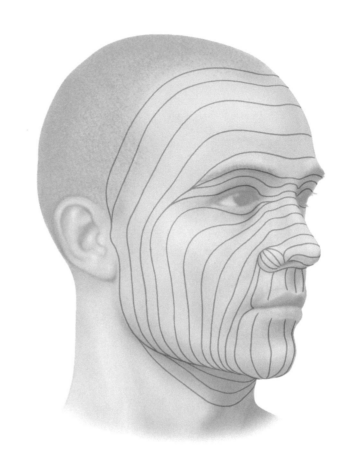

A Cleavage or tension lines
Anterior oblique view.
Skin and its subcutaneous tissue are under tension, explaining why a small, round needle hole can result in a small longish slit in the skin aligned along the tension lines in the area around the incision. To promote swift healing and reduce visible scarring, incisions in the head region are aligned along these tension lines. Knowledge of the tension line patterns in the face and neck are critically important in plastic surgery to minimize scarring in these highly visible areas.

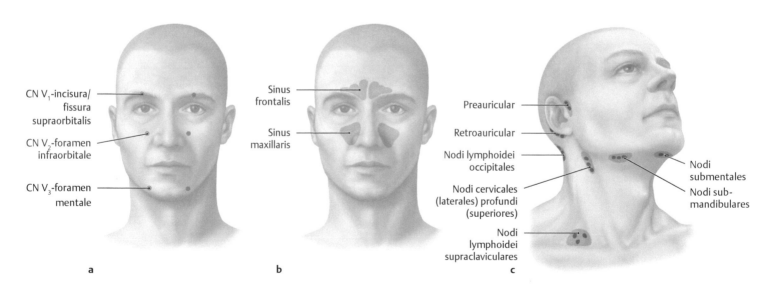

CN V₁-incisura/ fissura supraorbitalis

CN V₂-foramen infraorbitale

CN V₃-foramen mentale

Sinus frontalis

Sinus maxillaris

Preauricular

Retroauricular

Nodi lymphoidei occipitales

Nodi cervicales (laterales) profundi (superiores)

Nodi lymphoidei supraclaviculares

Nodi submentales

Nodi sub-mandibulares

a   b   c

B Projection of clinically important structures onto the head and neck
Frontal view (**a** and **b**) and right lateral view (**c**).

a Exit points of the n. trigeminus (CN V-sensory): These points are important for sensory testing of the head. If the pressure of a fingertip placed at these exit points causes pain, the respective branch of the n. trigeminus is stimulated.

b Skin areas above the sinus paranasales: When sinus paranasales are inflamed, the skin areas above them are sensitive to pressure, causing pain.

c Superficial lymph nodes at the junction between head and neck: The most important of lymph node groups are shown here. If the lymph nodes are enlarged, the cause can be related to inflammation or a tumor in the tributary area of the nodes. During a clinical examination of the head, these lymph node groups are always palpated.

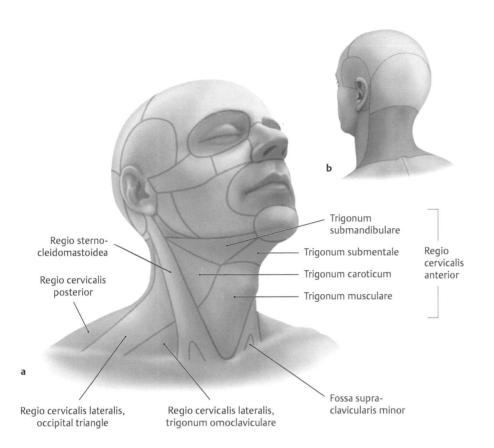

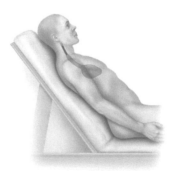

Regio sterno-
cleidomastoidea

Regio cervicalis
posterior

a

Regio cervicalis lateralis,
occipital triangle

Regio cervicalis lateralis,
trigonum omoclaviculare

b

Trigonum
submandibulare

Trigonum submentale

Trigonum caroticum

Trigonum musculare

Regio
cervicalis
anterior

Fossa supra-
clavicularis minor

Regio cervicalis anterior
- Trigonum submandibulare
  - Nll. submandibulares
  - Gl. submandibularis
  - N. hypoglossus
  - Gl. parotidea (posterior)
- Trigonum caroticum
  - Bifurcatio carotidis
  - Glomus caroticum
  - N. hypoglossus
- Trigonum musculare
  - Gl. thyroidea
  - Larynx
  - Trachea
  - Oesophagus
- Trigonum submentale
  - Nll. submentales

Regio sternocleidomastoidea
- M. sternocleidomastoideus
- A. carotis
- V. jugularis interna
- N. vagus
- Nll. cervicales laterales

Regio cervicalis lateralis
- Nll. cervicales laterales
- N. accessorius
- Plexus cervicalis
- Plexus brachialis

Regio cervicalis posterior
- Mm. colli
- Trigonum arteriae vertebralis

C Regions of the neck (cervical regions)
a Right lateral view; **b** Left posterior view.
Certain deeper structures of the neck project onto other regions. Conversely, pathological changes in one region can be referred to the underlying anatomical structure.

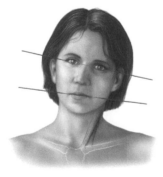

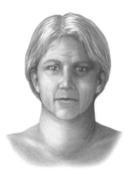

D Left-sided muscular torticollis
(after Anschütz)
Torticollis and struma (swellings of the neck-see **E**) can be readily diagnosed by visual examination. In the case of torticollis, the m. sternocleidomastoideus is shortened—most commonly as a result of intrauterine malposition in infants. The head is tilted toward the affected side and is slightly rotated toward the opposite side. Without therapy (physical therapy/surgery) torticollis secondarily leads to asymmetrical growth of spinal column and facial skeleton. The effects of the cranial asymmetry may include a convergence of the facial planes toward the affected side (see lines).

E Retrosternal goiter (after Hegglin)
A goiter that arises from the inferior poles (see p. 224) of the gl. thyroidea may extend to the apertura thoracis superior and compress the cervical veins at that level. The result of this is venous congestion and dilation in the head and neck region.

F Assessing the central venous pressure in the neck in a semi-upright position
Normally the cervical veins are collapsed in the sitting position. But in a patient with right-sided heart failure, there is diminished venous return to the right heart, causing distention of the vv. jugulares. The extent of the venous congestion is indicated by the level of pulsations in the v. jugularis externa (the "venous pulse," upper end of the blue line). The higher the level of jugular pulsation, the greater the backup of blood into the vein. This provides a means of assessing the severity of right-sided heart failure.

1.4 Embryology of the Face

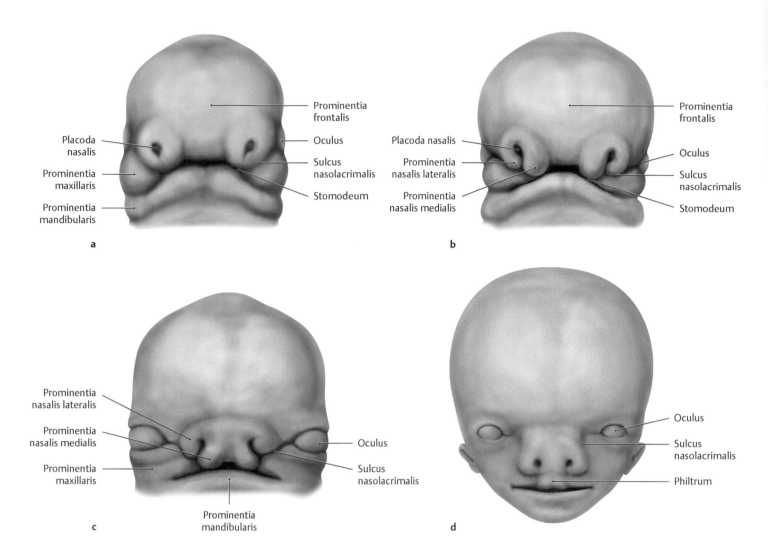

A Fusion of facial prominences (after Sadler)
Frontal view. Understanding the clinically important development of the cleft lip, jaw, and palatum (**c**) requires knowledge of facial development.

a Embryo at five weeks. The surface ectoderma of the arcus pharyngeus primus invaginates to form the stomodeum which later connects to the endodermal epithelium of the cavitas oris. The facial outline develops from facial prominences, the tissue of which arises from the arcus pharyngeus primus or mesenchyma cristae neuralis. The prominentiae mandibulares are located caudal to the stomodeum with the prominentiae maxillares located lateral to it.

Superomedial to the prominentiae maxillares are the prominentiae nasales mediales and laterales. Both prominentiae nasales mediales border the prominentia frontalis.

b Embryo at six weeks. A sulcus separates the prominentiae nasales from the prominentia maxillaris.
c Embryo at seven weeks. The prominentiae nasales mediales have fused along the midline and their inferolateral margins contact the prominentiae maxillares on either side.
d Embryo at ten weeks. Cell migration is completed.

B Facial prominences and their derivatives (after Sadler)

Facial prominence	Derivative
Prominentia frontalis	Forehead, bridge of nose, medial and lateral nasal process
Prominentia maxillaris	Cheeks, lateral parts of upper lip
Prominentia nasalis medialis	Philtrum, tip of the nose and ridge of the nose
Prominentia nasalis lateralis	Nasal wing
Prominentia mandibularis	Lower lip

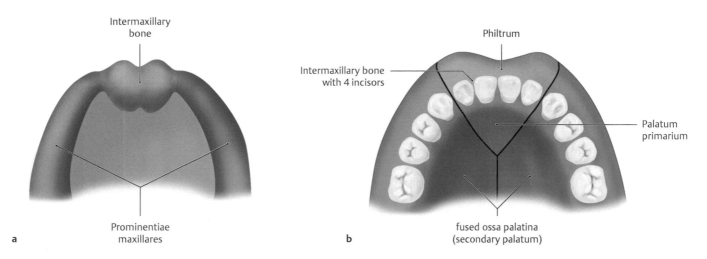

a **Prominentiae maxillares**

b **fused ossa palatina (secondary palatum)**

C Intermaxillary segment (after Sadler)
Caudal view of palatum.

a The prominentiae nasales mediales develop bone tissue that fuses along the midline and gives rise to a separate bone, the intermaxillary bone.

b The philtrum also arises from tissue of the proc. nasalis medialis along with intermaxillary bone and its four incisors. The bone of the primary palate fuses with the prominentiae maxillares (palatum secundarium) and is no longer a separate bone in adults.

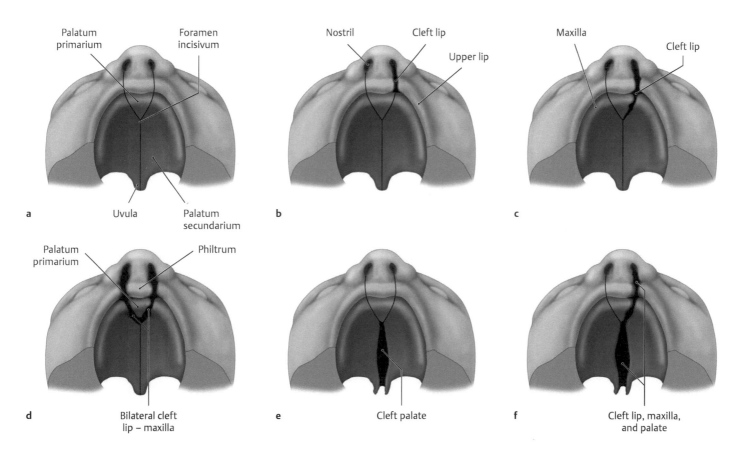

D Formation of facial clefts (after Sadler)
Caudal and ventral view.

a **Normal condition.** The ossa palatina and the prominentiae maxillares have fused with the palatum primarium. The surface epithelium forms oral mucosa that lines the roof of the cavitas oris. The palatum osseum (bony palate) beneath the oral mucosa separates the cavitates oris and nasi.

b **Cheiloschisis.** A cleft lip that extends up to the nose (harelip) occurs on the left side if the tissue of the upper lip does not fuse on the left side.

c **Cheilognathoschisis.** A cleft lip and maxilla occurs if the fusion of palata primaria and secundaria on the left side does not occur.

d Cleft formation can also occur bilaterally: bilateral cleft lip and maxilla.

e **Palatoschisis.** Incomplete fusion of the palata primaria and secundaria on both sides results in an isolated cleft palate.

f **Cheilognathopalatoschisis.** Combination of all three: unilateral cleft lip, maxilla, and palatum. If it occurs bilaterally it is known as cleft palate.

9

1.5 Embryology of the Neck

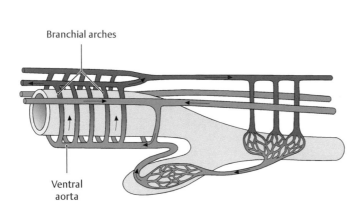

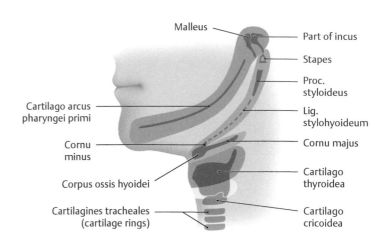

A The branchial arches of the lancelet
(after Romer, Parsons, and Frick)

Left lateral view. This simplified schematic of the circulatory system of a lancelet fish illustrates the basic relation between the vascular tree and the branchial arches in chordates, including the vertebrates. Oxygen-depleted blood (in blue) is pumped rostrally (toward the head) through a ventral aorta to a series of branchial arches, where it passes through gills, picks up oxygen (red), and then is distributed to the body (compare this paired, segmental arterial arch with the thoracic segment in humans). A similar anatomical organization and circulatory pattern is seen in the human embryo, where the gills and branchial arches are transformed into arcus pharyngei which develop into various structures in the head and neck. Errors during this developmental process give rise to a series of relatively common anatomical anomalies in the neck (see **G**).

C Derivation of musculoskeletal structures from the arcus pharyngei in the adult (after Sadler)

Left lateral view. Besides the cartilaginous rudiments of the skeleton (see labels), the muscles and their associated nerves can be traced embryologically to specific arcus pharyngei. The arcus pharyngeus primus gives rise to the mm. masticatorii, the m. mylohyoideus, the venter anterior m. digastrici, the m. tensor veli palatini, and the m. tensor tympani. The arcus pharyngeus secundus gives origin to the muscles of facial expression, the venter posterior m. digastrici, the m. stylohyoideus, and the m. stapedius. The m. stylopharyngeus is derived from the arcus pharyngeus tertius. The arcus pharyngei quartus and sixtus give rise to the m. cricothyroideus, m. levator veli palatini, mm. constrictores pharyngis, and the intrinsic muscles of the larynx. The nerve supply to the muscles can also be explained in terms of their embryologic origins (see **D**).

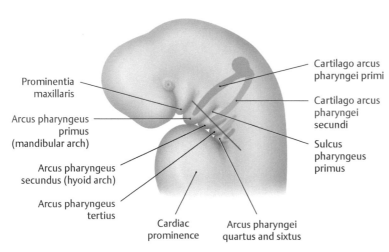

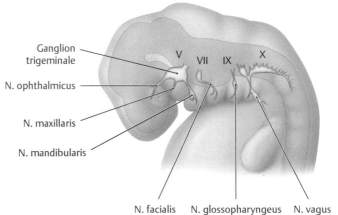

B Arcus pharyngei and sulci pharyngei of a 4-week-old embryo
(after Sadler)

Left lateral view. The human embryo has four arcus pharyngei separated by intervening sulci pharyngei. The cartilages of the four arcus pharyngei are shown in different colors. Like other tissues of the arcus pharyngei, they migrate with further development to form various skeletal and ligamentous elements in the adult (see **C**).

D Innervation of the arcus pharyngei
Left lateral view. Each of the arcus pharyngei is associated with a n. cranialis:

Arcus pharyngeus primus	N. trigeminus (CN V) (n. mandibularis)
Arcus pharyngeus secundus	N. facialis (CN VII)
Arcus pharyngeus tertius	N. glossopharyngeus (CN IX)
Arcus pharyngei quartus and sixtus	N. vagus (CN X) (nervi laryngeus superior and recurrens)

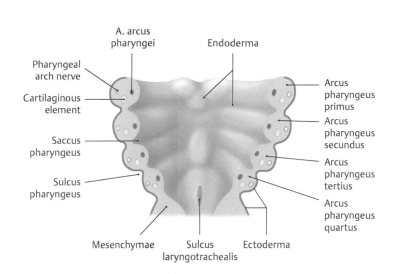

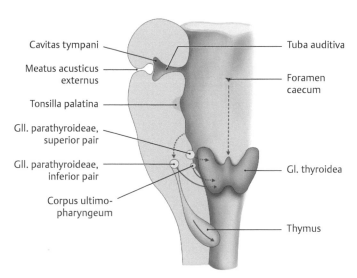

E Internal structure of the arcus pharyngei (after Sadler)

Anterior view (plane of section shown in **B**). The arcus pharyngei are covered externally by ectoderma and internally by endoderma. Each arcus pharyngeus contains an a. arcus pharyngei, an arch nerve, and a cartilaginous element, all of which are surrounded by mesodermal and muscular tissue. The external furrows are called the sulci pharyngei, and the internal furrows are called the sacci pharyngei. The endodermal lining of the sacci pharyngei develops into endocrine glands of the neck, a process which may involve significant migration of cells from their site of origin.

F Migratory movements of the arcus pharyngeus tissues
(after Sadler)

Anterior view. During embryonic development, the epithelium from which the gl. thyroidea is formed migrates from its site of origin on the basal midline of the tongue to the level of the first cartilago trachealis, where the gl. thyroidea is located in postnatal life. As the thyroid tissue buds off from the tongue base, it leaves a vestigial depression on the dorsum linguae, the foramen caecum. The gll. parathyroideae are derived from the arcus pharyngeus quartus (superior pair) or arcus pharyngeus tertius (inferior pair), which also gives origin to the thymus. The corpus ultimopharyngeum, whose cells migrate into the gl. thyroidea to form the calcitonin-producing C cells or parafollicular cells, is derived from the fifth, vestigial, arcus pharyngeus. The latter arch is the last to develop and is usually considered part of the arcus pharyngeus quartus. The meatus acusticus externus is derived from the sulcus pharyngeus primus, the cavitas tympani and tuba auditiva from the saccus pharyngeus primus, and the tonsilla palatina from the saccus pharyngeus secundus.

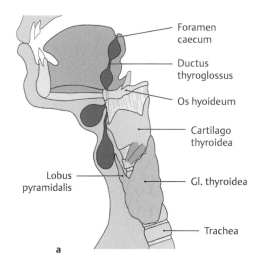

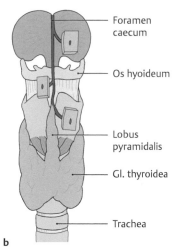

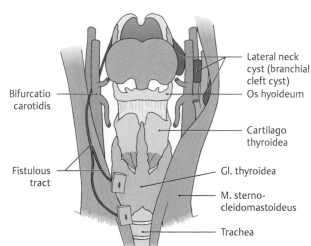

G Location of cysts and fistulas in the neck

a Median cysts, **b** median fistulas, **c** lateral fistulas and cysts.
Median cysts and fistulas in the neck (**a, b**) are remnants of the ductus thyroglossus. Failure of this duct to regress completely may lead to the formation of a mucus-filled cavity (cyst), which presents clinically as a firm neck mass.

Lateral cysts and fistulas in the neck are anomalous remnants of the ductal portions of the cervical sinus, which forms as a result of tissue migration during embryonic development. If epithelium-lined remnants persist, neck cysts (right) or fistulas (left) may appear in postnatal life (**c**). A complete fistula opens into the pharynx and onto the surface of the skin, whereas an incomplete (blind) fistula is open at one end only. The external orifice of a lateral cervical fistula is typically located at the anterior border of the m. sternocleidomastoideus.

2.1 Skull, Lateral View

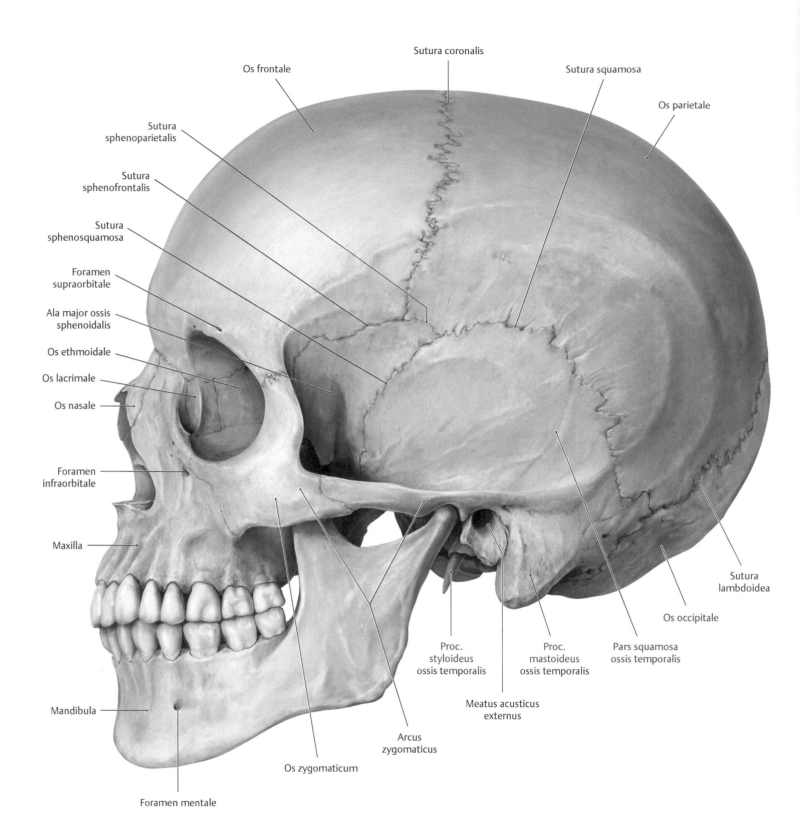

Sutura coronalis
Os frontale
Sutura squamosa
Os parietale
Sutura sphenoparietalis
Sutura sphenofrontalis
Sutura sphenosquamosa
Foramen supraorbitale
Ala major ossis sphenoidalis
Os ethmoidale
Os lacrimale
Os nasale
Foramen infraorbitale
Maxilla
Mandibula
Foramen mentale
Os zygomaticum
Arcus zygomaticus
Proc. styloideus ossis temporalis
Proc. mastoideus ossis temporalis
Meatus acusticus externus
Pars squamosa ossis temporalis
Os occipitale
Sutura lambdoidea

A Lateral view of the skull (cranium)
Left lateral view. This view was selected as an introduction to the skull because it displays the greatest number of cranial bones (indicated by different colors in **B**). The individual bones and their salient features as well as the suturae cranii and apertures are described in the units that follow. This unit reviews the principal structures of the lateral aspect of the skull. The chapter as a whole is intended to familiarize the reader with the names of the cranial bones before proceeding to finer anatomical details and the relationships of the bones to one another. The teeth are described in a separate unit (see p. 48 ff).

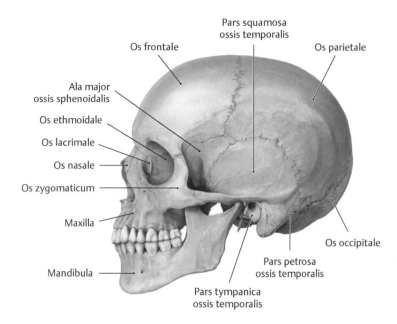

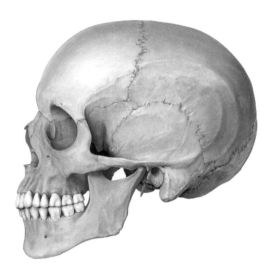

B Lateral view of the cranial bones
Left lateral view. The bones are shown in different colors to demonstrate more clearly their extents and boundaries.

C Bones of the neurocranium (gray) and viscerocranium (orange)
Left lateral view. The skull forms a bony capsule that encloses the brain, sensory organs, and viscera of the head. The greater size of the neurocranium (cranial vault) relative to the viscerocranium (facial skeleton) is a typical primate feature directly correlated with the larger primate brain.

E Bones of the neurocranium and viscerocranium

Neurocranium (gray)	Viscerocranium (orange)
• Os frontale • Os sphenoidale (excluding the proc. pterygoideus) • Os temporale (pars squamosa, pars petrosa) • Os parietale • Os occipitale • Os ethmoidale (lamina cribrosa) • Ossicula auditoria	• Os nasale • Os lacrimale • Os ethmoidale (excluding the lamina cribrosa) • Os sphenoidale (proc. pterygoideus) • Maxilla • Os zygomaticum • Os temporale (pars tympanica, proc. styloideus) • Mandibula • Vomer • Concha nasi inferior • Os palatinum • Os hyoideum (see p. 47)

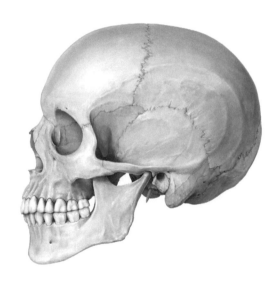

D Ossification of the cranial bones
Left lateral view. The bones of the skull either develop directly from mesenchymal connective tissue (intramembranous ossification, gray) or form indirectly by the ossification of a cartilaginous model (enchondral ossification, blue). Elements derived from intramembranous and endochondral ossification (desmocranium and chondrocranium respectively) may fuse together to form a single bone (e.g., the os occipitale, os temporale, and os sphenoidale).
The clavicula is the only tubular bone that undergoes intra membranous ossification. This explains why congenital defects of intramembranous ossification affect both the skull and clavicula *(cleidocranial dysostosis)*.

F Bones of the desmocranium and chondrocranium

Desmocranium (gray)	Chondrocranium (blue)
• Os hyoideum • Os lacrimale • Maxilla • Mandibula • Os zygomaticum • Os frontale • Os parietale • Os occipitale (upper part of the squama) • Os temporale (pars squamosa, pars tympanica) • Os palatinum • Vomer	• Os ethmoidale • Os sphenoidale (excluding the lamina medialis of the proc. pterygoideus) • Os temporale (partes petrosa and mastoidea, proc. styloideus) • Os occipitale (excluding the upper part of the squama) • Concha nasi inferior • Os hyoideum (see p. 47) • Ossicula auditoria

2.2 Skull, Anterior View

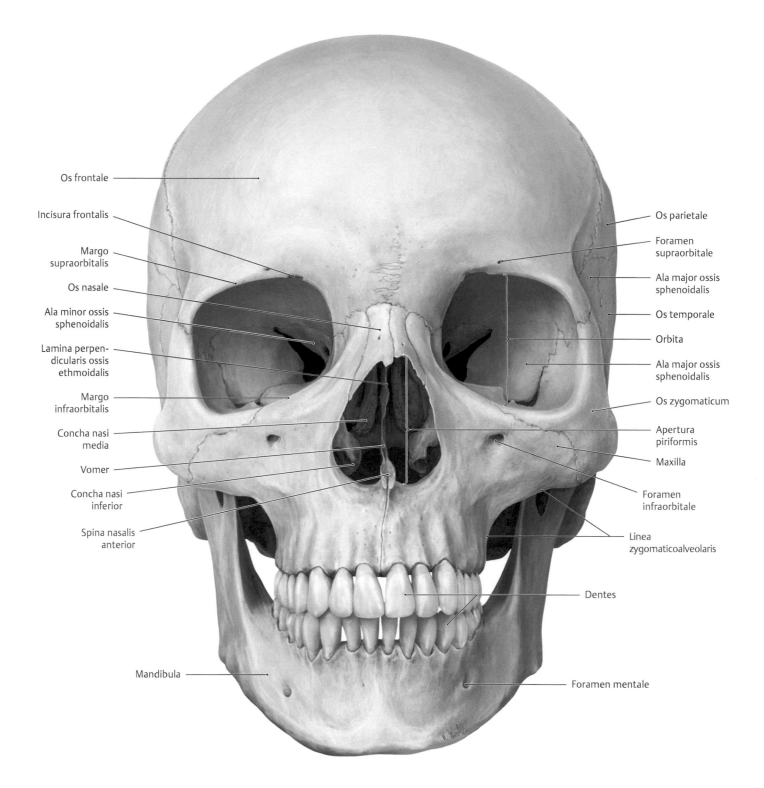

Os frontale

Incisura frontalis

Margo supraorbitalis

Os nasale

Ala minor ossis sphenoidalis

Lamina perpendicularis ossis ethmoidalis

Margo infraorbitalis

Concha nasi media

Vomer

Concha nasi inferior

Spina nasalis anterior

Mandibula

Os parietale

Foramen supraorbitale

Ala major ossis sphenoidalis

Os temporale

Orbita

Ala major ossis sphenoidalis

Os zygomaticum

Apertura piriformis

Maxilla

Foramen infraorbitale

Linea zygomaticoalveolaris

Dentes

Foramen mentale

A Anterior view of the skull

The boundaries of the facial skeleton (viscerocranium) can be clearly appreciated in this view (the individual bones are shown in **B**). The bony margins of the apertura piriformis mark the start of the respiratory tract in the skull. The cavitas nasi, like the orbitae, contains a sensory organ (the olfactory mucosa). The *sinus paranasales* are shown schematically in **C**. The anterior view of the skull also displays the three clinically

important openings through which sensory nerves pass to supply the face: the foramen supraorbitale, foramen infraorbitale, and foramen mentale (see p. 123 and 227).

Note: In cases of suspected midfacial fracture (mainly Le Fort I and II) intraoral palpation of the zygomatic-alveolar line is recommended for a possible step off and change in maxilla mobility against the skull in the case of dislodged os zygomaticum fractures.

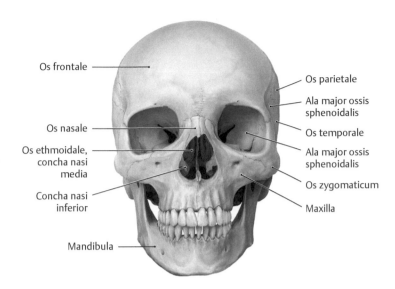

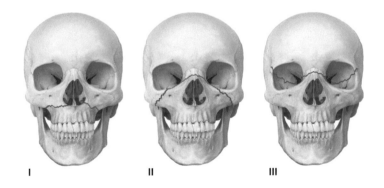

B Cranial bones, anterior view

C Sinus paranasales: pneumatization lightens the bone
Anterior view. Some of the bones of the facial skeleton are pneumatized (i.e., they contain air-filled cavities that reduce the total weight of the bone). These cavities, called the sinus paranasales, communicate with the cavitas nasi and, like it, are lined by ciliated respiratory epithelium. Inflammations of the sinus paranasales (sinusitis) and associated complaints are very common. Because some of the pain of sinusitis is projected to the skin overlying the sinuses, it is helpful to know the projections of the sinuses onto the surface of the skull.

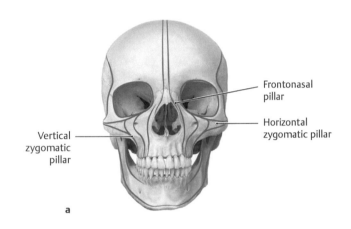

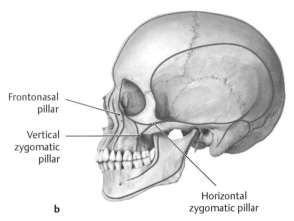

E LeFort classification of midfacial fractures
The frame-like construction of the facial skeleton leads to characteristic patterns of fracture lines in the midfacial region (LeFort I, II, and III).
LeFort I: This fracture line runs across the maxilla and above the palatum durum. The maxilla is separated from the upper facial skeleton, disrupting the integrity of the sinus maxillaris *(low transverse fracture)*.
LeFort II: The fracture line passes across the radix nasi, os ethmoidale, maxilla, and os zygomaticum, creating a *pyramid fracture* that disrupts the integrity of the orbit.
LeFort III: The facial skeleton is separated from the base of the skull. The main fracture line passes through the orbitae, and the fracture may additionally involve the os ethmoidale, sinus frontalis, sinus sphenoidalis, and ossa zygomatica.

D Principal lines of force (blue) in the facial skeleton
a Anterior view, **b** lateral view. The pneumatized sinus paranasales (**C**) have a mechanical counterpart in the thickened bony "pillars" of the facial skeleton, which partially bound the sinuses. These pillars develop along the principal lines of force in response to local mechanical stresses (e.g., masticatory pressures). In visual terms, the frame-like construction of the facial skeleton may be likened to that of a frame house: The sinus paranasales represent the rooms while the pillars (placed along major lines of force) represent the supporting columns.

2.3 Skull, Posterior View and Cranial Sutures (Suturae Cranii)

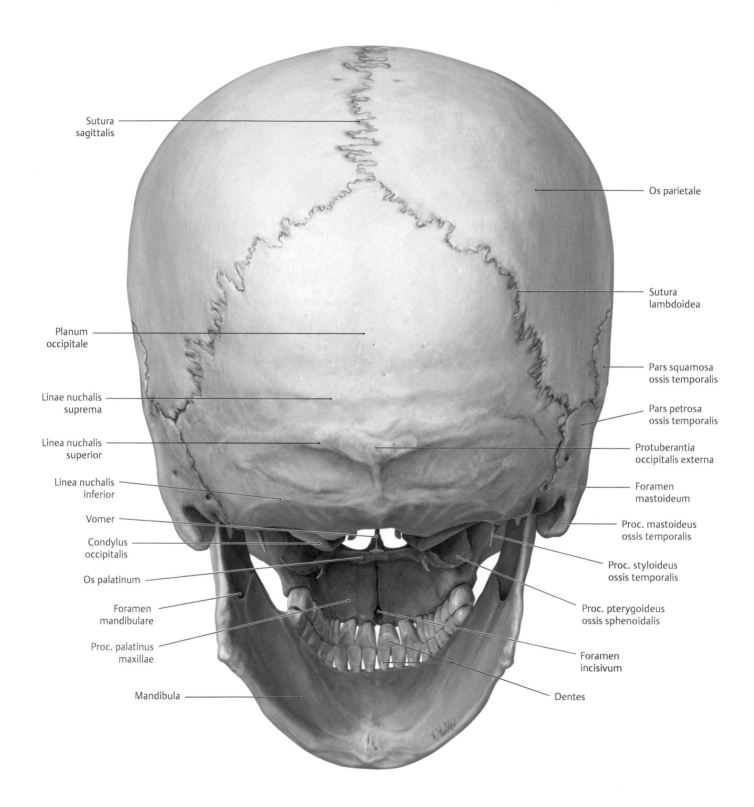

Sutura sagittalis

Os parietale

Sutura lambdoidea

Planum occipitale

Pars squamosa ossis temporalis

Linae nuchalis suprema

Pars petrosa ossis temporalis

Linea nuchalis superior

Protuberantia occipitalis externa

Linea nuchalis inferior

Foramen mastoideum

Vomer

Proc. mastoideus ossis temporalis

Condylus occipitalis

Os palatinum

Proc. styloideus ossis temporalis

Foramen mandibulare

Proc. pterygoideus ossis sphenoidalis

Proc. palatinus maxillae

Foramen incisivum

Mandibula

Dentes

A Posterior view of the skull

The os occipitale, which is dominant in this view, articulates with the ossa parietalia, to which it is connected by the sutura lambdoidea. The suturae cranii are a special type of syndesmosis (=ligamentous attachments that ossify with age, see **F**). The outer surface of the os occipitale is contoured by muscular origins and insertions: the lineae nuchales inferior, superior, and suprema. The protuberantia occipitalis externa serves as an anatomical reference point: It is palpable at the back of the head. The foramen mastoideum provides a point of an emergence of a vein (see p. 19).

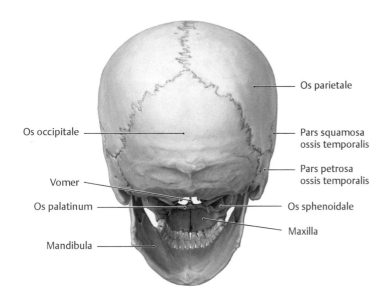

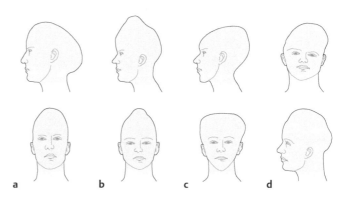

B Posterior view of the cranial bones

Note: The os temporale consists of two main parts based on its embryonic development: a pars squamosa and a pars petrosa (cf. p. 28).

D Cranial deformities due to the premature closure of suturae cranii

The premature closure of a cranial suture (craniosynostosis) may lead to characteristic cranial deformities, which are normal variants of no clinical significance. The following sutures may close prematurely, resulting in various cranial shapes:

a Sutura sagittalis: scaphocephaly (long, narrow skull)
b Sutura coronalis: oxycephaly (pointed skull)
c Sutura frontalis: trigonocephaly (triangular skull)
d Asymmetrical suture closure, usually involving the sutura coronalis: plagiocephaly (asymmetrical skull).

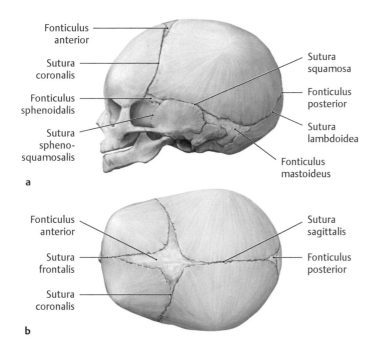

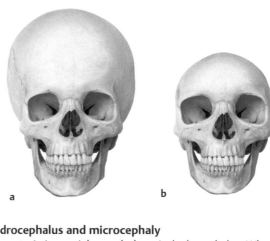

E Hydrocephalus and microcephaly

a Characteristic cranial morphology in *hydrocephalus*. When the brain becomes dilated due to liquor cerebrospinalis accumulation *before* the suturae cranii ossify (hydrocephalus, "water on the brain"), the neurocranium will expand while the facial skeleton remains unchanged.
b *Microcephaly* results from premature closure of the suturae cranii. It is characterized by a small neurocranium with relatively large orbitae.

C The neonatal skull

a Left lateral view, b superior view.

The flat cranial bones must grow as the brain expands, and so the sutures between them must remain open for some time (see **F**). In the neonate, there are areas between the still-growing cranial bones that are not occupied by bone: the fonticuli. They close at different times (the fonticulus sphenoidalis in about the 6th month of life, the fonticulus mastoideus in the 18th month, the fonticulus anterior in the 36th month). The *fonticulus posterior* provides a reference point for describing the position of the fetal head during childbirth, and the *fonticulus anterior* provides a possible access site for drawing a liquor cerebrospinalis sample in infants (e.g., in suspected meningitis).

F Age at which the principal sutures ossify

Sutura	Age at ossification
Sutura frontalis	Childhood
Sutura sagittalis	20–30 years of age
Sutura coronalis	30–40 years of age
Sutura lambdoidea	40–50 years of age

2.4 Exterior and Interior of the Calvarium

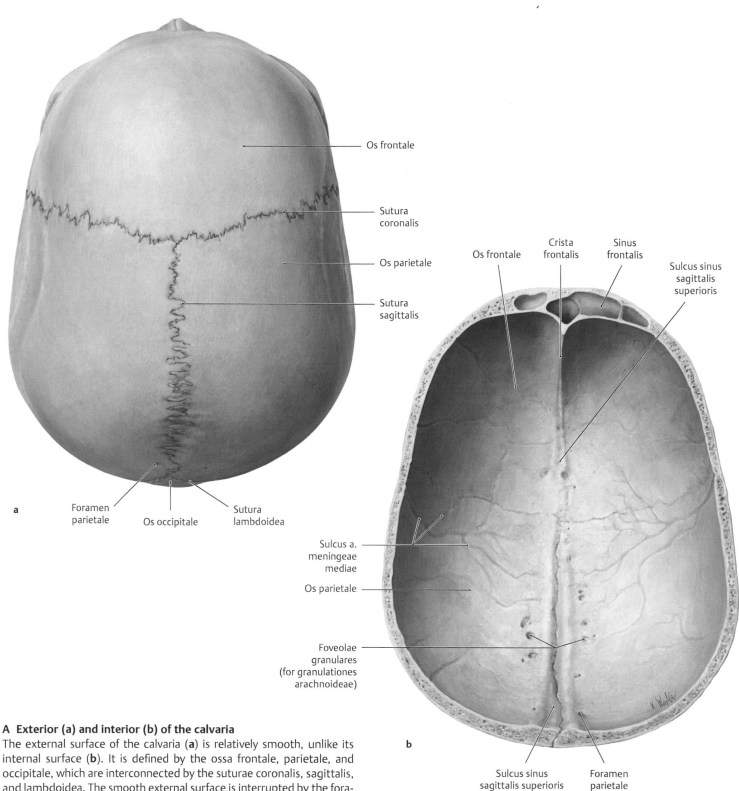

A Exterior (a) and interior (b) of the calvaria

The external surface of the calvaria (**a**) is relatively smooth, unlike its internal surface (**b**). It is defined by the ossa frontale, parietale, and occipitale, which are interconnected by the suturae coronalis, sagittalis, and lambdoidea. The smooth external surface is interrupted by the foramen parietale, which gives passage to the v. emissaria parietalis (see **F**). The internal surface of the calvaria also bears a number of pits and grooves:

- The foveolae granulares (small pits in the inner surface of the skull caused by saccular protrusions of the arachnoidea mater covering the brain)
- The sulcus sinus sagittalis superioris (a dural venous sinus of the brain)
- The sulci arteriosi (which mark the positions of the arterial vessels of the dura mater, such as the a. meningea media which supplies most of the dura mater and overlying bone)

- The crista frontalis (which gives attachment to the falx cerebri, a sickleshaped fold of dura mater between the hemispheria cerebri, see p. 308).

The sinus frontalis in the os frontale is also visible in the interior view.

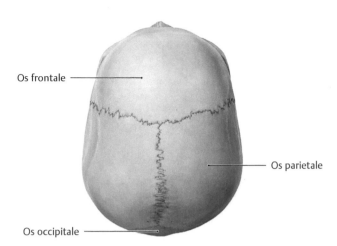

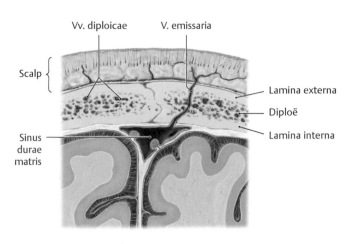

B Exterior of the calvaria viewed from above

C The scalp and calvaria

Note the three-layered structure of the calvaria, consisting of the lamina externa, the diploë, and the lamina interna.

The diploë has a spongy structure and contains red (blood-forming) bone marrow. With a plasmacytoma (malignant transformation of certain white blood cells), many small nests of tumor cells may destroy the surrounding bony trabeculae, and radiographs will demonstrate multiple lucent areas ("punched-out lesions") in the skull. Vessels called *venae emissariae* may pass through the calvaria to connect the venous sinuses of the brain with the veins of the scalp (see panels **E** and **F**).

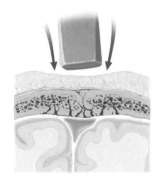

D Sensitivity of the lamina interna to trauma

The lamina interna of the calvaria is very sensitive to external trauma and may fracture even when the lamina externa remains intact (look for corresponding evidence on CT Images).

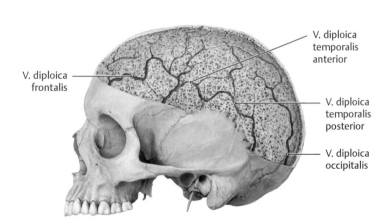

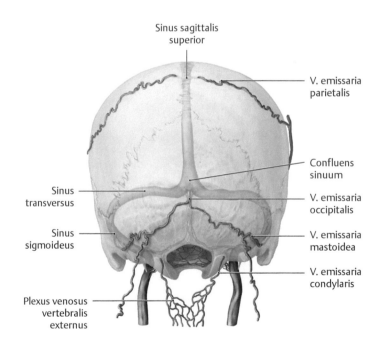

E Venae diploicae in the calvaria

The vv. diploicae are located in the cancellous or spongy tissue of the ossa cranii (the diploë) and are visible when the lamina externa is removed. The vv. diploicae communicate with the sinus durae matris and scalp veins by way of the vv. emissariae, which create a potential route for the spread of infection.

F Venae emissariae of the occiput

Venae emissariae establish a direct connection between the sinus durae matris and the extracranial veins. They pass through preformed cranial openings such as the foramen parietale and foramen mastoideum. The vv. emissariae are of clinical interest because they may allow bacteria from the scalp to enter the skull along these veins and infect the dura mater, causing meningitis.

2.5   Base of the Skull (Basis Cranii), External View

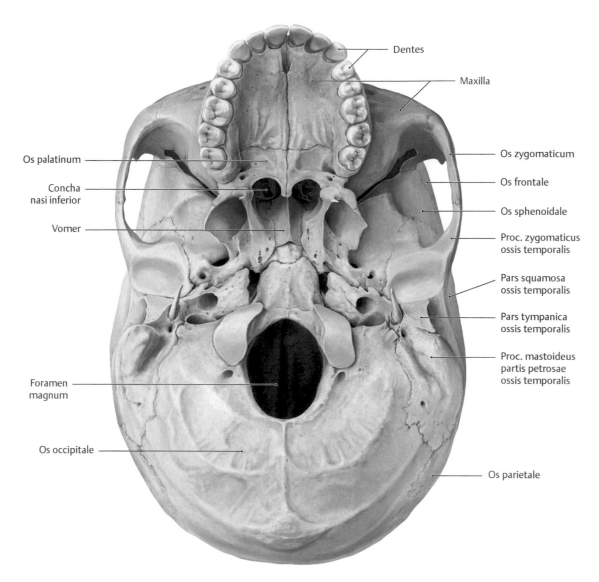

Dentes

Maxilla

Os palatinum

Concha
nasi inferior

Vomer

Foramen
magnum

Os occipitale

Os zygomaticum

Os frontale

Os sphenoidale

Proc. zygomaticus
ossis temporalis

Pars squamosa
ossis temporalis

Pars tympanica
ossis temporalis

Proc. mastoideus
partis petrosae
ossis temporalis

Os parietale

A Bones of the basis cranii
Inferior view. The basis cranii is composed of a mosaic-like assembly of
various bones. It is helpful to review the shape and location of these
bones before studying further details.

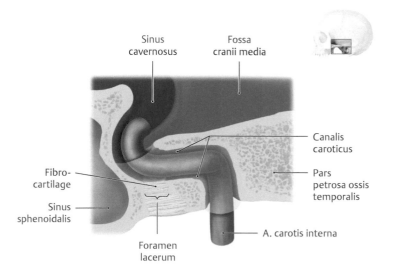

Sinus
cavernosus

Fossa
cranii media

Fibro-
cartilage

Sinus
sphenoidalis

Foramen
lacerum

Canalis
caroticus

Pars
petrosa ossis
temporalis

A. carotis interna

**B Relationship of the foramen lacerum to the canalis caroticus and
arteria carotis interna**
Left lateral view. The foramen lacerum is not a true aperture, being
occluded in life by a layer of fibrocartilage; it appears as an opening only
in the dried skull. The foramen lacerum is closely related to the canalis caroticus and to the a. carotis interna that traverses the canal. The n.
petrosus major and deep n. petrosus profundus through the foramen
lacerum (see pp. 127, 131, and 136).

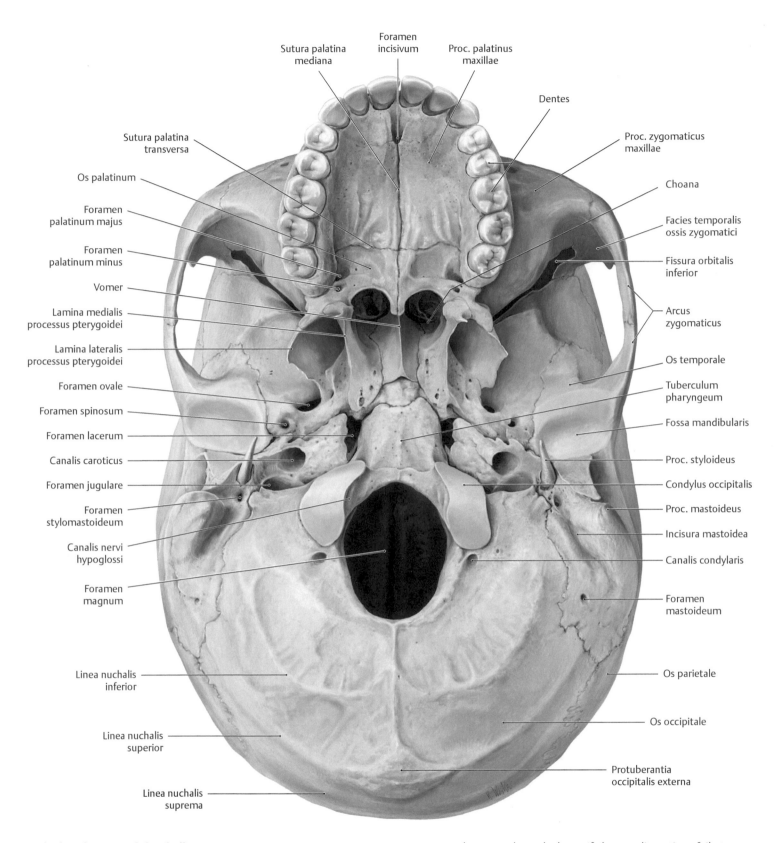

Foramen
incisivum

Sutura palatina
mediana

Proc. palatinus
maxillae

Dentes

Proc. zygomaticus
maxillae

Sutura palatina
transversa

Os palatinum

Choana

Facies temporalis
ossis zygomatici

Foramen
palatinum majus

Foramen
palatinum minus

Fissura orbitalis
inferior

Vomer

Arcus
zygomaticus

Lamina medialis
processus pterygoidei

Lamina lateralis
processus pterygoidei

Os temporale

Tuberculum
pharyngeum

Foramen ovale

Foramen spinosum

Fossa mandibularis

Foramen lacerum

Canalis caroticus

Proc. styloideus

Foramen jugulare

Condylus occipitalis

Foramen
stylomastoideum

Proc. mastoideus

Incisura mastoidea

Canalis nervi
hypoglossi

Canalis condylaris

Foramen
magnum

Foramen
mastoideum

Linea nuchalis
inferior

Os parietale

Os occipitale

Linea nuchalis
superior

Protuberantia
occipitalis externa

Linea nuchalis
suprema

C The basal aspect of the skull

Inferior view. The principal external features of the basis cranii are labeled. Note particularly the openings that transmit nerves and vessels. With abnormalities of bone growth, these openings may remain too small or may become narrowed, compressing the neurovascular structures that pass through them. If the canalis opticus fails to grow normally, it may compress and damage the nervus opticus, resulting in visual field defects. The symptoms associated with these lesions depend on the affected opening. All of the structures depicted here will be considered in more detail in subsequent pages.

2.6 Base of the Skull (Basis Cranii), Internal View

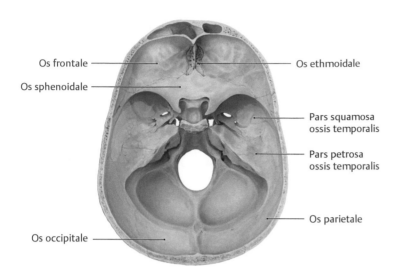

Os frontale
Os sphenoidale
Os ethmoidale
Pars squamosa ossis temporalis
Pars petrosa ossis temporalis
Os parietale
Os occipitale

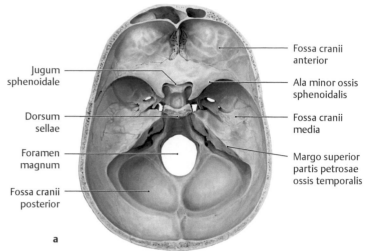

Jugum sphenoidale
Dorsum sellae
Foramen magnum
Fossa cranii posterior
Fossa cranii anterior
Ala minor ossis sphenoidalis
Fossa cranii media
Margo superior partis petrosae ossis temporalis

a

A Bones of the basis cranii, internal view
Different colors are used here to highlight the arrangement of bones in the basis cranii as seen from within the cranium.

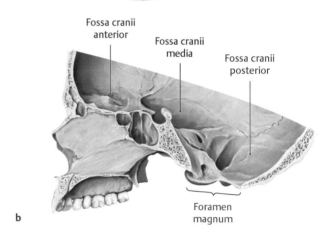

Fossa cranii anterior
Fossa cranii media
Fossa cranii posterior
Foramen magnum

b

B The fossae cranii
a Interior view, **b** midsagittal section. The interior of the basis cranii is not flat but is deepened to form three successive fossae: the fossae cranii anterior, media, and posterior. These depressions become progressively deeper in the frontal-to-occipital direction, forming a terraced arrangement that is displayed most clearly in **b**.
The fossae cranii are bounded by the following structures:

* Anterior to middle: the alae minores ossis sphenoidalis and the jugum sphenoidale.
* Middle to posterior: the margo superior partis petrosae ossis temporalis and the dorsum sellae.

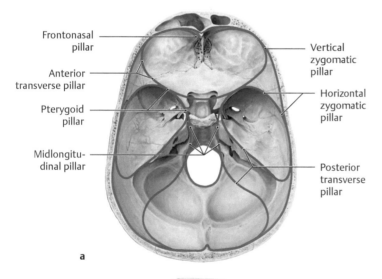

Frontonasal pillar
Anterior transverse pillar
Pterygoid pillar
Midlongitu-dinal pillar
Vertical zygomatic pillar
Horizontal zygomatic pillar
Posterior transverse pillar

a

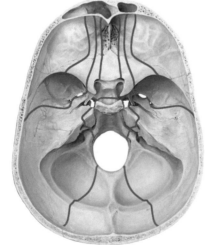

b

C Basis cranii: principal lines of force and common fracture lines
a Principal lines of force, **b** common fracture lines (interior views). In response to masticatory pressures and other mechanical stresses, the bones of the skull base are thickened to form "pillars" along the principal lines of force (compare with the force distribution in the anterior view on p. 15). The intervening areas that are not thickened are sites of predilection for bone fractures, resulting in the typical patterns of basal skull fracture lines shown here. An analogous phenomenon of typical fracture lines is found in the midfacial region (see the anterior views of LeFort fractures on p. 15).

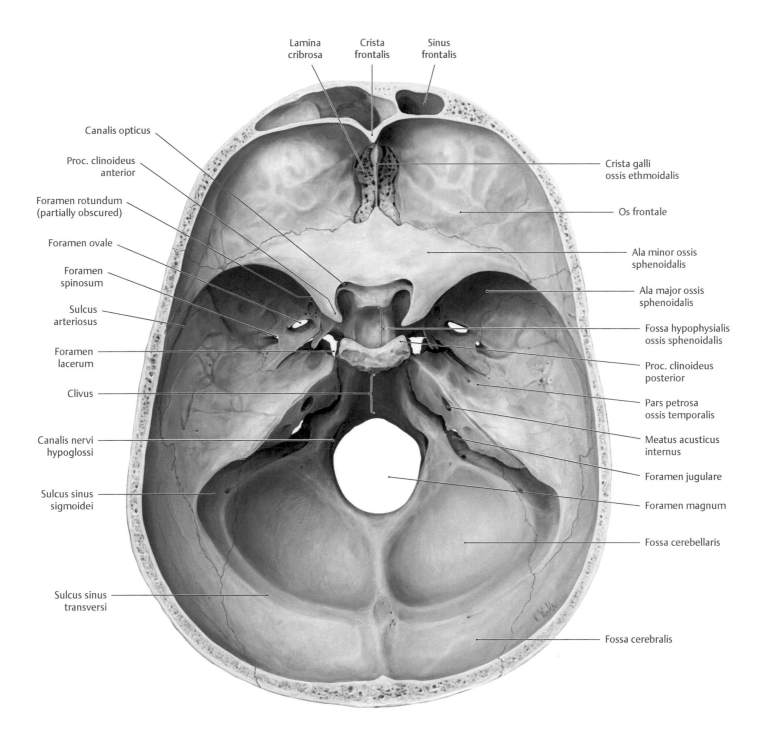

Lamina cribrosa
Crista frontalis
Sinus frontalis
Canalis opticus
Proc. clinoideus anterior
Foramen rotundum (partially obscured)
Foramen ovale
Foramen spinosum
Sulcus arteriosus
Foramen lacerum
Clivus
Canalis nervi hypoglossi
Sulcus sinus sigmoidei
Sulcus sinus transversi

Crista galli ossis ethmoidalis
Os frontale
Ala minor ossis sphenoidalis
Ala major ossis sphenoidalis
Fossa hypophysialis ossis sphenoidalis
Proc. clinoideus posterior
Pars petrosa ossis temporalis
Meatus acusticus internus
Foramen jugulare
Foramen magnum
Fossa cerebellaris
Fossa cerebralis

D Interior of the basis cranii

It is interesting to compare the openings in the interior of the basis cranii with the openings visible in the external view (see p. 21). These openings do not always coincide because some neurovascular structures change direction when passing through the bone or pursue a relatively long intraosseous course. An example of this is the meatus acusticus interior, through which the n. facialis, among other structures, passes from the interior of the skull into the pars petrosa ossis temporalis. Most of its fibers then leave the pars petrosa through the foramen stylomastoideum, which is visible from the external aspect (see pp. 126, 137, and 151).

In learning the sites where neurovascular structures pass through the basis cranii, it is helpful initially to note whether these sites are located in the fossa cranii anterior, media, or posterior. The arrangement of the fossae cranii is shown in **B**. The lamina cribrosa of the os ethmoidale connects the cavitas nasi with the fossa cranii anterior and is perforated by numerous foramina for the passage of the fila olfactoria (see p. 182). *Note:* Because the bone is so thin in this area, a frontal head injury may easily fracture the lamina cribrosa and lacerate the dura mater, allowing liquor cerebrospinalis to enter the nose. This poses a risk of meningitis, as bacteria from the nonsterile nasal cavity may enter the sterile liquor cerebrospinalis.

2.7 Occipital Bone (Os Occipitale) and Ethmoid Bone (Os Ethmoidale)

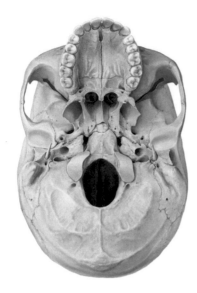

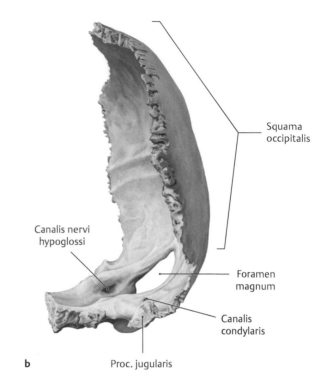

Squama occipitalis

Canalis nervi hypoglossi

Foramen magnum

Canalis condylaris

b Proc. jugularis

A Integration of the os occipitale into the external basis cranii
Inferior view. Note the relationship of the os occipitale to the adjacent bones.
The os occipitale fuses with the os sphenoidale during puberty to form the "tribasilar bone."

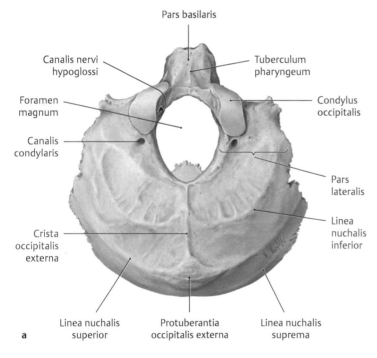

Pars basilaris

Canalis nervi hypoglossi

Tuberculum pharyngeum

Foramen magnum

Condylus occipitalis

Canalis condylaris

Pars lateralis

Crista occipitalis externa

Linea nuchalis inferior

Linea nuchalis superior

Protuberantia occipitalis externa

Linea nuchalis suprema

a

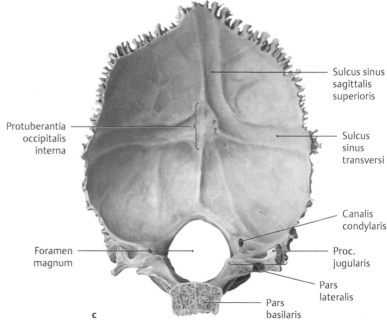

Protuberantia occipitalis interna

Sulcus sinus sagittalis superioris

Sulcus sinus transversi

Canalis condylaris

Foramen magnum

Proc. jugularis

Pars lateralis

Pars basilaris

c

B Isolated os occipitale

a Inferior view. This view shows the pars basilaris of the os occipitale, whose anterior portion is fused to the os sphenoidale. The canalis condylaris terminates posterior to the condyli occipitales, while the canalis nervi hypoglossi passes superior to the condyli occipitales. The former contains the v. emissaria condylaris, which begins in the sinus sigmoideus and ends in the plexus venosus vertebralis externus (vv. emissariae, see p. 19). The latter, in addition to the venous plexus, contains the n. hypoglossus (CN XII). The tuberculum pharyngeum gives attachment to the m. constrictor pharyngis superior while the protuberantia occipitalis externa provides a palpable bony landmark on the occiput.

b Left lateral view. The extent of the squama occipitalis, which lies above the foramen magnum, is clearly appreciated in this view. The internal openings of the canalis condylaris and canalis nervi hypoglossi are visible along with the proc. jugularis, which forms part of the wall of the foramen jugulare (see p. 21). This process is analogous to the proc. transversus of a vertebra.

c Internal surface. The grooves for the sinus durae matris of the brain can be identified in this view. The protuberantia occipitalis interna (eminentia cruciformis) overlies the confluence of the sinus sagittalis superior and sinus transversi. The configuration of the eminence shows that in some cases the sinus sagittalis superior drains predominantly into the left sinus transversus (see p. 384).

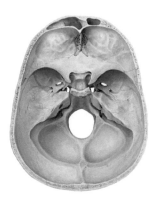

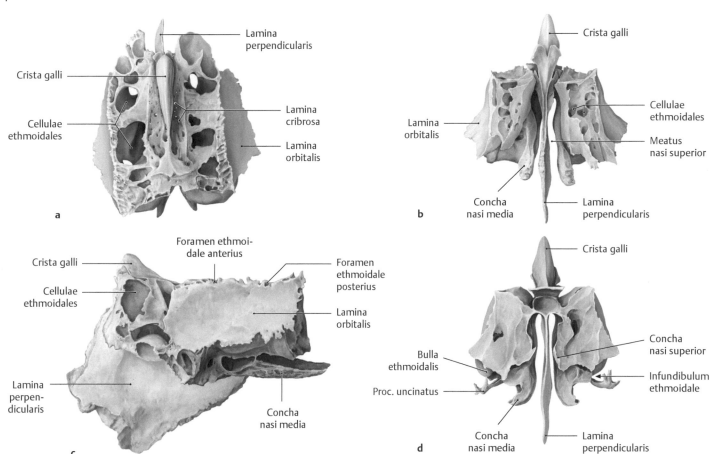

C Integration of the os ethmoidale into the internal base of the skull

Superior view. The upper portion of the os ethmoidale forms part of the fossa cranii anterior, while its lower portions contribute structurally to the cavitates nasi. The os ethmoidale is bordered by the ossa frontale and sphenoidale.

D Integration of the os ethmoidale into the facial skeleton

Anterior view. The os ethmoidale is the central bone of the nose and sinus paranasales.

a — Crista galli, Cellulae ethmoidales, Lamina perpendicularis, Lamina cribrosa, Lamina orbitalis

b — Lamina orbitalis, Concha nasi media, Crista galli, Cellulae ethmoidales, Meatus nasi superior, Lamina perpendicularis

c — Crista galli, Cellulae ethmoidales, Lamina perpendicularis, Foramen ethmoidale anterius, Foramen ethmoidale posterius, Lamina orbitalis, Concha nasi media

d — Bulla ethmoidalis, Proc. uncinatus, Concha nasi media, Crista galli, Concha nasi superior, Infundibulum ethmoidale, Lamina perpendicularis

E Isolated os ethmoidale

a Superior view. This view demonstrates the crista galli, which gives attachment to the falx cerebri (see p. 308) and the horizontally directed lamina cribrosa. The latter is perforated by foramina through which the fila olfactoria pass from the cavitas nasi into the fossa cranii anterior. With its numerous foramina, the lamina cribrosa is a mechanically weak structure that fractures easily in response to trauma. This type of fracture is manifested clinically by liquor cerebrospinalis leakage from the nose ("runny nose" in a patient with head injury).

b Anterior view. The anterior view displays the midline structure that separates the two cavitates nasi: the lamina perpendicularis (which resembles the pendulum of a grandfather clock). Note also the concha nasi media, which is part of the os ethmoidale (of the conchae, only the concha nasi inferior is a separate bone), and the cellulae ethmoidales, which are clustered on both sides of the conchae nasi mediae.

c Left lateral view. Viewing the bone from the left side, we observe the lamina perpendicularis and the opened cellulae ethmoidales anteriores. The orbita is separated from the cellulae ethmoidales by a thin sheet of bone called the lamina orbitalis.

d Posterior view. This is the only view that displays the proc. uncinatus, which is almost completely covered by the concha nasi media when in situ. It partially occludes the entrance to the sinus maxillaris, the hiatus semilunaris, and it is an important landmark during endoscopic surgery of the sinus maxillaris. The narrow depression between the concha nasi media and proc. uncinatus is called the infundibulum ethmoidale. The sinus frontalis, sinus maxillaris, and cellulae ethmoidales open into this "funnel." The concha nasi superior is located at the posterior end of the os ethmoidale.

25

2.8 Ossa Frontale and Parietale

A Os frontale

a Anterior view (external surface), **b** inferior view (orbital surface), and **c** posterior view (internal surface).

The **os frontale** forms the bony base of the pars anterior calvariae (see p. 14 and 34 for its position in the skull). It develops from two bones that fuse in the midline. The dividing line between the two bones is still detectable in adolescents as the sutura frontalis; in adults it is usually completely ossified, obliterating the suture. The os frontale comprises the following parts:

- squama frontalis (the bony base of the forehead),
- two partes horizontales orbitae (the pars major basis osseae parietis superioris orbitae), and
- the pars nasalis that lies between them and forms the pars superior (ossea) nasi.

The squama frontalis has external and internal surfaces; the latter forms part of the fossa cranii anterior. It curves to become the facies temporalis on both sides.

Clinically important features of the os frontale include the paired sinus frontales which are separated by a pars ossea septi nasi and form part of the parietes superiores orbitae. Infections can spread from this site (see **C**). Fractures play a role as well. They usually occur as a result of occupational and traffic accidents involving frontal trauma (for example when the skull hits the windshield in a rear-end collision). The result is a frontobasal or anterior skull base fracture. These fractures are classified after Escher according to the anatomic region involved (see **B**).

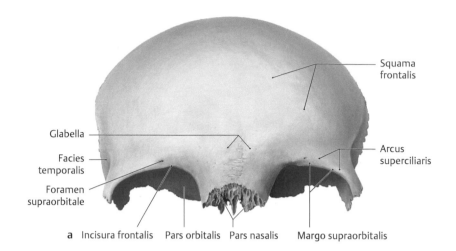

a Glabella, Facies temporalis, Foramen supraorbitale, Squama frontalis, Arcus superciliaris — Incisura frontalis Pars orbitalis Pars nasalis Margo supraorbitalis

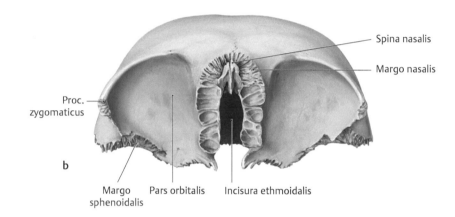

b Proc. zygomaticus, Spina nasalis, Margo nasalis — Margo sphenoidalis Pars orbitalis Incisura ethmoidalis

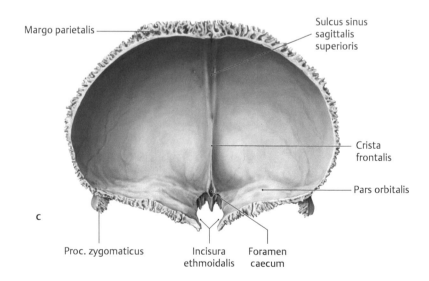

c Margo parietalis, Sulcus sinus sagittalis superioris, Crista frontalis, Pars orbitalis — Proc. zygomaticus Incisura ethmoidalis Foramen caecum

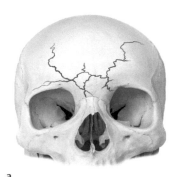 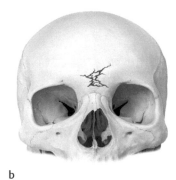 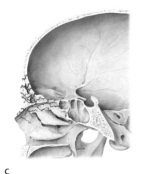 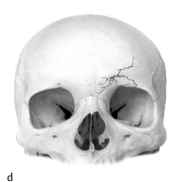

a   b   c   d

B Classification of frontobasal fractures after Escher

a Type I: High frontobasal fracture: force is directed against the superior portions of the squama frontalis. The fracture lines extend into the sinus frontales from above.

b Type II: Middle frontobasal fracture: Force directed against the forehead and base of the nose leads to an impression fracture of the sinus frontalis, the os ethmoidale, and in applicable cases the sinus

sphenoidalis as well. When the dura mater is torn, cerebrospinal fluid flows out facies interna.

c Type III: Deep frontobasal fracture: central anterior trauma. The midface is avulsed off the skull base, merging into vertical or transverse midface fractures (Le Fort III, see p. 15).

d Type IV: Lateral orbital fractures: These result from anterolateral incident force. The facies interna and orbital roof are involved.

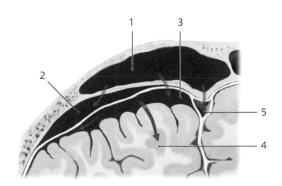

C Anatomic basis of complications involving bacterial frontal sinus infection.

Superior view of the os frontale (cut away). The close proximity of the sinus frontalis (as a part of the frontal bone) to the brain means that infections of the sinus frontalis can easily spread to vital structures. The sinus frontalis itself can fill with pus (empyema; 1). The pus can break through the bone to the dura mater (epidural abscess; 2). Penetration of the dura mater results in meningitis (3). If this infection enters the brain, it will lead to formation of an abscess (4). Spread of the infection to the sinus sagittalis superior leads to sagittal sinus thrombosis (5).

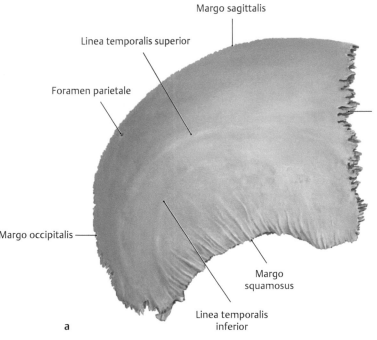

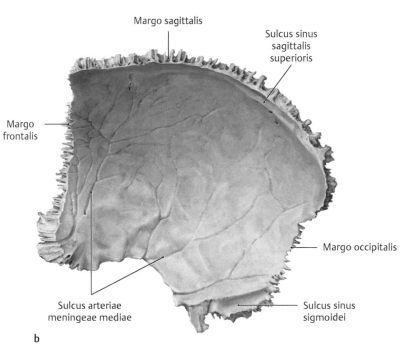

a   b

D Parietal bone

a Right os parietale, lateral view (external surface); **b** right os parietale, medial view (internal surface).

The two ossa parietalia form the middle portion of the calvaria with its highest portion, the apex. The os parietale is divided into a facies

interna and a facies externa. The sulcus arteriae meningeae mediae is visible on the facies interna. The a. meningea media plays an important role in epidural hematomas (see p. 390).

2.9 Temporal Bone (Os Temporale)

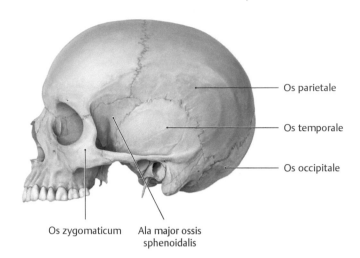

Os parietale

Os temporale

Os occipitale

Os zygomaticum

Ala major ossis sphenoidalis

A Position of the os temporale in the skull
Left lateral view. The os temporale is a major component of the base of the skull. It forms the bony housing for the auditory and vestibular apparatus and bears the fossa articularis of the art. temporomandibularis.

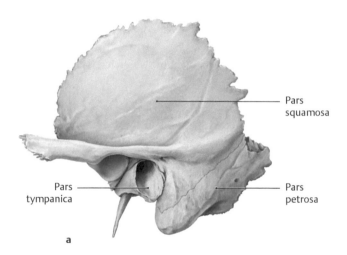

Pars squamosa

Pars tympanica

Pars petrosa

a

Fossa mandibularis

Proc. styloideus

Pars squamosa

Pars tympanica

Pars petrosa

b

B Ossification centers of the left os temporale
a Left lateral view; **b** Inferior view.
The os temporale develops from three centers that fuse to form a single bone:

- The pars squamosa, or temporal squama (light green), bears the fossa articularis of the art. temporomandibularis (fossa mandibularis).

- The pars petrosa, or petrous bone (pale green), contains the auditory and vestibular apparatus.
- The pars tympanicus (darker green) forms large portions of the meatus acusticus externus.

Note: The proc. styloideus appears to belong to the pars tympanica of the os temporale because of its location. Developmentally, however, it is part of the pars petrosa.

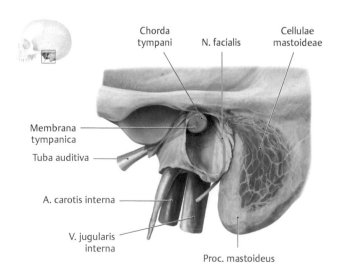

Chorda tympani

N. facialis

Cellulae mastoideae

Membrana tympanica

Tuba auditiva

A. carotis interna

V. jugularis interna

Proc. mastoideus

C Projection of clinically important structures onto the left os temporale
The membrana tympanica is shown translucent in this lateral view. Because the pars petrosa contains the auris media and inner ear and the membrana tympanica, a knowledge of its anatomy is of key importance in otological surgery. The internal surface of the pars petrosa has openings (see **D**) for the passage of the n. facialis, a. carotis interna, and v. jugularis interna. A small nerve, the chorda tympani, passes through the cavitas tympani, and lies medial to the membrana tympanica. The chorda tympani arises from the n. facialis, which is susceptible to injury during surgical procedures (cf. **A**, p. 126). The proc. mastoideus of the pars petrosa forms air-filled chambers, the cellulae mastoideae, that vary greatly in size. Because these chambers communicate with the auris media, which in turn communicates with the pars nasalis pharyngis via the tuba auditiva (also called eustachian tube), bacteria in the pars nasalis pharyngis may pass up the tuba auditiva and gain access to the auris media. From there they may pass to the cellulae mastoideae and finally enter the cavitas cranii, causing meningitis.

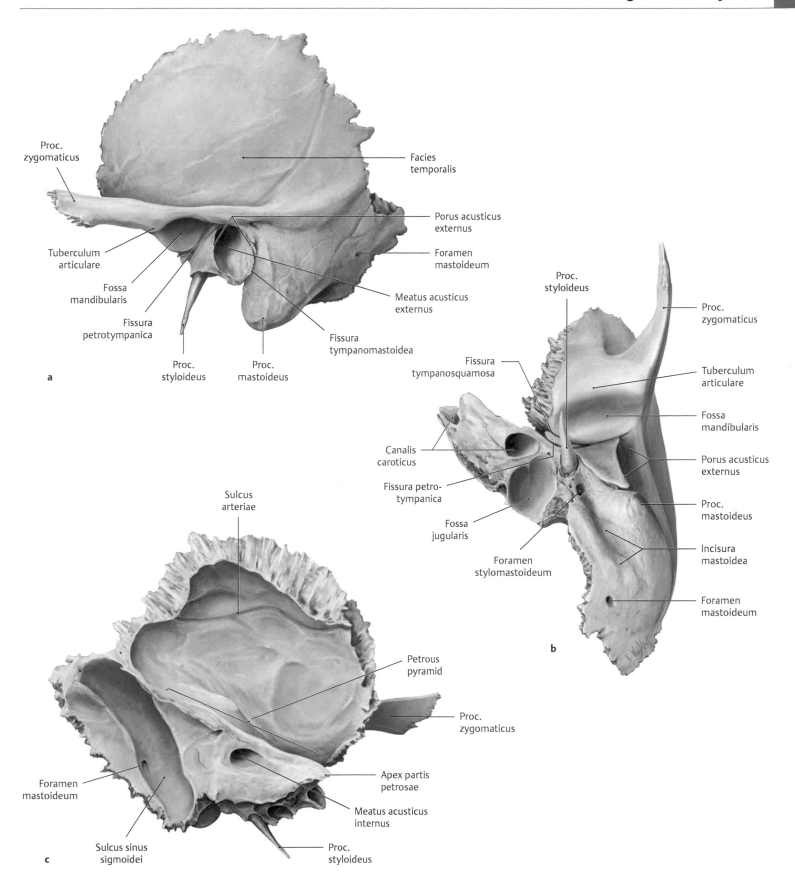

a

Proc. zygomaticus

Tuberculum articulare

Fossa mandibularis

Fissura petrotympanica

Proc. styloideus

Proc. mastoideus

Facies temporalis

Porus acusticus externus

Foramen mastoideum

Meatus acusticus externus

Fissura tympanomastoidea

Proc. styloideus

Fissura tympanosquamosa

Canalis caroticus

Fissura petro-tympanica

Fossa jugularis

Foramen stylomastoideum

Proc. zygomaticus

Tuberculum articulare

Fossa mandibularis

Porus acusticus externus

Proc. mastoideus

Incisura mastoidea

Foramen mastoideum

b

Sulcus arteriae

Foramen mastoideum

Sulcus sinus sigmoidei

Proc. styloideus

Petrous pyramid

Proc. zygomaticus

Apex partis petrosae

Meatus acusticus internus

c

D Left os temporale

a Lateral view. The principal structures of the os temporale are labeled in the diagram. A v. emissaria (see p. 19) passes through the foramen mastoideum (external orifice shown in **a**, internal orifice in **c**), and the chorda tympani passes through the medial part of the fissura petrotympanica (see p. 149). The proc. mastoideus develops gradually in life due to traction from the m. sternocleidomastoideus and is pneumatized from the inside (see **C**).

b Inferior view. The shallow fossa articularis of the art. temporomandibularis (the fossa mandibularis) is clearly seen from the inferior view. The n. facialis emerges from the basis cranii through the

foramen stylomastoideum. The initial part of the v. jugularis interna is adherent to the fossa jugularis, and the a. carotis interna passes through the canalis caroticus to enter the skull.

c Medial view. This view displays the internal orifice of the foramen mastoideum and the meatus acusticus internus. The n. facialis and n. vestibulocochlearis are among the structures that pass through the meatus acusticus internus to enter the pars petrosa. The part of the pars petrosa shown here is also called the *petrous pyramid*, whose apex (often called the "apex partis petrosae") lies on the interior of the base of the skull.

29

2.10 Maxilla

A Position of the two maxillae in the skull
Frontal view. The structure of the two maxillae largely determines the shape of the face. They support the superior row of teeth and transfer the pressure of chewing via the proc. frontalis and arcus zygomatici to the cranium. In their central position they form part of the orbitae (see p. 36) and the wall of the cavitas nasalis (see p. 40) as well as part of the palatum (see p. 44 f). The sinus maxillaris in the maxilla is an important sinus paranasalis (see p. 41 and 184).

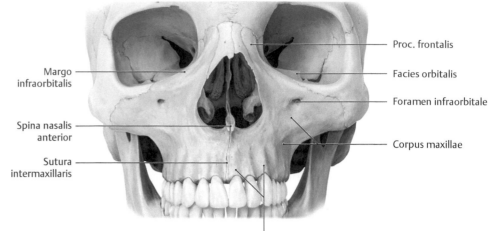

Margo infraorbitalis

Proc. frontalis

Facies orbitalis

Foramen infraorbitale

Spina nasalis anterior

Corpus maxillae

Sutura intermaxillaris

Proc. alveolaris

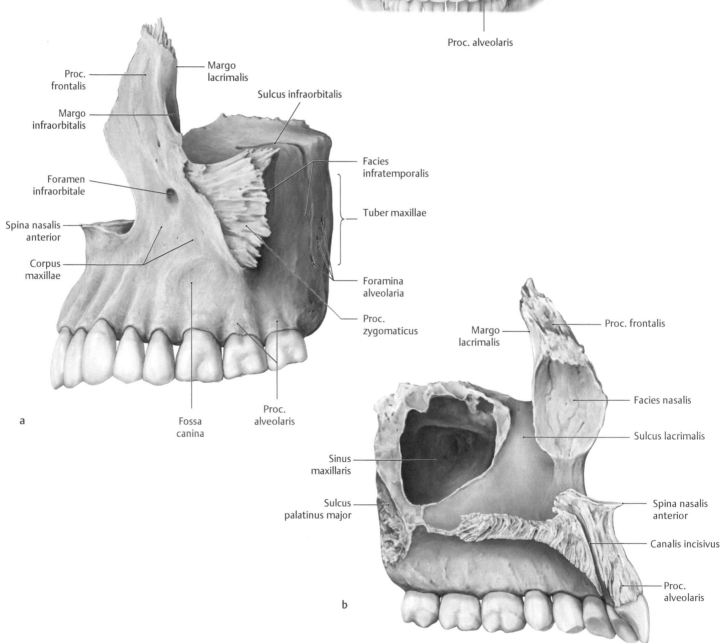

Proc. frontalis

Margo lacrimalis

Margo infraorbitalis

Sulcus infraorbitalis

Foramen infraorbitale

Facies infratemporalis

Tuber maxillae

Spina nasalis anterior

Corpus maxillae

Foramina alveolaria

Fossa canina

Proc. zygomaticus

Proc. alveolaris

a

Margo lacrimalis

Proc. frontalis

Facies nasalis

Sulcus lacrimalis

Sinus maxillaris

Sulcus palatinus major

Spina nasalis anterior

Canalis incisivus

Proc. alveolaris

b

B Isolated maxilla
Lateral view (**a**) and medial view (**b**) with the sinus maxillaris opened.

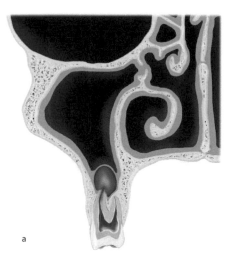

a

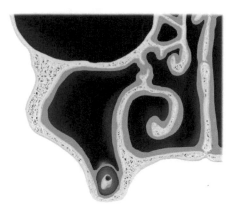

b

C Odontogenic cysts in the maxilla
Anterior view of a right sinus maxillaris. The roots of the superior teeth extend into the sinus maxillaris. This anatomic relationship is clinically important as pain referred to the sinus maxillaris can be caused by teeth. Conversely, inflammation in the sinus maxillaris can spread to the teeth of the upper jaw.
a Radicular cysts develop from the tip of the root of a tooth. Chronic inflammation in the root of the tooth then leads to development of a cyst in the sinus maxillaris.

b Follicular cysts occur as a result of expansion of the dental follicle in the coronal region of a tooth that is prevented from erupting (such as a dens serotinus). Thus, clinical evaluation of an inflammation of the sinus maxillaris sinus must always consider possible causes in the teeth. Because of this, disorders of the sinus maxillaris require close cooperation between ear, nose, and throat specialists and dentists.

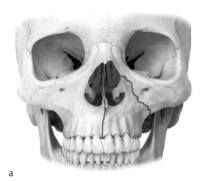

a

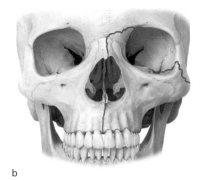

b

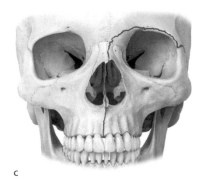

c

D Maxillary resections
Tumors in the sinus maxillaris can be removed surgically. The position and extent of the tumor determine how radical the operation will be.

The following procedures are differentiated: a partial resection of the maxilla (**a**), a total resection (**b**), and a total resection combined with removal of the orbit and its contents (orbital exenteration) (**c**).

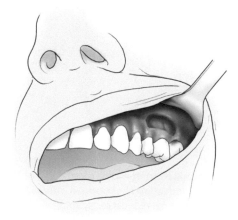

E Surgical approach to the sinus maxillaris
An approach through the vestibulum oris is often chosen for surgical removal of a tumor. The upper lip is reflected with a retractor and the anterior wall of the sinus maxillaris is removed. This exposes the sinus maxillaris. Where indicated, this procedure can be expanded into adjacent regions including the os ethmoidale, orbita, and sinus sphenoidalis. In chronic sinusitis, an endonasal approach is chosen (see **Ed**, p. 25 and **F**, p. 43).

31

2.11 Os Zygomaticum, Os Nasale, Vomer, and Os Palatinum

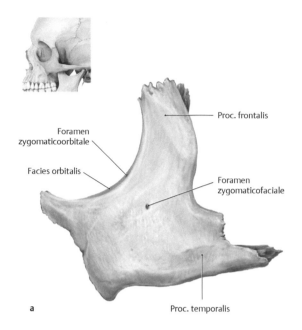

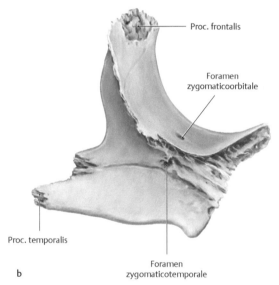

A Os zygomaticum

a Left lateral view (lateral surface) and **b** medial view (temporal surface).
The os zygomaticum forms a bridge between the lateral wall of the skull and the facial bones. It is the bony base of the cheek and as a result it often determines the shape of the face in slender persons. The os zygomaticum has a facies buccalis, facies lateralis, et facies orbitalis et temporalis.

The foramen zygmaticoorbitalis on the facies orbitalis represents the inlet of the canalis zygomaticus. It splits into two canals within the os zygomaticum which terminate at the foramina zygomaticofaciale et zygomaticotemporale. The n. zygomaticus (ramus nervi maxillaris) enters the canalis zygomaticus, where it splits and courses through the two canals.

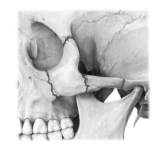
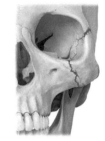

B Fractures of the os zygomaticum

Lateral view (**a**) and frontal view (**b**).
Fractures of the os zygomaticum are relatively common in *blunt trauma of the lateral midface.* Often the bone breaks at all three junctions with its two adjacent bones. Zygomatic fractures are occasionally obscured by soft-tissue swelling. Therefore, one should always determine whether a zygomatic fracture is present after blunt trauma. This is done by comparing both sides (shape of cheek, motility of the eyeball) and testing for sensory deficits (the zygomatic nerve, which courses through a bony canal, may be injured as well).

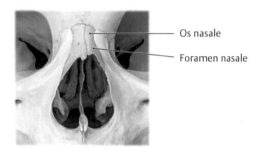

C Os nasale

The two ossa nasalia form the bony base of the bridge of the nose. Their superior borders articulate with the os frontale, their lateral borders with the maxilla. The margo inferior is part of the apertura nasi anterior (see p. 14). Fractures of the os nasale are common and often require reduction.

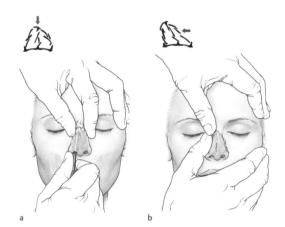

D Principle of the reduction of nasal fractures

In frontal trauma the reduction is performed internally with a retractor (**a**); in lateral trauma external manual reduction is performed (**b**).

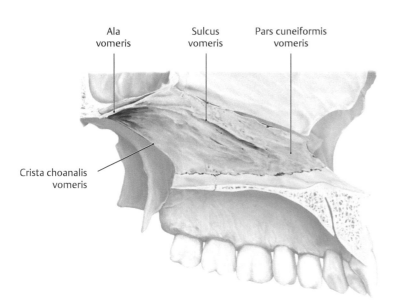

Ala vomeris — Sulcus vomeris — Pars cuneiformis vomeris

Crista choanalis vomeris

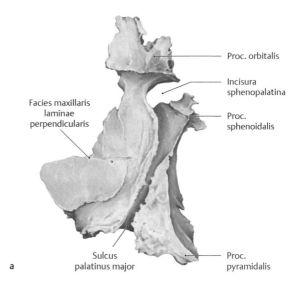

Proc. orbitalis

Incisura sphenopalatina

Facies maxillaris laminae perpendicularis

Proc. sphenoidalis

Sulcus palatinus major

Proc. pyramidalis

a

E Vomer

Lateral view. The vomer and the lamina perpendicularis ossis ethmoidalis together form the bony base of the septum nasi (see p. 14). Along its margo superior are two wings (alae vomeris) that form the junction with the corpus ossis sphenoidalis. As a midline structure, it helps to separate the two partes posteriores cavitatis nasi (choanae; see p. 44 and 185).

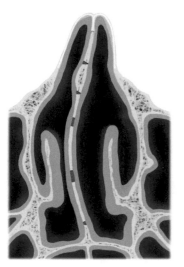
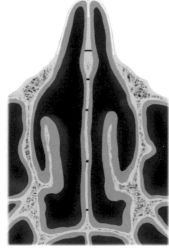

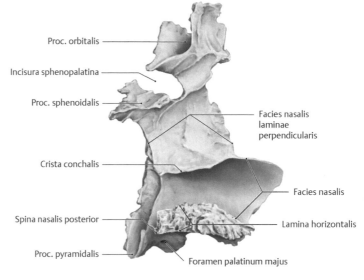

Proc. orbitalis

Incisura sphenopalatina

Proc. sphenoidalis

Crista conchalis

Spina nasalis posterior

Proc. pyramidalis

Facies nasalis laminae perpendicularis

Facies nasalis

Lamina horizontalis

Foramen palatinum majus

b

F Correction of the septum nasi

Superior view. Curved septa nasorum are a common cause of impaired nasal breathing. Surgical correction can involve removing the septum nasi, straightening it, and reimplanting it.

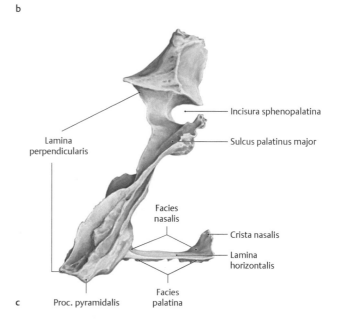

Lamina perpendicularis

Incisura sphenopalatina

Sulcus palatinus major

Facies nasalis

Crista nasalis

Lamina horizontalis

c Proc. pyramidalis — Facies palatina

G Os palatinum

a Lateral view of os palatinum, **b** medial view, and **c** posterior view. The os palatinum consists of a lamina horizontalis and lamina perpendicularis. The lamina horizontalis is the margo posterior palati ossei (see p. 41); the lamina perpendicularis is the portion of the pars lateralis cavitatis nasi that lies in front of the proc. pterygoideus. The os palatinum supplements the pars posterior maxillae and with this bone separates the cavitas oris from the cavitas nasi.

2.12　Sphenoid Bone (Os Sphenoidale)

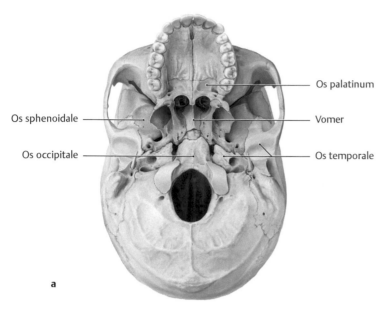

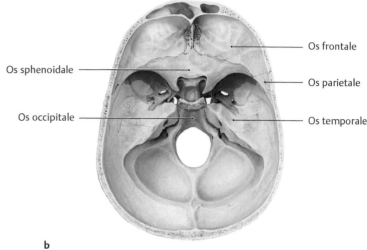

a

b

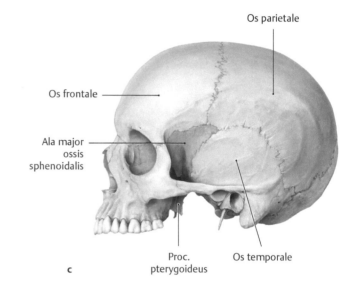

c

A Position of the os sphenoidale in the skull

The os sphenoidale is the most structurally complex bone in the human body. It must be viewed from various aspects in order to appreciate all its features (see also **B**):

a **Basis cranii, external aspect.** The os sphenoidale combines with the os occipitale to form the load-bearing midline structure of the basis cranii.

b **Basis cranii, internal aspect.** The os sphenoidale forms the boundary between the fossae cranii anterior and media. The openings for the passage of nerves and vessels are clearly displayed (see details in **B**).

c **Lateral view.** Portions of the ala major of the os sphenoidale can be seen above the arcus zygomaticus, and portions of the proc. pterygoideus can be seen below the arcus zygomaticus.

Note the bones that border on the os sphenoidale in each view.

B Isolated os sphenoidale

a **Inferior view** (its position in situ is shown in **A**). This view demonstrates the laminae medialis and lateralis of the proc. pterygoidea. Between them is the fossa pterygoidea, which is occupied by the m. pterygoideus medialis. The foramen spinosum and foramen rotundum provide pathways through the basis cranii.

b **Anterior view.** This view illustrates why the os sphenoidale was originally called the sphecoid bone ("wasp bone") before a transcription error turned it into the sphenoid ("wedge-shaped") bone. The apertures of the sinus sphenoidalis on each side resemble the eyes of the wasp, and the procc. pterygoidei of the os sphenoidale form its dangling legs, between which are the fossae pterygoideae. This view also displays the fissura orbitalis superior, which connects the fossa cranii media with the orbita on each side. The two sinus sphenoidales are separated by an internal septum (see p. 43).

c **Superior view.** The superior view displays the sella turcica, whose central depression, the fossa hypophysialis, contains the hypophysis. The foramen spinosum, foramen ovale, and foramen rotundum can be identified posteriorly.

d **Posterior view.** The fissura orbitalis superior is seen particularly clearly in this view, while the canalis opticus is almost completely obscured by the proc. clinoideus anterior. The foramen rotundum is open from the fossa cranii media to the external basis cranii (the foramen spinosum is not visible in this view; compare with **a**). Because the ossa sphenoidale and occipitale fuse together during puberty ("tribasilar bone"), a suture is no longer present between the two bones. The cancellous trabeculae are exposed and have a porous appearance.

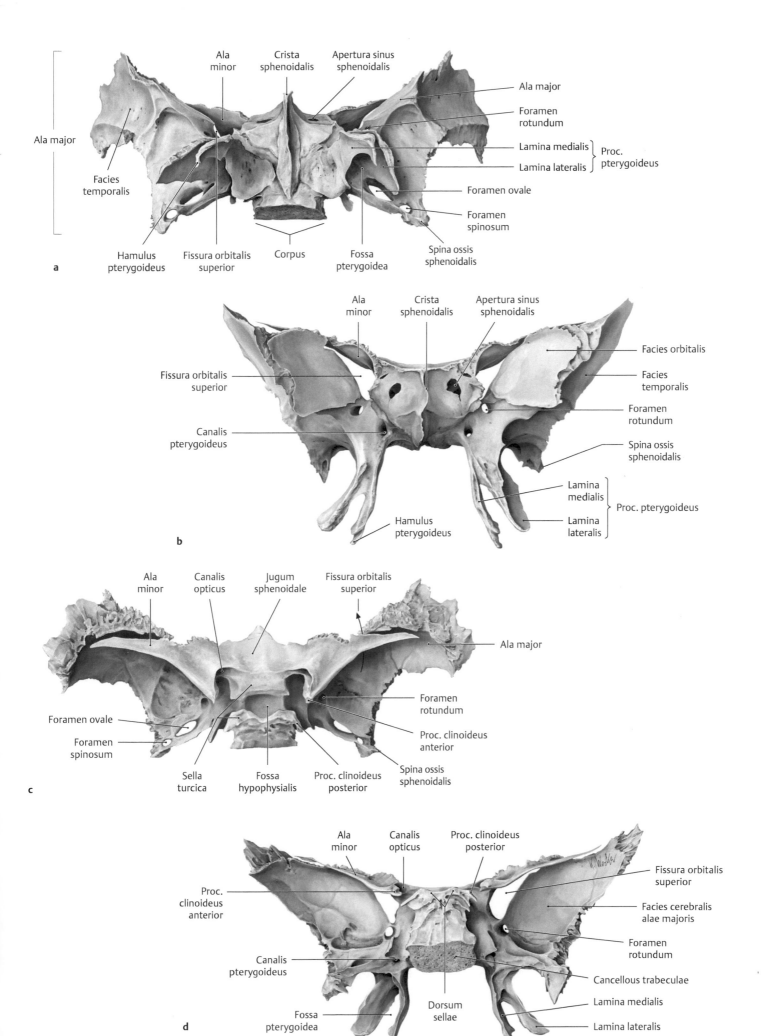

a

Ala major

Facies temporalis

Hamulus pterygoideus

Ala minor

Crista sphenoidalis

Apertura sinus sphenoidalis

Ala major

Foramen rotundum

Lamina medialis
Lamina lateralis } Proc. pterygoideus

Foramen ovale

Foramen spinosum

Spina ossis sphenoidalis

Fissura orbitalis superior

Corpus

Fossa pterygoidea

b

Fissura orbitalis superior

Canalis pterygoideus

Ala minor

Crista sphenoidalis

Apertura sinus sphenoidalis

Facies orbitalis

Facies temporalis

Foramen rotundum

Spina ossis sphenoidalis

Lamina medialis
Lamina lateralis } Proc. pterygoideus

Hamulus pterygoideus

c

Ala minor

Canalis opticus

Jugum sphenoidale

Fissura orbitalis superior

Ala major

Foramen ovale

Foramen spinosum

Sella turcica

Fossa hypophysialis

Proc. clinoideus posterior

Spina ossis sphenoidalis

Foramen rotundum

Proc. clinoideus anterior

d

Proc. clinoideus anterior

Canalis pterygoideus

Fossa pterygoidea

Ala minor

Canalis opticus

Proc. clinoideus posterior

Dorsum sellae

Fissura orbitalis superior

Facies cerebralis alae majoris

Foramen rotundum

Cancellous trabeculae

Lamina medialis

Lamina lateralis

2.13 Orbit (Orbita): Bones and Openings for Neurovascular Structures

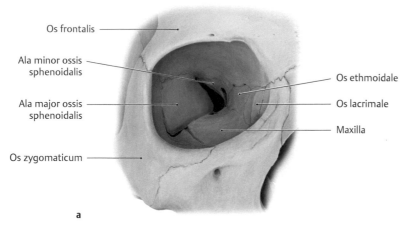

a

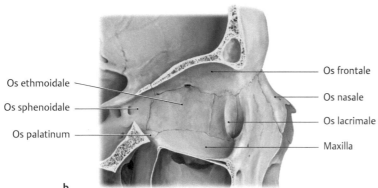

b

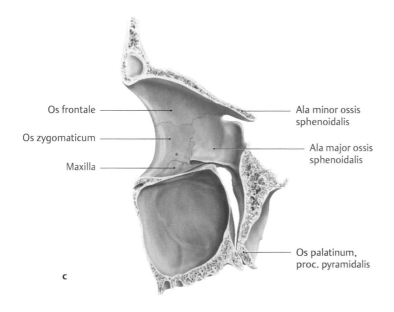

c

Os frontalis
Ala minor ossis sphenoidalis
Ala major ossis sphenoidalis
Os zygomaticum
Os ethmoidale
Os lacrimale
Maxilla

Os ethmoidale
Os sphenoidale
Os palatinum
Os frontale
Os nasale
Os lacrimale
Maxilla

Os frontale
Os zygomaticum
Maxilla
Ala minor ossis sphenoidalis
Ala major ossis sphenoidalis
Os palatinum, proc. pyramidalis

A Bones of the right orbita

Anterior view (**a**), lateral view (**b**), and medial view (**c**). The paries lateralis orbitae has been removed in **b**, and the paries medialis orbitae has been removed in **c**.

The orbita is formed by seven different bones (indicated here by color shading): the os frontale, os zygomaticum, maxilla, os ethmoidale, os sphenoidale (see **a** and **c**), and also the os lacrimale and os palatinum, which are visible only in the medial view (see **b**).

The present unit deals with the bony anatomy of the orbitae themselves. The relationships of the orbits to each other are described in the next unit.

B Openings in the orbita for neurovascular structures

Note: The supraorbital foramen is an important site in routine clinical examinations because the examiner presses on the supraorbital rim with the thumb to test the sensory function of the supraorbital nerve. The supraorbital nerve is a terminal branch of the first division of the trigeminal nerve (CN V_1, see p. 116). When pain is present in the distribution of the trigeminal nerve, tenderness to pressure may be noted at the supraorbital site.

Opening or passage	Neurovascular structures
Canalis opticus	• N. opticus (CN II) • A. ophthalmica

Fissura orbitalis superior	• N. oculomotorius (CN III)
	• N. trochlearis (CN IV)
	• N. ophthalmicus (CN V_1)
	  – N. lacrimalis
	  – N. frontalis
	  – N. nasociliaris
	• N. abducens (CN VI)
	• V. ophthalmica superior

Fissura orbitalis inferior	• N. infraorbitalis (of CN V_2) • A., v., and n. infraorbitalis (of CN V_2) • Rami orbitales (of CN V_2) • V. opthalmica inferior
Foramen ethmoidale anterius	• A., v., and n. ethmoidalis anterior
Foramen ethmoidale posterius	• A., v., and n. ethmoidalis posterior
Canalis infraorbitalis	• A., v., and n. infraorbitalis
Foramen supraorbitale	• A. supraorbitalis • N. supraorbitalis (ramus lateralis)
Incisura frontalis	• A. supratrochlearis • N. supraorbitalis (ramus medialis)
Foramen zygomatico-orbitale	• N. zygomaticus (of CN V_2)
Canalis naso-lacrimalis	• Ductus nasolacrimalis

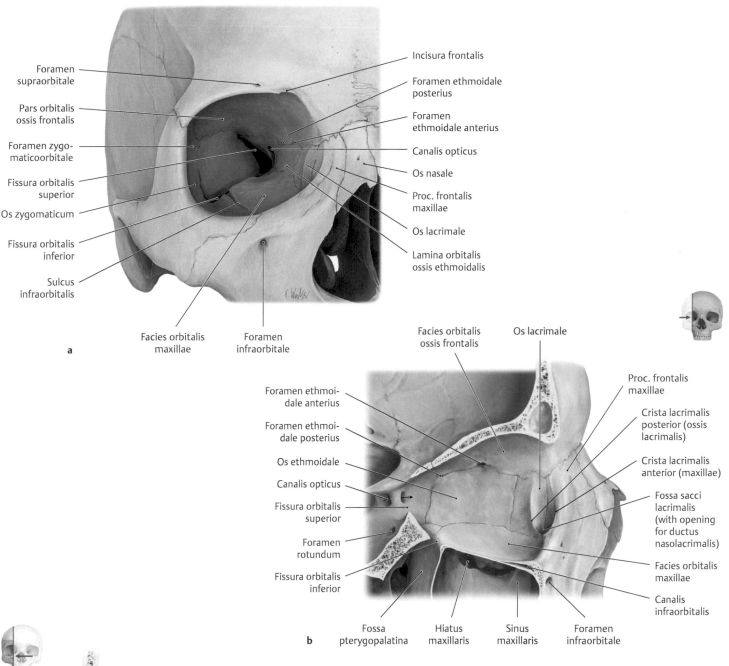

a

Foramen supraorbitale
Pars orbitalis ossis frontalis
Foramen zygomaticoorbitale
Fissura orbitalis superior
Os zygomaticum
Fissura orbitalis inferior
Sulcus infraorbitalis
Facies orbitalis maxillae
Foramen infraorbitale

Incisura frontalis
Foramen ethmoidale posterius
Foramen ethmoidale anterius
Canalis opticus
Os nasale
Proc. frontalis maxillae
Os lacrimale
Lamina orbitalis ossis ethmoidalis

b

Facies orbitalis ossis frontalis
Os lacrimale
Foramen ethmoidale anterius
Foramen ethmoidale posterius
Os ethmoidale
Canalis opticus
Fissura orbitalis superior
Foramen rotundum
Fissura orbitalis inferior
Fossa pterygopalatina
Hiatus maxillaris
Sinus maxillaris
Foramen infraorbitale
Proc. frontalis maxillae
Crista lacrimalis posterior (ossis lacrimalis)
Crista lacrimalis anterior (maxillae)
Fossa sacci lacrimalis (with opening for ductus nasolacrimalis)
Facies orbitalis maxillae
Canalis infraorbitalis

c

Facies orbitalis ossis frontalis
Sinus frontalis
Facies orbitalis ossis zygomatici
Foramen zygomaticoorbitale
Facies orbitalis maxillae
Canalis infraorbitalis
Fissura orbitalis inferior
Fissura orbitalis superior
Ala minor ossis sphenoidalis
Ala major ossis sphenoidalis
Sinus maxillaris
Proc. pyramidalis ossis palatini

C Openings and pathways for neurovascular structures

Right orbita, anterior view (**a**), lateral view (**b**), and medial view (**c**). The paries lateralis orbitae has been removed in **b**, the paries medialis orbitae in **c**. The following openings for the passage of neurovascular structures (see listing in **B**) can be identified: the fissurae orbitales superior and inferior (**a–c**), the canalis opticus (**a, b**), the foramina ethmoidalia anterius and posterius (**b, c**), the sulcus infraorbitalis (**a**), which merges into the canalis infraorbitalis (**b, c**) and ends in the foramen infraorbitale (**a, b**); Foramen supraorbitale and incisura frontalis (**a**); Foramen zygomaticoorbitale (**c**).

Diagram **b** shows the orifice of the ductus nasolacrimalis, by which lacrimal fluid is conveyed to the meatus nasi inferior (see p. 42).

The lateral view (**b**) demonstrates the funnel-like structure of the orbita, which functions like a socket to contain the bulbus oculi and constrain its movements. The fissura orbitalis inferior opens into the fossa pterygopalatina, which borders on the posterior wall of the sinus maxillaris. It contains the ganglion pterygopalatinum, an important component of the parasympathetic nervous system (see pp. 239 and 127). In the sinus maxillaris, which has been exposed, the elevated opening of the sinus maxillaris (hiatus maxillaris) is identifiable. It connects the sinus maxillaris located below the concha nasi media with the cavitas nasi.

2.14 Orbita and Neighboring Structures

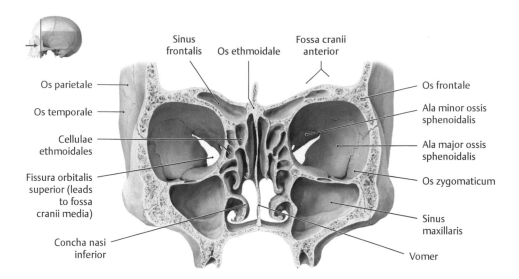

Sinus frontalis — Os ethmoidale — Fossa cranii anterior
Os parietale
Os temporale
Cellulae ethmoidales
Fissura orbitalis superior (leads to fossa cranii media)
Concha nasi inferior
Os frontale
Ala minor ossis sphenoidalis
Ala major ossis sphenoidalis
Os zygomaticum
Sinus maxillaris
Vomer

B Clinically important relationships between the orbitae and surrounding structures

Relationship to the orbit	Neighboring structures
Inferior	• Sinus maxillaris
Superior	• Sinus frontalis • Fossa cranii anterior (contains the lobus frontalis encephali)
Medial	• Cellulae ethmoidales

Deeper structures that have a clinically important relationship to the orbita:

- Sinus sphenoidalis
- Fossa cranii media
- Chiasma opticum
- Hypophysis
- Sinus cavernosus
- Fossa pterygopalatina

A Bones of the orbita and adjacent cavities

The color-coding here is the same as for the bones of the orbita on pp.14–15. These bones also form portions of the walls of neighboring cavities. The following adjacent structures are visible in the diagram:

- Fossa cranii anterior
- Sinus frontalis
- Fossa cranii media

- Cellulae ethmoidales*
- Sinus maxillaris

Disease processes may originate in the orbita and spread to these cavities, or originate in these cavities and spread to the orbita.

* The *Terminologia Anatomica* has dropped the term "sinus ethmoidalis" in favor of "cellulae ethmoidales."

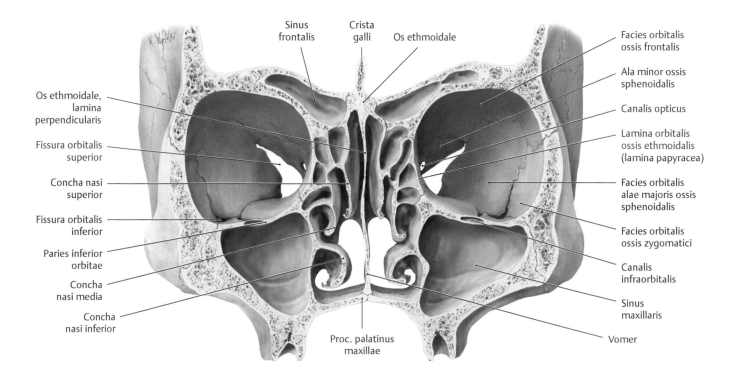

Sinus frontalis — Crista galli — Os ethmoidale
Os ethmoidale, lamina perpendicularis
Fissura orbitalis superior
Concha nasi superior
Fissura orbitalis inferior
Paries inferior orbitae
Concha nasi media
Concha nasi inferior
Proc. palatinus maxillae
Facies orbitalis ossis frontalis
Ala minor ossis sphenoidalis
Canalis opticus
Lamina orbitalis ossis ethmoidalis (lamina papyracea)
Facies orbitalis alae majoris ossis sphenoidalis
Facies orbitalis ossis zygomatici
Canalis infraorbitalis
Sinus maxillaris
Vomer

C Orbitae and neighboring structures

Coronal section through both orbitae, viewed from the front. The walls separating the orbit from the cellulae ethmoidales (0.3 mm, lamina papyracea) and from the sinus maxillaris (0.5 mm, paries inferior orbitae) are very thin. Thus, both of these walls are susceptible to frac-tures and provide routes for the spread of tumors and inflammatory processes into or out of the orbita. The fissura orbitalis superior com-municates with the fossa cranii media, and so several structures that are not pictured here—the sinus sphenoidalis, hypophysis, and chiasma opticum—are also closely related to the orbita.

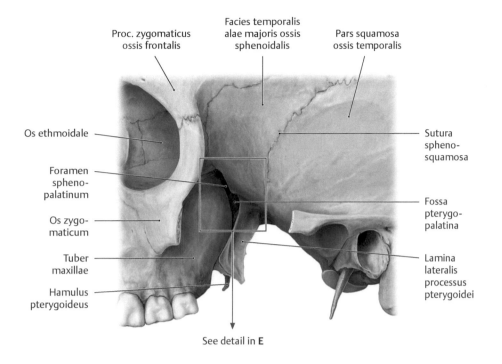

Proc. zygomaticus ossis frontalis

Facies temporalis alae majoris ossis sphenoidalis

Pars squamosa ossis temporalis

Os ethmoidale

Foramen spheno-palatinum

Os zygo-maticum

Tuber maxillae

Hamulus pterygoideus

Sutura spheno-squamosa

Fossa pterygo-palatina

Lamina lateralis processus pterygoidei

See detail in **E**

D Close-up view of the left fossa pterygo-palatina

Lateral view. The fossa pterygopalatina is a crossroads between the fossa cranii media, orbita, and cavitas nasi, being traversed by many nerves and vessels that supply these regions. The fossa pterygopalatina is continuous laterally with the fossa infratemporalis. This diagram shows the lateral approach to the fossa pterygopalatina through the fossa infratemporalis, which is utilized in surgical approaches to tumors in this region (e.g., nasopharyngeal fibroma).

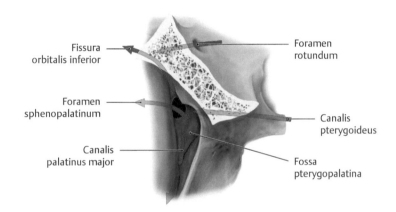

Fissura orbitalis inferior

Foramen sphenopalatinum

Canalis palatinus major

Foramen rotundum

Canalis pterygoideus

Fossa pterygopalatina

E Connections of the left fossa pterygopalatina with adjacent regions

Detail from **D**. The contents of the fossa pterygopalatina include the ganglion pterygopalatinum (see pp. 239 and 127), which is an important parasympathetic ganglion in the autonomic nervous system.

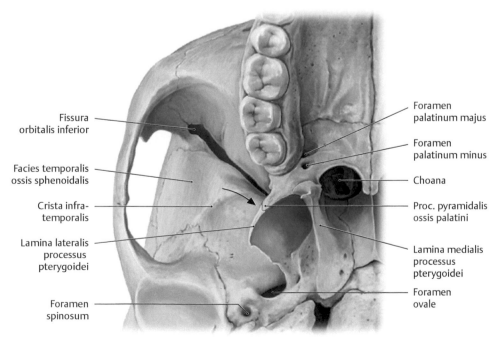

Fissura orbitalis inferior

Facies temporalis ossis sphenoidalis

Crista infra-temporalis

Lamina lateralis processus pterygoidei

Foramen spinosum

Foramen palatinum majus

Foramen palatinum minus

Choana

Proc. pyramidalis ossis palatini

Lamina medialis processus pterygoidei

Foramen ovale

F Structures adjacent to the right fossa pterygopalatina

Inferior view. The arrow indicates the approach to the fossa pterygopalatina via the fossa infratemporalis as viewed from the basis cranii. The fossa itself (not visible in this view) is lateral to the lamina lateralis of the proc. pterygoideus of the os sphenoidale. In this image the os sphenoidale is shaded green.

For borders of the fossa pterygopalatina as well as access routes and neurovascular structures see p. 238 f.

2.15 Nose: Nasal Skeleton

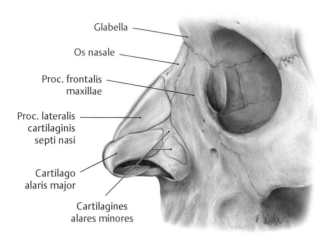

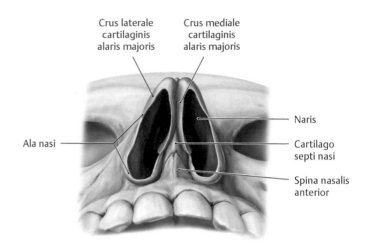

A Skeleton of the external nose
Left lateral view. The skeleton of the nose is composed of bone, cartilage, and connective tissue. Its upper portion is bony and frequently involved in midfacial fractures, while its lower, distal portion is cartilaginous and therefore more elastic and less susceptible to injury. The proximal lower portion of the nostrils (alae nasi) is composed of connective tissue with small embedded pieces of cartilage. The proc. lateralis is a winglike lateral expansion of the cartilago septi nasi rather than a separate piece of cartilage.

B Nasal cartilage
Inferior view. Viewed from below, each of the cartilagines alares majores is seen to consist of a crus mediale and laterale. This view also displays the two nares, which open into the cavitates nasi. The right and left cavitates nasi are separated by the septum nasi, whose inferior pars cartilaginea is just visible in the diagram. The wall structure of a single cavitas nasi will be described in this unit, and the relationship of the cavitas nasi to the sinus paranasales will be explored in the next unit.

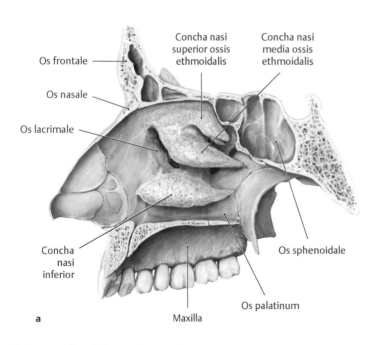

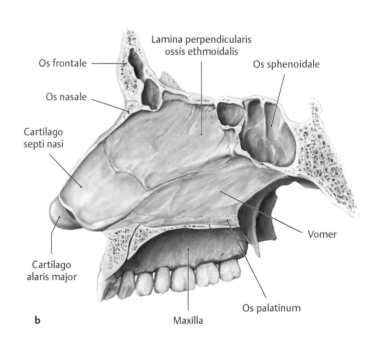

C Bony walls of the cavitas nasi
a Right cavitas nasi, left lateral view; septum nasi has been removed.
b Paramedian section, left lateral view.
The cavitas nasi has four walls:

- the roof (ossa nasale, frontale and ethmoidale),
- the floor (maxilla and os palatinum),

- the lateral wall including maxilla, os nasale, os lacrimale, os ethmoidale, and os palatinum, and the concha nasi inferior.
- the medial wall (septum nasi, see **b** and **E**), which is composed of cartilage and the following bones: os nasale, os ethmoidale, vomer, and os sphenoidale, os palatinum, and maxilla, these latter three contributing only small bony projections to the septum nasi.

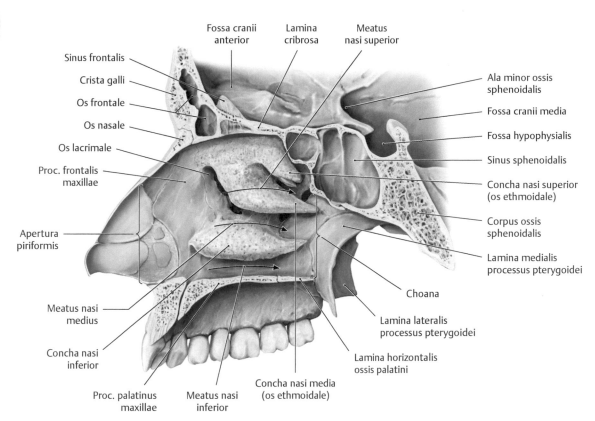

Sinus frontalis

Crista galli

Os frontale

Os nasale

Os lacrimale

Proc. frontalis maxillae

Apertura piriformis

Meatus nasi medius

Concha nasi inferior

Proc. palatinus maxillae

Meatus nasi inferior

Fossa cranii anterior

Lamina cribrosa

Meatus nasi superior

Concha nasi media (os ethmoidale)

Ala minor ossis sphenoidalis

Fossa cranii media

Fossa hypophysialis

Sinus sphenoidalis

Concha nasi superior (os ethmoidale)

Corpus ossis sphenoidalis

Lamina medialis processus pterygoidei

Choana

Lamina lateralis processus pterygoidei

Lamina horizontalis ossis palatini

D Cavitas nasi with illustration of airflow around the three conchae nasi

Left lateral view. Air enters the bony concha nasi through the apertura piriformis and passes over the three conchae nasi as well as through the spaces under each concha—the meatus nasi inferior, medius, and superior. Air leaves the nose through the choanae, entering the pars nasalis pharyngis.

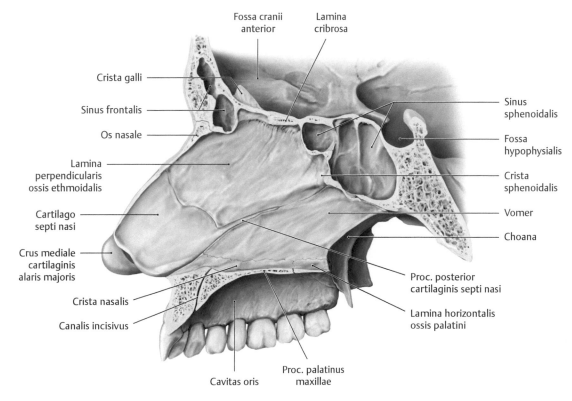

Crista galli

Sinus frontalis

Os nasale

Lamina perpendicularis ossis ethmoidalis

Cartilago septi nasi

Crus mediale cartilaginis alaris majoris

Crista nasalis

Canalis incisivus

Fossa cranii anterior

Lamina cribrosa

Sinus sphenoidalis

Fossa hypophysialis

Crista sphenoidalis

Vomer

Choana

Proc. posterior cartilaginis septi nasi

Lamina horizontalis ossis palatini

Cavitas oris

Proc. palatinus maxillae

E Septum nasi

Parasagittal section viewed from the left side. The left lateral wall of the cavitas nasi has been removed with the adjacent bones. The septum nasi consists of an anterior cartilaginous part, the septal cartilage, and a posterior bony part (see **Cb**). The posterior process of the cartilaginous septum extends deep into the bony septum. Deviations of the septum nasi are common and may involve the cartilaginous part of the septum, the bony part, or both. Cases in which the septal deviation is sufficient to cause obstruction of nasal breathing can be surgically corrected.

41

2.16   Nose: Paranasal Sinuses (Sinus Paranasales)

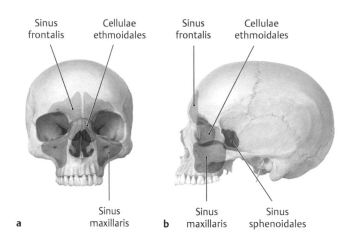

a — Sinus frontalis · Cellulae ethmoidales · Sinus maxillaris
b — Sinus frontalis · Cellulae ethmoidales · Sinus maxillaris · Sinus sphenoidales

Age 1 · Age 4 · Age 8 · Age 12 · Age 20 · Age 60+
Age 20 · Age 12 · Age 8 · Age 4 · Age 1

A Projection of the sinus paranasales onto the skull
a Anterior view, **b** lateral view.
The sinus paranasales are air-filled cavities that reduce the weight of the skull. Because they are subject to inflammation that may cause pain over the affected sinus (e.g., frontal headache due to frontal sinusitis), knowing the location of the sinuses is helpful in making the correct diagnosis.
Note: The term "cellulae ethmoidales" has replaced the formerly used term "sinus ethmoidalis."

B Pneumatization of the sinus maxillaris and frontalis
Anterior view. The sinus frontalis and maxillaris develop gradually during the course of cranial growth (pneumatization)—unlike the cellulae ethmoidales which are already pneumatized at birth. As a result, sinusitis in children is most likely to involve the cellulae ethmoidales (with risk of orbital penetration: red, swollen eye; see **D**).

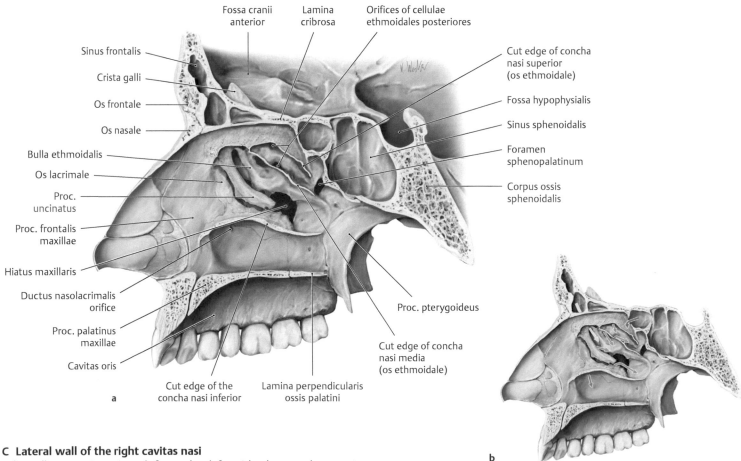

C Lateral wall of the right cavitas nasi
a,b Midline section viewed from the left with the conchae nasi removed to display the openings in the underlying meatal regions, i.e., the ductus nasolacrimalis and sinus paranasales emptying into the cavitas nasi (see colored arrows in **b**: red = ductus nasolacrimalis, yellow = sinus frontalis, orange = sinus maxillaris, green = cellulae ethmoidales anteriores and posteriores, blue = sinus sphenoidalis; drainage routes are described in **E**).

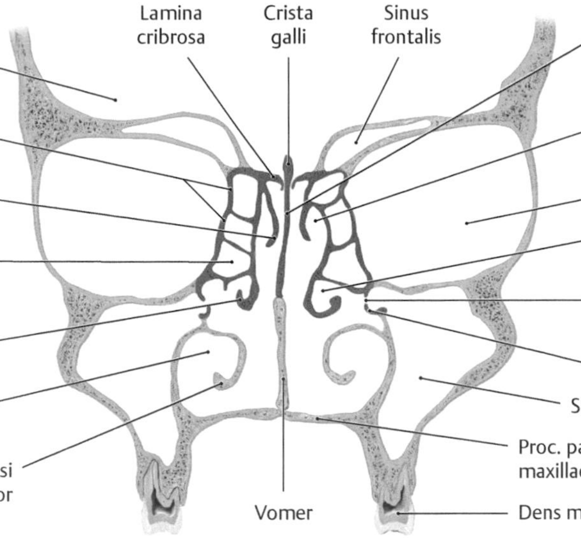

Lamina cribrosa
Crista galli
Sinus frontalis
Fossa cranii anterior
Lamina orbitalis ossis ethmoidalis
Concha nasi superior
Cellulae ethmoidales mediae
Concha nasi media
Meatus nasi inferior
Concha nasi inferior
a
Vomer
Lamina perpendicularis ossis ethmoidalis
Meatus nasi superior
Orbita
Meatus nasi medius
Ostium of sinus maxillaris
Proc. uncinatus
Sinus maxillaris
Proc. palatinus maxillae
Dens molaris maxillaris

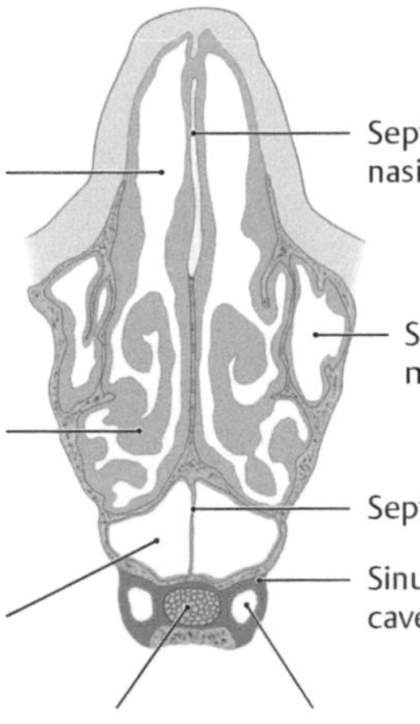

Cavitas nasi
Septum nasi
Sinus maxillaris
Mucosal folds on the concha nasi media
Septum nasi
Sinus cavernosus
Sinus sphenoidalis
Hypophysis
A. carotis interna
b

D Bony structure of the sinus paranasales

a Frontal section; **b** transverse section, mucosa has been left intact, superior view.

The central structure of the sinus paranasales is the os ethmoidale (red). Its cribriform plate forms a portion of the anterior basis cranii. The sinus frontalis and maxillares are grouped around the os ethmoidale. In the cavitas nasi, the meatus nasales inferior, medius and superior are visible. They are each bounded by its analogously-named concha. The concha *media* is a useful landmark in surgical procedures on the anterior os ethmoidale and the sinus maxillaris, the bony ostium of which is located lateral to the concha nasi media, and opens into the meatus nasi medius. *Below* this concha, located cranially is the largest chamber in the os ethmoidale, the bulla ethmoidalis. At its anterior margin a bony hook is visible. It bounds the sinus maxillaris opening anteriorly as the proc. uncinatus. The lateral wall separating the os ethmoidale from the orbita is paper-thin (lamina papyracea) so inflammatory processes and tumors may penetrate this thin plate in either direction.

Note: The deepest point of the sinus maxillaris is located in the root area of the dentes maxillares molares (in 30% of people, the distance between sinus maxillaris and radix dentis buccalis is less than 1 mm). Thus, periapical inflammation in this area can extend to the sinus floor. When extracting an upper molar, opening the sinus maxillaris is the most likely procedure.

The transverse section (**b**), shows the hypophysis, located behind the sinus sphenoidalis in the fossa hypophysialis (see **C**), is accessible to transnasal surgical procedures. The surface of the mucosa has been left intact to show how narrow the entire cavitas nasi is and how swelling can quickly obstruct it (see **E**).

E Sites where the ductus nasolacrimalis and sinus paranasales open into the cavitas nasi

Nasal passage	Structures that open into the passage
Meatus nasi inferior	• Ductus nasolacrimalis
Meatus nasi medius	• Sinus frontalis • Sinus maxillaris • Cellulae ethmoidales anteriores • Cellulae ethmoidales mediae
Meatus nasi superior	• Cellulae ethmoidales posteriores
Recessus sphenoethmoidalis	• Sinus sphenoidalis

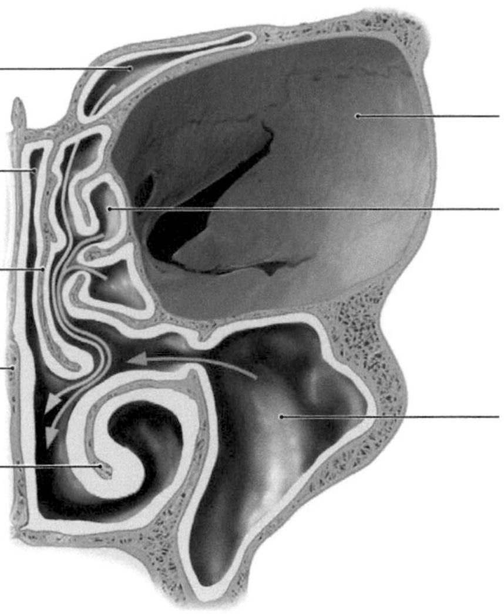

Sinus frontalis
Cavitas nasi
Concha nasi media
Septum nasi
Concha nasi inferioris
Orbita
Cellulae ethmoidales
Sinus maxillaris

F Ostiomeatal unit on the left side of the cavitas nasi

Coronal section. When the mucosa (ciliated respiratory epithelium) in the cellulae ethmoidales (green) becomes swollen due to inflammation (sinusitis), it blocks the flow of secretions (see arrows) from the sinus frontalis (yellow) and sinus maxillaris (orange) in the ostiomeatal unit (red). Because of this blockage, micro-organisms also become trapped in the other sinuses, where they may incite inflammation. Thus, while the anatomical focus of the disease lies in the cellulae ethmoidales, inflammatory symptoms are also manifested in the sinus frontalis and maxillaris. In patients with *chronic sinusitis*, the narrow sites can be surgically widened to establish an effective drainage route, alleviating the condition.

2.17 Hard Palate (Palatum Durum)

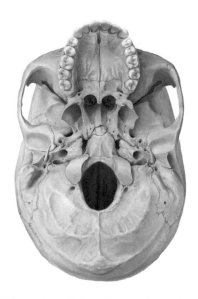

A Integration of the palatum durum into the basis cranii
Inferior view.

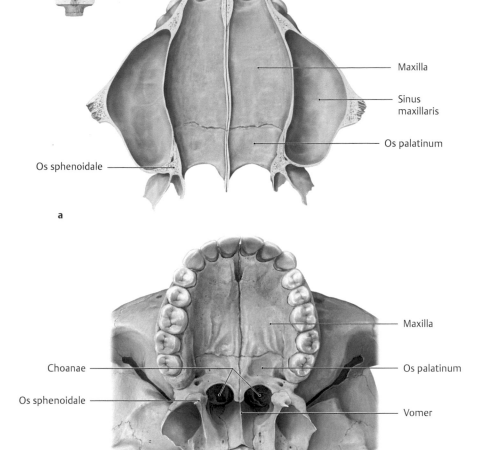

a

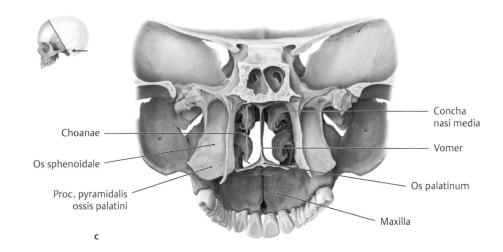

b

c

B Bones of the palatum durum

a Superior view. The palatum durum is a horizontal bony plate formed by parts of the maxilla and os palatinum. It serves as a partition between the cavitates oris and nasi. In this view we are looking down at the floor of the cavitatis nasi, whose inferior surface forms the roof of the cavitas oris. The upper portion of the maxilla has been removed. The os palatinum is bordered posteriorly by the os sphenoidale.

b Inferior view. The choanae, the posterior openings of the cavitas nasi, begin at the posterior border of the palatum durum.

c Oblique posterior view. This view demonstrates the close relationship between the cavitates oris and nasi.
Note how the proc. pyramidalis of the os palatinum is integrated into the lamina lateralis of the proc. pterygoideus of the os sphenoidale.

Labels in figure a: Maxilla, Sinus maxillaris, Os palatinum, Os sphenoidale

Labels in figure b: Maxilla, Os palatinum, Vomer, Choanae, Os sphenoidale

Labels in figure c: Concha nasi media, Vomer, Os palatinum, Maxilla, Choanae, Os sphenoidale, Proc. pyramidalis ossis palatini

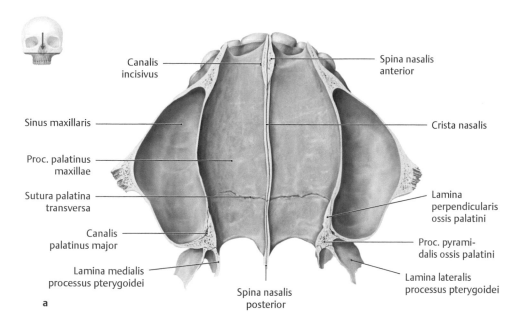

Canalis incisivus

Spina nasalis anterior

Sinus maxillaris

Crista nasalis

Proc. palatinus maxillae

Sutura palatina transversa

Lamina perpendicularis ossis palatini

Canalis palatinus major

Proc. pyramidalis ossis palatini

Lamina medialis processus pterygoidei

Lamina lateralis processus pterygoidei

Spina nasalis posterior

a

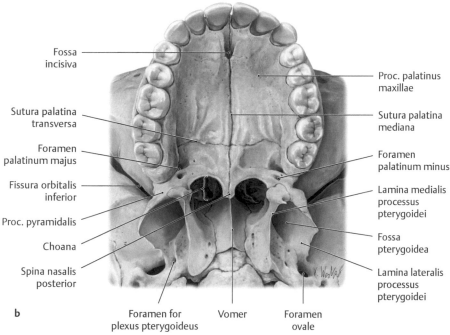

Fossa incisiva

Proc. palatinus maxillae

Sutura palatina transversa

Sutura palatina mediana

Foramen palatinum majus

Foramen palatinum minus

Fissura orbitalis inferior

Lamina medialis processus pterygoidei

Proc. pyramidalis

Choana

Fossa pterygoidea

Spina nasalis posterior

Lamina lateralis processus pterygoidei

b

Foramen for plexus pterygoideus

Vomer

Foramen ovale

Proc. clinoideus anterior

Septum sinuum sphenoidalium

Canalis opticus

Apertura sinus sphenoidalis

Fissura orbitalis superior

Fossa pterygoidea

Concha nasi media

Fissura orbitalis inferior

Vomer

Choana

Concha nasi inferior

Os palatinum

Lamina lateralis processus pterygoidei

Sutura palatina mediana

Lamina medialis processus pterygoidei

Foramen incisivum

Proc. palatinus maxillae

c

C Palatum durum

a **Superior view** of the floor of the cavitas nasi (=upper portion of palatum durum) with the upper part of the maxilla removed. The palatum durum separates the cavitas oris from the cavitates nasi. The small canal that links the cavitates oris and nasi, the canalis incisivus (present here on both sides), merges within the bone to form one canal, which opens on the inferior surface by a single orifice, the foramen incisivum (see **b**).

b **Inferior view.** The two horizontal processes of the maxilla, the procc. palatini, grow together during development and become fused at the sutura palatina mediana. Failure of this fusion results in a *cleft palate*. The boundary line between anterior clefts (cleft lip, alone or combined with a cleft alveolus) and posterior clefts (cleft palate) is the foramen incisivum. These anomalies may also take the form of cleft lip and palate (with a defect involving the lip, alveolus, and palate).

Note: The cavitas nasi (whose floor is formed by the palatum durum) communicates with the pars nasalis pharyngis by way of the choanae.

c **Oblique posterior view** of the posterior part of the os sphenoidale at the level of the corpus ossis sphenoidalis, displaying both sinus sphenoidales separated by a septum. The close topographical relationship between the cavitas nasi and palatum durum can be appreciated in this view. If the palatum durum is unfused in a nursing infant due to a cleft anomaly (cf. **b**), some of the ingested milk will be diverted from the cavitas oris and will enter the nose. This defect should be closed with a plate immediately after birth to permit satisfactory oral nutrition.

45

2.18 Mandible (Mandibula) and Hyoid Bone (Os Hyoideum)

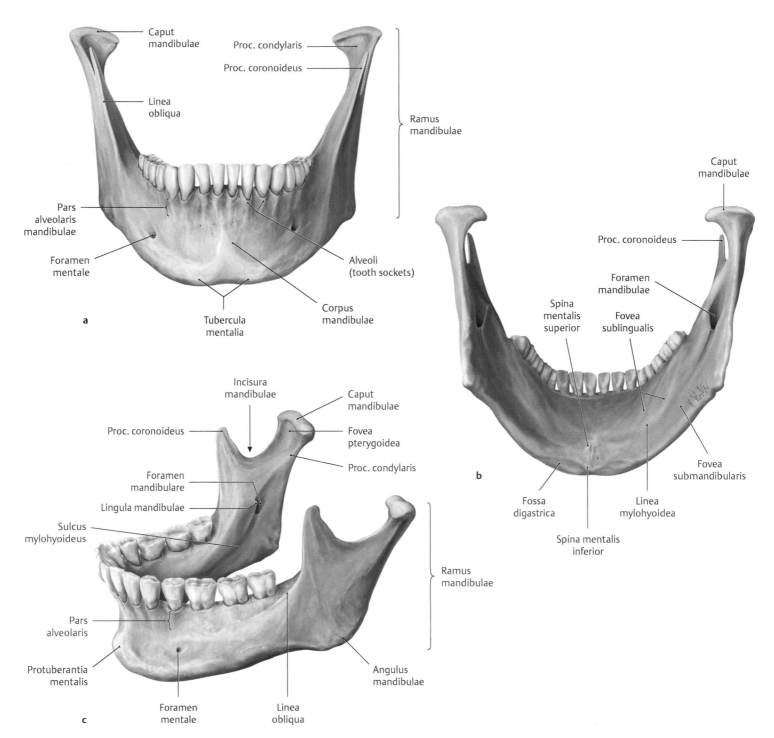

A Mandibula

a Anterior view. The mandibula is connected to the viscerocranium at the art. temporomandibularis, whose convex surface is the head of the condylus mandibulae. This "caput mandibulae" is situated atop the vertical (ascending) ramus mandibulae, which joins with the corpus mandibulae at the angulus mandibulae. The dentes are set in the pars alveolaris along the upper border of the corpus mandibulae. This part of the mandibula is subject to typical agerelated changes as a result of dental development (see **B**). The n. mentalis branch of the n. trigeminus exits through the foramen mentale to enter its bony canal. The location of this foramen is important in clinical examinations, as the tenderness of the nerve to pressure can be tested at that location (e.g., in trigeminal neuralgia, p. 123).

b Posterior view. The foramen mandibulae is particularly well displayed in this view. It transmits the n. alveolaris inferior, which supplies sensory innervation to the mandibular teeth. Its terminal branch emerges from the foramen mentale. The two mandibular foramina are interconnected by the canalis mandibularis.

c Oblique left lateral view. This view displays the proc. coronoideus, the proc. condylaris, and the incisura mandibulae between them. The proc. coronoideus is a site for muscular attachments, while the proc. condylaris bears the caput mandibulae, which articulates with the fossa mandibularis of the os temporale. A depression on the medial side of the proc. condylaris, the fovea pterygoidea, gives attachment to portions of the m. pterygoideus lateralis.

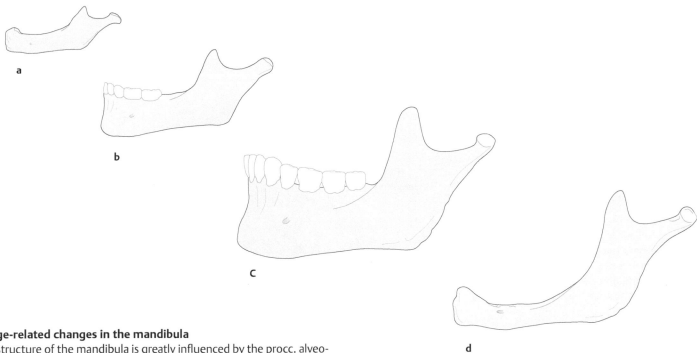

B Age-related changes in the mandibula

The structure of the mandibula is greatly influenced by the procc. alveolares of the teeth. Because the angulus mandibulae adapts to changes in the pars alveolaris, the angle between the corpus and ramus mandibulae also varies with age-related changes in the dentition. The angle measures approximately 150° at birth, and approximately 120—130° in adults, increasing to 140° in the edentulous mandibula of old age.

a At birth, the mandibula is without teeth and the pars alveolaris has not yet formed.
b In children, the mandibula bears the dentes decidui. The pars alveolaris is still relatively poorly developed because the dentes decidui are considerably smaller than the dentes permanentes.

c In adults, the mandibula bears the dentes permanentes, and the pars alveolaris of the bone is fully developed.
d Old age is characterized by an edentulous mandibula with resorption of the pars alveolaris.

Note: The resorption of the pars alveolaris with advanced age leads to a change in the position of the foramen mentale (which is normally located below the second dens premolaris, as in **c**). This change must be taken into account in surgery or dissections involving the n. mentalis.

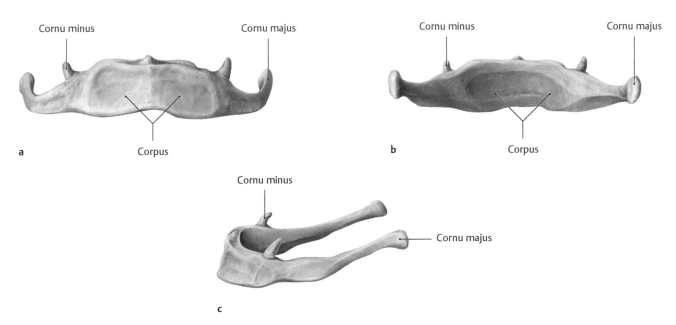

C Os hyoideum

a Anterior view; **b** Posterior view; **c** Oblique left lateral view. The os hyoideum is suspended by muscles between the oral floor and larynx in the neck (see p. 189), although it is listed among the ossa cranii in the *Terminologia Anatomica*. The cornu majus and corpus of the os hyoideum are palpable in the neck. The physiological movement of the os hyoideum during swallowing is also palpable.

2.19 Teeth (Dentes) in situ

A Characteristics of teeth

Human teeth are the result of a long phylogenetic evolution in vertebrates. The typical dentition of a mammal is as follows:

- **heterodont** = four different forms of teeth (incisors, canine, premolars, molars)
- **diphyodont** = two successive sets of teeth
- **thecodont** = teeth set in sockets composed of alveolar bone and held in place by a resilient attachment apparatus.

Note: In humans diphyodonty pertains only to dentes decidui (1. tooth generation) and their replacement teeth (2. tooth generation). The accessional teeth (1., 2., and 3. molar), which come through at the back of the gum are monophyodont since they do not have primary predecessors.

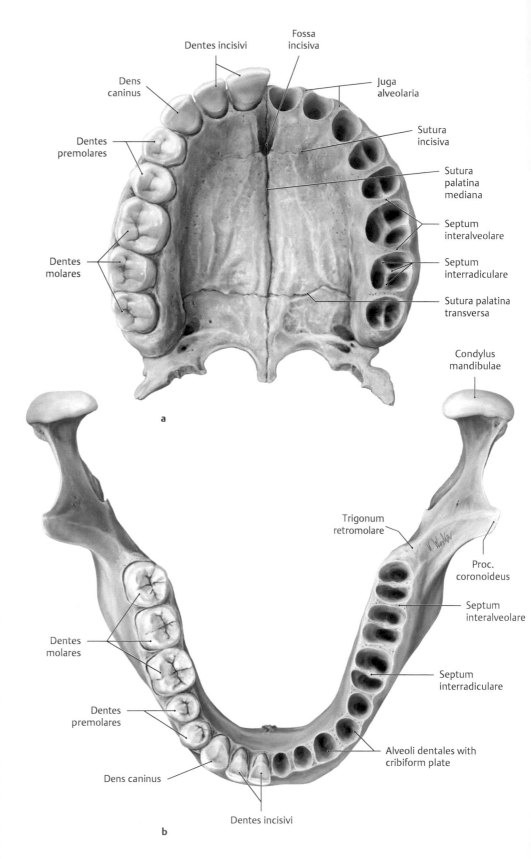

a

b

B Permanent teeth (dentes permanentes) in adults

a Maxilla. Caudal view showing the chewing surfaces.

b Mandibula. Cranial view; right side of both images shows the proc. alveolaris of maxilla and mandibula after removal of teeth.

In human dentition, both the maxilla and mandibula each contain 16 teeth, which are aligned in a bilateral-symmetrical fashion and are adjusted to different chewing functions. Each half of both maxilla and mandibula consists of

- **Front Teeth:** two dentes incisivi and one dens caninus,
- **Side Teeth:** two dentes premolares and three dentes molares.

Note: While the front teeth grab the food and bite off pieces for mastication, it is the side teeth that actually perform mastication. They function in mincing and grinding the food. After removal of teeth (see left side in each image) the proc. alveolaris, which holds the teeth, becomes visible. Particularly in the front teeth area, the dental roots in the alveoli curve the jawbone in parts heavily to the vestibular to the extent that they become palpable as so-called Juga alveolaria. At these points, the adjacent substantia compacta is extremely thin (approximately 0.1 mm). The septum interalveolare separates the alveoles of two adjacent teeth. The septum interradiculare separates the tooth chambers of multi-rooted teeth (for structure of the alveolar bone see p. 57).

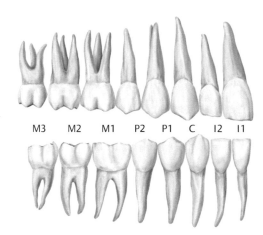

C Tooth shapes of the permanent dentition

The dentition of an adult consists of 8 different shapes of teeth in both the maxilla and mandibula. Starting from the front of the jaw, the teeth are arraigned successively to lateral-posterior and without any gaps:

- I1 - dens incisivus medialis
- I2 - dens incisivus lateralis
- C - dens caninus
- P1 - dens premolaris primus
- P2 - dens premolaris secundus
- M1 - dens molaris primus
- M2 - dens molaris secundus
- M3 - dens molaris tertius

Note: Dentes molares are the human's largest teeth. They have distinct cuspides (tubercula) and fossae. The dens molaris primus often possesses an additional cuspis, the tuberculum anomale (see **E** for comparison). For build-up of occlusal surfaces cf. p. 45.

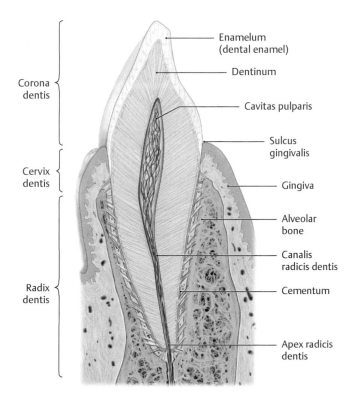

Enamelum (dental enamel)

Dentinum

Corona dentis

Cavitas pulparis

Sulcus gingivalis

Cervix dentis

Gingiva

Alveolar bone

Canalis radicis dentis

Cementum

Radix dentis

Apex radicis dentis

D Histology of a tooth

A dens incisivus mandibularis serves as an example in this image, which depicts both hard substance (dentinum, enamelum, cementum) and soft tissue (pulp).

E Number of cuspides, radices, and canales radicum of the dentes permanentes of the maxilla and mandibula

Data about the frequency was taken from Lehmann et al. (2009) and Strup et al. (2003). The area where a root is divided into two branches is called bifurcation and trifurcation for three root branches.

Dens Maxillaris	Number of Cuspides	Number of Radices	Number of Canales Radicum
I1 (11/21)*	incisal edge	1	1
I2 (12/22)	incisal edge	1	1
C (13/23)	1 (cutting edge)	1	1
P1 (14/24)	2	2 (ca. 60 %) 1 (ca. 40 %) 3 (rare)	2 (ca. 80 %) 1 (ca. 20 %) 3 (rare)
P2 (15/25)	2	1 (ca. 90 %) 2 (ca. 10 %)	1 (ca. 60 %) 2 (ca. 40 %)
M1 (16/26)	4 (without tuberculum anomale = additional cusp located on mesio-palatine cusp)	3	3 (ca. 45 %) 4 (ca. 55 %)
M2 (17/27)	4	3	3 (ca. 55 %) 4 (ca. 45 %)
M3 (18/28)	mostly 3 (extremely inconsistent in shape)	Roots often intermingled (so-called taproots)	irregular

Mandibular Tooth	Number of Cusps	Number of Roots	Number of Root Canals
I1 (31/41)	incisal edge	1	1 (ca. 70 %) 2 (ca. 30 %) 3 (rare)
I2 (32/42)	incisal edge	1	1 (ca. 70 %) 2 (ca. 30 %)
C (33/43)	cutting edge	1	1 (ca. 80 %) 2 (ca. 20 %)
P1 (34/44)	2 (75 %) 3 (25 %)	1	1 (ca. 75 %) 2 (ca. 25 %) 3 (rare)
P2 (35/45)	3 (cuspis lingualis often divided into 2)	1	1 (ca. 95 %) 2 (ca. 5 %) 3 (rare)
M1 (36/46)	5	2	3 (ca. 75 %) 2 (ca. 25 %) 4 (rare)
M2 (37/47)	4	2	3 (ca. 70 %) 2 (ca. 30 %) 4 (rare)
M3 (38/48)	usually 4 (very variable)	usually 2 (very variable)	irregular

* For identification of teeth with 2-digit numbers see **D**. p. 50

2.20 Terminology, Dental Schema, and Dental Characteristics

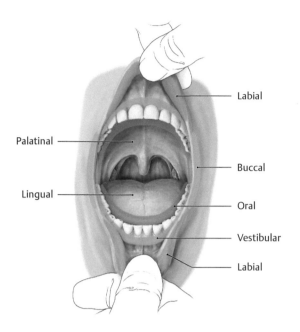

A Directions of the cavitas oris

Labial

Palatinal

Lingual

Buccal

Oral

Vestibular

Labial

B Anatomical terms of the tooth

Term	Description
mesial	in the arcus dentalis toward the midline
distal	toward the end of arcus dentalis
oral	toward cavitas oris
facial	toward the cheek or lips
lingual	toward the tongue
labial	toward the inside of the lip
buccal	toward the inside of the cheek
palatal	toward the palatum (only with maxillary teeth)
vestibular	toward vestibulum oris
approximal	between two teeth crowns
incisal	toward biting edge
occlusal	on the chewing surface
cervical	toward cervix dentis
coronal	toward corona dentis
apical	toward apex radicis dentis
pulpal	toward pulpa dentis

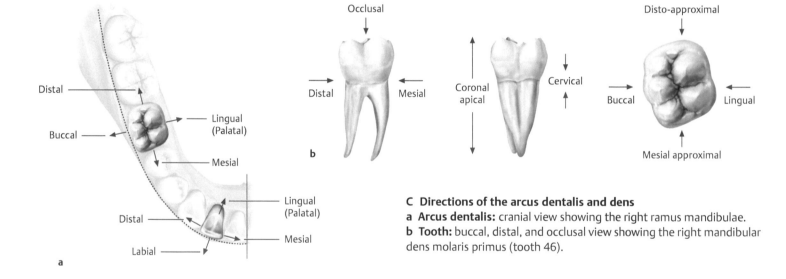

C Directions of the arcus dentalis and dens
a Arcus dentalis: cranial view showing the right ramus mandibulae.
b Tooth: buccal, distal, and occlusal view showing the right mandibular dens molaris primus (tooth 46).

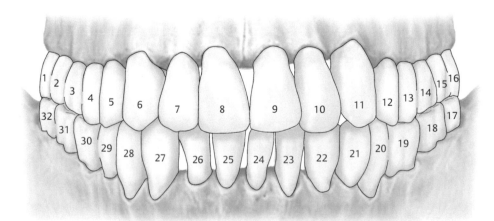

D Coding the dentes permanentes
In the United States, the dentes permanentes are numbered sequentially, not assigned to quadrants. Progressing in a clockwise fashion (from the perspective of the dentist), the teeth of the arcus dentalis superior are numbered 1 to 16, and those of the arcus dentalis inferior are considered 17 to 32.
Note: The dens molaris tertius maxillaris (dens serotinus) on the patient's right is considered 1.

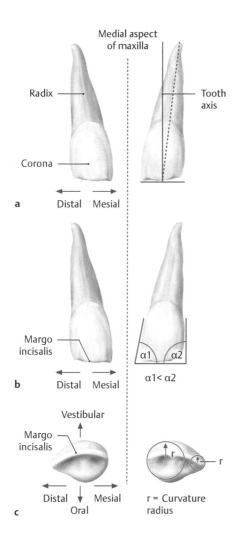

Medial aspect
of maxilla

Radix — Tooth axis

Corona —

a Distal | Mesial

Margo
incisalis

α1 α2

α1 < α2

b Distal | Mesial

Vestibular

Margo
incisalis

Distal | Mesial
Oral

r = Curvature
radius

c

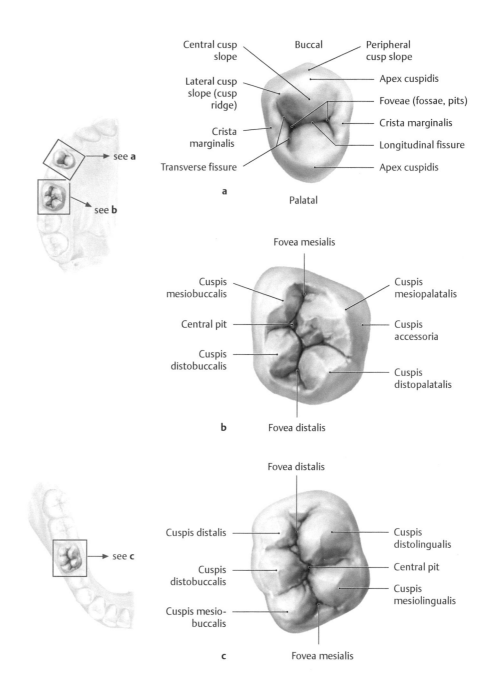

see **a**

see **b**

Central cusp slope — Buccal — Peripheral cusp slope

Lateral cusp slope (cusp ridge) — Apex cuspidis

Foveae (fossae, pits)

Crista marginalis — Crista marginalis

Transverse fissure — Longitudinal fissure

Apex cuspidis

a Palatal

Fovea mesialis

Cuspis mesiobuccalis — Cuspis mesiopalatalis

Central pit — Cuspis accessoria

Cuspis distobuccalis — Cuspis distopalatalis

b Fovea distalis

Fovea distalis

Cuspis distalis — Cuspis distolingualis

Central pit

Cuspis distobuccalis — Cuspis mesiolingualis

Cuspis mesio-buccalis

c Fovea mesialis

see **c**

E Common dental characteristics

As early as 1870, Felix Muehlreiter described certain dental characteristics, which all teeth have in common and with the help of which the same teeth can be safely assigned to either the left or the right side respectively:

a Root surface characteristic: Evaluation of tooth from vestibular. It refers to the course of the radix dentis, which bends distally and thus slightly deviates from the axis of the tooth.

b Tooth angle characteristic: Evaluation of tooth from vestibular. It is particularly pronounced in dentes canini. The angle formed by the margo incisalis and the sides of the corona is shorter on the facies mesialis compared to the facies distalis.

c Curvature characteristic: Evaluation from incisal or occlusal. It shows that the proximal surface radius of curvature is longer on the facies mesialis than on the facies distalis, meaning teeth are significantly more dense mesially.

Further distinguishing features include the **cervical line of a tooth** (course of the cementoenamel junction), the **tooth equator** (anatomical equator), the **crown escape** (particularly pronounced in mandibular teeth) as well as the **root cross-section.**

F Structure of the chewing surface

a components of the chewing surface illustrated with the help of an upper right dens premolaris (P1 or Tooth 14 respectively), occlusal view

b nomenclature of the cusp of the dens molaris primus (M1) and the right maxilla (tooth 16), cranial view

c nomenclature of the cusp of the dens molaris primus (M1) of the right mandibula (tooth 46), cranial view

With the exception of both the upper and lower incisors (dentes incisivi), the chewing surfaces of the human permanent dentition have up to 5 cusps (cuspides dentis). While the canines (dentes canini) have a split incisal edge in the shape of a biting edge composed of a single large cusp, the molars (dentes premolares and molares) all have at least two biting

edges (see p. 53). On an individual basis, one distinguishes between apex cuspidis, cusp ridge, fossae, fissures, and crista marginalis (**a**). Horizontal and vertical fissures separate the individual tooth cusps. Dents at cross points and junctions of the tooth have a predilection to become decayed. Inside the cusps of a chewing surface one distinguishes between supporting and non-supporting cusps (see p. 47). Cuspides accessoriae, so-called tubercula anomalia, are not rare (for example tuberculum of carabelli at the cuspis mesiopalatalis of the dens molaris maxillaris primus).

Note: While the anatomical chewing surface is defined by both the cristae marginales as well as the ridge of the cusp edge, the functional chewing surface overlaps with the outside surface of the supporting cusps.

2.21 Position of Teeth in Permanent Dentition: Orientation of the Skull and Dental Occlusion

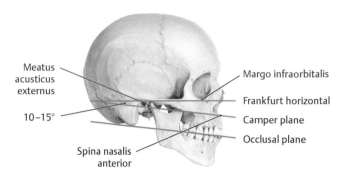

A Occlusal planes of the skull

The following planes help to evaluate the position of teeth in the jaw and orientation of the skull:

- **Frankfurt Horizontal Plane** = passing from the upper edge of the porus acusticus to the lowest point of the margo infraorbitalis.
- **Camper Plane** = according to Camper (1792), running from lower rim of the porus acusticus externus to spina nasalis anterior. Nowadays, its clinical definition describes the plane extending between both the dorsal soft tissue points (left and right tragus) and the anterior subnasale.
- **Occlusal Plane** = running through margo incisalis (see **B**) and the highest point of the apices cuspidum distobuccalium (see **B**) of the 2. left and right dentes molares mandibulares.

Note: While the Camper and Frankfurt planes form an angle of 10–15°, the Camper and occlusal planes run parallel.

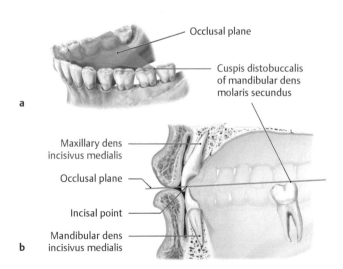

a

b

B Occlusal plane

a Left-front and above view of occlusal plane; **b** vestibular view of occlusal plane. The occlusal plane is marked by three reference points in the tooth-bearing region of the mandibula:

- Incisal point (where the margines incisales of the two lower dentes incisivi mediales touch)
- Tip of the cuspis distobuccalis of the 2. mandibular right dens molaris (tooth 47)
- Tip of the cuspis distobuccalis of the 2. mandibular left dens molaris (tooth 37)

Thus, the occlusal plane is situated at the height of lip closure line and runs parallel to the Camper plane (see **A**).

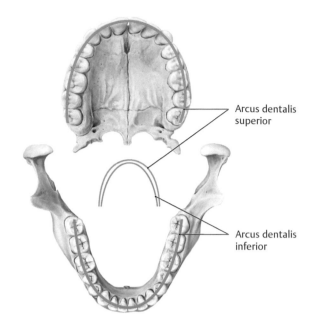

C Arcus dentales superior and inferior

In the maxilla and mandibula, the teeth are positioned in the shape of an arch (so-called dental arches: arcus dentales superior and inferior respectively). The arcus dentales relate to the curve formed by the cutting edges of the dentes incisivi, apices coronarum of the canines and apices cuspidum buccalium of the dentes premolares and molares. The arcus dentalis superior forms a semi-ellipse and the arcus dentalis inferior a parable. Due to the different shapes of the two arcus dentales, both the maxillary dentes incisivi and molares overhang their mandibular counterparts, thereby covering the margines incisales and the cuspides buccales.

Note: Due to the convex proximate surfaces, the teeth forming the arcus dentales touch only at certain points (so-called proximal contact points). The contact points are usually situated in the upper third of the corona dentis and help to give interdental support and stabilization of two adjacent teeth (see **B**).

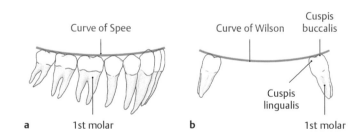

a   1st molar   **b**   1st molar

D Sagittal and transversal curveae occlusales

a Sagittal curvea occlusalis (so-called curve of Spee), vestibular view; **b** Transversal curvea occlusalis (so-called curve of Wilson), distal view. If looking at the apices cuspidum of the mandibular toothrow from vestibular, the line connecting the apices cuspidum buccalium forms a convex curve the lowest point of which is situated in the area around the dens molaris primus. According to Spee (1870), that curve touches the anterior area of the capsula art. temporomandibularis; its center is supposed to be situated in the middle of the orbita. The course of the transversal curvea occlusalis is the result of the cuspides linguales of the mandibular teeth lying lower than the cuspides buccales.

Note: Both the sagittal and transversal curveae occlusales are important when installing artificial teeth.

E Different types of occlusal forms

Occlusion means the contact of teeth of the maxilla and mandibula. In more detail, one distinguishes between

- **static occlusion** = contacts of teeth when the jaw is not moving,
- **dynamic occlusion** = contacts made when the jaw is moving,
- **habitual occlusion** = alignment of the teeth of the upper and lower jaw when brought together.

Maximal intercuspation refers to the position of the maxilla and mandibula when brought into maximum contact, meaning the cusps of the teeth of both arches fully interpose themselves with one another.

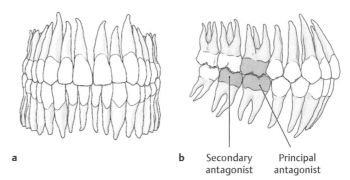

a   b   Secondary   Principal
                 antagonist   antagonist

F Occlusion of tooth rows at normal occlusion
a Frontal view; **b** Vestibular view.
At normal occlusion, two phenomena become visible:

- Due to the differing sizes of both arcus dentales, the margines incisales of the upper dentes incisivi overlap the lower dentes incisivi by approximately 3–4 mm on the vestibular (see **b** and **Ga**). The overlapping of the cuspides buccales of the maxillary teeth with the mandibular teeth is attributable to the same cause. It is however not visible (see **Gc** and **d**).
- The upper dens incisivus medialis is wider than the lower dens incisivus medialis, which results in a mesiodistal shift, which extends to the posterior region (see **b** and **Gb**).

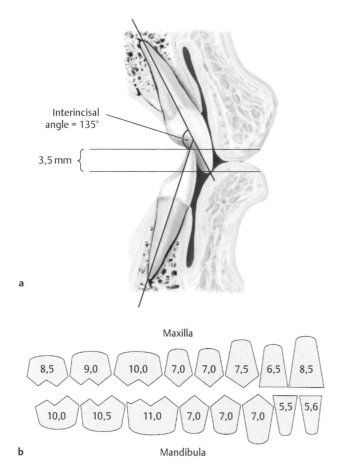

a

Interincisal angle = 135°

3,5 mm

Maxilla

| 8,5 | 9,0 | 10,0 | 7,0 | 7,0 | 7,5 | 6,5 | 8,5 |

| 10,0 | 10,5 | 11,0 | 7,0 | 7,0 | 7,0 | 5,5 | 5,6 |

b   Mandibula

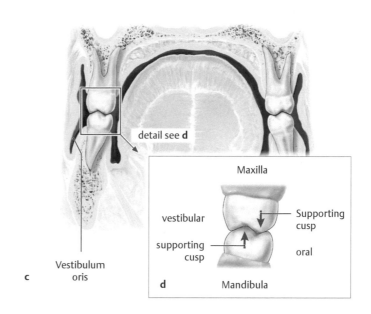

detail see **d**

Maxilla

vestibular

supporting cusp

Supporting cusp

oral

c   Vestibulum oris   d   Mandibula

G Position of teeth at normal occlusion
a Occlusion of the upper and lower incisors; **b** Schema of the teeth's position in the maxilla and mandibula (according to Schuhmacher). Stated is the medium mesiodistal width of the teeth in millimeters (according to Carlsson et al.); **c** Normal occlusion, distal view; **d** Enlarged section from image **c**.

a In the lateral view, the so-called incisor overbite (see **F**), also known as scissors bite, is clearly visible. The occlusal contacts between the lower incisors and the palatal surfaces of the upper incisors and the axes of the upper and lower incisors are at a 135° angle (interincisal angle) to each other.

b In the sagittal direction—with the exception of two teeth (1. lower incisor, and 3. upper molar)—every tooth is in contact with two teeth of the opposing jaw, the primary and secondary antagonist (= **one-tooth to two-teeth relationship in the posterior region,** cf. **F**). The tip of the upper dens caninus is situated between the lower dens

caninus and the following lower dens premolaris, the cuspis mesiobuccalis of the dens molaris maxillaris primus points toward the mesiobuccal fissure of the dens molaris mandibularis primus. This tooth position is called neutral occlusion.

c and **d** In transversal direction, the maxillary and mandibular cuspides buccales overlap on the vestibular. The cusps, which reach into the fissure and fossa of their antagonists respectively, are called supporting and working cusp respectively and have a rather round shape unlike the non-supporting cusps. The maxillary supporting cusps are cuspides palatales and cuspides buccales in the mandibula.

Note: The primary function of the chewing surfaces in the posterior tooth region is chopping and grinding food between the cusps. The fissures serve as drain channels for the crushed food and at the same time offer space for the cusps to grind.

2.22 Permanent Teeth (Dentes Permanentes) Morphology

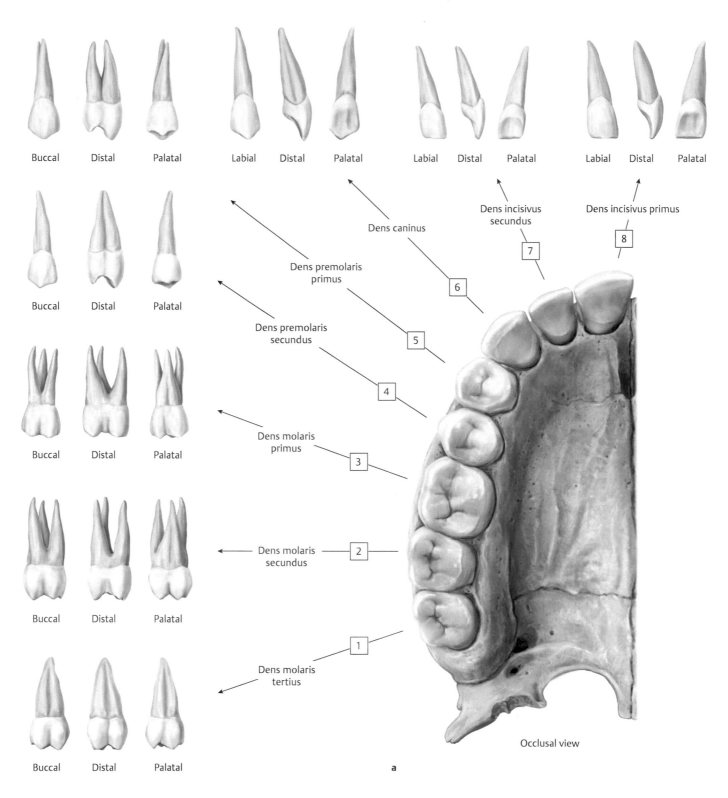

| Buccal | Distal | Palatal |

| Labial | Distal | Palatal |

| Labial | Distal | Palatal |

| Labial | Distal | Palatal |

Dens incisivus secundus

Dens incisivus primus

Dens caninus

7

8

Dens premolaris primus

6

Dens premolaris secundus

5

| Buccal | Distal | Palatal |

4

Dens molaris primus

3

| Buccal | Distal | Palatal |

Dens molaris secundus 2

| Buccal | Distal | Palatal |

1

Dens molaris tertius

| Buccal | Distal | Palatal |

Occlusal view

a

A Morphology of the dentes permanentes of the maxilla and mandibula

a Right maxilla, occlusal view; **b** Right mandibula, occlusal view Isolated teeth shown in various views; for numeration of individual teeth cf. Dental formula, p. 50)

Incisors (dentes incisivi): Incisors are used for cutting off chunks of food. Accordingly, they are sharp-edged (scoop-shaped). In addition, they largely determine the esthetic appearance of the oral region. In general, all incisors are single-rooted. The upper medial incisor is the largest, the lower medial the smallest. The palatal surfaces of the two upper incisors have two cristae marginales each, in between which a tuberculum dentis is located in the dens incisivus medialis and a foramen cecum in the dens incisivus lateralis. Similar characteristics are considerably less distinct in both the lower incisors.

Canines (dentes canini): Canines are the most shape-consistent teeth. Their common characteristic is a single cusp formed by a divided incisal surface. Usually, canines are single-rooted, have a relatively long root and support the incisors (longer and more pointed canines in mammals are considered fangs). While the labial surface has two facets, the oral

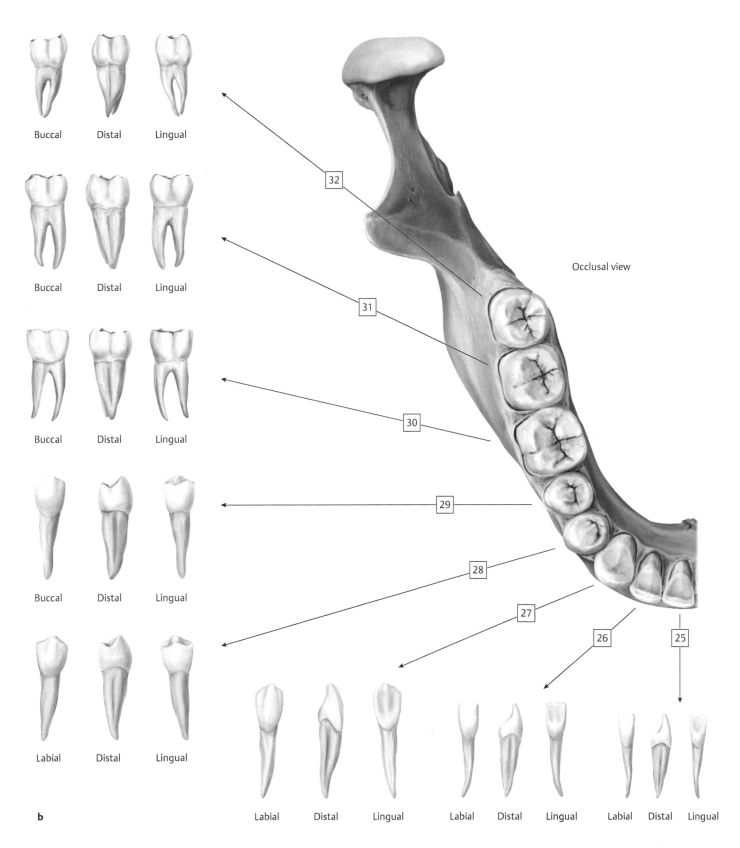

Buccal Distal Lingual

Buccal Distal Lingual

Buccal Distal Lingual

Buccal Distal Lingual

Labial Distal Lingual

Occlusal view

b Labial Distal Lingual Labial Distal Lingual Labial Distal Lingual Labial Distal Lingual

surface has two well pronounced cristae marginales, a median line and a tuberculum dentis. Root surface and curvature characteristic are well defined.

Premolars (dentes premolares): Their common characteristic is a two-cusp morsal surface with a vestibular cusp alignment. Except for the 1. upper dens premolaris, they have a single root. The dentes premolares represent a transitional form from dentes incisivi to molares and have cusps and fissures. That is a sign that now it is all about grinding rather than biting off food.

Molars (dentes molares): They are the largest teeth of the permanent dentition and have a morsal suface with multiple cusps. In order to absorb the powerful chewing pressure, the maxillary molars have three roots, compared with usually two in the mandibula. Only the roots of the third molars (dentes serotini, which usually erupt not before age 16—if at all) are often fused together (see **E**, p. 49).

55

2.23 Periodontium

A Elements and functions of the periodontium

What holds teeth to the jaw bone is a particular form of syndesmosis, the gomphosis (dentoalveolar syndesmosis). The periodontium's functional unit includes all structures that bind the tooth to its bony socket:

- gum (gingiva)
- cementum
- periodontal membrane
- alveolar bone

Essential functions of the periodontium:

- anchoring of the tooth in the bone and transforming chewing pressure into tensile stress
- mediating sensation of pain and regulating chewing pressure through nerve fibers and sensitive nerve endings
- defending against infection through efficient separation of cavitas oris and dental root region and large number of defense cells
- rapid metabolism and high regenerative capacity (adapting to functional and topographic changes for example in position of teeth as a result of orthodontic treatment) through a generous blood supply.

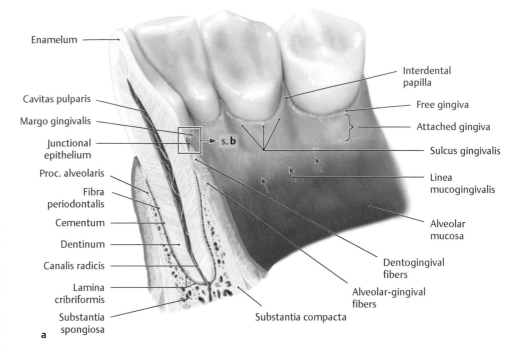

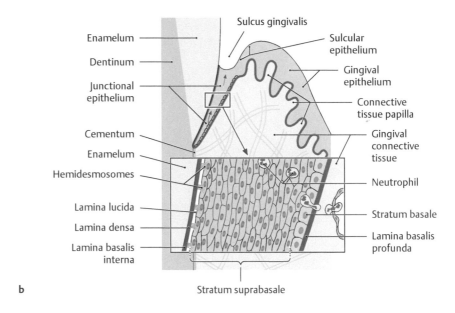

B Gingiva

a Gingiva at a glance; **b** Junctional epithelium.

a Gingiva is part of the oral mucosa and extends from the margo gingivalis to the mucogingival border. There, the gingival epithelium (multi-layered, usually parakeratinized stratified squamous epithelium), which has a light pink shade, blends into the considerably more reddish alveolar epithelium (multi-layered, not parakeratinized stratified squamous epithelium). There is a clinical distinction between two sections:

- free gingiva (1–2 mm wide) = margo gingivalis, surrounds the neck of the tooth like a cuff and is attached to the cervical enamel. The sulcus gingivalis is a 0.5–1 mm deep channel that extends around the tooth. At the bottom edge of the sulcus is the junctional epithelium (see **b**);
- attached gingiva (3–7 mm wide): begins at the height of the sulcus gingivalis and extends to the mucogingival border. Since it is attached to both the neck of the tooth and the alveolar crest (part of the proc. alveolaris) through dentogingival fibers, which run horizontally, it often has a speckled texture.

b The junctional epithelium attaches to the cementum surface by hemidesmosomes and lamina basalis thereby ensuring a complete attachment of the tunica mucosa oris to the tooth surface. It becomes broader in the apical-coronal direction. The deep outer layer of lamina basalis represents the border to the gingival connective tissue and further extends to the lamina basalis of the oral sulcus epithelium. The junctional epithelium differs from the other epitheliums in the cavitas oris in several aspects:

- it consists of only two layers: stratum basale and stratum suprabasale;
- at its base, it lacks connective tissue papillae;
- it has a high cell turnover (formation of new cells every 4–6 days): While the cuboid basal cells are responsible for cell replenishment, the daughter cells differentiate into flattened cells, which are aligned parallel to the tooth surface. Further toward the sulcus gingivalis where they are rejected, these cell layers constantly form new hemidesmosomes while dissolving old ones;
- it has a particular immune defense (neutrophil granulocytes constantly move around the junctional epithelium).

Note: The integrity of the junctional epithelium is a precondition for the health of the entire periodontium. If bacterial colonization leads to inflammation of the neck of the tooth (typical plaque formation as a result of poor oral hygiene), the junctional epithelium loses its attachment to the tooth and gingival pockets form in the area around the sulcus gingivalis (periodontosis).

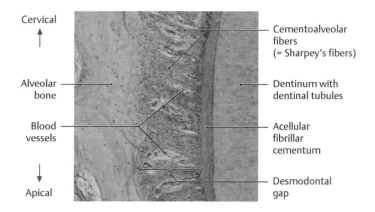

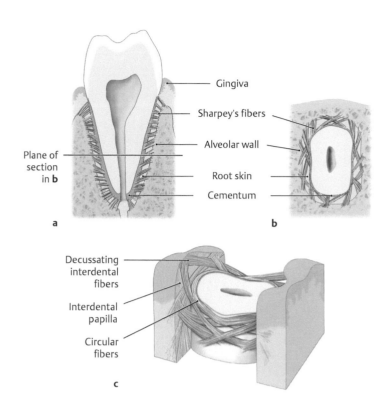

C Periodontal ligament (desmodontium)

The periodontal ligament is a highly vascularized, cell- and fiber-rich connective tissue, which fills the 200μm wide gap between cementum-covered root element and alveolar bone. It consists of a complex system of collagen fibers (cementum or dental alveolar collagen fiber bundles), which holds the tooth in place in the bony socket in a spring-like manner. The collagen fibers, also known as Sharpey's fibers, are attached to both the cementum and alveolar bone. The fibers run in different directions (see **D**), which enables them to counteract all movements of the tooth (axial pressure, lateral tilt, and torsional motion) and develop tension. The tensile stress, which is constantly present during the chewing process, helps stimulate permanent regeneration in bones and collagen fibers. In addition, highly active fibroblasts are responsible for a high turnover of collagen fibers in the periodontal ligament. Their collagen synthesis, which is dependent on vitamin C, occurs four times faster compared to skin synthesis (which explains rapid fiber loss as a result of vitamin C deficiency). In a toothless jaw, the pars alveolaris gradually atrophies, a fact that further underscores the significance of masticatory forces for the bone.

D Course of collagen fibers in the periodontal ligament and gingiva

a and **b** Longitudinal and cross-section of the tooth; **c** Schematic course of gingival fibers

While the cementoalveolar fiber bundles in the periodontal ligament are usually oriented obliquely (slanted downwards) (**a**), the supra-alveolar fiber apparatus consists mainly of bundles that run in a circular direction around the circumference of the tooth (**c**).

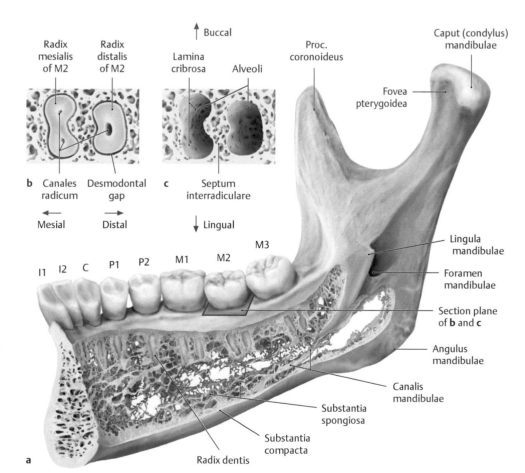

E Structure of the alveolar bone

a Right side of a human mandibula, oral view (the layer of substantia compacta on the mandibula is removed); **b** and **c** Horizontal section of alveoli dentales with (**b**) and without radices dentum (**c**). Cranial view (based on prepared specimen slides part of the anatomical collection of the University of Kiel).

With regard to their structure, the proc. alveolaris maxillae and mandibula are lamellar bones with an inner (lingual/palatal) and outer (vestibular/buccal) compact layer as well as a central spongy layer, which lies in between. An additional component is the alveolar bone, which forms part of the alveolar pocket (socket). The alveolar sockets resemble cups with numerous holes in their bony walls, the cribriform layer of bone. Blood and lymphatic vessels enter the periodontal ligament through these holes into the desmodontal gap where they form a dense latticework surrounding the dental roots.

2.24 Deciduous Teeth (Dentes Decidui)

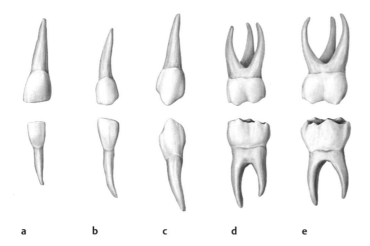

a   b   c   d   e

A Dentes decidui of the left maxilla and mandibula
The deciduous dentition consists of 20 teeth. We distinguish between

a dens incisivus medialis
b dens incisivus lateralis
c dens caninus
d dens molaris primus
e dens molaris secundus

B Average age of eruption of teeth (according to Rauber/Kopsch)
Eruption of the dentes decidui is called primary (1.) dentition and the eruption of the permanent teeth is called dentition. The last column lists the chronological order in which the teeth erupt. For instance: For the 2. dentition, the dens molaris primus (tooth 6) is the first to erupt (six-year molar).
Note: Dentes decidui are given Roman numerals and the dentes permanentes Arabic numbers.

1. Dentition	Tooth	Eruption	Order	
	I	6–8 months	1	
	II	8–12 months	2	
	III	15–20 months	4	
	IV	12–16 months	3	"1st milk molar"
	V	20–40 months	5	"2nd milk molar"

2. Dentition	Tooth	Eruption	Order	
	1	6–9 years	2	
	2	7–10 years	3	
	3	9–14 years	5	
	4	9–13 years	4	
	5	11–14 years	6	
	6	6–8 years	1	"six-year molar"
	7	10–14 years	7	"twelve-year molar"
	8	16–30 years	8	"wisdom tooth"

Birth

6 months

1 year

2 ½ years

4 years

6 years

8 years

10 years

12 years

C Eruption of dentes decidui and permanentes
(according to Meyer)
The left maxilla serves as an example to show the tooth eruption pattern (dentes decidui in black, dentes permanentes in red). Knowledge of the eruption pattern is clinically important since corresponding data helps to diagnose growth delay in children.

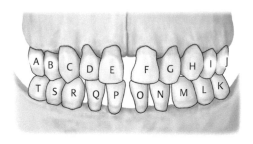

D Dental chart of the deciduous dentition

E Dentes decidui and underlying dentes permanentes in the maxilla and mandibula of a 6 year old

a and **b** Frontal view; **c** and **d** Left view. The anterior bone lamella above the roots of the dentes decidui has been removed, the underlying dentes permanentes are visible.

A six year old was chosen because at that age all dentes decidui have erupted and are all still present. Yet, at the same time, the dens molaris primus has started to erupt as the first permanent tooth (see **C**).

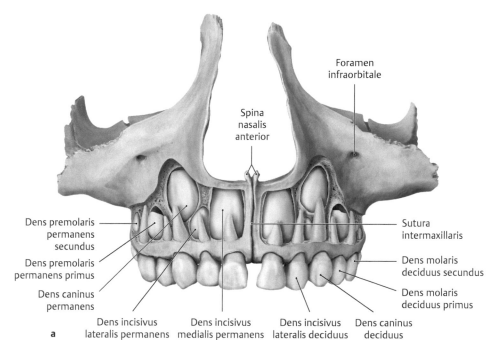

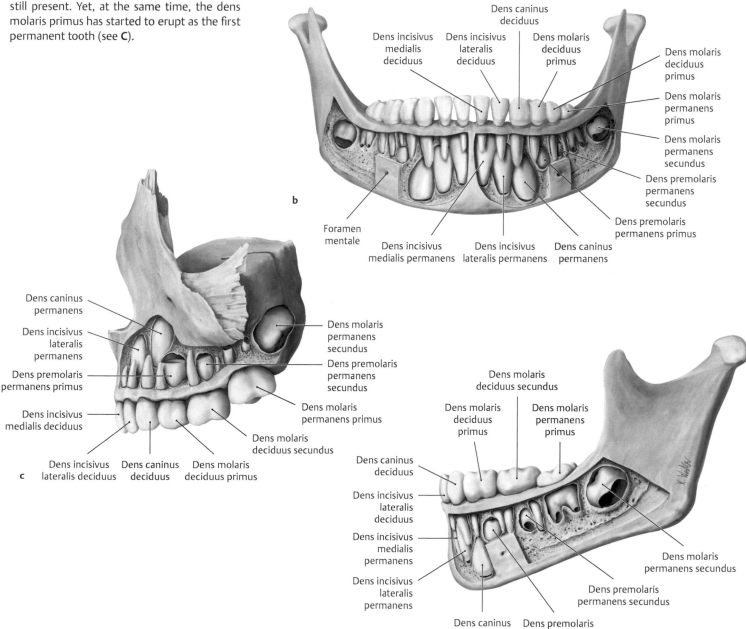

2.25 Tooth Development (Odontogenesis)

A Early stage of tooth development in the mandibula of a human embryo (according to Schumacher and Schmidt)

View of a mandibula at the beginning of the 7th week of embryonic development (with the coronal cut at the height of the enamel caps of the dens molaris primarius secundus). Localized epithelial thickening presents the first morphologically verifiable sign of the start of tooth development. They run in a horseshoe-shape parallel to the lip line and grow into the mesenchyme of the maxilla and mandibula of a five-week old human embryo (cf. **Ba**). In mesial-distal direction, the free margins on both sides of the general dental lamina thickens to form 5 tooth buds each, equal to the 10 primary teeth in both lower and upper jaw. Subsequently, each of these tooth epithelial buds transforms first into cap-shaped and later bell-shaped organa enamelea (cf. **Bb** and **c**).

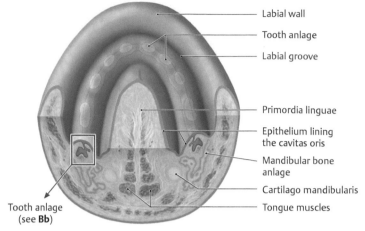

Labial wall
Tooth anlage
Labial groove
Primordia linguae
Epithelium lining the cavitas oris
Mandibular bone anlage
Cartilago mandibularis
Tongue muscles

Tooth anlage (see **Bb**)

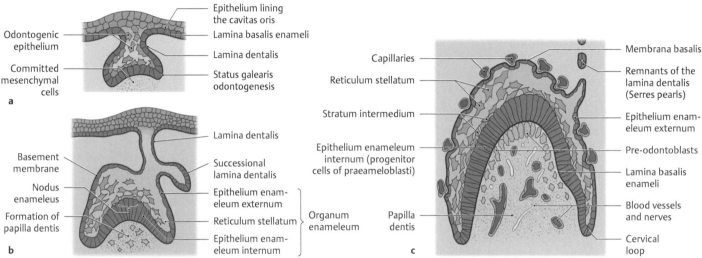

Epithelium lining the cavitas oris
Odontogenic epithelium
Lamina basalis enameli
Lamina dentalis
Committed mesenchymal cells
Status galearis odontogenesis

a

Lamina dentalis
Basement membrane
Successional lamina dentalis
Nodus enameleus
Epithelium enameleum externum
Formation of papilla dentis
Reticulum stellatum ⎫ Organum enameleum
Epithelium enameleum internum ⎭

b

Capillaries
Reticulum stellatum
Stratum intermedium
Epithelium enameleum internum (progenitor cells of praeameloblasti)
Papilla dentis

Membrana basalis
Remnants of the lamina dentalis (Serres pearls)
Epithelium enameleum externum
Pre-odontoblasts
Lamina basalis enameli
Blood vessels and nerves
Cervical loop

c

B Early stage of tooth development and formation of tooth germs
a Status galearis; **b** Status campanalis; **c** Status serus campanalis (according to Weiss).

In the human embryo, dentes decidui begin to develop in the 5th week. At around 3 months of gestation (15th–19th embryonic week), the hard tissue that surrounds the teeth starts to form.

Status galearis odontogenesis: Bud- and cap-shaped collections of cells develop as a result of intensive cell proliferation in the odontogenic epithelium. Their concavity deepens at the far side of the epithelium and starting from the margin they grow around the mesenchyme (see **C**).

Status campanalis:
- The organum enameleum is composed of an epithelium enameleum internum and externum and the reticulum stellatum, which lies in between. The cells of the epithelium enameleum internum grow increasingly columnar-shaped on the lamina basalis enameli particularly around the nodus enameleus. Increasing extracellular matrix production (reticulum stellatum) leads to further separation of the epithelium enameleum externum and internum. Cells of the epithelium enameleum externum spread further apart in the reticulum stellatum.
- Starting from the palatal (maxilla) and lingual (mandibula) margin of the lamina dentalis, the permanent (successional) lamina dentalis starts to develop and forms the basis for the formation of the dentes permanentes of the secondary dentition.

Note: The permanent teeth (molars of the permanent dentition), which are located distally from the primary dentition result from the dental lamina, which elongates distally.

Status serus campanalis:
- The reticulum stellatum becomes increasingly more voluminous and divides into a loose mid-zone (reticulum stellatum proper) and a cellular layer (stratum intermedium) immediately next to the epithelium enameleum internum.
- The organum enameleum surrounds the mesenchymal tissue, which thickens toward the papilla dentis. Blood vessels and nerve fibers grow into the papilla dentis where the pulpa dentis later develops.
- The cells of the epithelium enameleum internum develop into precursor cells for the praeameloblasti. Their secretions are responsible for the formation of the adjacent mesenchymal cells into the future pre-odontoblasts.
- The thickening of the basement membrane located between praeameloblasti and pre-odontoblasts leads to the transformation of the membrana perforata. In the area around the cervical loop, the basement membrane of the epithelium enameleum internum continues into the basement membrane of the epithelium enameleum externum thereby covering the entire surface of the organum enameleum. Capillaries on the outer layer of the basement membrane provide its nourishment.
- The connection of the developing organum enameleum to the lamina dentalis becomes increasingly weaker until the lamina almost completely dissolves.
- With increasing expansion of the growing tooth bud the loose mesenchymal tissue, which surrounds the organum enameleum and papilla dentis, thickens into the saccus dentis from which the periodontium later develops (see **E**).

Shortly before the hard tissue starts to develop (cf. **D**), the tooth bud consists of a bell-shaped organum enameleum, papilla dentis, and the saccus dentis.

C Epithelial-mesenchymal interaction (according to Schroeder)

The development of dentes decidui results from the interaction of surface ectoderm (epithelium of the primitive cavitas oris) and mesenchyme (of the cranial crista neuralis), which lies underneath. This interaction leads to clusters of highly specialized cells, the odontoblasti and ameloblasti. They in turn, induce secretion of dental hard tissue praedentinum and enamelum matrix through growth and differentiation factors (e.g., BMPs = bone morphogenetic proteins, FGFs = fibroblast growth factors, SHh = sonic hedgehog) (see **D**).

Note: The growth and differentiation factors are concentrated in the nodus enameleus primarius (see **Bb**), which are the localized thickenings of the lamina dentis where the dentes decidui will later develop. Thus, nodi enamelei have a signaling function for tooth development (e.g., for shape of crowns and number of cusps) and resemble the ectodermal ridges, which regulate gemma membri development.

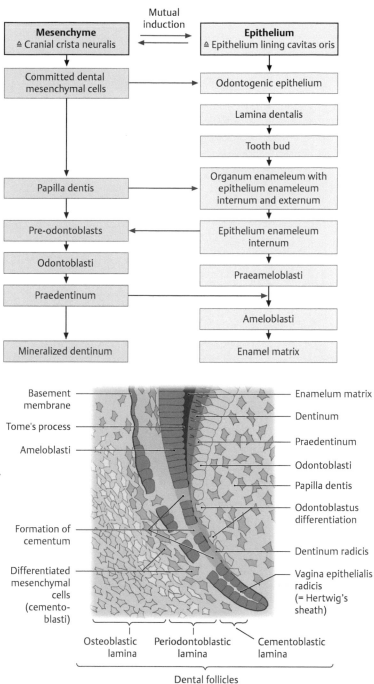

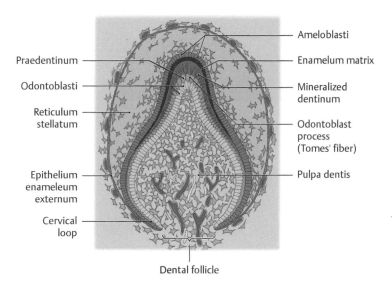

D Formation of dental hard tissues forming the corona dentis

The formation of dental hard tissue around the forming corona dentis is—similar to the early development stages—the result of a series of processes of mutual induction (see **Ba–c**). The thickening of the basement membrane (membrana perforata, see **Bc**) leads to the transformation of pre-odontoblasts into odontoblasti and the start of the synthesis of praedentinum, which is deposited in the area of the basement membrane. This process, in turn, induces differentiation of praeameloblasti into secretory ameloblasti. With the layer of praedentinum deposited, the ameloblasti start releasing organic enamel matrix. With the dissolution of the basement membrane (membrana perforata), the enamelum is now directly adjacent to the dentinum and the deposition gradually spreads toward the cervix (neck) of the corona dentis. With the two dental hard tissues continuing to form, the odontoblasti and ameloblasti move further apart in opposite directions. The ameloblasti secrete column-shaped enamelum rods, which will later mineralize and extend from the enamelum-dentinum junction to the enamelum surface. The ameloblasts will become inactive when the enamel layer is completed and are eventually sloughed when the tooth erupts. As a result, enamelum is cell-free and cannot repair itself. The odontoblasti also recede with increasing formation of dentinum, yet leave behind a thin process (odontoblastic process or "Tomes fiber") in a small channel within the dentinum (dentinal tubule), which permeates the entire dentinum layer. The odontoblastus cell bodies are positioned at the pulpa-dentinum junction and are able to continually form dentinum throughout the life of the tooth.

Note: While the corona dentis formation of the primary teeth is complete by the time a baby is between 2 and 6 months old, the formation of the root in the primary dentition takes approximately 2–3 years from the time the tooth erupts.

E Radix dentis formation and differentiation of the saccus dentis

The formation of the root begins once enamelum and dentinum have developed in the area of the corona dentis. It organizes along the vagina epithelialis radicis (Hertwig epithelial root sheath)—a two-layered epithelium (epithelium enameleum internum and externum lie directly on top of each other, the reticulum stellatum is absent). The vagina epithelialis radicis grows from the cervical loop in an apical direction. In teeth with multiple roots, the vagina epithelialis radicis induces differentiation of odontoblasti, which in turn start to synthesize dentinum. The resulting cavitas pulpae increasingly narrows in an apical direction creating one or more canales radicum so nerves and vessels can enter and exit the pulpa dentis. With progressing dissolution of the vagina epithelialis radicis (from cervical to apical), the mesenchyme cells of the saccus dentis contact the root dentin and start forming cementum (lamina cementoblastica). Further peripheral in the adjacent mesenchyme of the saccus dentis, the root dentinum induces formation of the future periodontal ligament and alveolar bone.

2.26 Dental Radiology

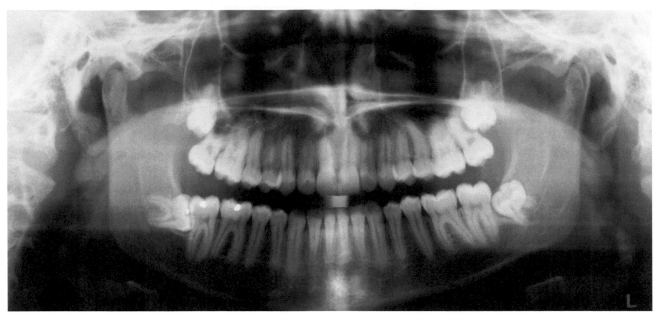

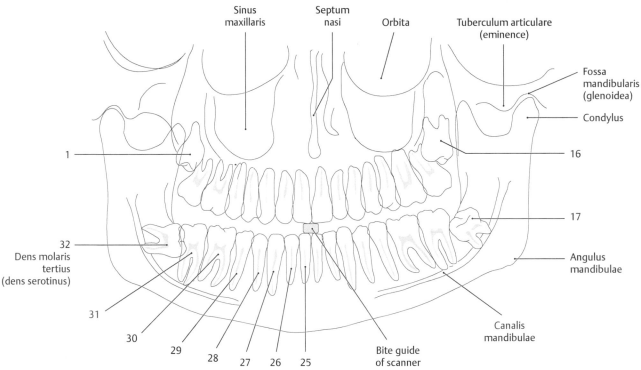

Sinus maxillaris · Septum nasi · Orbita · Tuberculum articulare (eminence) · Fossa mandibularis (glenoidea) · Condylus · 1 · 16 · 17 · 32 · Dens molaris tertius (dens serotinus) · 31 · 30 · 29 · 28 · 27 · 26 · 25 · Bite guide of scanner · Canalis mandibulae · Angulus mandibulae

A Panoramic tomogram and orthopanotomogram

The panoramic tomogram is a topogram, which provides a first overview of the artt. temporomandibulares, cavities and bones as well as the condition of the teeth (carious lesions, position of dentes serotini). In this imaging technique, X-ray tube and film move around the planes to be shown while blurring the images of the structures lying outside of the focal zone. Corresponding to the shape of the jaw, the plane in the panoramic tomogram is parabolic. The image of the dentition shown here indicates that removal of the dentes serotini is advisable since they either have not yet fully erupted (1, 16, and 17) or are in transverse position and thus cannot erupt (32). If based on the panoramic tomogram, caries can be suspected, single tooth radiographs of the affected region are taken. Their higher resolution allows for a more refined diagnosis (see **C–H**).

In addition to the conventional (analog) technique, which uses an X-ray film as image receptor, digital X-ray technology is increasingly used, in which a sensor transforms the absorbed X-rays into digital signals and displays them on a computer screen. A substantial advantage of this technology is the lower level of radiation exposure through shorter exposure time and the easy transfer of data.

(Our thanks to Prof. Dr. med. Dent. U.J. Rother, Director of the Polyclinic for Dental Radiology for permission to use the X-ray image.)

Note: The dentes incisivi maxillares are wider than the dentes incisivi mandibulares leading to the interlocking of cusps and fissures (see p. 53).

B Single tooth radiographs

Single tooth radiographs are detailed X-rays of an individual tooth and its neighboring teeth. Generally, orthoradial images are taken in which the X-ray beam is directed vertically to the tangent to the dental arch or, to put in simpler terms, linearly from outside toward the tooth. Thus, the X-ray shows all structures that follow each other in the beam path consecutively so that they overlap. Thus, in teeth with multiple roots, the individual root canals cannot be clearly evaluated (see **C**). This is only possible with the help of so-called eccentric images, in which the X-ray beam is directed to the tangent in a particular angle,

so that consecutive structures are clearly distinguishable. One particular type of single tooth radiograph is the so-called bitewing X-ray (see **H**), in which only an image of the crown is taken instead of the entire tooth. The patient bites the teeth together on a small piece of film, allowing for the display of maxillary and mandibular teeth at the same time, which helps detection of tooth decay underneath fillings or on the contact surfaces.

(Our thanks to Dr. med. Dent. Christian Friedrichs for his permission to use the X-rays on this page.)

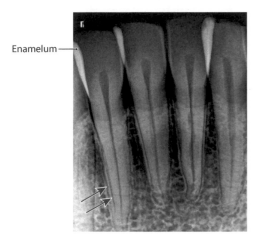

Enamelum

C Mandible front, teeth 23–26

Single-rooted teeth, like the incisors shown here, have two root canals in a third of all cases. The orthoradial image shows a cross section of the dental root and a double periodontal space (see arrows). If the tooth has in fact two root canals, it cannot be determined with the help of the orthoradial image (see **B**).

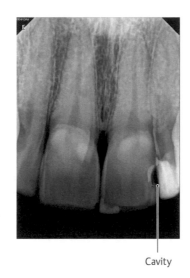

Cavity

D Maxilla front, teeth 7–10

The bright spots shown here in tooth 9 distal can indicate caries, open cavities or such as in this case, old, non X-ray opaque filling material. Underfilling material is slightly X-ray opaque.

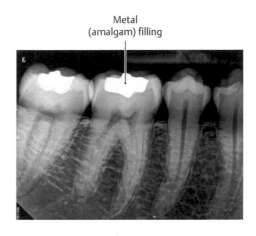

Metal (amalgam) filling

E Mandible side teeth, 28–31

Metal-dense X-ray shadows as those shown here near the crowns of teeth 30 and 31 can be the result of metal inlays, crowns, amalgam fillings, or modern zinc oxide ceramics.

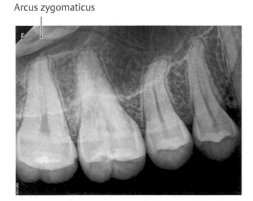

Arcus zygomaticus

F Maxilla side teeth, 2–5

In the lateral tooth area of the maxilla, superimposition of teeth and arcus zygomaticus frequently occurs, shown here in the upper left margin. The roots of the molars are less clearly visible.

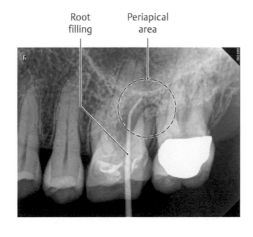

Root filling   Periapical area

G Maxilla side teeth with pathological finding, teeth 12–15

An infection of the canalis radicis system, which has spread to the periapical bone can lead to the formation of a fistula. In order to be able to exactly locate the infection, a guttapercha root-filling peg is inserted into the fistula from outside. Around the distobuccal dental root of tooth 14, a bright spot indicating the infection is visible. Tooth 15 has been capped with a crown.

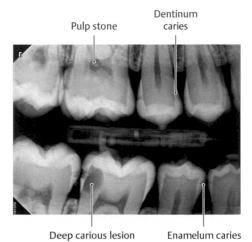

Pulp stone   Dentinum caries

Deep carious lesion   Enamelum caries

H Bitewing image for caries diagnosis

Massive carious damage at tooth 30 distal. Enamel caries and partial beginning of dentinal caries at the contact points of almost all teeth. In addition to the occlusal planes, the contact points represent typical caries predilection sites. Partly visible in the lumen of the pulp chambers are pulp stones.

2.27 Dental Local Anesthesia

A Anatomical facts and local anesthesia technique

Knowledge of the topographic anatomy of the head and neck is crucial when administering local anesthesia for dental procedures. Of particular significance here is the course of the nervus trigeminus. As the largest cranial nerve, it provides sensory innervation to the tooth-supporting parts of the maxilla and mandibula (alveolar bone, teeth and gingiva). In addition, a thorough understanding of the topography of the osseous structures is indispensable because they are of greater importance for needle direction than the soft tissue is. Two of the most popular injection techniques are infiltration and block anesthesia (see below). Vasoconstrictor is an additional component of local anesthetic solutions (for example adrenaline), which prolongs the local anesthetic duration, prevents increased plasma levels and greater risk of toxicity reactions, and decreases the risk of bleeding. In order to eliminate the risk of an accidental intravascular injection it is important to always aspirate when performing infiltration and block anesthesia. Among the most serious side effects in case of an accidental vascular puncture are cardiovascular and anaphylactic reactions.

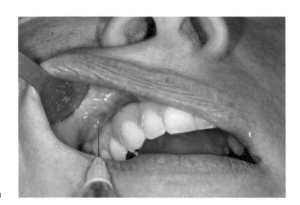

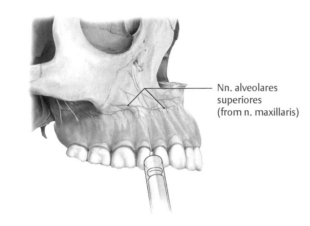

Nn. alveolares superiores (from n. maxillaris)

B Principle of infiltration anesthesia

a Injection technique performed on patient; **b** Schematic diagram illustrating loss of sensation.

Infiltration anesthesia is the technique most commonly used in odontology (see **C** for injection technique). It is particularly suitable for a range of maxilla procedures. The maxilla is predominantly substantia spongiosa with an extremely thin layer of substantia compacta facilitating diffusion of the anesthetic through the bone to the apex of the tooth. When administering infiltration anesthesia, local anesthetic solution floods the terminal nerve endings thus blocking them. The anesthetic is usually deposited supraperiosteally in the apical area of the affected tooth.

Note: Due to the significantly thicker cortical bone of the mandibula, the diffusion rate surrounding the mandibular molar areas is considerably lower. This is the main reason why block anesthesia is used for mandibular procedures (see **D** and **E**).

C Infiltration anesthesia technique

(According to Daublaender in van Aken and Wulf)

- penetrate tunica mucosa oris in the area near the apex
- place needle toward bone
- advance the needle until you can feel it meet bony resistance, parallel to the tooth axis in a 30 degree angle to the bone surface
- aspirate area
- slowly inject local anesthetic solution (1mL/30s) while maintaining bone contact
- remove needle from cavitas oris
- wait for anesthetic to diffuse while monitoring the patient

D Frequently used methods of block anesthesia in oral and maxillofacial surgery
(From Daublaender M. Lokalanesthesie in der Zahn, Mundund Kieferheilkunde. In van Aken H, Wulf H. Lokalanaesthesie, Regionalanaesthesie, Regionale Schmerztherapie. 3. Aufl. Stuttgart: Thieme: 2010)

The goal of block anesthesia is the complete and reversible blockage of an entire sensitive peripheral nerve. What is crucial is the exact deposition of a sufficient volume of anesthetic (solution) in an area with close topographical connection to the relevant nerve—for example where the nerve enters or exits the bone channel.

Nerve	Innervation Area	Injection Site	Volume
Maxilla			
N. infra-orbitalis	Alveolar extension/appendage, vestibular mucosa and maxillary front teeth, upper lip, lateral aspect of the nose and anterior cheek	Foramen infraorbitale	1–1.5 mL
N. naso-palatinus	Palatal mucosa in area surrounding front teeth	Foramen incisum	0.1–0.2 mL
N. palatinus major	Palatal mucosa running up to the canine teeth of relevant side	Foramen palatinum majus	0.3–0.5 mL
Nn. alveolares superiores posteriores	Alveolar extension, vestibular mucosa and molar teeth	Tuber maxillae	1–1.8 mL
Mandibula			
N. alveolaris inferior	Alveolar extension. Lingual mucosa and mandible teeth of respective side, vestibular mucosa in area around front teeth	Foramen mandibulare	1.5–2 mL
N. buccalis	Vestibular mucosa in molar area		0.5 mL
N. mentalis	Vestibular mucosa in front teeth area	Foramen mentale	0.5–1 mL

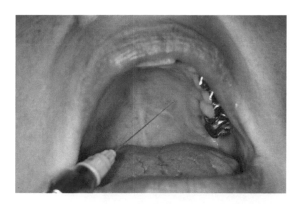

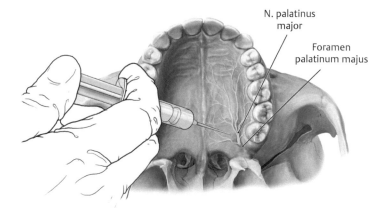

N. palatinus major

Foramen palatinum majus

a

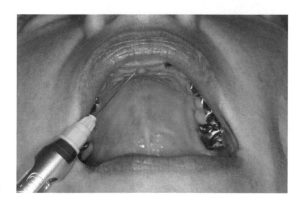

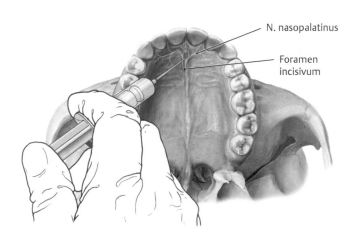

N. nasopalatinus

Foramen incisivum

b

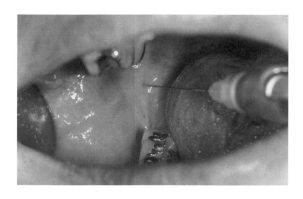

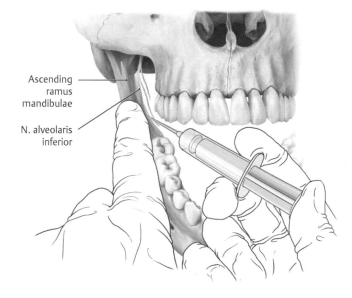

Ascending ramus mandibulae

N. alveolaris inferior

c

E Site of a typical injection for the anesthetic block of maxilla and mandibula (Photos Daubländer M. Lokalanästhesie in der Zahn-, Mund- und Kieferheilkunde. In van Aken H, Wulf H. Lokalanästhesie, Regionalanästhesie, Regionale Schmerztherapie. 3. Aufl. Stuttgart: Thieme; 2010)

a Foramen palatinum majus (n. palatinus major)

Indication: Painful treatment in the area surrounding the palatal mucosa and the bones in the molar and premolar area of one side of the maxilla.

Technique: Local anesthetic needs to be deposited as close as possible to the foramen palatinum majus (area of insertion in children is near the dens molaris primus; in adults: more distal near the dentes molares secundus and tertius). With the mouth opened wide and the head reclined, the needle—approaching from the premolar area of the contralateral side—is advanced in a 45 degree angle to the palatal surface until it touches the bone.

Clinical considerations: As a result of the injection placed/positioned too far distal, the ipsilateral palatum molle is anesthetized, which causes the patient discomfort (difficulty swallowing).

b Foramen incisivum (n. nasopalatinus)

Indication: Painful treatment in the area of the anterior third of the palatum (stretching from the left to the right dens caninus).

Technique: With the mouth wide open and the head reclined, the needle—advancing from a lateral direction—is inserted directly next to the papilla incisiva, approximately 1cm palatal off the gingival edge and further advanced in a medial-distal direction.

Clinical considerations: Compact mucosa requires high injection pressure.

c Foramen mandibulae (n. alveolaris inferior)

Indication: Painful treatment in the area around mandibular teeth as well as the buccal mucosa mesial of the foramen mentale.

Technique: In the wide-open mouth, the therapist palpates with his index finger the leading edge of the ascending ramus mandibulae. Approaching from the premolar area of the opposite side, the needle is inserted approximately 1 cm above occlusal plane, lateral to the pterygomandibular fold and reaches the foramen mandibulae after advancing another 2.5 cm cranial to the lingula mandibulae.

Clinical considerations: In children, the foramen mandibulae is on level with the occlusal plane.

2.28 Temporomandibular Joint (Articulatio Temporomandibularis)

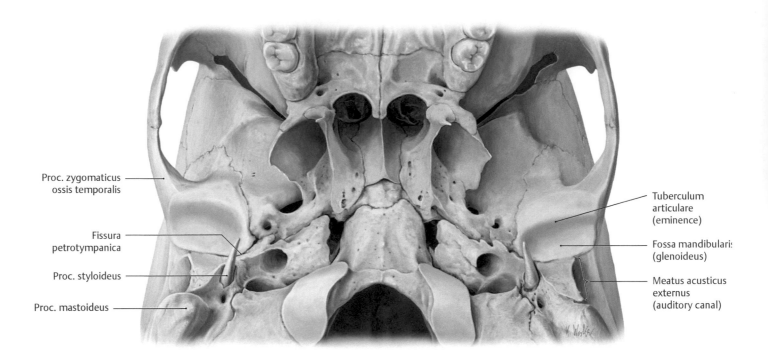

Proc. zygomaticus ossis temporalis

Fissura petrotympanica

Proc. styloideus

Proc. mastoideus

Tuberculum articulare (eminence)

Fossa mandibularis (glenoideus)

Meatus acusticus externus (auditory canal)

A Fossa mandibularis of the art. temporomandibularis on the outer basis cranii

View from below. In the art. temporomandibularis, the caput mandibulae of the lower jaw articulates with the socket, the fossa mandibularis as shown here. It is part of the pars squamosa of the os temporale. The tuberculum articulare, or eminence, is located at the anterior part of the fossa mandibularis. Since the capsula articularis (see **B**) is considerably smaller than the fossa, sufficient motility of the art. temporomandibularis is ensured. Unlike other joint surfaces, the fossa mandibularis is covered with fibrous cartilage and not hyaline cartilage. The meatus acusticus externus is located behind the fossa of the art. temporomandibularis. This proximity explains blunt force jaw trauma causing damage to the meatus acusticus externus.

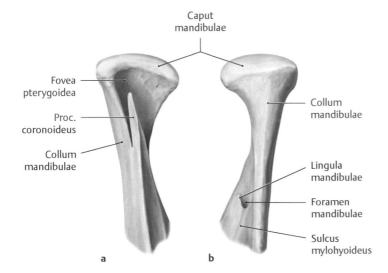

Caput mandibulae

Fovea pterygoidea

Proc. coronoideus

Collum mandibulae

Collum mandibulae

Lingula mandibulae

Foramen mandibulae

Sulcus mylohyoideus

a   b

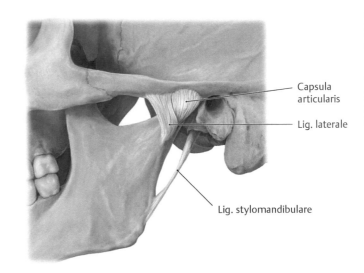

Capsula articularis

Lig. laterale

Lig. stylomandibulare

B Caput mandibulae of the right art. temporomandibularis

Frontal view (**a**) and dorsal view (**b**). The capsula articularis of the caput mandibularis is not only considerably smaller than the socket but it is also cylindrical. This cylinder shape increases head mobility given that it allows rotation around a vertical axis.

C Left art. temporomandibularis with ligamentous apparatus

Lateral view. The art. temporomandibularis is surrounded by a relatively atonic capsule (danger of luxation), which extends dorsally up to the fissura petrotympanica (see **A**). It is secured by three ligaments. This lateral view shows the strongest ligament, the lig. laterale, which lies on the capsule and with which it is connected as well as the weaker lig. stylomandibulare.

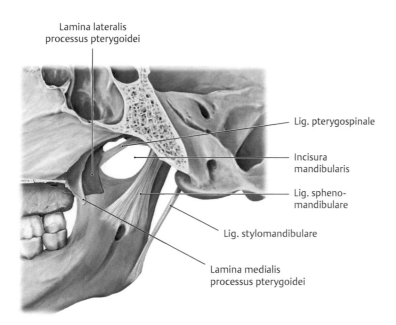

Lamina lateralis
processus pterygoidei

Lig. pterygospinale

Incisura
mandibularis

Lig. spheno-
mandibulare

Lig. stylomandibulare

Lamina medialis
processus pterygoidei

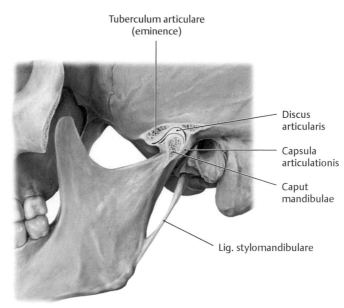

Tuberculum articulare
(eminence)

Discus
articularis

Capsula
articulationis

Caput
mandibulae

Lig. stylomandibulare

D Right art. temporomandibularis with ligamentous apparatus
Medial view. From a medial view, the lig. sphenomandibulare is visible.

E Opened, left art. temporomandibularis
Lateral view. Sagittal section through joint. The capsule extends dorsally to the fissura petrotympanica (not shown here). The discus articularis, which is located between head and fossa, is visible creating separate superior and inferior synovial cavities. It is attached to the capsule on all sides.

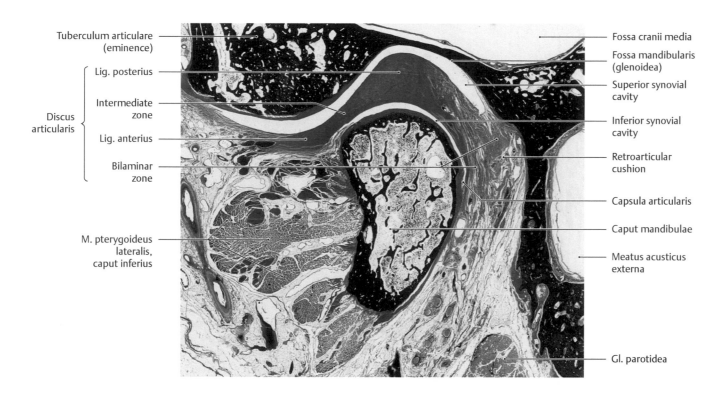

Tuberculum articulare
(eminence)

Discus
articularis
{
Lig. posterius

Intermediate
zone

Lig. anterius

Bilaminar
zone
}

M. pterygoideus
lateralis,
caput inferius

Fossa cranii media

Fossa mandibularis
(glenoidea)

Superior synovial
cavity

Inferior synovial
cavity

Retroarticular
cushion

Capsula articularis

Caput mandibulae

Meatus acusticus
externa

Gl. parotidea

F Histology of the art. temporomandibularis
Sagittal cut showing the lateral area of a human art. temporomandibularis, lateral view (sections stained with azan, 10 μm).
The discus articularis divides the art. temporomandibularis in two com- pletely separate synovial joint cavities. We distinguish between an anterior, avascular, and collagen rich fiber section and one posterior and vascularized section. While the front section in its entirety shows a biconcave shape, a lig. posterius and anterius and an intermediary zone, the back section is divided into two leaves (called the bilaminar zone).

The superior leaf contains elastic fibers and inserts in the area around the fissura petrosquamosa, the inferior leaf extends to the collum mandibulae. Located between the two leaves lies the retroarticular cushion. The capsula is rather weak, laterally and is secured medially by collateral ligaments (see **C**).
Note: While the caput inferius of the m. pterygoideus lateralis inserts at the proc. condylaris (collum mandibulae), the caput superius of the muscle inserts into the discus articularis and pulls on it (not shown here).

2.29 Biomechanics of the Temporomandibular Joint (Articulatio Temporomandibularis)

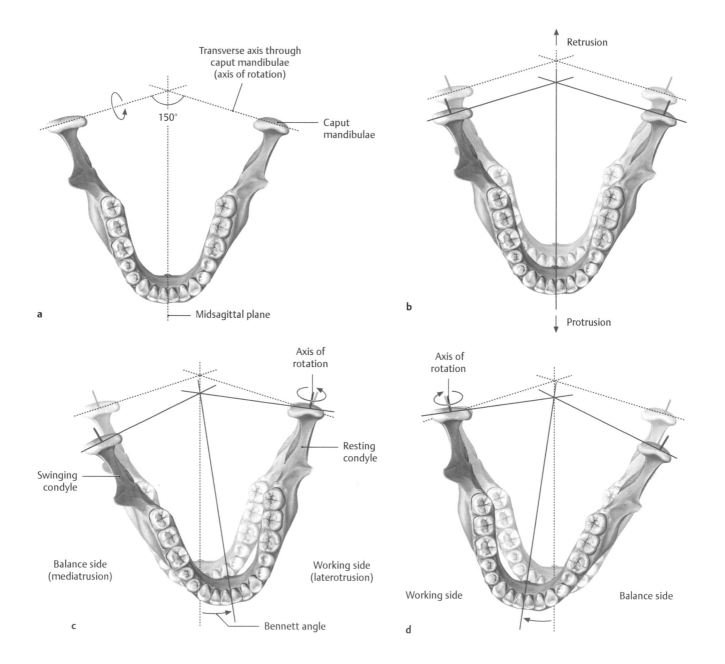

A Movement options of the art. temporomandibularis, mandibula
View from above. Most of the motions of the art. temporomandibularis are combined motions. They can be attributed to three basic motions:

- rotary motion (opening and closing of the mouth)
- translatory motion (feeding motion)
- grinding motion

a Rotary motion. During the rotary motion the joint axis crosses diagonally through both capita mandibulae. Both joint axes intersect in an individually variable angle of about 150° (margin of deviation 110–180°). During this motion the art. temporomandibularis is a hinge joint (abduction, lowering, bond abduction lifting, of the mandibula). Such a clean rotary motion usually happens when asleep, when the mouth is slightly open (angle of up to approximately 15°, s. **Bb**). During every additional opening of the mouth of more than 15° it is combined with a translatory motion (rotary gliding).

b Translatory motion. During this motion the mandibula is pushed forward and pulled back (protrusion and retrusion respectively). The axes during this motion run parallel to the median axis through the center of the mandibular capsulae articulares.

c Grinding motion in the left art. temporomandibularis. During the grinding motion one differentiates the resting and the swinging condylus. The resting condylus on the left working side rotates around a nearly vertical axis (also a rotary axis) through the caput mandibulae, while the swinging condylus of the right balancing side pans to the front, inner side in the sense of a translatory motion. The extent of the mandibula panning is measured in degrees and is called a Bennett angle. During the panning of the mandibula a laterotrusion is carried out on the working side and a mediotrusion on the balancing side.

d Grinding motion of the right art. temporomandibularis. Now the right art. temporomandibularis is the working side, the right resting condylus turns around the nearly vertical rotation axis, while the left condylus pans to the front, inner side: balancing side.

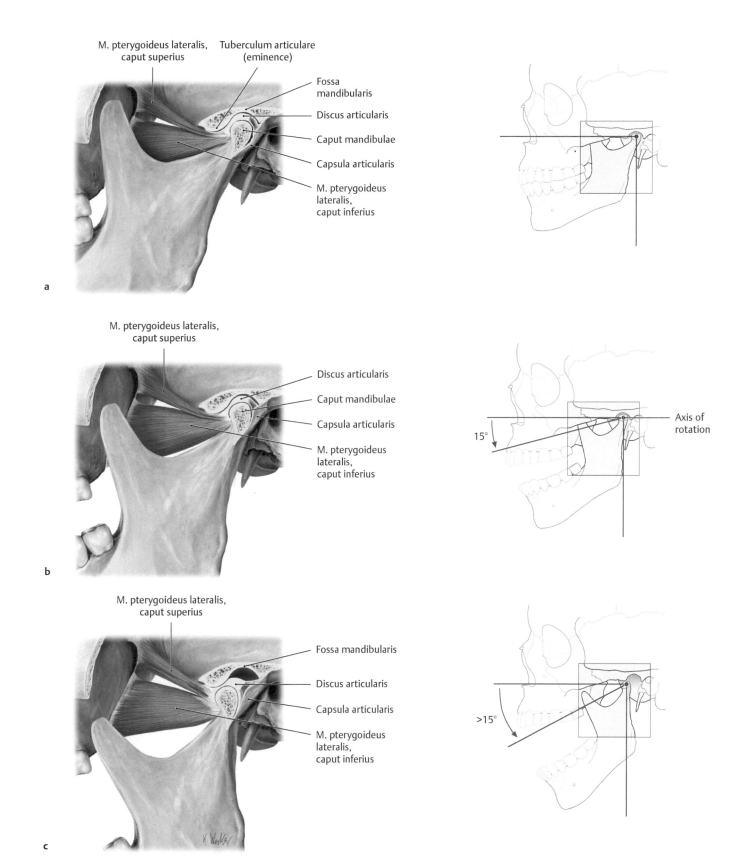

M. pterygoideus lateralis, caput superius   Tuberculum articulare (eminence)

Fossa mandibularis

Discus articularis

Caput mandibulae

Capsula articularis

M. pterygoideus lateralis, caput inferius

a

M. pterygoideus lateralis, caput superius

Discus articularis

Caput mandibulae

Capsula articularis

M. pterygoideus lateralis, caput inferius

15°

Axis of rotation

b

M. pterygoideus lateralis, caput superius

Fossa mandibularis

Discus articularis

Capsula articularis

M. pterygoideus lateralis, caput inferius

>15°

c

B Art. temporomandibularis motions
View from the left lateral side. Depicted on the left side is the joint with the discus articularis and the capsula articularis as well as the m. pterygoideus lateralis respectively, and on the right side schematic the course of the axis. Muscle, capsule, and disk build a functionally combined musculo-disco-capsulo system that works closely together during the opening and closing of the mouth.

a Closed mouth. In idle position with the mouth closed the caput mandibulae rests in the fossa mandibularis of the os temporale.

b Mouth opening up to 15°. The capita mandibulae stay in the man-fossa mandibularis up to this degree of abduction.

c Mouth opening more than 15°. The capita mandibulae shift to the front of the tuberculum articulare; as a result the joint axis that runs diagonally through the capita mandibulae shifts ventrally. The discus articularis is pulled forward by the caput superius of the m. ptery-goideus lateralis The caput inferius of the m. pterygoideus lateralis inserts onto the neck of the proc. condylaris of the mandibula.

69

2.30 The Cervical Spine

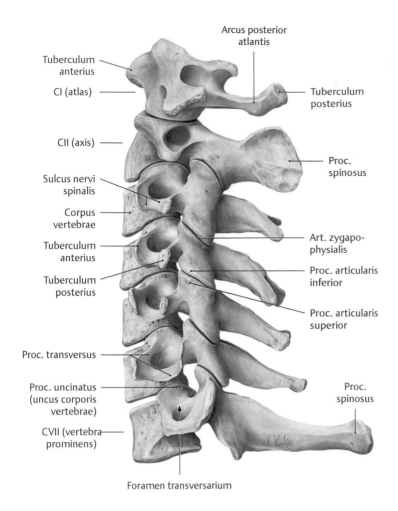

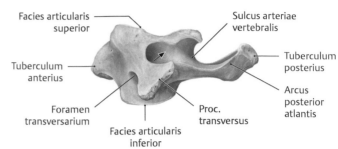

a Vertebra cervicalis prima (CI, atlas)

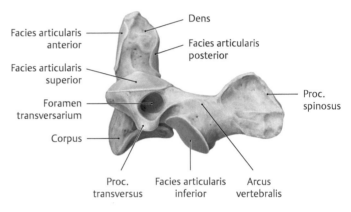

b Vertebra cervicalis secunda (CII, axis)

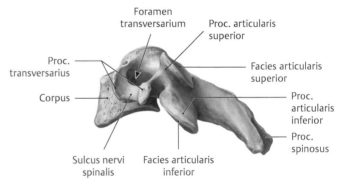

c Vertebra cervicalis quarta (CIV)

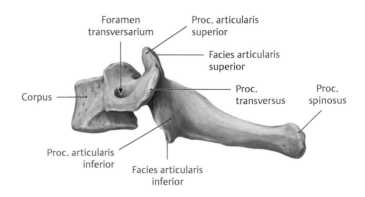

d Vertebra cervicalis septima (CVII, vertebra prominens)

B Vertebrae cervicales, left lateral view

A Cervical spine, left lateral view

The cervical spine consists of seven vertebrae, the upper two of which, the atlas (CI) and axis (CII), differ markedly from the other five vertebrae. They form the artt. atlantooccipitalis and atlantoaxialis which will be dicussed in the next unit. The remaining five vertebrae are made up of the following components:

- One corpus vertebrae,
- One arcus vertebrae,
- One proc. spinosus,
- Two procc. transversi,
- Four procc. articulares.

Vertebrae cervicales have the following characteristics:

- Bifid procc. spinosi,
- Foramen transversarium on proc. transversus,
- Large, triangular foramen vertebrale as well as
- Uncovertebral joints (see p. 76 f).

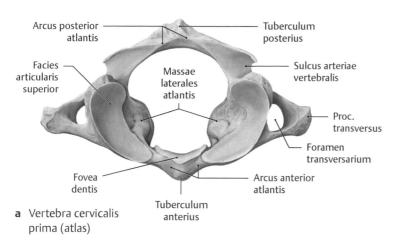

Arcus posterior atlantis
Tuberculum posterius
Facies articularis superior
Massae laterales atlantis
Sulcus arteriae vertebralis
Proc. transversus
Foramen transversarium
Arcus anterior atlantis
Fovea dentis
Tuberculum anterius

a Vertebra cervicalis prima (atlas)

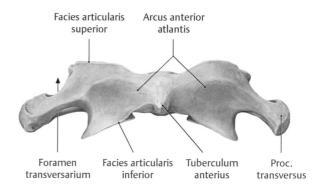

Facies articularis superior
Arcus anterior atlantis
Foramen transversarium
Facies articularis inferior
Tuberculum anterius
Proc. transversus

a Vertebra cervicalis prima (atlas)

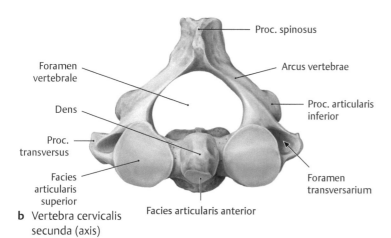

Proc. spinosus
Foramen vertebrale
Arcus vertebrae
Dens
Proc. articularis inferior
Proc. transversus
Facies articularis superior
Facies articularis anterior
Foramen transversarium

b Vertebra cervicalis secunda (axis)

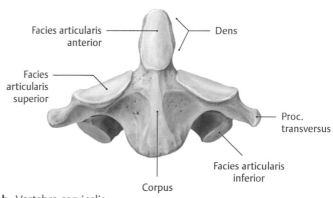

Facies articularis anterior
Dens
Facies articularis superior
Proc. transversus
Facies articularis inferior
Corpus

b Vertebra cervicalis secunda (axis)

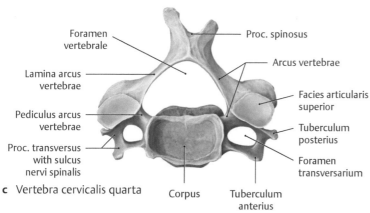

Foramen vertebrale
Proc. spinosus
Lamina arcus vertebrae
Arcus vertebrae
Facies articularis superior
Pediculus arcus vertebrae
Tuberculum posterius
Proc. transversus with sulcus nervi spinalis
Foramen transversarium
Corpus
Tuberculum anterius

c Vertebra cervicalis quarta

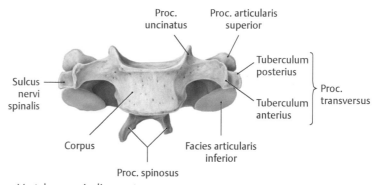

Proc. uncinatus
Proc. articularis superior
Sulcus nervi spinalis
Tuberculum posterius
Proc. transversus
Tuberculum anterius
Corpus
Facies articularis inferior
Proc. spinosus

c Vertebra cervicalis quarta

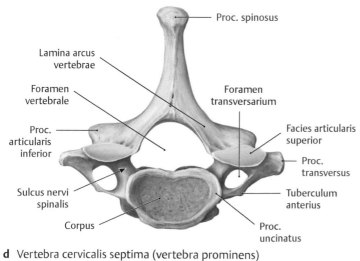

Proc. spinosus
Lamina arcus vertebrae
Foramen vertebrale
Foramen transversarium
Proc. articularis inferior
Facies articularis superior
Proc. transversus
Sulcus nervi spinalis
Tuberculum anterius
Corpus
Proc. uncinatus

d Vertebra cervicalis septima (vertebra prominens)

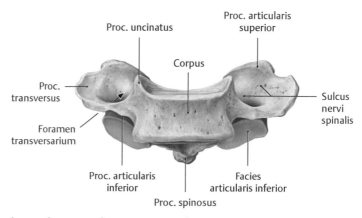

Proc. uncinatus
Corpus
Proc. articularis superior
Proc. transversus
Sulcus nervi spinalis
Foramen transversarium
Proc. articularis inferior
Facies articularis inferior
Proc. spinosus

d Vertebra cervicalis septima (vertebra prominens)

C Vertebrae cervicales, superior view

D Vertebrae cervicales, anterior view

2.31 Overview of the Ligaments of the Cervical Spine

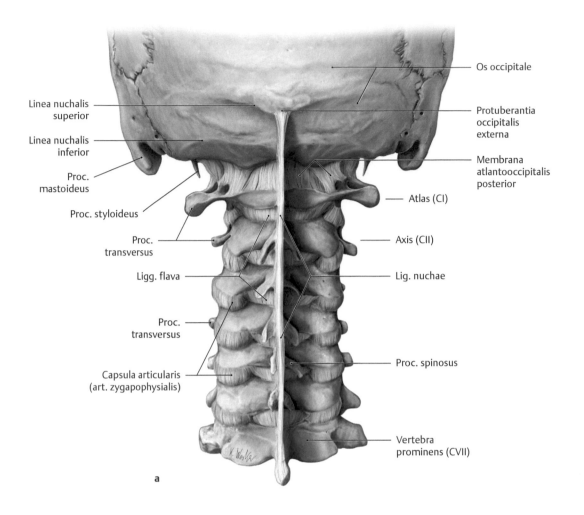

Linea nuchalis superior

Linea nuchalis inferior

Proc. mastoideus

Proc. styloideus

Proc. transversus

Ligg. flava

Proc. transversus

Capsula articularis (art. zygapophysialis)

Os occipitale

Protuberantia occipitalis externa

Membrana atlantooccipitalis posterior

Atlas (CI)

Axis (CII)

Lig. nuchae

Proc. spinosus

Vertebra prominens (CVII)

a

b → ← a

A The ligaments of the cervical spine
a Posterior view
b Anterior view after removal of the anterior skull base (see p. 68 for the ligaments of the upper cervical spine, especially the craniovertebral joints).

B The craniovertebral joints

The craniovertebral joints are the articulations between the atlas (CI) and os occipitale (artt. atlantooccipitales) and between the atlas and axis (CII, artt. atlantoaxiales). While these joints, which number six in all, are anatomically distinct, they are mechanically interlinked and comprise a functional unit (cf.p. 68).

Atlanto-occipital joints

Paired articulationes condyloideae where the oval, slightly concave superior articular facets of the atlas articulate with the convex occipital condyles

Artt. atlantoaxiales

- *Art. atlantoaxialis lateralis* = paired articulation between the facies articulares inferiores of the atlas and the facies articulares superiores of the axis
- *Art. atlantoaxialis mediana* = unpaired articulation (comprising an anterior and posterior compartment) between the dens of the axis, the fovea dentis of the atlas, and the cartilage-covered anterior surface of the lig. transversum atlantis (see p. 74)

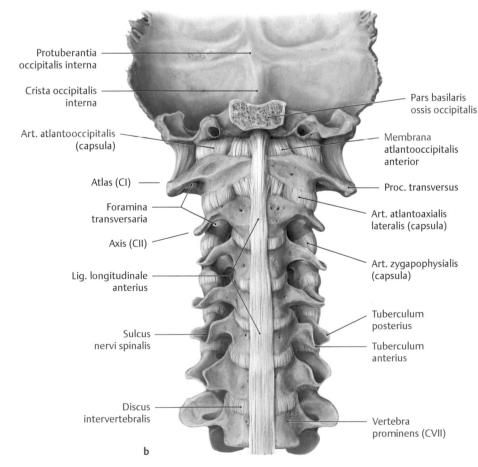

Protuberantia occipitalis interna

Crista occipitalis interna

Art. atlantooccipitalis (capsula)

Atlas (CI)

Foramina transversaria

Axis (CII)

Lig. longitudinale anterius

Sulcus nervi spinalis

Discus intervertebralis

Pars basilaris ossis occipitalis

Membrana atlantooccipitalis anterior

Proc. transversus

Art. atlantoaxialis lateralis (capsula)

Art. zygapophysialis (capsula)

Tuberculum posterius

Tuberculum anterius

Vertebra prominens (CVII)

b

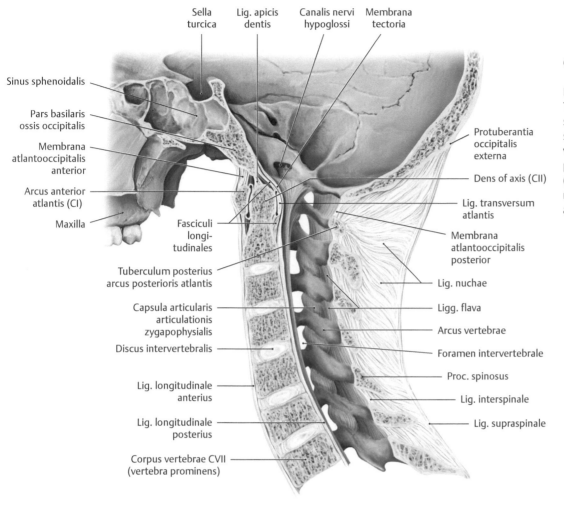

Sella turcica

Lig. apicis dentis

Canalis nervi hypoglossi

Membrana tectoria

Sinus sphenoidalis

Pars basilaris ossis occipitalis

Membrana atlantooccipitalis anterior

Arcus anterior atlantis (CI)

Maxilla

Fasciculi longitudinales

Tuberculum posterius arcus posterioris atlantis

Capsula articularis articulationis zygapophysialis

Discus intervertebralis

Lig. longitudinale anterius

Lig. longitudinale posterius

Corpus vertebrae CVII (vertebra prominens)

Protuberantia occipitalis externa

Dens of axis (CII)

Lig. transversum atlantis

Membrana atlantooccipitalis posterior

Lig. nuchae

Ligg. flava

Arcus vertebrae

Foramen intervertebrale

Proc. spinosus

Lig. interspinale

Lig. supraspinale

C The ligaments of the cervical spine: lig. nuchae
Midsagittal section, left lateral view. The lig. nuchae is the broadened, sagittally oriented part of the lig. supraspinale that extends from the vertebra prominens (CVII) to the protuberantia occipitalis externa (see **A**; see also p. 74 for the ligaments of the artt. atlantooccipitalis and atlantoaxialis).

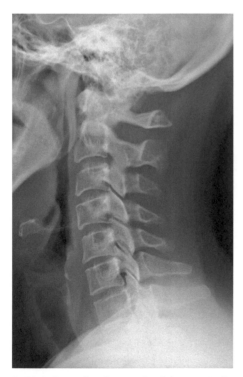

D Plain lateral radiograph of the cervical spine

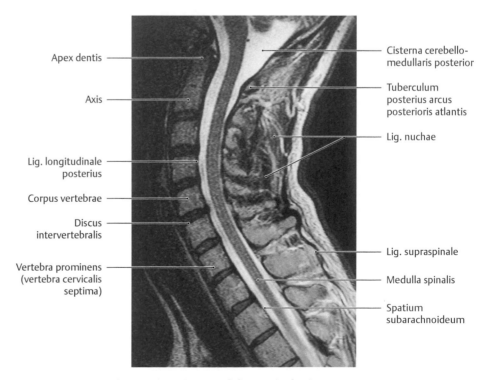

Apex dentis

Axis

Lig. longitudinale posterius

Corpus vertebrae

Discus intervertebralis

Vertebra prominens (vertebra cervicalis septima)

Cisterna cerebellomedullaris posterior

Tuberculum posterius arcus posterioris atlantis

Lig. nuchae

Lig. supraspinale

Medulla spinalis

Spatium subarachnoideum

E Magnetic resonance image of the cervical spine
Midsagittal section, left lateral view T2-weighted TSE sequence (from Vahlensieck M, Reiser M. MRT des Bewegungsapparates. 2nd ed. Stuttgart: Thieme; 2001).

2.32 The Ligaments of the Upper Cervical Spine (Articulationes Atlantooccipitalis and Atlantoaxialis)

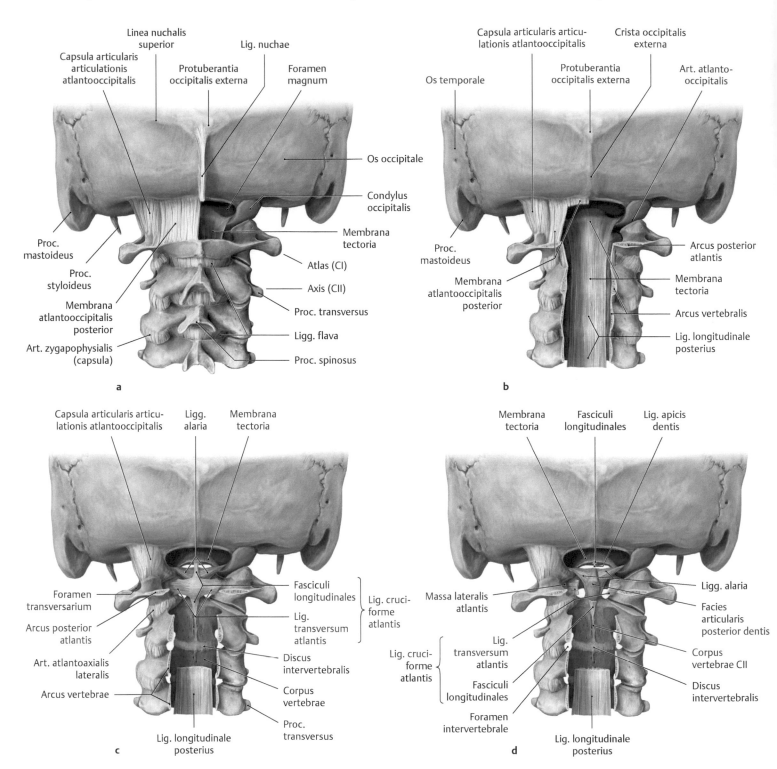

A The ligaments of the craniovertebral joints
Skull and upper cervical spine, posterior view.

a The membrana atlantooccipitalis posterior—the "ligamentum flavum" between the atlas and os occipitale (see p. 66)—stretches from the arcus posterior atlantis to the posterior rim of the foramen magnum. This membrane has been removed on the right side.

b With the canalis vertebralis opened and the medulla spinalis removed, the membrana tectoria, a broadened expansion of the lig. longitudinale posterius, is seen to form the anterior boundary of the canalis vertebralis at the level of the craniovertebral joints.

c With the membrana tectoria removed, the lig. cruciforme atlantis can be seen. The lig. transversum atlantis forms the thick horizontal bar of the cross, and the fasciculi longitudinales form the thinner vertical bar.

d The lig. transversum atlantis and fasciculi longitudinales have been partially removed to demonstrate the paired ligg. alaria, which extend from the lateral surfaces of the dens to the corresponding inner surfaces of the condyli occipitales, and the unpaired lig. apicis dentis, which passes from the apex dentis to the anterior rim of the foramen magnum.

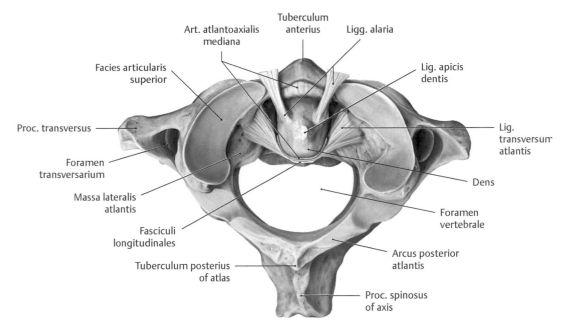

B The ligaments of the articulatio atlantoaxialis mediana
Atlas and axis, superior view. (The fovea dentis, while part of the art. atlantoaxialis mediana, is hidden by the capsula articularis.)

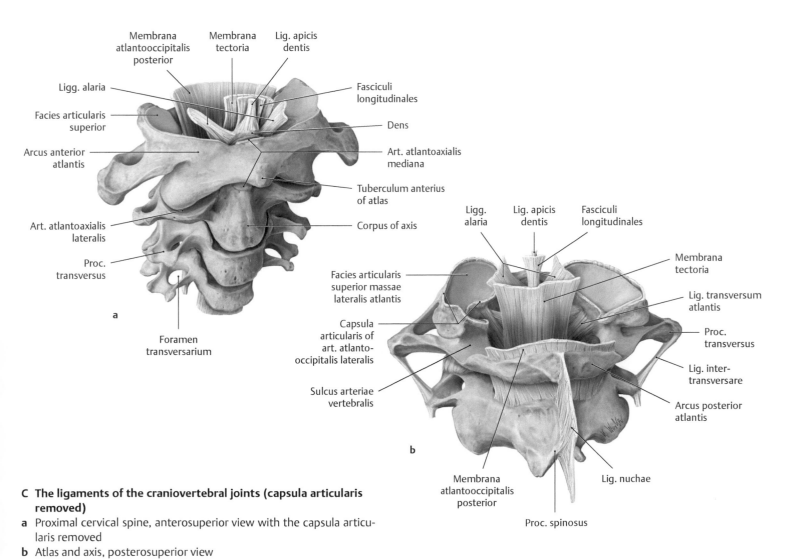

C The ligaments of the craniovertebral joints (capsula articularis removed)
a Proximal cervical spine, anterosuperior view with the capsula articularis removed
b Atlas and axis, posterosuperior view

2.33 The Uncovertebral Joints of the Cervical Spine

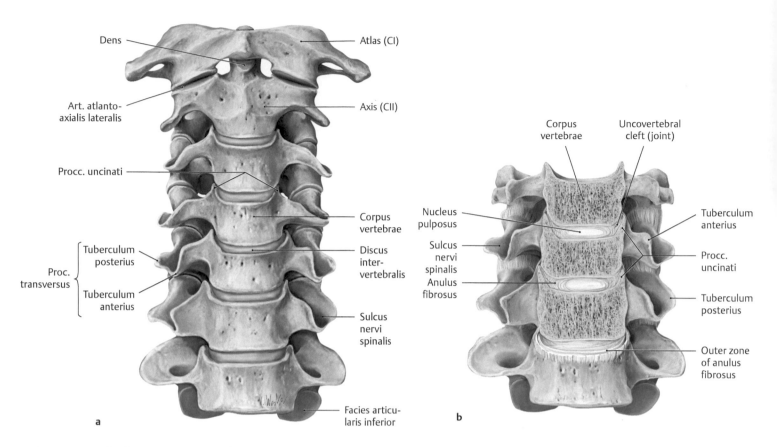

a

b

A The uncovertebral joints in a young adult
Cervical spine of an 18-year-old man, anterior view

a The upper end plates of the corpora vertebrarum CIII–CVII have lateral projections (procc. uncinati) that develop during childhood. Starting at about 10 years of age, the procc. uncinati gradually come into contact with the oblique, crescent-shaped margin on the undersurface of the next higher corpus vertebrae. This results in the formation of lateral clefts (uncovertebral clefts or joints, see **b**) in the outer portions of the disci intervertebrales.

b Vertebrae CIV through CVII. The corpora vertebrarum CIV–CVI have been sectioned in the coronal plane to demonstrate more clearly the uncovertebral joints or clefts. These clefts are bounded laterally by a connective tissue structure, a kind of joint capsule, which causes them to resemble true joint spaces. These clefts or fissures in the discus intervertebralis were first described by the anatomist Hubert von Luschka in 1858, who called them *lateral hemiarthroses*. He interpreted them as primary mechanisms designed to enhance the flexibility of the cervical spine and confer a functional advantage (drawings based on specimens from the Anatomical Collection at Kiel University).

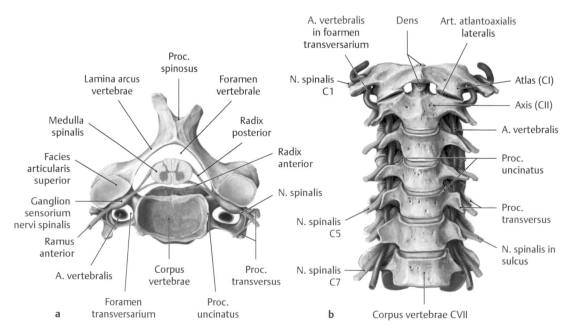

a

b

B Topographical relationship of the n. spinalis and a. vertebralis to the proc. uncinatus
a Vertebra cervicalis quarta with medulla spinalis, spinal roots, nn. spinales, and aa. vertebrales, superior view;

b Cervical spine with both aa. vertebrales and the emerging nn. spinales, anterior view.

Note the course of the a. vertebralis through the foramina transversaria and the course of the n. spinalis at the level of the foramina intervertebralia. Given their close proximity, both the artery and nerve may be compressed by osteophytes (bony outgrowths) caused by uncovertebral arthrosis (cf. **D**).

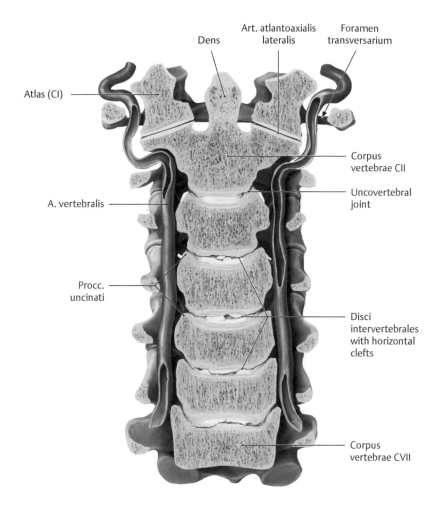

Dens · Art. atlantoaxialis lateralis · Foramen transversarium

Atlas (CI)

A. vertebralis

Procc. uncinati

Corpus vertebrae CII

Uncovertebral joint

Disci intervertebrales with horizontal clefts

Corpus vertebrae CVII

C Degenerative changes in the cervical spine (uncovertebral arthrosis)

Coronal section through the cervical spine of a 35-year-old man, anterior view. Note the course of the aa. vertebrales on both sides of the corpora vertebrarum.

The development of the uncovertebral joints at approximately 10 years of age initiates a process of cleft formation in the disci intervertebrales. This process spreads toward the center of the disk with aging, eventually resulting in the formation of complete transverse clefts that subdivide the disci intervertebrales into two slabs of roughly equal thickness. The result is a progressive degenerative process marked by flattening of the disks and consequent instability of the motion segments (drawing based on specimens from the Anatomical Collection at Kiel University).

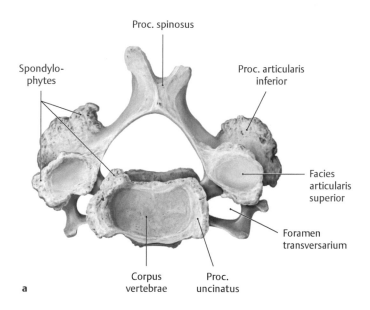

Proc. spinosus

Spondylo-phytes

Proc. articularis inferior

Facies articularis superior

Foramen transversarium

Corpus vertebrae · Proc. uncinatus

a

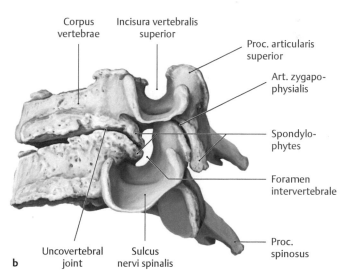

Corpus vertebrae · Incisura vertebralis superior

Proc. articularis superior

Art. zygapophysialis

Spondylophytes

Foramen intervertebrale

Uncovertebral joint · Sulcus nervi spinalis

Proc. spinosus

b

D Advanced uncovertebral arthrosis of the cervical spine

a Vertebra cervicalis quarta, superior view; **b** Vertebrae cervicales quarta and quinta, lateral view (drawings based on specimens from the Anatomical Collection at Kiel University).

The uncovertebral joints undergo degenerative changes comparable to those seen in other joints, including the formation of osteophytes (called spondylophytes when they occur on corpora vertebrarum). These sites of new bone formation serve to distribute the imposed forces over a larger area, thereby reducing the pressure on the joint. With progressive destabilization of the corresponding motion segment, the facet joints undergo osteoarthritic changes leading to osteophyte formation. Osteophytes of the uncovertebral joints have major clinical importance because of their relation to the foramen intervertebrale and a. vertebralis (uncovertebral arthrosis). They cause a progressive narrowing of the foramen intervertebrale, with increasing compression of the nervus spinalis and often of the a. vertebralis as well (cf. **C**). Meanwhile, the canalis spinalis itself may become significantly narrowed (spinal stenosis) by the same process.

3.1 Muscles of Facial Expression (Musculi Faciei): Overview

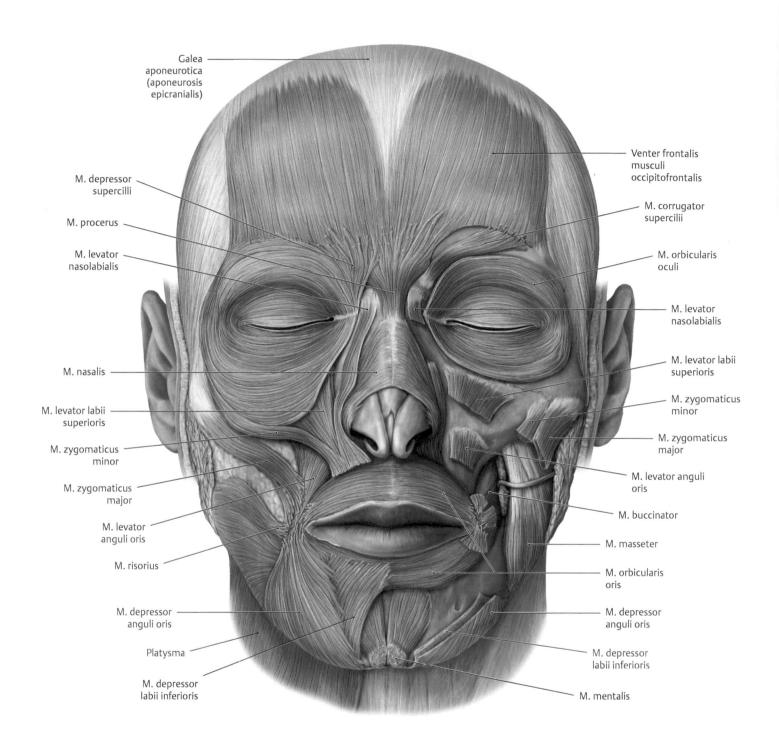

A Musculi faciei

Anterior view. The superficial layer of muscles is shown on the right half of the face, the deep layer on the left half. The mm. faciei represent the superficial muscle layer in the face and vary greatly in their development among different individuals. They arise either directly from the periosteum or from adjacent muscles to which they are connected, and they insert either onto other facial muscles or directly into the connective tissue of the skin. The classic scheme of classifying the other somatic muscles by their origins and insertions is not so easily adapted to the facial muscles. Because the mm. faciei terminate directly in the subcutaneous fat and the superficial body fascia is absent in the face, the surgeon must be particularly careful when dissecting in this region. Due to their cutaneous attachments, the facial muscles are able to move the facial skin (e.g., they can wrinkle the skin, an action temporarily abolished by botulinum toxin injection) and produce a variety of facial expressions. They also serve a protective function (especially for the eyes) through their sphincter-like action and are active during food ingestion (closing the mouth for swallowing). All of the mm. faciei are innervated by branches of the n. facialis, while the mm. masticatorii (see p. 82) are supplied by motor fibers from the n. trigeminus (the m. masseter has been left in place to represent these muscles). A thorough understanding of muscular anatomy in this region is facilitated by dividing the muscles into different groups (see p. 80).

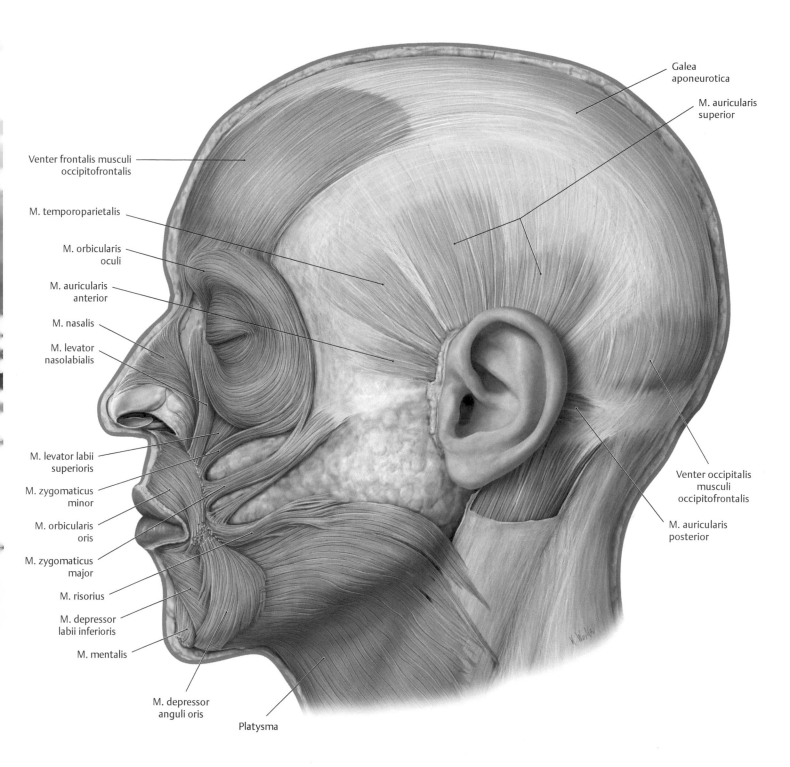

Galea
aponeurotica

M. auricularis
superior

Venter frontalis musculi
occipitofrontalis

M. temporoparietalis

M. orbicularis
oculi

M. auricularis
anterior

M. nasalis

M. levator
nasolabialis

M. levator labii
superioris

M. zygomaticus
minor

M. orbicularis
oris

M. zygomaticus
major

M. risorius

M. depressor
labii inferioris

M. mentalis

M. depressor
anguli oris

Platysma

Venter occipitalis
musculi
occipitofrontalis

M. auricularis
posterior

B Musculi faciei
Left lateral view. The superficial muscles of the ear and neck are particularly well displayed from this perspective. A tough tendinous sheet, the galea aponeurotica, stretches over the calvaria and is loosely attached to the periosteum. The muscles of the calvaria that arise from the galea aponeurotica are known collectively as the "m. epicranius." The two bellies of the m. occipitofrontalis (ventres frontalis and occipital) can be clearly identified. The m. temporoparietalis, whose posterior part is called the m. auricularis superior, arises from the lateral part of the galea aponeurotica. The m. levator anguli oris is not visible here because it is covered by the m. levator labii superioris located above it.

79

3.2 Muscles of Facial Expression: Actions

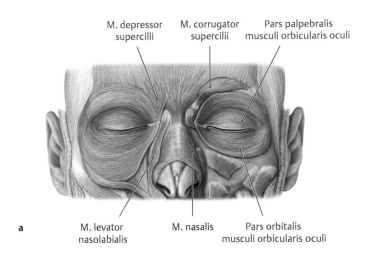

M. depressor supercilli   M. corrugator supercilii   Pars palpebralis musculi orbicularis oculi

M. levator nasolabialis   M. nasalis   Pars orbitalis musculi orbicularis oculi

a

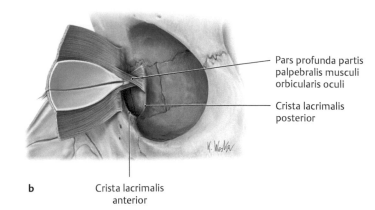

Pars profunda partis palpebralis musculi orbicularis oculi

Crista lacrimalis posterior

Crista lacrimalis anterior

b

A Musculi faciei: rima palpebrarum and nose

a Anterior view. The most functionally important muscle is the *m. orbicularis oculi*, which closes the rima palpebralis as a protective reflex against foreign matter. If the action of the m. orbicularis oculi is lost because of n. facialis paralysis (see also **D**), the loss of this protective reflex will be accompanied by drying of the eye from prolonged exposure to air without the lubricating nature of being able to blink.

The function of the m. orbicularis oculi is tested by asking the patient to squeeze the eyelids tightly shut.

b The m. orbicularis oculi has been dissected from the left orbita to the medial canthus of the eye and reflected anteriorly to demonstrate its pars profunda partis palpebralis. This part of the m. orbicularis oculi arises mainly from the crista lacrimalis posterior, and its action is a subject of debate (expand or empty the saccus lacrimalis).

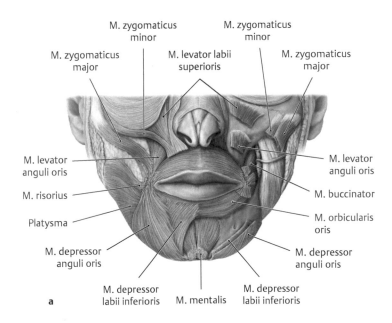

M. zygomaticus minor   M. zygomaticus minor

M. zygomaticus major   M. levator labii superioris   M. zygomaticus major

M. levator anguli oris

M. risorius

Platysma

M. depressor anguli oris

M. levator anguli oris

M. buccinator

M. orbicularis oris

M. depressor anguli oris

M. depressor labii inferioris   M. mentalis   M. depressor labii inferioris

a

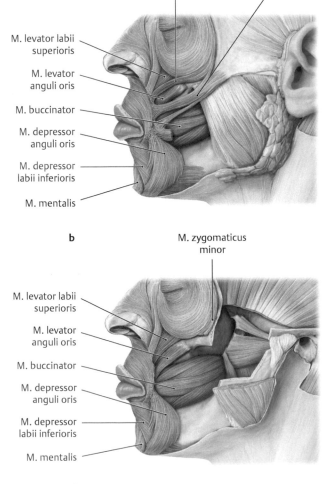

M. zygomaticus minor   M. zygomaticus major

M. levator labii superioris

M. levator anguli oris

M. buccinator

M. depressor anguli oris

M. depressor labii inferioris

M. mentalis

b

M. zygomaticus minor

M. levator labii superioris

M. levator anguli oris

M. buccinator

M. depressor anguli oris

M. depressor labii inferioris

M. mentalis

c

B Musculi faciei: mouth

a Anterior view, **b** left lateral view, **c** left lateral view of the deeper lateral layer.

The *m. orbicularis oris* forms the muscular foundation of the lips, and its contraction closes the oral aperture. Its function can be tested by asking the patient to whistle. N. facialis caralysis may lead to drinking difficulties because the liquid will trickle back out of the unclosed mouth during swallowing. The *m. buccinator* lies at a deeper level and forms the foundation of the cheek. During mastication, this muscle moves food between the dental arches from the oral vestibule.

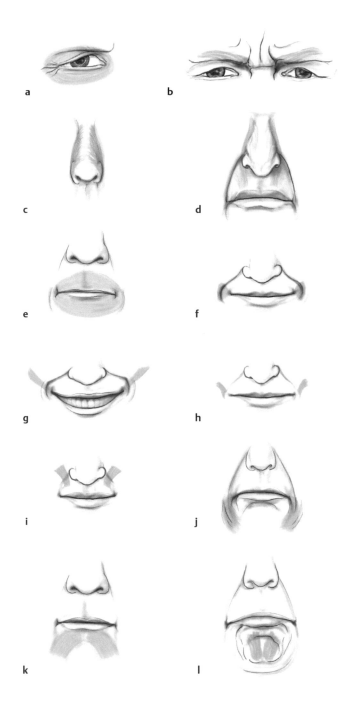

C Changes of facial expression

a Contraction of the m. orbicularis oculi at the lateral canthus of the eye expresses concern.

b Contraction of the m. corrugator supercilii occurs in response to bright sunlight: "thoughtful brow."

c Contraction of the m. nasalis constricts the naris and produces a cheery or lustful facial expression.

d Forceful contraction of the m. levator nasolabialis on both sides is a sign of disapproval.

e Contraction of the m. orbicularis oris expresses determination.

f Contraction of the m. buccinator signals satisfaction.

g The m. zygomaticus major contracts during smiling.

h Contraction of the m. risorius reflects purposeful action.

i Contraction of the m. levator anguli oris signals self-satisfaction.

j Contraction of the m. depressor anguli oris signals sadness.

k Contraction of the m. depressor labii inferioris depresses the lower lip and expresses perseverence.

l Contraction of the m. mentalis expresses indecision.

D Musculi faciei: functional groups

The various mimetic muscles are easier to learn when they are studied by regions. It is useful clinically to distinguish between the muscles of the forehead and rima palpebrarum and the rest of the mimetic muscles. The muscles of the forehead and rima palpebrarum are innervated by the superior branch of the n. facialis, while all the other mimetic muscles are supplied by other n. facialis branches. As a result, patients with central n. facialis paralysis can still close their eyes while patients with peripheral n. facialis paralysis cannot (see p. 125 for further details).

Region	Muscle	Remarks
Calvarium	M. epicranius, consisting of	Muscle of the calvarium
	– M. occipitofrontalis (ventres frontalis and occipitalis)	Wrinkles the forehead
	– M. temporoparietalis	Has no mimetic function
Rima palpebrarum	M. orbicularis oculi, consisting of	Closes the eyelid (**a**)
	– Pars orbitalis	Tightly contracts the skin around the eye
	– Pars palpebralis	Palpebral reflex
	– Pars profunda partis palpebralis	Acts on the saccus lacrimalis
	M. corrugator supercilii	Wrinkles the eyebrow (**b**)
	M. depressor supercilii	Lowers the eyebrow
Nose	M. procerus	Wrinkles the root of the nose
	M. nasalis	Narrows the naris (**c**)
	M. levator nasolabialis	Elevates the upper lip and nasal alae (**d**)
Mouth	M. orbicularis oris	Closes the mouth (**e**)
	M. buccinator	Muscle of the cheek (important during eating and drinking) (**f**)
	M. zygomaticus major	Large muscle of the arcus zygomaticus (**g**)
	M. zygomaticus minor	Small muscle of the arcus zygomaticus
	M. risorius	Muscle of smiling/grinning (**h**)
	M. levator labii superioris	Elevates the upper lip
	M. levator anguli oris	Pulls the corner of the mouth upward (**i**)
	M. depressor anguli oris	Pulls the corner of the mouth downward (**j**)
	M. depressor labii inferioris	Pulls the lower lip downward (**k**)
	M. mentalis	Pulls the skin of the chin upward (**l**)
Ear	M. auricularis anterior	Anterior muscle of the auricula
	M. auricularis superior	Superior muscle of the auricula
	M. auricularis posterior	Posterior muscle of the auricula
Neck	Platysma	Cutaneous muscle of the neck

3.3 Muscles of Mastication (Musculi Masticatorii): Overview and Superficial Muscles

Overview of the musculi masticatorii

The musculi masticatorii in the strict sense consist of four muscles: the m. masseter, m. temporalis, m. pterygoideus medialis, and m. pterygoideus lateralis.

The primary function of all these muscles is to close the mouth and move the upper teeth against the lower teeth in a grinding action during mastication. The m. pterygoideus lateralis assists in opening the mouth. The two pterygoid muscles are also active during mastication (for the individual muscle actions, see **A–C**).

The mouth is opened primarily by the suprahyoid muscles and the force of gravity. The m. masseter and m. pterygoideus medialis form a muscular sling in which the mandibula is suspended (see p. 84).

Note: All muscles of mastication are innervated by the n. mandibularis (third division of the n. trigeminus), while the muscles of facial expression are innervated by the n. facialis.

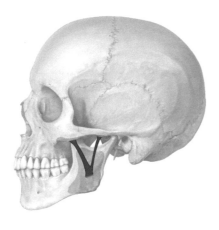

A Schematic of the musculus masseter

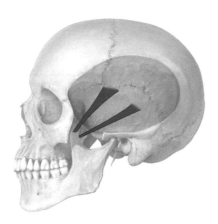

B Schematic of the musculus temporalis

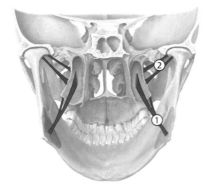

C Schematic of the musculi pterygoidei medialis and lateralis

---

Musculus masseter

Origin:	• Pars superficialis: arcus zygomaticus (anterior two-thirds)
	• Pars profunda: arcus zygomaticus (posterior third)
Insertion:	• Tuberositas masseterica on the angulus mandibulae
Actions:	• Elevates the mandibula
	• Protrudes the mandibula
Innervation:	N. massetericus, a branch of the n. mandibularis division of the n. trigeminus (CN V_3)

Musculus temporalis

Origin:	• Linea temporalis inferior of the fossa temporalis
Insertion:	• Apex and medial surface of the proc. coronoideus of the mandibula
Actions:	• Elevates the mandibula, chiefly with its vertical fibers
	• Retracts the protruded mandibula with its horizontal posterior fibers
	• Unilateral contraction: mastication (moves the caput mandibulae on the balance side forward)
Innervation:	Nn. temporales profundi, branches of the n. mandibularis division of the n. trigeminus (CN V_3)

① Musculus pterygoideus medialis

Origin:	Fossa pterygoidea and medial surface of the lamina lateralis of the proc. pterygoideus
Insertion:	Medial surface of the angulus mandibulae (tuberositas pterygoidea)
Actions:	Elevates the mandibula
Innervation:	N. pterygoideus medialis, a branch of the n. mandibularis division of the n. trigeminus (CN V_3)

② Musculus pterygoideus lateralis

Origin:	• Caput superius: crista infratemporalis of ala major ossis sphenoidalis
	• Caput inferius: lateral surface of the lamina lateralis processus pterygoidei
Insertion:	• Caput superius: discus articularis of the art. temporomandibularis
	• Caput inferius: neck of the proc. condylaris of the mandibula
Actions:	• Bilateral contraction: initiates mouth opening by protruding the mandibula and moving the discus articularis forward
	• Unilateral contraction: elevates the mandibula to the opposite side during mastication
Innervation:	N. pterygoideus lateralis, a branch of the n. mandibularis division of the n. trigeminus (CN V_3)

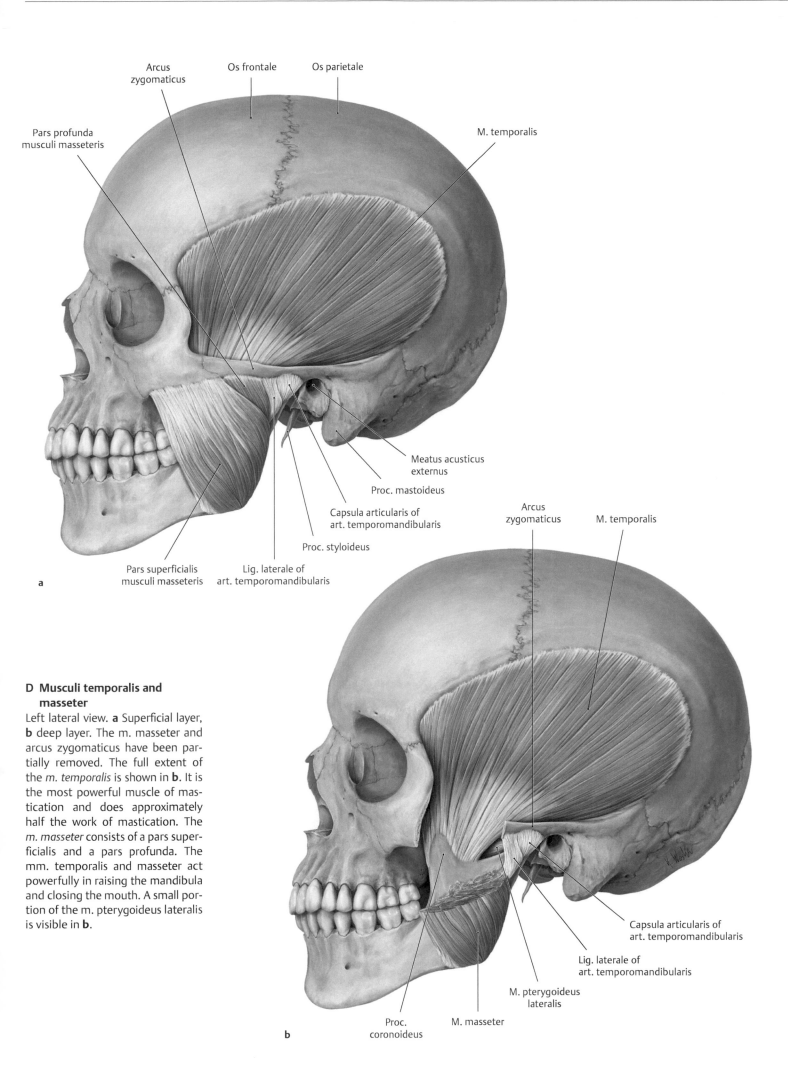

Arcus zygomaticus

Os frontale

Os parietale

M. temporalis

Pars profunda musculi masseteris

Meatus acusticus externus

Proc. mastoideus

Capsula articularis of art. temporomandibularis

Arcus zygomaticus

M. temporalis

Proc. styloideus

a

Pars superficialis musculi masseteris

Lig. laterale of art. temporomandibularis

D Musculi temporalis and masseter

Left lateral view. **a** Superficial layer, **b** deep layer. The m. masseter and arcus zygomaticus have been partially removed. The full extent of the *m. temporalis* is shown in **b**. It is the most powerful muscle of mastication and does approximately half the work of mastication. The *m. masseter* consists of a pars superficialis and a pars profunda. The mm. temporalis and masseter act powerfully in raising the mandibula and closing the mouth. A small portion of the m. pterygoideus lateralis is visible in **b**.

Capsula articularis of art. temporomandibularis

Lig. laterale of art. temporomandibularis

M. pterygoideus lateralis

Proc. coronoideus

M. masseter

b

3.4 Muscles of Mastication (Musculi Masticatorii): Deep Muscles

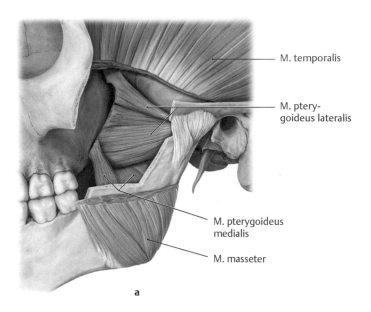

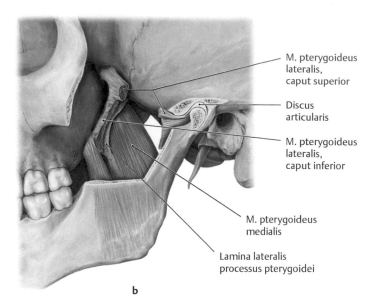

a

b

A Musculi pterygoidei lateralis and medialis
Left lateral views.

a The proc. coronoideus of the mandibula has been removed here along with the lower part of the m. temporalis so that both pterygoid muscles can be seen.

b The m. temporalis has been completely removed, and the inferior part of the m. pterygoideus lateralis has been windowed. The m. pterygoideus lateralis initiates mouth opening, which is then continued by the suprahyoid muscles. With the art. temporomandibularis

opened, we can see that fibers from the m. pterygoideus lateralis blend with the discus articularis of the art. temporomandibularis. The m. pterygoideus lateralis functions as the guide muscle of the joint. Because its various parts (capita superius and inferius) are active during all movements, its actions are more complex than those of the other mm. masticatorii. The m. pterygoideus medialis runs almost perpendicular to the m. pterygoideus lateralis and contributes to the formation of a muscular sling that partially encompasses the mandibula (see **B**).

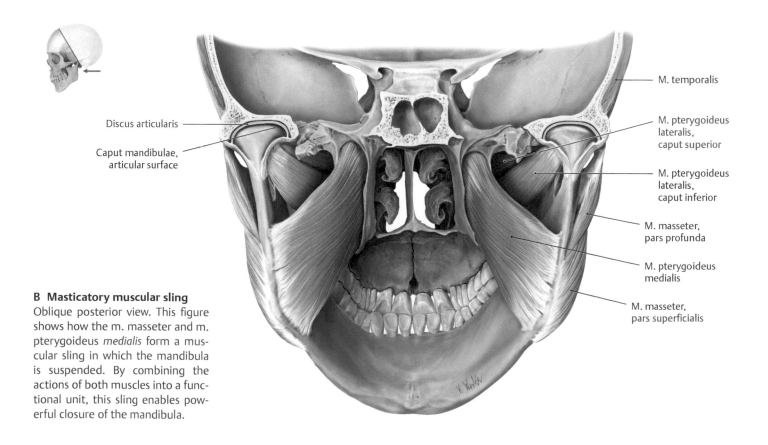

B Masticatory muscular sling
Oblique posterior view. This figure shows how the m. masseter and m. pterygoideus *medialis* form a muscular sling in which the mandibula is suspended. By combining the actions of both muscles into a functional unit, this sling enables powerful closure of the mandibula.

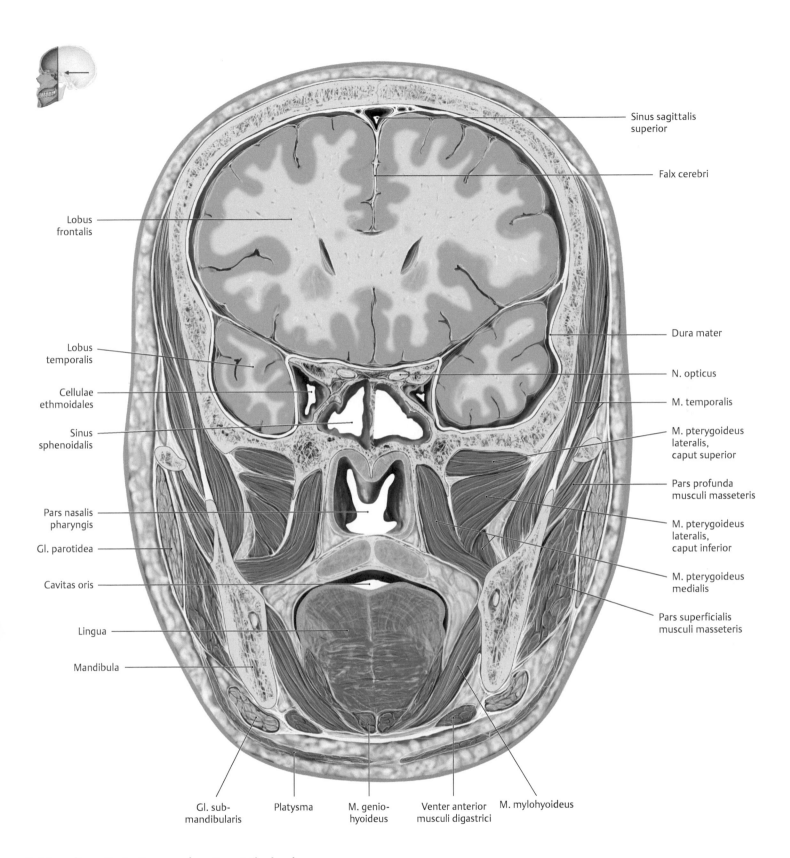

Sinus sagittalis superior

Falx cerebri

Dura mater

N. opticus

M. temporalis

M. pterygoideus lateralis, caput superior

Pars profunda musculi masseteris

M. pterygoideus lateralis, caput inferior

M. pterygoideus medialis

Pars superficialis musculi masseteris

Lobus frontalis

Lobus temporalis

Cellulae ethmoidales

Sinus sphenoidalis

Pars nasalis pharyngis

Gl. parotidea

Cavitas oris

Lingua

Mandibula

Gl. sub-mandibularis

Platysma

M. genio-hyoideus

Venter anterior musculi digastrici

M. mylohyoideus

C Musculi masticatorii, coronal section at the level of the sinus sphenoidalis

Posterior view. The topography of the mm. masticatorii and neighboring structures is particularly well displayed in this section.

3.5 Muscles of the Head: Origins and Insertions

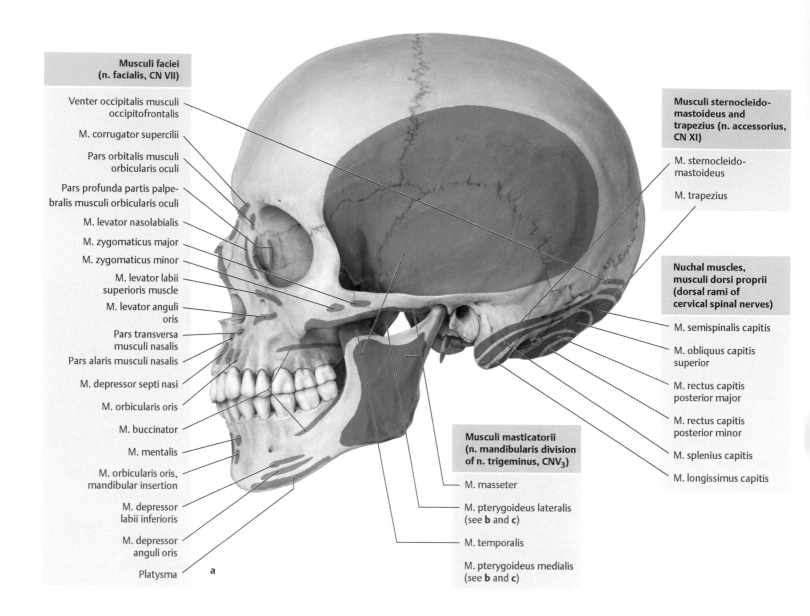

**Musculi faciei
(n. facialis, CN VII)**

Venter occipitalis musculi occipitofrontalis

M. corrugator supercilii

Pars orbitalis musculi orbicularis oculi

Pars profunda partis palpebralis musculi orbicularis oculi

M. levator nasolabialis

M. zygomaticus major

M. zygomaticus minor

M. levator labii superioris muscle

M. levator anguli oris

Pars transversa musculi nasalis

Pars alaris musculi nasalis

M. depressor septi nasi

M. orbicularis oris

M. buccinator

M. mentalis

M. orbicularis oris, mandibular insertion

M. depressor labii inferioris

M. depressor anguli oris

Platysma

Musculi sternocleido-mastoideus and trapezius (n. accessorius, CN XI)

M. sternocleido-mastoideus

M. trapezius

Nuchal muscles, musculi dorsi proprii (dorsal rami of cervical spinal nerves)

M. semispinalis capitis

M. obliquus capitis superior

M. rectus capitis posterior major

M. rectus capitis posterior minor

M. splenius capitis

M. longissimus capitis

**Musculi masticatorii
(n. mandibularis division of n. trigeminus, CNV₃)**

M. masseter

M. pterygoideus lateralis (see **b** and **c**)

M. temporalis

M. pterygoideus medialis (see **b** and **c**)

a

A Muscle origins and insertions on the skull

a Left lateral view, **b** View of the inner surface of the right hemimandible, **c** inferior view of the basis cranii.

The origins and insertions of the muscles are indicated by color shading (origin: red, insertion: blue).

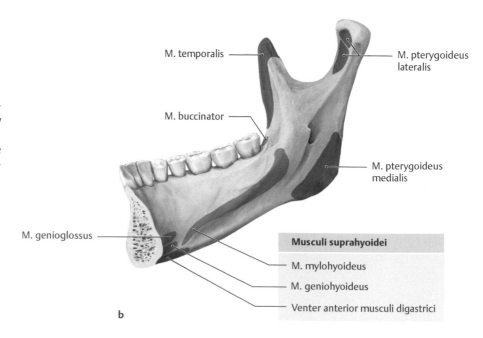

M. temporalis

M. pterygoideus lateralis

M. buccinator

M. pterygoideus medialis

M. genioglossus

Musculi suprahyoidei

M. mylohyoideus

M. geniohyoideus

Venter anterior musculi digastrici

b

Musculi masticatorii (n. mandibularis division of n. trigeminus, CN V₃)

M. masseter

M. pterygoideus medialis

M. pterygoideus lateralis

M. temporalis

Muscles of tongue (n. hypoglossus, CN XII)

M. hyoglossus (not shown)

M. genioglossus (not shown)

M. styloglossus

M. stylohyoid

Venter anterior musculi digastrici

Nuchal muscles, musculi dorsi proprii (dorsal rami of cervical spinal nerves)

M. splenius capitis

M. longissimus capitis

M. obliquus capitis superior

M. rectus capitis posterior major

M. rectus capitis posterior minor

M. semispinalis capitis

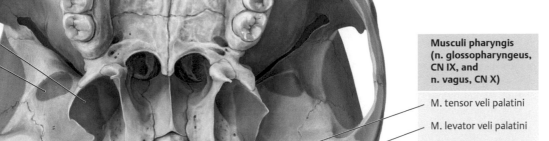

Musculi pharyngis (n. glossopharyngeus, CN IX, and n. vagus, CN X)

M. tensor veli palatini

M. levator veli palatini

M. stylopharyngeus

M. constrictor pharyngis medius (not shown)

Prevertebral muscles (ventral cervical nerve rami and cervical plexus)

M. rectus capitis lateralis

M. longus capitis

M. rectus capitis anterior

Musculi sternocleidomastoideus and trapezius (n. accessorius, CN XI)

M. sternocleidomastoideus

M. trapezius

c

3.6 Neck Muscles: Overview and Superficial Muscles

A Scheme used for classifying the neck muscles into groups

The next few sections follow the outline below, which is based on the topographical anatomy of the neck. Various schemes may be used, however. While the nuchal muscles are classified as neck muscles from a topographical standpoint, they belong functionally to the category of intrinsic back muscles (musculi dorsi proprii, which are not described here).

Superficial neck muscles
- Platysma
- M. sternocleidomastoideus
- M. trapezius*

Musculi suprahyoidei
- M. digastricus
- M. geniohyoideus
- M. mylohyoideus
- M. stylohyoideus

Musculi infrahyoidei
- M. sternohyoideus
- M. sternothyroideus
- M. thyrohyoideus
- M. omohyoideus

* Not a neck muscle in the strict sense, but included here owing to its topographical importance

Prevertebral muscles (deep strap muscles)
- M. longus capitis
- M. longus colli
- M. rectus capitis anterior
- M. rectus capitis lateralis

Lateral (deep) neck muscles
- M. scalenus anterior
- M. scalenus medius
- M. scalenus posterior

Nuchal muscles (intrinsic back muscles)
- M. semispinalis capitis
- M. semispinalis cervicis
- M. splenius capitis
- M. splenius cervicis
- M. longissimus capitis
- M. iliocostalis cervicis
- Mm. suboccipitales

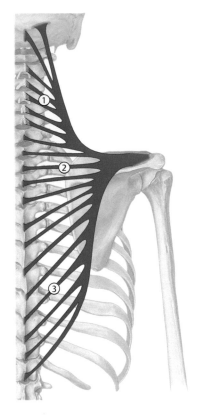

C Schematic of the musculus trapezius

Origin:	① Pars descendens: • Os occipitale (linea nuchalis superior and protuberantia occipitalis externa) • The procc. spinosi of all vertebrae cervicales via the lig. nuchae ② Pars transversa: Broad aponeurosis at the level of the procc. spinosi T1–T4 ③ Pars ascendens: Procc. spinosi T5–T12
Insertion:	• Lateral third of the clavicula (pars descendens) • Acromion (pars transversalis) • Spina scapulae (pars ascendens)
Actions:	• Pars descendens: – Draws the scapula obliquely upward and rotates it externally (acting with the inferior part of the m. serratus anterior) – Tilts the head to the same side and rotates it to the opposite side (with the shoulder girdle fixed) • Pars transversalis: draws the scapula medially • Pars ascendens: draws the scapula medially downward (supports the rotating action of the pars descendens) • Entire muscle: stabilizes the scapula on the thorax
Innervation:	N. accessorius (CN XI) and plexus cervicalis (C2–C4)

Caput laterale of m. sternocleidomastoideus

Caput mediale of m. sternocleidomastoideus

B Schematic of the musculus sternocleidomastoideus

Origin:	• Caput mediale: manubrium sterni • Caput laterale: medial third of the clavicula
Insertion:	Proc. mastoideus and linea nuchalis superior
Actions:	• Unilateral: – Tilts the head to the same side – Rotates the head to the opposite side • Bilateral: – Extends the head – Assists in respiration when the head is fixed
Innervation:	N. accessorius (cranial nerve XI [CN XI] and direct branches from the plexus cervicalis (C1–C2)

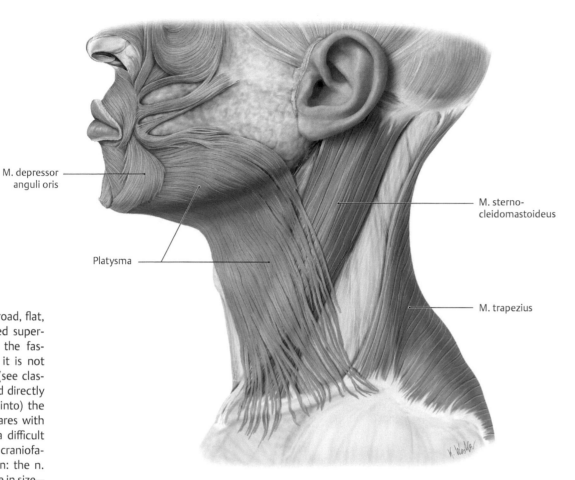

M. depressor
anguli oris

M. sterno-
cleidomastoideus

Platysma

M. trapezius

D Cutaneous muscle of the neck (platysma)

Left lateral view. The platysma is a broad, flat, subcutaneous muscular sheet located superficial to the lamina superficialis of the fascia cervicalis. Unlike most muscles, it is not enveloped in its own fascial sheath (see classification scheme in **A**), but is instead directly associated with (and in part inserts into) the skin. This characteristic, which it shares with the mm. faciei, makes the platysma difficult to dissect. It also shares with those craniofacial muscles its source of innervation: the n. facialis. The platysma is highly variable in size—its fibers may reach from the lower part of the face to the upper thorax.

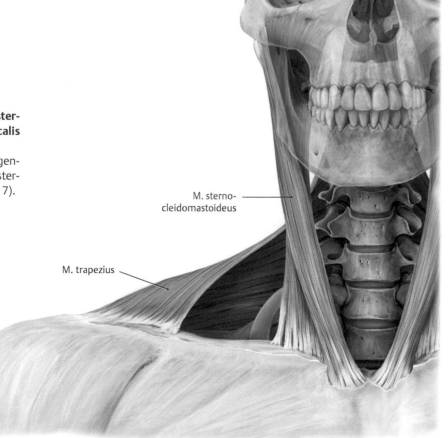

M. sterno-
cleidomastoideus

M. trapezius

E Superficial neck muscles: musculus sternocleidomastoideus and pars cervicalis of musculus trapezius, anterior view

Congenital muscular torticollis involves degenerative scarring and shortening of the m. sternocleidomastoideus on one side (see **D**, p. 7).

89

3.7 Neck Muscles: Suprahyoid and Infrahyoid Muscles

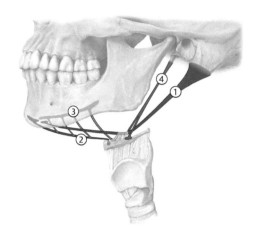

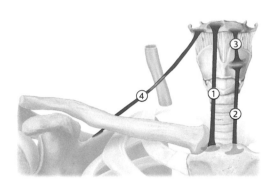

A Overview of the musculi suprahyoidei

B Schematic of the musculi infrahyoidei

---

① M. digastricus

Origin:	• Venter anterior: fossa digastrica of the mandibula
	• Venter posterior: medial to the proc. mastoideus (incisura mastoidea)
Insertion:	Corpus of the os hyoideum via an intermediate tendon with a fibrous loop
Actions:	• Elevates the os hyoideum (during swallowing)
	• Assists in opening the mandibula
Innervation:	• Venter anterior: n. mylohyoideus (from the n. mandibularis of CN V – n. trigeminus)
	• Venter posterior: n. facialis (CN VII)

② M. geniohyoideus

Origin:	Spina mentalis inferior of the mandibula
Insertion:	Corpus of the os hyoideum
Actions:	• Draws the os hyoideum forward (during swallowing)
	• Assists in opening the mandibula
Innervation:	Ramus ventralis of C1

③ M. mylohyoideus

Origin:	Linea mylohyoidea of the mandibula
Insertion:	Body of the os hyoideum by a median tendon of insertion (mylohyoid raphe)
Actions:	• Tightens and elevates the oral floor
	• Draws the os hyoideum forward (during swallowing)
	• Assists in opening the mandibulae and moving it from side to side (mastication)
Innervation:	N. mylohyoideus (from the n. mandibularis, a division of CN V)

④ M. stylohyoideus

Origin:	Proc. styloideus of the os temporale
Insertion:	Corpus of the os hyoideum by a split tendon
Actions:	• Elevates the os hyoideum (during swallowing)
	• Assists in opening the mandibula
Innervation:	N. facialis (CN VII)

① M. sternohyoideus

Origin:	Posterior surface of the manubrium of the sternum and art. sternoclavicularis
Insertion:	Corpus of the os hyoideum
Actions:	• Depresses (fixes) the os hyoideum
	• Depresses the larynx and os hyoideum (for phonation and the terminal phase of swallowing)
Innervation:	Ansa cervicalis of the plexus cervicalis (C1–C3) as well as C4

② M. sternothyroideus

Origin:	Posterior surface of the manubrium of the sternum
Insertion:	Linea obliqua of the cartilago thyroidea
Actions:	• Draws the larynx and os hyoideum downward (fixes the os hyoideum)
	• Depresses the larynx and os hyoideum (for phonation and the terminal phase of swallowing)
Innervation:	Ansa cervicalis of the plexus cervicalis (C1–C3) as well as C4

③ M. thyrohyoideus

Origin:	Linea obliqua of the cartilago thyroidea
Insertion:	Corpus of the os hyoideum
Actions:	• Depresses and fixes the os hyoideum
	• Raises the larynx during swallowing
Innervation:	Ramus ventralis of C1 as well as C4

④ M. omohyoideus

Origin:	Margo superior of the scapula
Insertion:	Corpus of the os hyoideum
Actions:	• Depresses (fixes) the os hyoideum
	• Draws the larynx and os hyoideum downward (for phonation and the terminal phase of swallowing)
	• Tenses the fascia cervicalis with its intermediate tendon and maintains patency of the v. jugularis interna
Innervation:	Ansa cervicalis of the plexus cervicalis (C1–C3) as well as C4

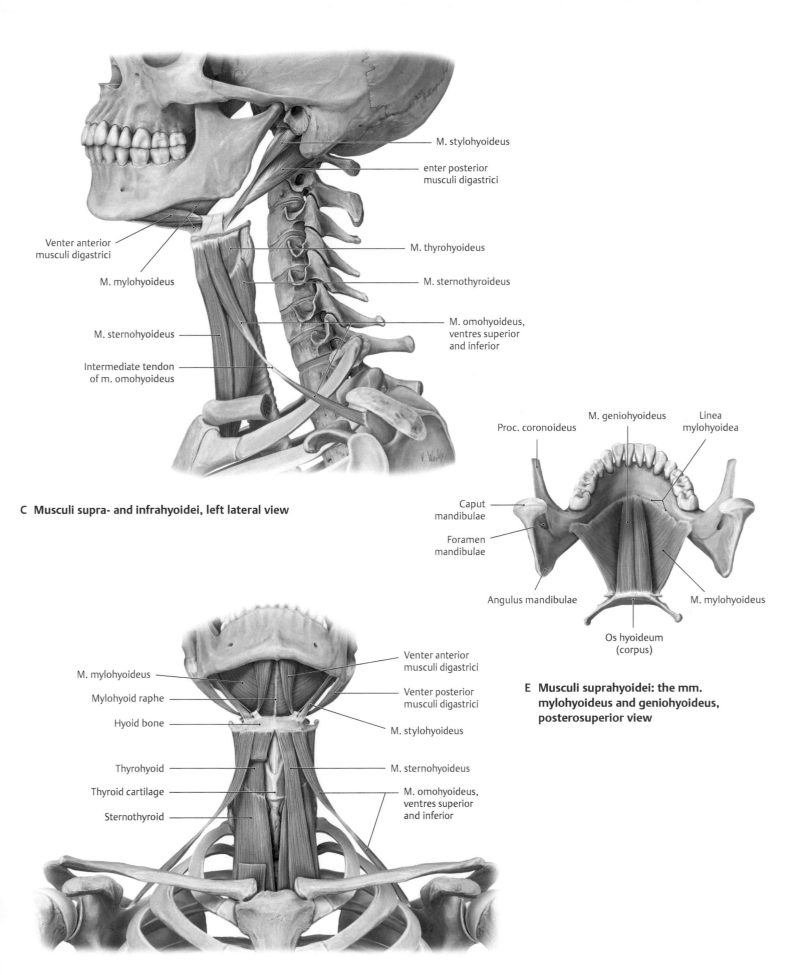

M. stylohyoideus

enter posterior
musculi digastrici

M. thyrohyoideus

M. sternothyroideus

M. omohyoideus,
ventres superior
and inferior

Venter anterior
musculi digastrici

M. mylohyoideus

M. sternohyoideus

Intermediate tendon
of m. omohyoideus

C Musculi supra- and infrahyoidei, left lateral view

Proc. coronoideus

M. geniohyoideus

Linea
mylohyoidea

Caput
mandibulae

Foramen
mandibulae

Angulus mandibulae

M. mylohyoideus

Os hyoideum
(corpus)

**E Musculi suprahyoidei: the mm.
mylohyoideus and geniohyoideus,
posterosuperior view**

M. mylohyoideus

Mylohyoid raphe

Hyoid bone

Thyrohyoid

Thyroid cartilage

Sternothyroid

Venter anterior
musculi digastrici

Venter posterior
musculi digastrici

M. stylohyoideus

M. sternohyoideus

M. omohyoideus,
ventres superior
and inferior

D Musculi supra- and infrahyoidei, anterior view
Part of the m. sternohyoideus has been removed on the right side.

91

3.8 Neck Muscles: Prevertebral and Lateral (Deep) Muscles

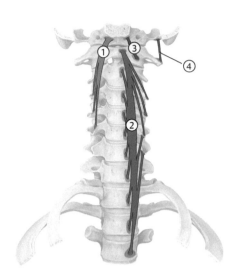

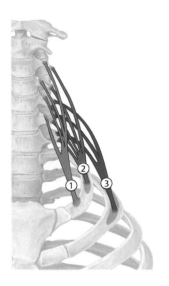

A Schematic of the prevertebral muscles

B Schematic of the lateral (deep) neck muscles

① **M. longus capitis**

Origin:	Tubercula anteriora of the procc. tranversi of the C3–C6 vertebrae
Insertion:	Pars basilaris of the os occipitale
Actions:	• Unilateral: tilts and slightly rotates the head to the same side
	• Bilateral: flexes the head
Innervation:	Direct branches from the plexus cervicalis (C1–C4)

② **M. longus colli**

Origin:	• Pars verticalis (intermediate): anterior surfaces of the C5–C7 and T1–T3 vertebral bodies
	• Pars obliqua superior: tubercula anteriora of the procc. transversi of the C3–C5 vertebrae
	• Pars obliqua inferior: anterior surfaces of the T1–T3 vertebral bodies
Insertion:	• Pars verticalis: anterior surfaces of the C2–C4 vertebrae
	• Pars obliqua superior: tuberculum anterius of the atlas
	• Pars obliqua inferior: tubercula anteriora of the procc. transversi of the C5 and C6 vertebrae
Actions:	• Unilateral: tilts and rotates and cervical spine to the same side
	• Bilateral: flexes the cervical spine
Innervation:	Direct branches from the plexus cervicalis (C2–C4) as well as direct branches from C5, C6

③ **M. rectus capitis anterior**

Origin:	Massa lateralis of the atlas
Insertion:	Pars basilaris of the os occipitale
Actions:	• Unilateral: lateral flexion at the art. atlantooccipitalis
	• Bilateral: flexion at the art. atlantooccipitalis
Innervation:	Rami ventrales of C1

④ **M. rectus capitis lateralis**

Origin:	Proc. transversus of the atlas
Insertion:	Pars basilaris of the os occipitale (lateral to the condyli occipitales)
Actions:	• Unilateral: lateral flexion at the art. atlantooccipitalis
	• Bilateral: flexion at the art. atlantooccipitalis
Innervation:	Rami ventrales of C1

Mm. scaleni

Origin:	① M. scalenus anterior: tubercula anteriora transversi of the procc. transversi of the C3–C6 vertebrae
	② M. scalenus medius: procc. transversi of atlas and axis; tubercula posteriora of the procc. transversi of the C3–C7 vertebrae
	③ M. scalenus posterior: tubercula posteriora of the procc. transversi of the C5–C7 vertebrae
Insertion:	• M. scalenus anterior: tuberculum musculi scaleni anterioris on the costa prima
	• M. scalenus medius: costa prima (posterior to the sulcus arteriae subclaviae)
	• M. scalenus posterior: outer surface of the costa secunda
Actions:	• With the ribs mobile: inspiration (elevates the upper ribs)
	• With the ribs fixed: bends the cervical spine to the same side (with unilateral contraction)
	• Flexes the neck (with bilateral contraction)
Innervation:	Direct branches from the plexus cervicalis and Mm. scaleni (C3–C6)

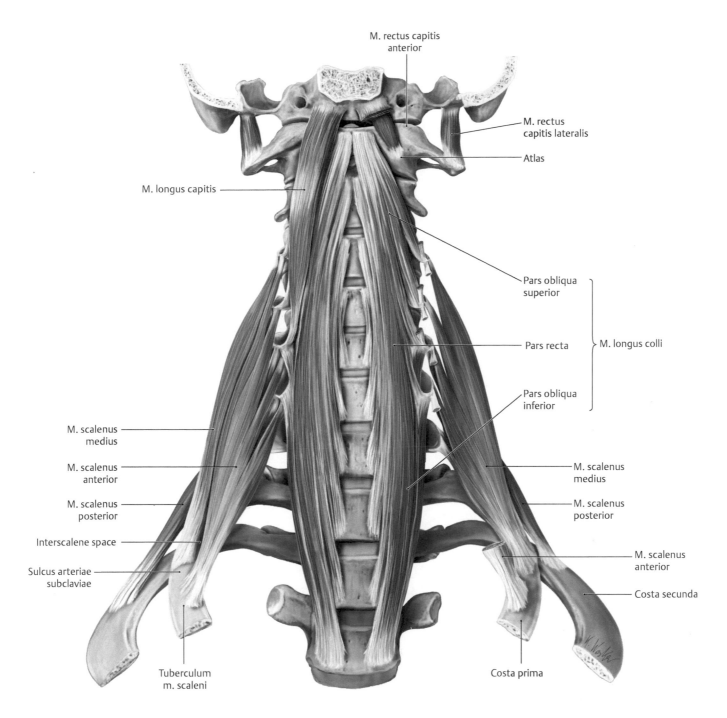

M. rectus capitis anterior

M. rectus capitis lateralis

Atlas

M. longus capitis

Pars obliqua superior

Pars recta — M. longus colli

Pars obliqua inferior

M. scalenus medius

M. scalenus anterior

M. scalenus medius

M. scalenus posterior

M. scalenus posterior

Interscalene space

M. scalenus anterior

Sulcus arteriae subclaviae

Costa secunda

Tuberculum m. scaleni

Costa prima

C Prevertebral and lateral (deep) neck muscles, anterior view
The mm. longus capitis and scalenus anterior have been partially removed on the left side. The prevertebral muscles stretch between the cervical spine and skull, acting upon both. The three overlapping scalene muscles are classified as lateral (deep) neck muscles. As they pass between the cervical spine and the upper two ribs, they also assist in respiration. The m. scalenus anterior and m. scalenus medius are separated by the *interscalene space*—a topographically important interval that is traversed by the plexus brachialis and a. subclavia.

4.1 Classification of the Arteries Supplying the Head and Neck

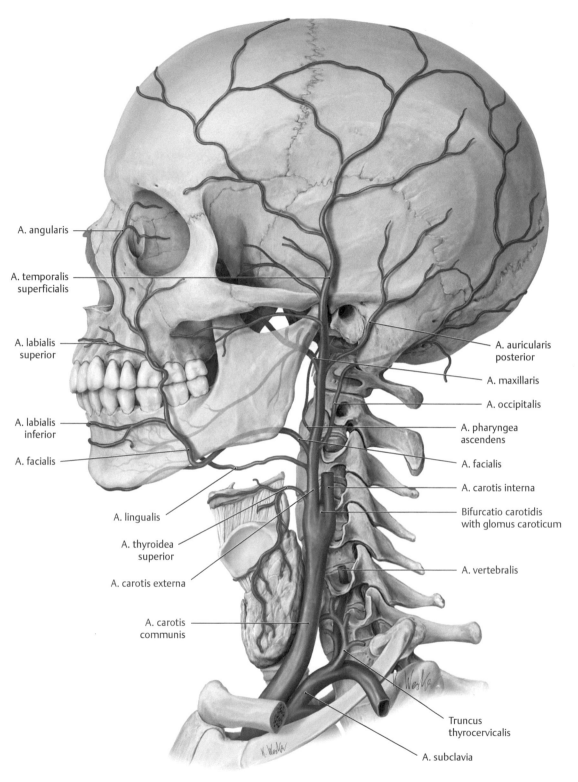

A. angularis

A. temporalis superficialis

A. labialis superior

A. labialis inferior

A. facialis

A. lingualis

A. thyroidea superior

A. carotis externa

A. carotis communis

A. auricularis posterior

A. maxillaris

A. occipitalis

A. pharyngea ascendens

A. facialis

A. carotis interna

Bifurcatio carotidis with glomus caroticum

A. vertebralis

Truncus thyrocervicalis

A. subclavia

Classification of the arteries supplying the head and neck

Branches of the arteria carotis externa

Anterior branches
- a. thyroidea superior
  - r. infrahyoideus
  - a. laryngea superior
  - r. cricothyroideus
  - r. sternocleidomastoideus
  - r. glandularis
- a. lingualis
- a. facialis

Medial branch
- a. pharyngea ascendens

Posterior branches
- a. occipitalis
- a. auricularis posterior

Terminal branches
- a. maxillaris
- a. temporalis superficialis

Branches of the arteria subclavia

A. thoracica interna
- rr. mediastinales
- rr. thymici
- a. pericardiacophrenica
- rr. mammarii mediales
- rr. intercostales anteriores
- a. musculophrenica
- a. epigastrica superior

A. vertebralis
- rr. spinales
- rr. meningei
- a. spinalis posterior
- a. spinalis anterior
- a. inferior posterior cerebelli
- a. basilaris

Truncus thyrocervicalis
- a. thyroidea inferior
  a. cervicalis ascendens
- a. transversa cervicis
  - r. superficialis (superficial cervical artery)
  - r. profundus (a. dorsalis scapulae)
- a. suprascapularis

Truncus costocervicalis
- a. cervicalis profunda
- a. intercostalis suprema

A Overview of the arteries of the head and neck

Left lateral view. The head and neck are mainly supplied by the aa. carotides interna and externa. They arise from the a. carotis communis, which bifurcates in the neck after originating from the arcus aortae. The internal and external arteries are connected with each other through anastomoses (see **D**). The a. carotis interna mainly—but not exclusively—supplies the intracranial structures (brain). The a. carotis externa

supplies the neck and head. In the neck region, the a. carotis communis and the a. carotis externa give off smaller branches. Additionally, areas near the thorax are also supplied by branches of the a. subclavia. The glomus caroticum is situated in the bifurcatio carotidis. It detects hypoxia and pH changes, which is important for the regulation of respiration.

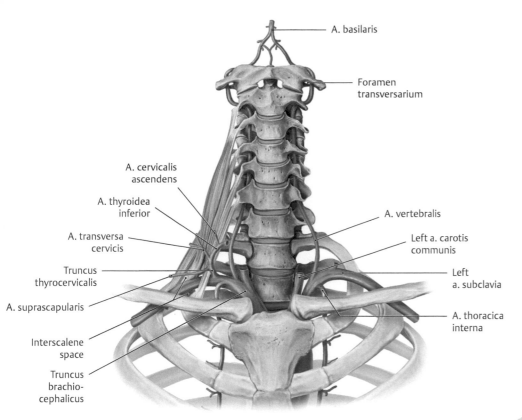

- A. basilaris
- Foramen transversarium
- A. cervicalis ascendens
- A. thyroidea inferior
- A. transversa cervicis
- Truncus thyrocervicalis
- A. suprascapularis
- Interscalene space
- Truncus brachio-cephalicus
- A. vertebralis
- Left a. carotis communis
- Left a. subclavia
- A. thoracica interna

B Arteria subclavia and its branches

Anterior view. The a. subclavia distributes a number of branches to structures located at the base of the neck and about the apertura thoracis superior. Two branches of special importance are the truncus thyrocervicalis, which gives origin to the a. transversa cervicis, and the truncus costocervicalis (see **C**).

Note: The branches of the a. subclavia may arise in a variable sequence. After emerging from the apertura thoracis superior, the a. subclavia passes through the interscalene space (between the scalenus anterior and medius, see p. 93), to the upper limb. The *a. vertebralis* arises from the posterior aspect of the a. subclavia on each side and ascends through the foramina in the procc. transversi of the vertebrae cervicales. After entering the skull, both aa. vertebrales fuse into a single a. basilaris, which will anastomose with the two aa. carotides internae, forming the circulus arteriosus cerebri (circle of Willis), which has a major clinical importance in supplying blood to the brain.

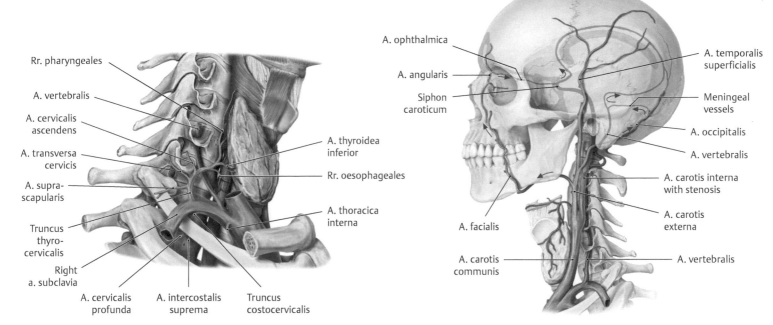

- Rr. pharyngeales
- A. vertebralis
- A. cervicalis ascendens
- A. transversa cervicis
- A. supra-scapularis
- Truncus thyro-cervicalis
- Right a. subclavia
- A. cervicalis profunda
- A. intercostalis suprema
- Truncus costocervicalis
- A. thyroidea inferior
- Rr. oesophageales
- A. thoracica interna

- A. ophthalmica
- A. angularis
- Siphon caroticum
- A. facialis
- A. carotis communis
- A. temporalis superficialis
- Meningeal vessels
- A. occipitalis
- A. vertebralis
- A. carotis interna with stenosis
- A. carotis externa
- A. vertebralis

C Truncus thyrocervicalis, truncus costocervicalis, and their branches

Right lateral view. The truncus thyrocervicalis arises from the a. subclavia and divides into the a. thyroidea inferior, a. transversa cervicis, and a. suprascapularis. It mainly supplies structures located at the lateral base of the neck and is variable in its development.

The truncus costocervicalis arises posteriorly from the a. subclavia at the level of the m. scalenus anterior. It divides into the a. cervicalis profunda and a. intercostalis suprema, supplying blood to the posterior neck muscles and the first spatium intercostale.

D Collateral pathways that develop in response to arteria carotis interna stenosis

Atherosclerosis of the a. carotis interna is a frequent clinical problem. Narrowing of the carotid lumen (stenosis) eventually results in decreased blood flow to the brain. If the lumen is occluded suddenly, the result is a stroke. But if the stenosis develops over time, blood can still reach the brain through the gradual recruitment of collateral channels. As this occurs, the direction of blood flow may become reversed in anastomotic areas close to the brain (see arrows). As long as an adequate collateral circulation is maintained, the stenosis does not produce clinical manifestations.

The principal collateral pathways are as follows:

- Ophthalmic collaterals: a. carotis externa → a. facialis → a. angularis → a. ophthalmica → siphon caroticum
- Occipital anastomosis: a. carotis externa → a. occipitalis → small meningeal arteries → a. vertebralis

4.2 Arteria Carotis Interna and Classification of the Branches of the Arteria Carotis Externa

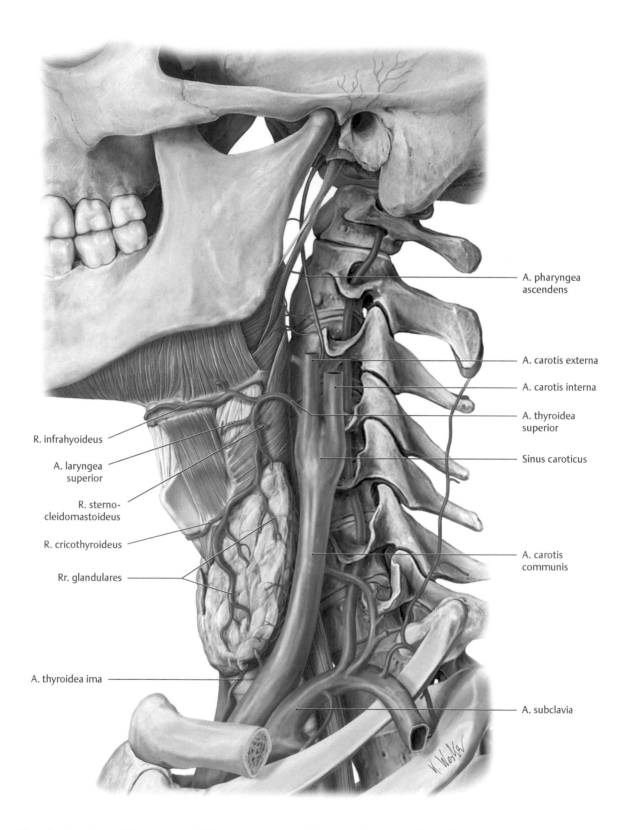

A. pharyngea ascendens

A. carotis externa

A. carotis interna

A. thyroidea superior

Sinus caroticus

A. carotis communis

A. subclavia

R. infrahyoideus

A. laryngea superior

R. sterno-cleidomastoideus

R. cricothyroideus

Rr. glandulares

A. thyroidea ima

A Common carotid and external carotid arteries and their branches in the neck

Left view. The head and neck are supplied by the a. carotis communis. It arises from the truncus brachiocephalicus, directly to the left of the arcus aortae. The aa. carotides communes dextra and sinistra bifurcate at approximately the level of the CIV vertebral body into the aa. carotides internae (dextra and sinstra) and the aa. carotides externae (dextra and sinistra). The a. carotis interna supplies the brain and orbit (see p. 102 f), giving off no branches in the neck.

The a. carotis externa gives off numerous branches in the head and neck (see **B**). In the neck, it primarily supplies the anterior structures including the cervical viscera. The two aa. carotides are invested in a connective-tissue layer of the fascia cervicalis, the vagina carotica (**B**, p. 4). *Note:* The brain is supplied exclusively by the aa. carotides internae and the aa. vertebrales.

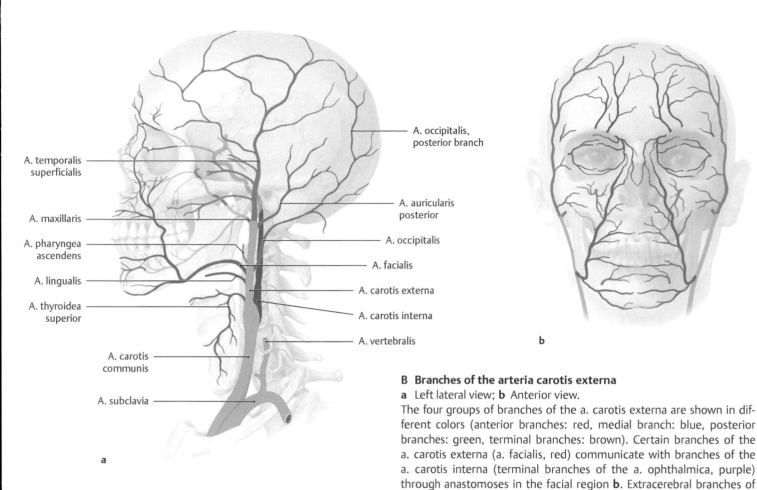

A. temporalis superficialis

A. maxillaris

A. pharyngea ascendens

A. lingualis

A. thyroidea superior

A. carotis communis

A. subclavia

A. occipitalis, posterior branch

A. auricularis posterior

A. occipitalis

A. facialis

A. carotis externa

A. carotis interna

A. vertebralis

a

b

B Branches of the arteria carotis externa

a Left lateral view; **b** Anterior view.

The four groups of branches of the a. carotis externa are shown in different colors (anterior branches: red, medial branch: blue, posterior branches: green, terminal branches: brown). Certain branches of the a. carotis externa (a. facialis, red) communicate with branches of the a. carotis interna (terminal branches of the a. ophthalmica, purple) through anastomoses in the facial region **b**. Extracerebral branches of the a. carotis interna are described on p. 102 f.

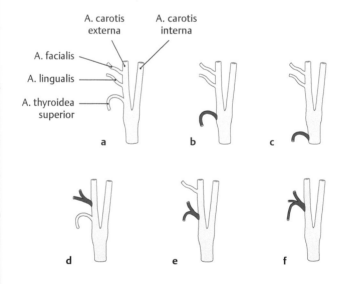

A. carotis externa

A. carotis interna

A. facialis

A. lingualis

A. thyroidea superior

a   b   c

d   e   f

C Branches of the artera carotis externa: typical anatomy and variants (after Lippert and Pabst)

a In **typical cases** (50 %) the a. facialis, a. lingualis, and a. thyroidea superior arise from the a. carotis externa above the bifurcatio carotidis.

b–f   Variants:

b, c The a. thyroidea superior arises at the level of the bifurcatio carotidis (20 %) or from the a. carotis communis (10 %).

d–f Two or three branches combine to form a common trunk: linguofacial trunk (18 %), thyrolingual trunk (2 %), or thyrolinguofacial trunk (1 %).

D Overview of the branches of the arteria carotis externa
(more distal branches are described in the units below)

Subsequent units deal with the arteries of the head as they are grouped in the table below, followed by the branches of the a. carotis interna and the veins.

External carotid branches	Distribution
Anterior:	
• A. thyroidea superior	• Larynx, gl. thyroidea
• A. lingualis	• Oral floor, tongue
• A. facialis	• Superficial facial region
Medial:	
• A. pharyngea ascendens	• Plexus to the skull base
Posterior:	
• A. occipitalis	• Occiput
• A. auricularis posterior	• Ear
Terminal:	
• A. maxillaris	• Mm. masticatorii, posteromedial part of the facial skeleton, meninges
• A. temporalis superficialis	• Temporal region, part of the ear

4.3 Arteria Carotis Externa: Anterior, Medial, and Posterior Branches

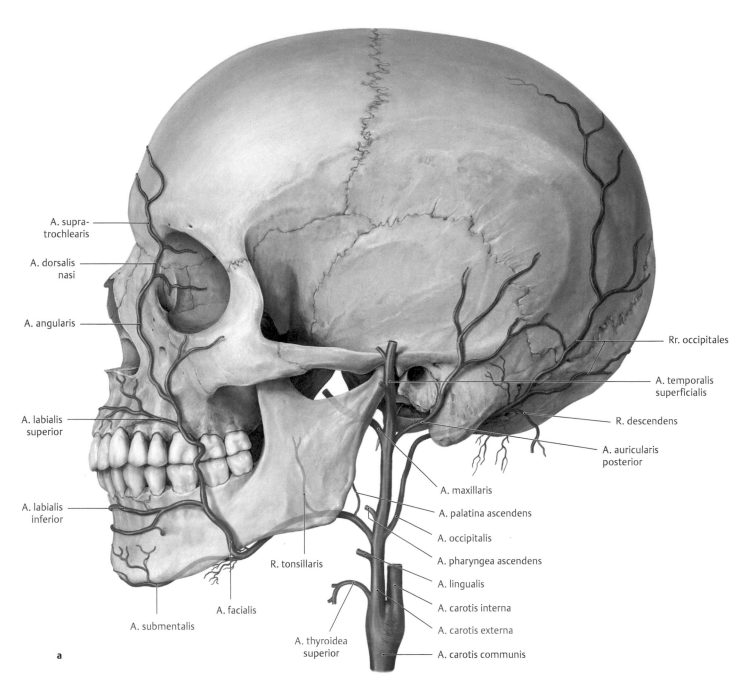

A. supra-trochlearis

A. dorsalis nasi

A. angularis

A. labialis superior

A. labialis inferior

R. tonsillaris

A. facialis

A. submentalis

A. thyroidea superior

Rr. occipitales

A. temporalis superficialis

R. descendens

A. auricularis posterior

A. maxillaris

A. palatina ascendens

A. occipitalis

A. pharyngea ascendens

A. lingualis

A. carotis interna

A. carotis externa

A. carotis communis

a

A Arteria facialis, arteria occipitalis, and arteria auricularis posterior and their branches

Left lateral view. An important anterior branch of the a. carotis externa is the **a. facialis**, which gives off branches in the neck and face. The principal *cervical branch* is the a. palatina ascendens; the *r. tonsillaris* is ligated during tonsillectomy. Of the *facial branches*, the superior and inferior combine to form an arterial circle around the mouth. The *terminal branch* of the a. facialis, the a. angularis, anastomoses with the a. dorsalis nasi. The latter vessel is the terminal branch of the a. ophthalmica, which arises from the a. carotis interna. Because there are extensive arterial anastomoses, facial injuries have a tendency to bleed profusely but also tend to heal quickly and well owing to the copious blood supply. The pulse of the a. facialis is palpable at the anterior border of the m. masseter insertion on the r. mandibulae. The principal branches of the **a. auricularis posterior** include the a. tympanica posterior and the r. parotideus. Alternatively, the a. tympanica posterior can arise as a ramus arteriae stylomastoideae, see **A**, p. 156, and **B**, p. 137.

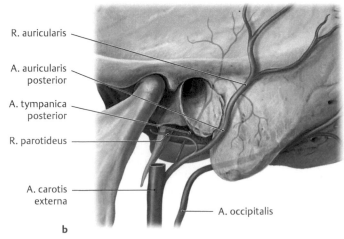

R. auricularis

A. auricularis posterior

A. tympanica posterior

R. parotideus

A. carotis externa

A. occipitalis

b

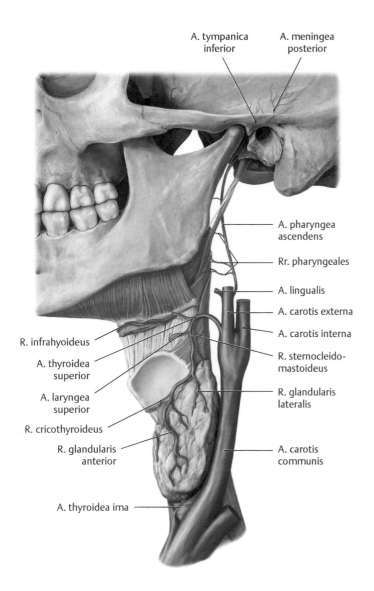

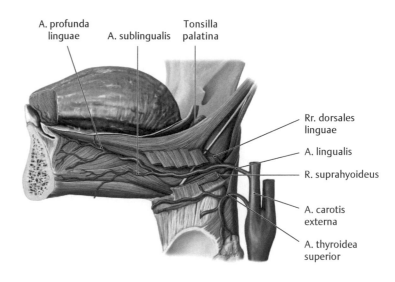

D Arteria lingualis and its branches
Left lateral view. The a. lingualis is the second anterior branch of the a. carotis externa. It has a relatively large caliber, providing the tongue with its rich blood supply. It also gives off branches to the pharynx and tonsils.

B Arteria thyroidea superior, arteria pharyngea ascendens and their branches
Left lateral view. The a. thyroidea superior is typically the first branch to arise from the a. carotis externa. One of the anterior branches, it supplies the larynx and gl. thyroidea. The a. pharyngea ascendens arises from the medial side of the a. carotis externa, usually above the level of the a. thyroidea superior. The level at which a vessel branches from the a. carotis externa does not necessarily correlate with the course of the vessel.

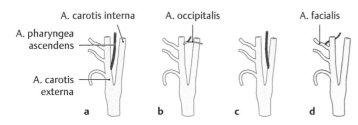

C Origin of the arteria pharyngea ascendens: typical case and variants (after Lippert and Pabst)
a In **typical cases** (70%) the a. pharyngea ascendens arises from the a. carotis externa.

b–d Variants:
b The a. pharyngea ascendens arises from **b** the a. occipitalis (20%), **c** the a. carotis interna (8%), or **d** the a. facialis (2%).

E Branches of the arteria carotis externa and their distribution: anterior, medial, and posterior branches with their principal distal branches

Branches of arteria carotis externa	Distribution
Anterior:	
• A. thyroidea superior (see **B**)	
– Rr. glandulares	• Gl. thyroidea
– A. laryngea superior	• Larynx
– R. sternocleidomastoideus	• M. sternocleidomastoideus
• A. lingualis (see **D**)	
– Rr. dorsales linguae	• Base of tongue, epiglottis
– A. sublingualis	• Gl. sublingualis, tongue, oral floor, cavitas oris
– A. profunda linguae	• Tongue
• A. facialis (see **A**)	
– A. palatina ascendens	• Pharyngeal wall, palatum molle, tuba auditiva
– R. tonsillaris	• Tonsilla palatina (main branch)
– A. submentalis	• Oral floor, gl. submandibularis
– Aa. labiales	• Lips
– A. angularis	• Radix nasi
Medial:	
• A. pharyngea ascendens (see **B**)	• Pharyngeal wall
– Rr. pharyngeales	• Mucosa of auris media
– A. tympanica inferior	• Dura, fossa cranii posterior
– A. meningea posterior	
Posterior:	
• A. occipitalis (see **A**)	
– Rr. occipitales	• Scalp, occipital region
– R. descendens	• Posterior neck muscles
• A. auricularis posterior (see **A**)	
– A. stylomastoidea	• N. facialis in the canalis nervi facialis
– A. tympanica posterior	• Cavitas tympani
– R. auricularis	• Posterior side of auricula
– R. occipitalis	• Occiput
– R. parotideus	• Gl. parotidea

4.4 Arteria Carotis Externa: Terminal Branches

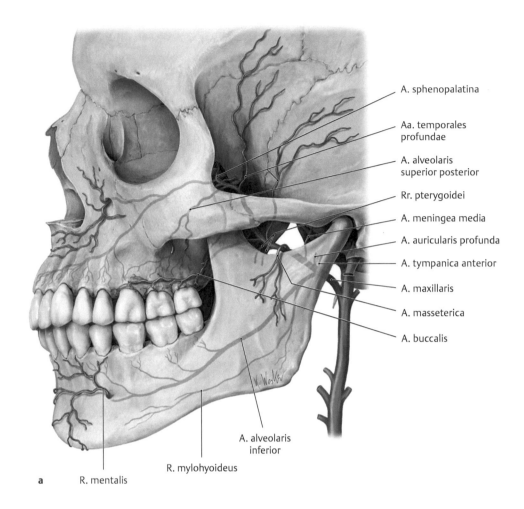

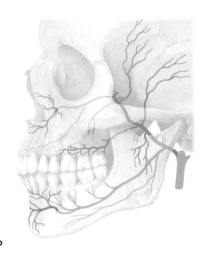

A. sphenopalatina

Aa. temporales profundae

A. alveolaris superior posterior

Rr. pterygoidei

A. meningea media

A. auricularis profunda

A. tympanica anterior

A. maxillaris

A. masseterica

A. buccalis

A. alveolaris inferior

R. mylohyoideus

a R. mentalis

b

A Arteria maxillaris and its branches
Left lateral view. The a. maxillaris is the larger of the two terminal branches of the a. carotis externa. Its origin lies deep to the ramus mandibulae (important landmark for locating the vessel). The a. maxillaris consists of three parts:

- Mandibular part (blue)
- Pterygoid part (green)
- Pterygopalatine part (yellow)

B The two terminal branches of the arteria carotis externa with their principal branches

Branch		Distribution
A. maxillaris		
Mandibular part:	• A. alveolaris inferior	• Mandibula, teeth, gingiva (the r. mentalis is its terminal branch)
		• Calvaria, dura, fossae cranii anterior and media
	• A. meningea media (see **C**)	• Art. temporomandibularis, meatus acusticus externus
	• A. auricularis profunda	• Cavitas tympani
	• A. tympanica anterior	
Pterygoid part:	• A. masseterica	• M. masseter
	• Aa. temporales profundae	• M. temporalis
	• Rr. pterygoidei	• Mm. pterygoidei
	• A. buccalis	• Buccal mucosa
Pterygopalatine part:	• A. alveolaris superior posterior	• Dentes molares maxillares, sinus maxillaris, gingiva
	• A. infraorbitalis	• Alveoli dentales maxillares
	• A. palatina descendens	
	– A. palatina major	• Palatum durum
	– Aa. palatinae minores	• Palatum molle, tonsilla palatina, pharyngeal wall
	• A. sphenopalatina	
	– Aa. nasales posteriores laterales	• Lateral wall of the cavitas oris, conchae nasi
	– Rr. septales posteriores	• Septum nasi
A. temporalis superficialis	• A. transversa faciei	• Soft tissues below the arcus zygomaticus
	• Rr. frontalis and parietalis	• Scalp of the forehead and vertex
	• A. zygomaticoorbitalis	• Paries lateralis orbitae

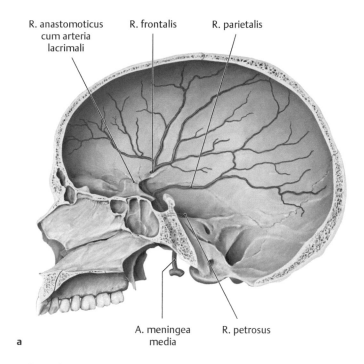

R. anastomoticus cum arteria lacrimali   R. frontalis   R. parietalis

A. meningea media   R. petrosus

a

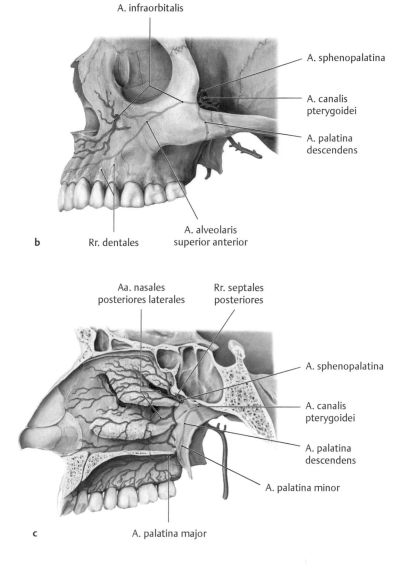

A. infraorbitalis

A. sphenopalatina

A. canalis pterygoidei

A. palatina descendens

A. alveolaris superior anterior

b   Rr. dentales

Aa. nasales posteriores laterales   Rr. septales posteriores

A. sphenopalatina

A. canalis pterygoidei

A. palatina descendens

A. palatina minor

c   A. palatina major

C Selected clinically important branches of the arteria maxillaris

a Right a. meningea media, **b** left a. infraorbitalis, **c** right a. sphenopalatina with its branches that supply the cavitas nasi.

The **a. meningea media** passes through the foramen spinosum into the fossa cranii media. Despite its name, it supplies blood not just to the meninges but also to the overlying calvarium. Rupture of the a. meningea media by head trauma results in an epidural hematoma (see p. 390). The **a. infraorbitalis** is a branch of the a. maxillaris and thus of the a. carotis externa, while the a. supraorbitalis (a branch of the a. ophthalmica) is a terminal branch of the a. carotis interna. These vessels provide a path for a potential anastomosis between the aa. carotides externa and interna. When severe nasopharyngeal bleeding occurs from branches of the **a. sphenopalatina** (a branch of the a. maxillaris), it may be necessary to ligate the a. maxillaris in the fossa pterygopalatina (see pp. 238, 103; see also **Gb**, p. 185).

D Arteria temporalis superficialis

Left lateral view. Particularly in elderly or cachectic patients, the often tortuous course of the r. frontalis of this vessel can easily be traced across the temple. The a. temporalis superficialis may be involved in an inflammatory autoimmune disease (temporal arteritis), which can be confirmed by biopsy of the vessel. The patients, usually elderly males, complain of severe headaches.

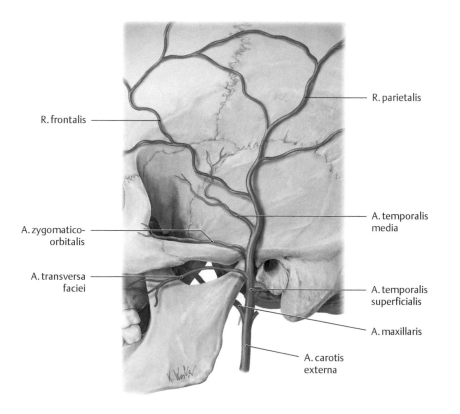

R. frontalis

R. parietalis

A. zygomatico-orbitalis

A. temporalis media

A. transversa faciei

A. temporalis superficialis

A. maxillaris

A. carotis externa

101

4.5 Arteria Carotis Interna: Branches to Extracerebral Structures

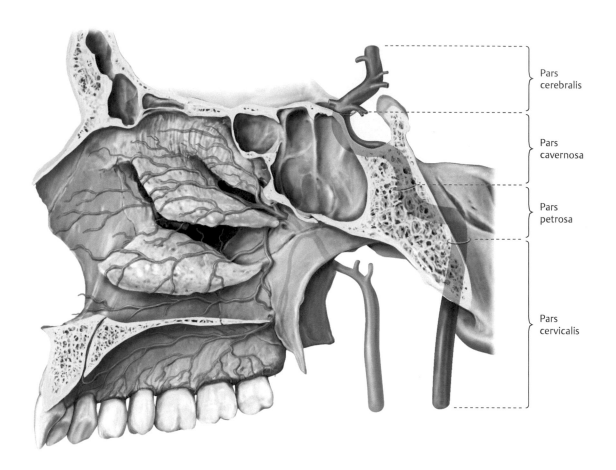

Pars cerebralis

Pars cavernosa

Pars petrosa

Pars cervicalis

a

A Subdivisions of the arteria carotis interna and branches that supply extracerebral structures of the head

a Medial view of the right a. carotis interna in its passage through the bones of the skull. **b** Anatomical segments of the a. carotis interna and their branches.

The a. carotis interna is distributed chiefly to the brain but also supplies extracerebral regions of the head. It consists of four parts (listed from bottom to top):

- Pars cervicalis
- Pars petrosa
- Pars cavernosa
- Pars cerebralis

The pars petrosa of the a. carotis interna (traversing the canalis caroticus) and the pars cavernosa (traversing the sinus cavernosus) have a role in supplying extracerebral structures of the head. They give off additional small branches that supply local structures and are usually named for the areas they supply. Only specialists may be expected to have a detailed knowledge of these branches. Of special importance is the a. ophthalmica, which arises from the pars cerebralis of the a. carotis interna (see **B**).

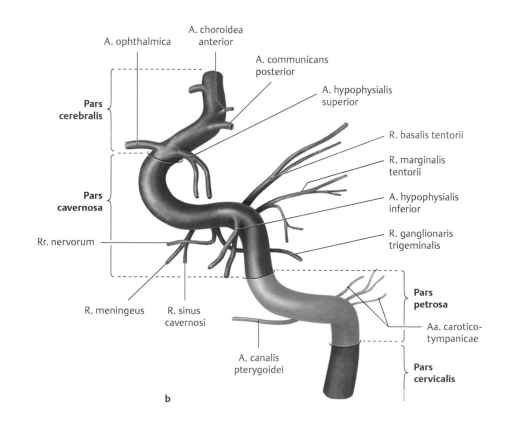

A. ophthalmica

A. choroidea anterior

A. communicans posterior

A. hypophysialis superior

R. basalis tentorii

R. marginalis tentorii

A. hypophysialis inferior

R. ganglionaris trigeminalis

Pars cerebralis

Pars cavernosa

Rr. nervorum

R. meningeus

R. sinus cavernosi

A. canalis pterygoidei

Pars petrosa

Aa. carotico-tympanicae

Pars cervicalis

b

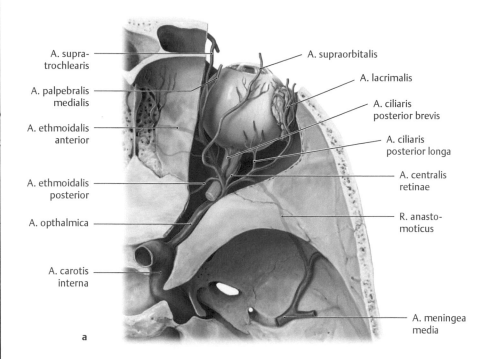

A. supra-
trochlearis

A. palpebralis
medialis

A. ethmoidalis
anterior

A. ethmoidalis
posterior

A. opthalmica

A. carotis
interna

A. supraorbitalis

A. lacrimalis

A. ciliaris
posterior brevis

A. ciliaris
posterior longa

A. centralis
retinae

R. anasto-
moticus

A. meningea
media

a

Arcus palpebralis
superior

A. palpebralis
lateralis

Arcus palpebralis
inferior

A. supraorbitalis

A. supra-
trochlearis

A. palpebralis
media

A. dorsalis
nasi

b

B Arteria ophthalmica

a Superior view of the right orbita. **b** Anterior view of the facial branches of the right a. ophthalmica.

Figure **a** shows the origin of the a. ophthalmica from the arteria carotis interna. The a. ophthalmica supplies blood to the eyeball (bulbus oculi) itself and to orbital structures. Some of its terminal branches are distributed to the eyelid (palpebra) and portions of the forehead (**b**). Other terminal branches (aa. ethmoidales anterior and posterior) contribute to the supply of the septum nasi (see **C**).

Note: Branches of the aa. palpebrales laterales and a. supraorbitalis (**b**) may form an anastomosis with the r. frontalis of the a. temporalis superficialis (territory of the a. carotis externa) (see p. 91). With atherosclerosis of the a. carotis interna, this anastomosis may become an important alternative route for blood to the brain.

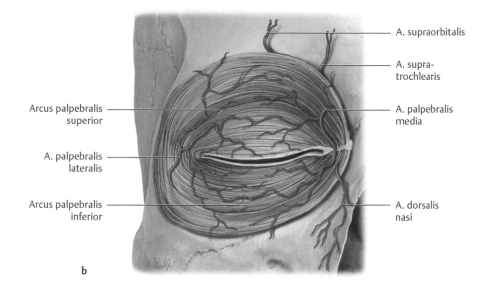

A. ethmoidalis
posterior

A. ophthalmica

A. ethmoidalis
anterior

Kiesselbach's
area

A. sphenopalatina

A. maxillaris

A. carotis
interna

A. carotis
externa

C Vascular supply of the septum nasi

Left lateral view. The septum nasi is another region in which the a. carotis interna (aa. ethmoidales anteriores and posteriores green) anastomoses with the a. carotis externa (a. sphenopalatina, yellow). A richly vascularized area on the anterior part of the septum nasi, called Kiesselbach's area (blue), is the most common site of nosebleed. Since Kiesselbach's area is an area of anastamosis, it may be necessary to ligate the r. sphenopalatina/maxillares and/or the aa. ethmoidales through an orbital approach, depending on the source of the bleeding.

4.6 Veins of the Head and Neck: Superficial Veins

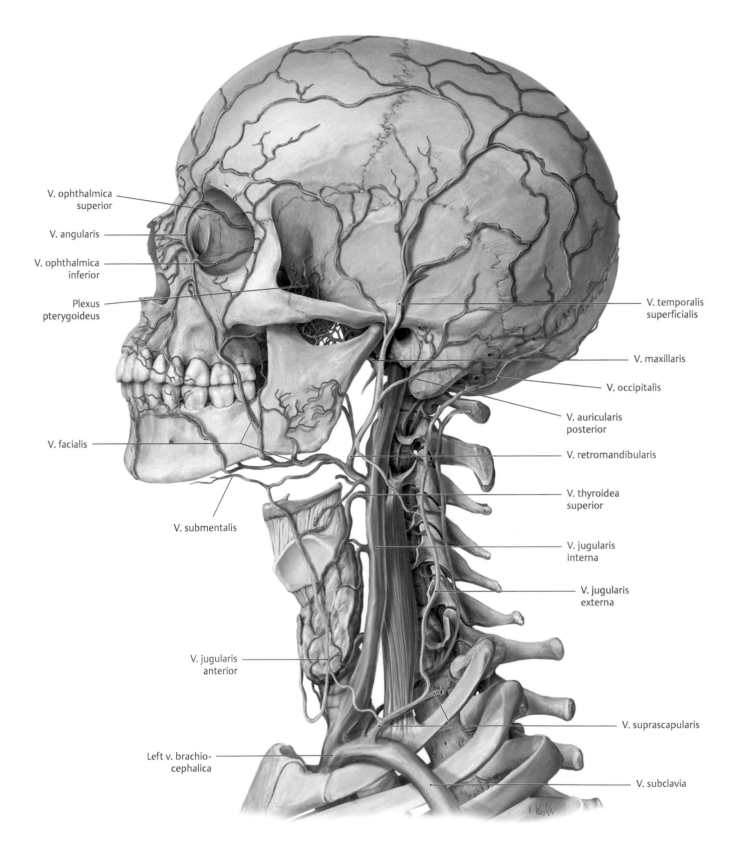

V. ophthalmica superior

V. angularis

V. ophthalmica inferior

Plexus pterygoideus

V. facialis

V. submentalis

V. jugularis anterior

Left v. brachio-cephalica

V. temporalis superficialis

V. maxillaris

V. occipitalis

V. auricularis posterior

V. retromandibularis

V. thyroidea superior

V. jugularis interna

V. jugularis externa

V. suprascapularis

V. subclavia

A Superficial head and neck veins and their drainage to the vena brachiocephalica

Left lateral view. The principal vein of the neck is the *v. jugularis interna*, which drains blood from the interior of the skull (including the brain). Enclosed in the vagina carotica, the left v. jugularis interna descends from the foramen jugulare to its union with the v. subclavia to form the v. brachiocephalica. The main tributaries of the v. jugularis interna in the head region are the vv. facialis and thyroideae. The *v. jugularis externa*

drains blood from the occiput (v. occipitalis) and nuchal regions to the v. subclavia, while the *v. jugularis anterior* drains the superficial anterior neck region. Besides these superficial veins, there are more deeply situated venous plexuses (orbita, plexus pterygoideus, fossa cranii media) that are described in the next unit.

Note: The superficial veins are most closely related to the deep veins in the area of the v. angularis, with an associated risk of spreading infectious organisms intracranially (see p. 107).

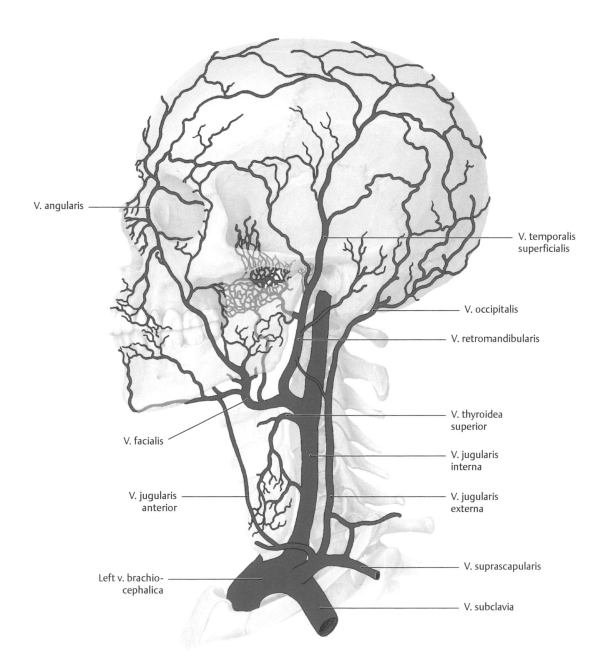

V. angularis

V. temporalis superficialis

V. occipitalis

V. retromandibularis

V. thyroidea superior

V. facialis

V. jugularis interna

V. jugularis anterior

V. jugularis externa

V. suprascapularis

Left v. brachio- cephalica

V. subclavia

B Overview of the principal veins in the head and neck
Left lateral view. Only the more important veins are labeled in the diagram. As at many other sites in the body, the course and caliber of the veins in the head and neck are variable to a certain degree, except for the largest venous trunk. The veins interconnect to form extensive anastomoses, some of which extend to the deep veins (see **A**, plexus pterygoideus).

C Drainage of blood from the head and neck
Blood from the head and neck is drained chiefly by three vv. jugulares: the interna, externa, and anterior. These veins have a variable size and course, but the v. jugularis interna is usually the smallest and most variable of the three. The vv. jugulares externa and interna communicate by valveless anastomoses that allow blood to drain from the v. jugularis externa back into the v. jugularis interna. This reflux is clinically significant because it provides a route by which bacteria from the skin of the head may gain access to the meninges (see p. 107 for details). The neck is subdivided into spaces by multiple layers of fascia cervicalis. One fascia-enclosed space is the vagina carotica, whose contents include the v. jugularis interna. The other two vv. jugulares lie within the lamina superficialis fasciae cervicalis.

Vein	Region drained	Relationship to deep cervical fasciae
• V. jugularis interna	• Interior of the skull (including the brain)	• Within the vagina carotica
• V. jugularis externa	• Head (superficial)	• Initially, it runs above the lamina superficialis of the fascia cervicalis then between superficial and middle layers of the fascia cervicalis
• V. jugularis anterior	• Neck, portions of the head	• Penetrates the lamina superficialis of fascia cervicalis at the posterior edge of the m. sternocleidomastoideus, and then runs above the middle layer of fascia cervicalis

105

4.7   Veins of the Head and Neck: Deep Veins

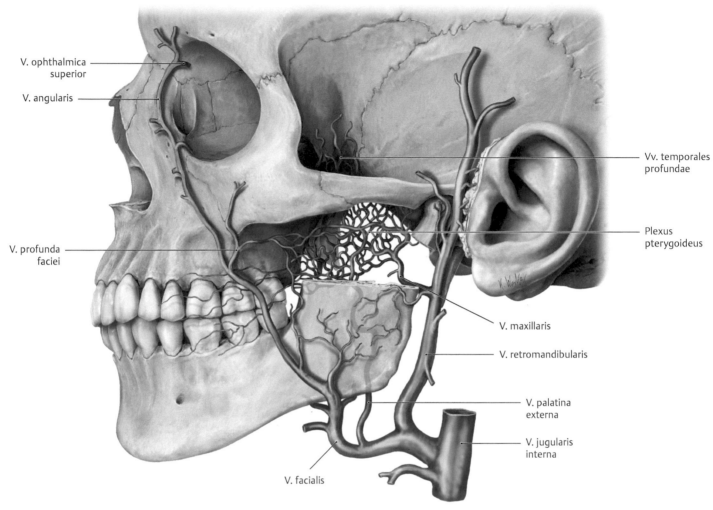

V. ophthalmica superior

V. angularis

V. profunda faciei

Vv. temporales profundae

Plexus pterygoideus

V. maxillaris

V. retromandibularis

V. palatina externa

V. jugularis interna

V. facialis

A   Deep veins of the head: plexus pterygoideus
Left lateral view. The plexus pterygoideus is a venous network situated within the fossa infratemporalis, behind the ramus mandibulae
between the mm. masticatorii. It has extensive connections with the
adjacent veins.

**B   Deep veins of the head: orbita and fossa
    cranii media**
Left lateral view. There are two relatively large
venous trunks in the orbita, the vv. ophthalmicae superior and inferior. They do not run
parallel to the arteries. The veins of the orbita
drain predominantly into the sinus cavernosus.
Orbital blood can also drain externally via the
v. angularis and v. faciei. Because the veins are
valveless, extracranial bacteria may migrate to
the sinus cavernosus and cause thrombosis in
that venous channel (see **E** and p. 217).

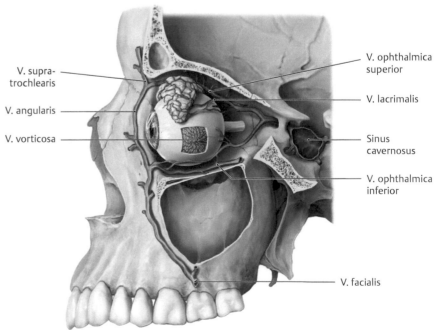

V. supra-trochlearis

V. angularis

V. vorticosa

V. ophthalmica superior

V. lacrimalis

Sinus cavernosus

V. ophthalmica inferior

V. facialis

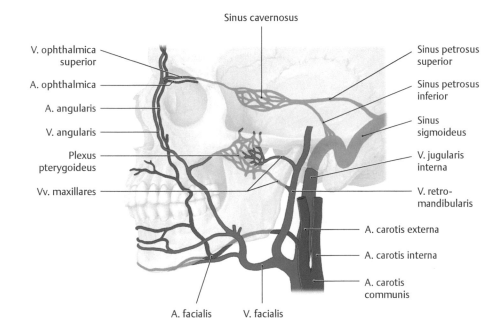

V. emissaria parietalis

Sinus sagittalis superior

Confluens sinuum

Sinus transversus

Sinus sigmoideus

V. emissaria occipitalis

V. emissaria mastoidea

Venous plexus around the foramen magnum

V. emissaria condylaris

Venous plexus of the canalis nervi hypoglossi

V. jugularis interna

Plexus venosus vertebralis externus

V. occipitalis

C Veins of the occiput

Posterior view. The superficial veins of the occiput communicate with the sinus durae matris by way of the vv. diploicae. These vessels, called vv. emissariae, provide a potential route for the spread of infectious organisms into the sinus durae matris.

Sinus cavernosus

V. ophthalmica superior

A. ophthalmica

A. angularis

V. angularis

Plexus pterygoideus

Vv. maxillares

Sinus petrosus superior

Sinus petrosus inferior

Sinus sigmoideus

V. jugularis interna

V. retro-mandibularis

A. carotis externa

A. carotis interna

A. carotis communis

A. facialis   V. facialis

D Clinically important vascular relation-ships in the facial region

The a. facialis and its branches and the terminal branch of the a. ophthalmica, the a. dorsalis nasi, are clinically important vessels in the facial region because they may bleed profusely in patients who sustain midfacial fractures. The veins in this region are clinically important because they may allow infectious organisms to enter the cavitas cranii. Bacteria from furuncles (boils) on the upper lip or nose may gain access to the sinus cavernosus by way of the v. angularis (see **E**).

E Venous anastomoses as portals of infection

* Very important clinically because the deep spread of bacterial infection from the facial region may result in sinus cavernosus thrombosis (infection leading to clot formation that may occlude the sinus). Bacterial thrombosis is less common at other sites.

Extracranial vein	Connecting vein	Venous sinus
• V. angularis	• V. ophthalmica superior	• Sinus cavernosus*
• Veins of tonsilla palatina	• Plexus pterygoideus, v. ophthalmica inferior	• Sinus cavernosus*
• V. temporalis superficialis	• V. emissaria parietalis	• Sinus sagittalis superior
• V. occipitalis	• V. emissaria occipitalis	• Sinus transversus, confluens sinuum
• V. occipitalis, v. auricularis posterior	• V. emissaria mastoidea	• Sinus sigmoideus
• Plexus venosus vertebralis externus	• V. emissaria condylaris	• Sinus sigmoideus

4.8   Veins of the Neck

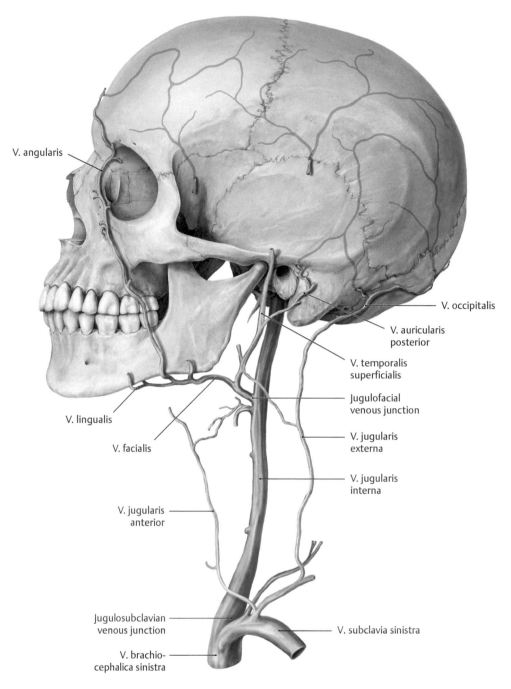

V. angularis

V. occipitalis

V. auricularis posterior

V. temporalis superficialis

Jugulofacial venous junction

V. lingualis

V. jugularis externa

V. facialis

V. jugularis interna

V. jugularis anterior

Jugulosubclavian venous junction

V. subclavia sinistra

V. brachio-cephalica sinistra

A Principal venous trunks in the neck

Left lateral view. Three vv. jugulares return blood to the v. cava superior from the head and neck region:

- The large v. jugularis interna (located in the vagina carotica) drains blood from the cavitas cranii and brain, face, and gl. thyroidea to the v. subclavia.
- The v. jugularis externa (smaller than v. jugularis interna and may be absent in around 25% of the population) at first lies over the lamina superficialis of fascia cervicalis but beneath the platysma. It perforates the

fascia to join the v. subclavia draining the superficial area located behind the ear.
- The v. jugularis anterior (smallest of the three vv. jugulares, not always present) begins below the os hyoideum and usually terminates at the v. jugularis externa. It drains the superficial anterior wall of the neck.

The v. jugularis interna and v. subclavia on each side unite to form the v. brachiocephalica (see **D**). The veins on the right and left sides may communicate via the arcus venosus jugularis (see **D**).

B Principal veins in the neck, their tributaries and anastomoses

In addition to the veins listed below, there are a number of smaller veins that drain blood from adjacent structures. Since they are highly variable in their development, they are not listed here.

The cervical veins are interconnected by extensive anastomoses (not all of which are shown here, in some cases because they are too small). As a result, the ligation of one vein will not cause a serious impairment of venous return. A *venous junction* is a site where two larger veins join at an approximately 90° angle. The two principal venous junctions in the neck are the jugulofacial and the jugulosubclavian. The jugulofacial venous junction is smaller than the jugulosubclavian venous junction, which also marks the termination of the ductus thoracicus (see **A** p. 232).

Tributaries of the v. cava superior
- V. brachiocephalica dextra
- V. brachiocephalica sinistra

Tributaries of the v. brachiocephalica
- V. jugularis interna
- V. subclavia
  - V. jugularis externa
- Plexus thyroideus impar (usually drains to left v. brachiocephalica)
- V. vertebralis
- Vv. thoracicae internae

Tributaries of the v. jugularis interna
- Sinus durae matris
- V. lingualis
- V. thyroidea superior
- V. facialis
  - V. lingualis
  - V. angularis (anastomosis with v. ophthalmica)
  - V. auricularis posterior (over the v. retromandibularis)
  - Vv. temporales superficiales (anastomoses with plexus pterygoideus)
- V. auricularis posterior

Tributaries of the v. jugularis externa
- V. occipitalis
- V. auricularis posterior

V. ophthalmica superior

V. angularis

Sinus cavernosus

Plexus pterygoideus

V. lingualis

V. facialis

V. thyroidea superior

V. jugularis anterior

V. jugularis interna

Arcus venosus jugularis

Left v. brachio-cephalica

Sinus sagittalis superior

Vv. temporales superficiales

Sinus transversus

V. temporalis superficialis

V. occipitalis

V. auricularis posterior

Vv. maxillares

V. cervicalis profunda

V. jugularis externa

V. vertebralis

V. subclavia

C Cervical veins and their relationship to the veins of the skull and sinus durae matris

Left lateral view. The sinus durae matris collect venous blood from the brain and channel it to the v. jugularis interna. When the nodi lymphoidei are removed in a neck dissection for a head and neck malignancy, the v. jugularis interna should be ligated on *one* side only to avoid causing a potentially lethal venous stasis in the brain.

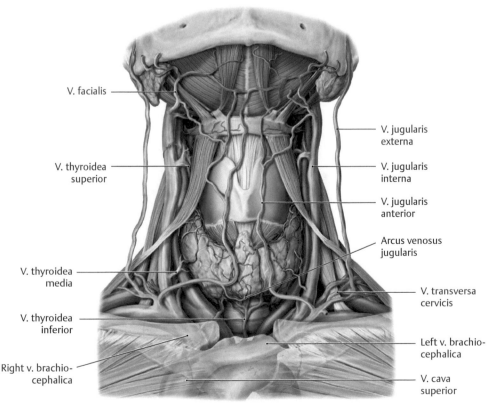

V. facialis

V. thyroidea superior

V. thyroidea media

V. thyroidea inferior

Right v. brachio-cephalica

V. jugularis externa

V. jugularis interna

V. jugularis anterior

Arcus venosus jugularis

V. transversa cervicis

Left v. brachio-cephalica

V. cava superior

D Cervical veins

Anterior view. Most veins in the neck are valveless "thoroughfares" that drain blood from the head. They are minimally distended and not readily visible above the plane of the heart in both the standing and sitting positions. In the supine position, however, the veins become engorged and are visible even in a healthy individual. Visible distention of cervical veins, specifically the vv. jugulares, in the standing position is a sign of right-sided heart failure, in which blood collects proximal to the right heart, generally due to improper functioning of the ventriculus dexter. The v. jugularis interna is large and is frequently used as an access site for the placement of a central venous catheter in intensive care medicine, making it possible to infuse greater fluid volumes than with a peripheral venous line. The arcus venosus jugularis forms a connecting trunk between the vv. jugulares anteriores on each side, which creates a potential hazard for hemorrhage in tracheostomies.

109

4.9 Lymph Nodes (Nodi Lymphoidei) and Lymphatic Drainage of the Head and Neck

Lymphatic system of the head and neck

A distinction is made between nodi lymphoidei regionales, which are associated with a particular organ or region and constitute primary filtering stations, and collecting lymph nodes, which usually receive lymph from multiple nodus lymphoideus regionalis groups. Lymph from the head and neck region, gathered in scattered nodi regionales, flows through its system of deep cervical collecting nodi lymphoidei, into the right and left trunci jugulares, each closely associated with its corresponding v. jugularis interna. The truncus jugularis on the right side drains into the ductus lymphaticus dexter, which terminates at the right jugulosubclavian junction. The truncus jugularis on the left side terminates at the ductus thoracicus, which empties into the left jugulosubclavian junction (cf. **D**).

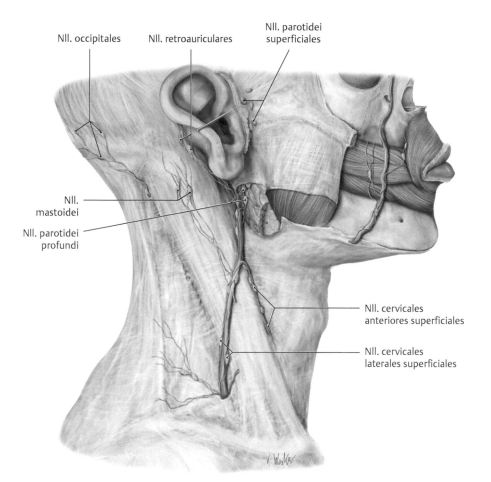

Nll. occipitales — Nll. retroauriculares — Nll. parotidei superficiales

Nll. mastoidei

Nll. parotidei profundi

Nll. cervicales anteriores superficiales

Nll. cervicales laterales superficiales

A Nodi lymphoidei superficiales in the neck
Right lateral view. It is extremely important to know the distribution of the lymph nodes in the neck because enlarged cervical lymph nodes are a common finding at physical examination. The enlargement of cervical lymph nodes may be caused by inflammation (usually a *painful* enlargement) or neoplasia (usually a *painless* enlargement) in the area drained by the nodes. The nll. cervicales superficiales are primary drainage locations for lymph from adjacent areas or organs.
Note: Lymph from superficial lymph vessels in the head region drain into lymph nodes in the neck located close to the head.

B Deep cervical lymph nodes

Right lateral view. The deep lymph nodes in the neck consist mainly of collecting nodes. They have major clinical importance as potential sites of metastasis from head and neck tumors (see **D** and **E**). One or more nodi lymphoidei prelaryngei that lie deep to the fascia musculi cricothyroidei are of particular clinical significance. As metastases can develop in them early, this group of nodes can be regarded as early warning nodi lymphoidei for laryngeal and thyroid carcinoma. Palpation of the thyroid also includes the nodus lymphoideus prelaryngeus. Normally it is too small to be palpated. It is only detectable when it becomes pathologically enlarged.

Affected deep cervical lymph nodes may be surgically removed (neck dissection) or may be treated by regional irradiation. For this purpose the American Academy of Otolaryngology, Head and Neck Surgery has grouped the deep cervical lymph nodes into six levels (Robbins 1991):

I Nll. submentales and submandibulares
II–IV Nll. cervicales profundi distributed along the v. jugularis interna (nll. cervicales laterales):
– II Nll. cervicales profundi (superiores laterales)
– III Nll. cervicales profundi (middle lateral group)
– IV Nll. cervicales profundi (inferiores laterales)
V Nll. in the posterior cervical triangle
VI Nll. cervicales anteriores

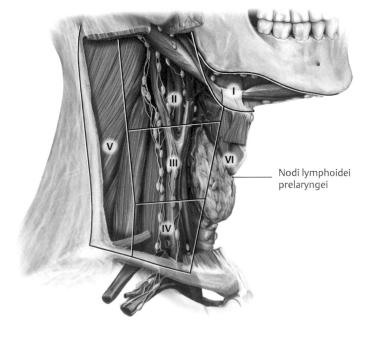

Nodi lymphoidei prelaryngei

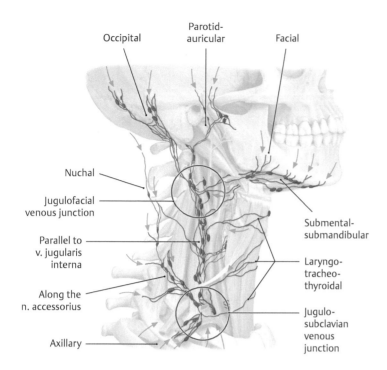

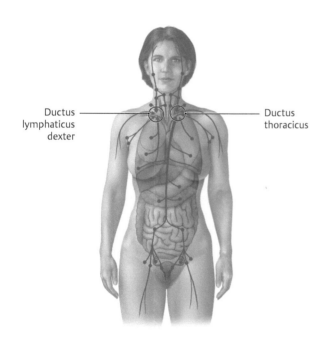

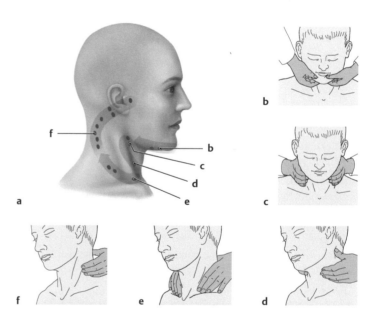

C Directions of lymphatic drainage in the neck

Right lateral view. The principal pattern of lymphatic flow in the neck is depicted. Understanding this pattern is critical to identifying the location of a potential cause of enlarged nll. cervicales. There are two main sites in the neck where the lymphatic pathways intersect:

- The jugulofacial venous junction: Lymphatics from the head pass obliquely downward to this site, where the lymph is redirected vertically downward in the neck.
- The jugulosubclavian venous junction: The main truncus lymphaticus, the ductus thoracicus, terminates at this central location, where lymph collected from the left side of the head and neck region is combined with lymph draining from the rest of the body.

If only peripheral nodal groups are affected, this suggests a localized disease process. If the central groups (e.g., those at the venous junctions) are affected, this usually signifies an extensive disease process. Central lymph nodes can be obtained for diagnostic evaluation by prescalene biopsy.

D Relationship of the cervical nodes to the systemic lymphatic circulation

Anterior view. The nll. cervicales may be involved by diseases that are not primary to the head and neck region, because lymph from the entire body is channeled to the left and right jugulosubclavian junctions (red circles). This can lead to retrograde involvement of the nll. cervicales. The ductus lymphaticus dexter terminates at the right jugulosubclavian junction, the ductus thoracicus at the left jugulosubclavian junction. Besides cranial and cervical tributaries, the lymph from nll. thoracis (mediastinal and tracheobronchial) and from nll. abdominis and caudal may reach the cervical nodes by way of the ductus thoracicus. As a result, diseases in those organs may lead to nl. cervicalis enlargement.

Note: Gastric carcinoma may metastasize to the left supraclavicular group of lymph nodes, producing an enlarged *sentinel node* that suggests an abdominal tumor. Systemic lymphomas may also spread to the nll. cervicales by this pathway.

E Systematic palpation of the nodi lymphoidei cervicales

The nll. cervicales are systematically palpated during the physical examination to ensure the detection of any enlarged nodes (see **D** for the special diagnostic significance of nll. cervicales).

Figure **a** shows the sequence in which the various nodal groups are successively palpated, **b – f** illustrate how each of the groups are palpated. The examiner usually palpates the submental-submandibular group first (**b**), including the angulus mandibulae (**c**), then proceeds along the anterior border of the m. sternocleidomastoideus (**d**). The supraclavicular lymph nodes are palpated next (**e**), followed by the lymph nodes along the n. accessorii and the nuchal group of nodes (**f**).

4.10 Overview of the Nervi Craniales

A Functional components of the cranial nerves

The twelve pairs of cranial nerves are designated by Roman numerals according to the order of their emergence from the brainstem (see topographical organization).

Note: The n. opticus and the n. olfactorius have special status among the cranial nerves. The n. opticus is an extension of the brain enveloped in meninges and containing cells found only in the CNS: oligodendrocytes and microglia cells. Thus, it is actually a component of the CNS and not a peripheral nerve. The tractus olfactorius and bulbus olfactorius, which together with the n. olfactorius form the externally visible portion of the olfactory system, are also components of the CNS by this definition. However, the n. olfactorius (composed of the fila olfactoria, which themselves are composed of fibers of the olfactory cells) does not belong to the CNS as the olfactory cells develop from the ectodermal olfactory placode and not the crista neuralis. Its embryologic origin from the placode epithelium gives this structure a special status as well. Like the spinal nerves, the cranial nerves may contain both *afferent* and *efferent* axons. These axons belong either to the somatic nervous system, which enables the organism to interact with its environment (*somatic fibers*), or to the autonomic nervous system, which regulates the activity of the internal organs (*visceral fibers*). The combinations of these different *general* fiber types in spinal nerves result in four possible compositions that are found chiefly in spinal nerves but also occur in cranial nerves (see functional organization):

- ☐ **General somatic afferents (somatic sensation):**
  → E.g., fibers convey impulses from the skin and skeletal muscle spindles

- ☐ **General visceral afferents (visceral sensation):**
  → E.g., fibers convey impulses from the viscera and blood vessels

- ☐ **General somatic efferents (somatomotor function):**
  → Fibers innervate skeletal muscles

- ☐ **General visceral efferents (visceromotor function):**
  → Fibers (in the cranial nerves only parasympathetic fibers) innervate the smooth muscle of the viscera, intraocular muscles, heart, gll. salivariae, etc.

Additionally, nervi craniales may contain special fiber types that are associated with particular structures in the head:

- ☐ **Special somatic afferents:**
  → E.g., fibers conduct impulses from the retina and from the auditory and vestibular apparatus

- ☐ **Special visceral afferents:**
  → E.g., fibers conduct impulses from the gemmae gustatoriae of the tongue and from the olfactory mucosa

- ☐ **Special visceral efferents:**
  → E.g., fibers innervate skeletal muscles derived from the arcus pharyngei *(branchiogenic efferents and branchiogenic muscles)*

C Topographical and functional organization of the nervi craniales

Topographical origin	Name	Functional fiber type
Telencephalon	• N. olfactorius (CN I)	• Special visceral afferent
Diencephalon	• N. opticus (CN II)	• Special somatic afferent
Mesencephalon	• N. oculomotorius (CN III)*	• Somatic efferent • Visceral efferent (parasympathetic)
	• N. trochlearis (CN IV)*	• Somatic efferent
Pons	• N. trigeminus (CN V)	• Special visceral efferent *(arcus pharyngeus primus)* • Somatic afferent
	• N. abducens (CN VI)*	• Somatic efferent
	• N. facialis (CN VII)	• Special visceral efferent *(arcus pharyngeus secundus)* • Special visceral afferent • Visceral efferent (parasympathetic) • Somatic afferent
Medulla oblongata	• N. vestibulocochlearis (CN VIII)	• Special somatic afferent
	• N. glossopharyngeus (CN IX)	• Special visceral efferent *(arcus pharyngeus tertius)* • Special visceral afferent • Visceral afferent (parasympathetic) • Somatic afferent
	• N. vagus (CN X)	• Special visceral efferent *(arcus pharyngeus quartus)* • Special visceral afferent • Visceral efferent (parasympathetic) • Visceral afferent • Somatic afferent
	• N. accessorius (CN XI)*	• Special visceral efferent *(arcus pharyngeus quintus)* • Somatic efferent
	• N. hypoglossus (CN XII)*	• Somatic efferent

* *Note:* Nn. craniales with somatic efferent fibers innervating skeletal muscles also have somatic afferent fibers that conduct proprioceptive impulses from the muscle spindles and other structures (for clarity, not listed above).

A characteristic feature of the nn. craniales is that their sensory and motor fibers enter and exit the truncus encephali at the same sites. This differs from the nn. spinales, in which the sensory fibers enter the medulla spinalis through the posterior (dorsal) roots while the motor fibers leave the medulla spinalis through the anterior (ventral) roots.

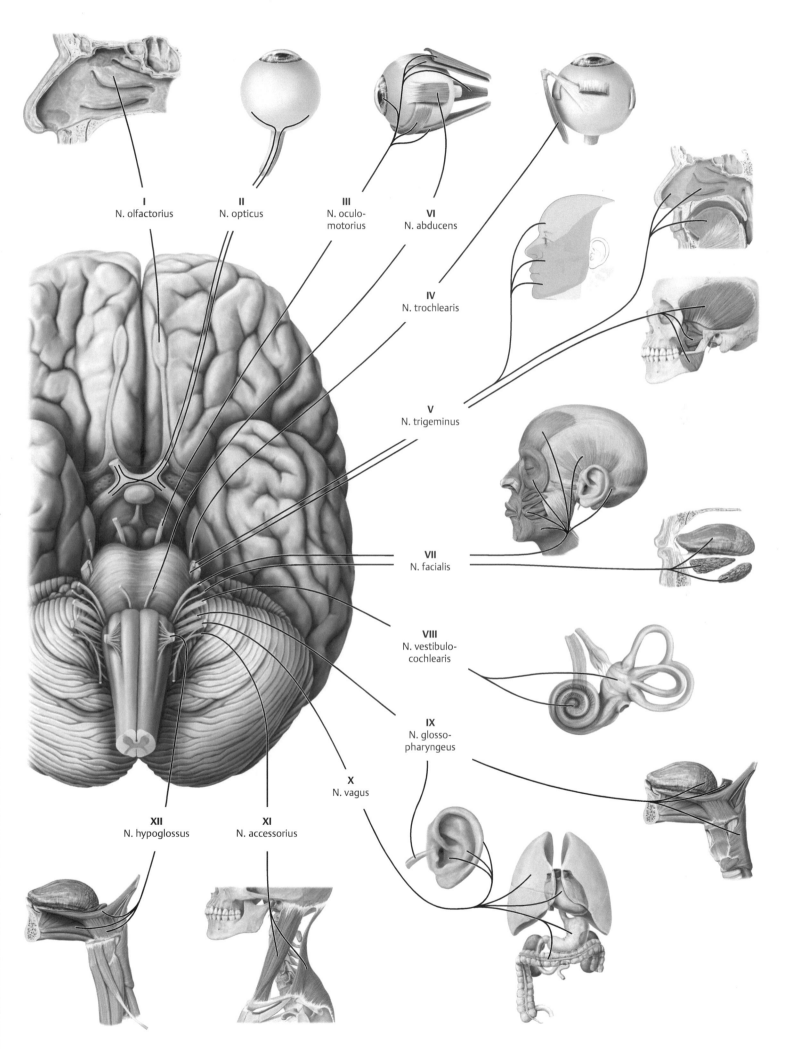

I
N. olfactorius

II
N. opticus

III
N. oculo-
motorius

VI
N. abducens

IV
N. trochlearis

V
N. trigeminus

VII
N. facialis

VIII
N. vestibulo-
cochlearis

IX
N. glosso-
pharyngeus

X
N. vagus

XII
N. hypoglossus

XI
N. accessorius

4.11 Nervi Craniales: Brainstem (Truncus Encephali) Nuclei and Peripheral Ganglia

A Overview of the nuclei of nervi craniales III – XII

Just as different fiber types can be distinguished in the nn. craniales (see C, p. 112), the nuclei of origin and nuclei of termination of the nervi craniales can also be classified according to different sensory and motor types and modalities. According to this scheme, the nuclei that belong to the parasympathetic nervous system are classified as *general* visceral efferent nuclei, while the nuclei of the arcus pharyngeus nerves are classified as *special* visceral efferent nuclei. The visceral afferent nuclei are considered either *general* (lower part of the nuclei tractus solitarii) or *special* (upper part, gustatory fibers). The somatic afferent nuclei can be differentiated in a similar way: the nucleus principalis nervi trigemini is classified as *general* somatic afferent, while the nuclei of the n. vestibulocochlearis are *special* somatic afferent.

Motor nuclei: (give rise to efferent [motor] fibers, left in **C**)

Somatic efferent (somatic motor) nuclei (red):
- Nucleus nervi oculomotorii (CN III: eye muscles)
- Nucleus nervi trochlearis (CN IV: eye muscles)
- Nucleus nervi abducentis (CN VI: eye muscles)
- Nucleus nervi accessorii (CN XI, spinal root: shoulder muscles)
- Nucleus nervi hypoglossi (CN XII: lingual muscles)

Visceral efferent (visceral motor) nuclei (blue):
Nuclei associated with the parasympathetic nervous system (light blue):
- Nucleus accessorius visceralis nervi oculomotorii (Edinger-Westphal nucleus) (CN III: m. sphincter pupillae and m. ciliaris)
- Nucleus salivatorius superior (CN VII, facial nerve: submandibular and sublingual glands)
- Nucleus salivatorius inferior (CN IX, glossopharyngeal nerve: parotid gland)
- Nucleus dorsalis nervi vagi (CN X: viscera)

Nuclei of the arcus pharyngeus nerves (dark blue):
- Nucleus motorius nervi trigemini (CN V: muscles of mastication)
- Nucleus nervi facialis (CN VII: facial muscles)
- Nucleus ambiguus (CN IX, n. glossopharyngeus; CN X, n. vagus; CN XI, n. accessorii [cranial root]: mm. pharyngis and laryngis)

Sensory nuclei: (where afferent [sensory] fibers terminate, right in **B**)

Somatic afferent (somatic sensory) and vestibulocochlear nuclei (yellow):
Sensory nuclei associated with the n. trigeminus (CN V, dark yellow):
- Nucleus mesencephalicus nervi trigemini (proprioceptive afferents from muscles of mastication)
- Nucleus principalis nervi trigemini (touch, vibration, joint position)
- Nucleus spinalis nervi trigemini (pain and temperature sensation in the head)

Nuclei of the n. vestibulocochlearis (CN VIII, light yellow):
- Vestibular part (sense of balance):
  - Nucleus vestibularis superior
  - Nucleus vestibularis lateralis
  - Nucleus vestibularis medialis
  - Nucleus vestibularis inferior
- Cochlear part (hearing, light yellow):
  - Nucleus cochlearis anterior
  - Nucleus cochlearis posterior

Visceral afferent (visceral sensory) nuclei (light or dark green):
- Nucleus tractus solitarii (nuclear complex):
  - Superior part (special visceral afferents [taste] from CN VII [n. facialis], CN IX [n. glossopharyngeus], and CN X [n. vagus]) (dark green)
  - Inferior part (general visceral afferents from CN IX [n. glossopharyngeus] and CN X [n. vagus]) (light green)

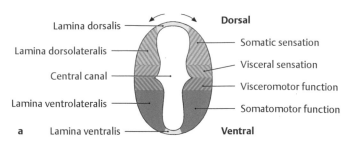

a Lamina dorsalis — Dorsal; Lamina dorsolateralis; Central canal; Lamina ventrolateralis; Lamina ventralis — Ventral; Somatic sensation; Visceral sensation; Visceromotor function; Somatomotor function

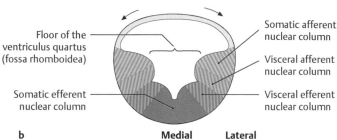

b Floor of the ventriculus quartus (fossa rhomboidea); Somatic efferent nuclear column; Somatic afferent nuclear column; Visceral afferent nuclear column; Visceral efferent nuclear column; Medial — Lateral

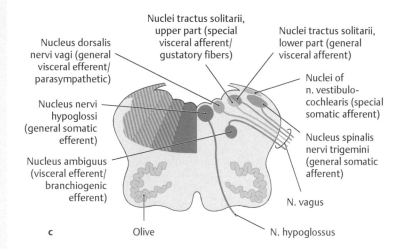

c Nucleus dorsalis nervi vagi (general visceral efferent/parasympathetic); Nuclei tractus solitarii, upper part (special visceral afferent/gustatory fibers); Nuclei tractus solitarii, lower part (general visceral afferent); Nuclei of n. vestibulocochlearis (special somatic afferent); Nucleus nervi hypoglossi (general somatic efferent); Nucleus ambiguus (visceral efferent/branchiogenic efferent); Nucleus spinalis nervi trigemini (general somatic afferent); N. vagus; Olive; N. hypoglossus

B Arrangement of truncus encephali nuclear columns during embryonic development (after Herrick)

Cross-sections through the medulla spinalis and btruncus encephali, superior view. The functional organization of the truncus encephali is determined by the location of the n. cranialis nuclei, which can be explained in terms of the embryonic migration of neuron populations.

a Initial form as seen in the medulla spinalis: The motor (efferent) neurons are ventral, and the sensory (afferent) neurons are dorsal (= dorsoventral arrangement).

b Early embryonic stage of truncus encephali development: the neurons of the lamina dorsolateralis (sensory nuclei) migrate laterally while the neurons of the lamina ventrolateralis (motor nuclei) migrate medially. This gives rise to a general mediolateral arrangement of the nuclear columns. The arrows indicate the directions of cell migration.

c Adult truncus encephali: features a medial to lateral arrangement of four longitudinal nuclear columns (one *somatic efferent*, one *visceral efferent*, one *visceral afferent*, and one *somatic afferent*). In each of these columns, nuclei that have the same function are arranged one above the other in a craniocaudal direction (see **C**). The nuclei in the *somatic afferent* and *visceral afferent* columns are differentiated into general and special afferent nuclei. Similarly, the *visceral efferent nuclear column* is differentiated into general (parasympathetic) and special (branchiogenic) efferent nuclei. This general/special subdivision is not present in the *somatic efferent nuclear column*.

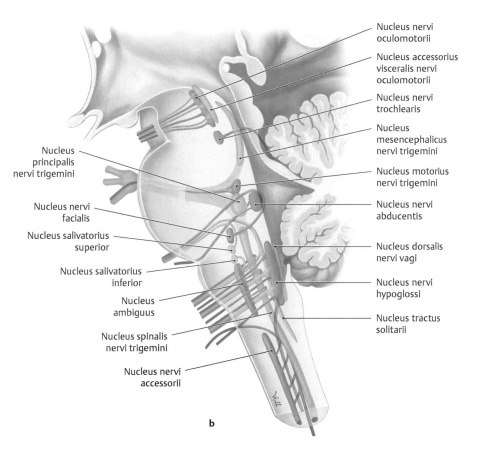

a

Nucleus nervi oculomotorii
Nucleus nervi trochlearis
Nucleus motorius nervi trigemini
Nucleus nervi abducentis
Nucleus nervi facialis
Nucleus salivatorius superior
Nucleus salivatorius inferior
Nucleus ambiguus
Nucleus dorsalis nervi vagi
Nucleus nervi hypoglossi
Nucleus nervi accessorii

Nucleus accessorius visceralis nervi oculomotorii
Nucleus mesencephalicus nervi trigemini
Nucleus principalis nervi trigemini
Nuclei vestibulares
Nuclei cochleares
Nucleus spinalis nervi trigemini
Nucleus tractus solitarii (special visceral afferent nucleus)

b

Nucleus principalis nervi trigemini
Nucleus nervi facialis
Nucleus salivatorius superior
Nucleus salivatorius inferior
Nucleus ambiguus
Nucleus spinalis nervi trigemini
Nucleus nervi accessorii

Nucleus nervi oculomotorii
Nucleus accessorius visceralis nervi oculomotorii
Nucleus nervi trochlearis
Nucleus mesencephalicus nervi trigemini
Nucleus motorius nervi trigemini
Nucleus nervi abducentis
Nucleus dorsalis nervi vagi
Nucleus nervi hypoglossi
Nucleus tractus solitarii

- ▉ General somatic afferent nuclei
- ▉ General visceral afferent nuclei
- ▉ General somatic efferent nuclei
- ▉ General visceral efferent nuclei
- ▉ Special somatic afferent nuclei
- ▉ Special visceral afferent nuclei
- ▉ Special visceral efferent nuclei

D Ganglia associated with nervi craniales

Ganglia fall into two main categories: sensory and autonomic (parasympathetic). The **ganglia sensoria** are analogous to the ganglia sensoria nervorum spinalium in the radices posteriores of the medulla spinalis. They contain the cell bodies of the *pseudounipolar* neurons (= primary afferent neuron). Their peripheral process comes from a receptor, and their central process terminates in the CNS. Synaptic relays do not occur in the ganglia sensoria. The **ganglia autonomica** in the head are entirely parasympathetic. They contain the cell bodies of the *multipolar* neurons (= second efferent, or postsynaptic, neuron). Unlike the ganglia sensoria, these ganglia synapse with parasympathetic fibers from the truncus encephali (= first efferent, or *preganglionic*, neuron). Specifically they synapse with the cell bodies of the second efferent (or *postsynaptic*) neuron, whose fibers are distributed to the target organ.

Nervi craniales	Ganglia sensoria	Ganglia autonomica
N. oculo-motorius (CN III)		• Ganglion ciliare
N. trigeminus (CN V)	• Ganglion trigeminale	
N. facialis (CN VII)	• Ganglion geniculi	• Ganglion pterygopalatinum • Ganglion submandibulare
N. vestibulo-cochlearis (CN VIII)	• Ganglion spirale • Ganglion vestibulare	
N. glosso-pharyngeus (CN IX)	• Ganglion superius • Ganglion inferius	• Ganglion oticum
N. vagus (CN X)	• Ganglion superius • Ganglion inferius	• Prevertebral and intramural ganglia of thoracic and abdominal viscera

C Location of nervi craniales III – XII in the brainstem

a Posterior view (with cerebellum removed).
b Midsagittal section, left lateral view.

Except for nervi craniales I and II, which are extensions of the brain rather than true nerves, all pairs of nervi craniales are associated with corresponding nuclei in the brainstem. The diagrams show the nerve pathways leading *to* and *from* these nuclei. The arrangement of the cranial nerve nuclei is easier to understand when they are classified them into functional nuclear columns (see **B**). The *efferent (motor) nuclei* where the *efferent* fibers arise are shown on the left side in **a**. The *afferent (sensory) nuclei* where the *afferent* fibers end are shown on the right side.

115

4.12 Nervi Craniales: Nervus Olfactorius (CN I) and Nervus Opticus (CN II)

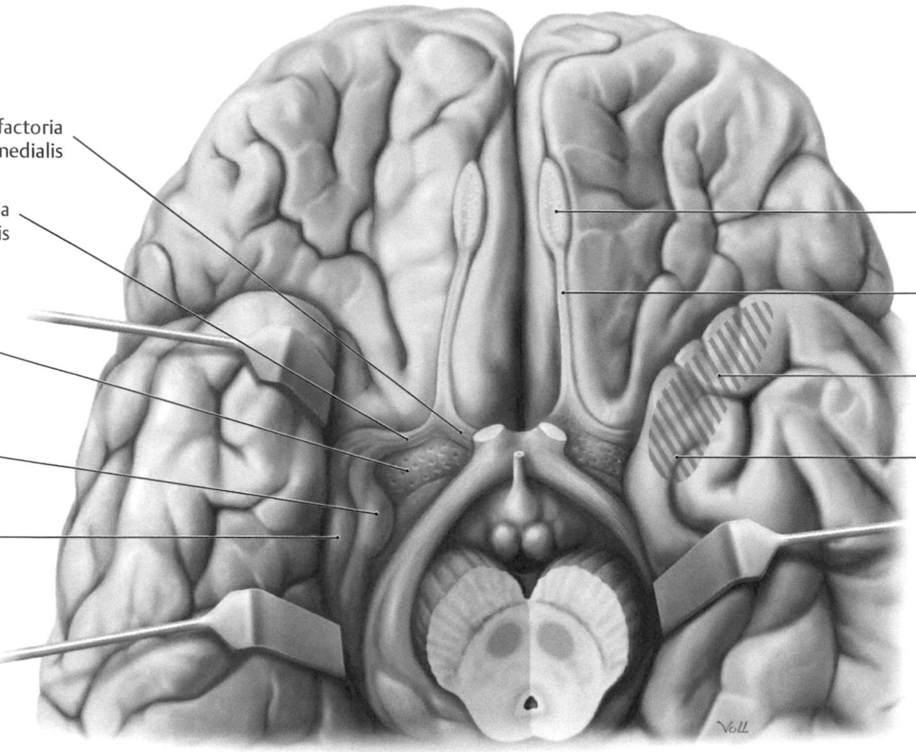

Stria olfactoria medialis
Stria olfactoria lateralis
Substantia perforata anterior
Gyrus semilunaris
Gyrus ambiens
Bulbus olfactorius
Tractus olfactorius
Area praepiriformis*
Corpus amygdaloideum*

A Bulbus olfactorius and tractus olfactorius on the basal surface of the frontal lobes of the brain

The unmyelinated axons of the primary bipolar sensory neurons in the olfactory mucosa are collected into approximately 20 fiber bundles—the fila olfactoria (see **B**), which are referred to collectively as the *nervus olfactorius*. These axon bundles pass from the nasal cavity through the lamina cribrosa of the os ethmoidale into the fossa cranii anterior (see **B**), and synapse in the *bulbus olfactorius*. The bulbus olfactorius is a club-like extension on the frontal end of the tractus olfactorius. Whereas the bulbus olfactorius has a cortical structure (allocortex, paleocortex), the tractus olfactorius exhibits the structure of a tract and contains CNS-specific glia such as oligodendrocytes and microglia. The bulbus olfactorius and tractus olfactorius have a meningeal covering and are components of the central nervous system. In contrast, the n. olfactorius develops from the ectodermal olfactory placode and does not belong to the CNS. Before it enters the telencephalon, the tractus olfactorius splits into the striae olfactoriae medialis and lateralis. Many of the axons of the tractus end directly in the cortex (without joining a nucleus) in the area praepiriformis or in the corpus amygdaloideum. The n. olfactorius transmits sensory information from the olfactory mucosa, an area on the roof of the nasal cavity measuring approximately 2–4 cm^2 (concha nasi superior and septum nasi, see **B**). The first neuron of the tractus olfactorius is the bipolar olfactory cell in the pars olfactoria tunicae mucosae nasi.

Note: Injuries to the lamina cribrosa may damage the meningeal covering of the olfactory fibers, resulting in olfactory disturbances and cerebrospinal fluid leakage from the nose ("runny nose" after head trauma). There is an associated risk of ascending bacterial infection causing meningitis.

Olfactory cells can divide throughout their life. Functionally, they are primary sensory cells. As they have their own axon, they are also neurons. Olfactory cells are thus an example of neurons that can divide throughout their life.

* The shaded structures are deep to the basal surface of the brain.

B Extent of the pars olfactoria tunicae mucosae nasi (olfactory region)

Portion of the left septum nasi and lateral wall of the right nasal cavity, viewed from the left side. The olfactory fibers on the septum nasi and concha nasi superior define the extent of the olfactory region (2–4 cm^2). The thin, unmyelinated olfactory fibers enter the skull through the lamina cribrosa of the os ethmoidale (see p. 25) and pass to the bulbus olfactorius (see also pp. 182, 330, and 490).

* In the new anatomic nomenclature, the regio olfactoria is described as the pars olfactoria tunicae mucosae nasi.

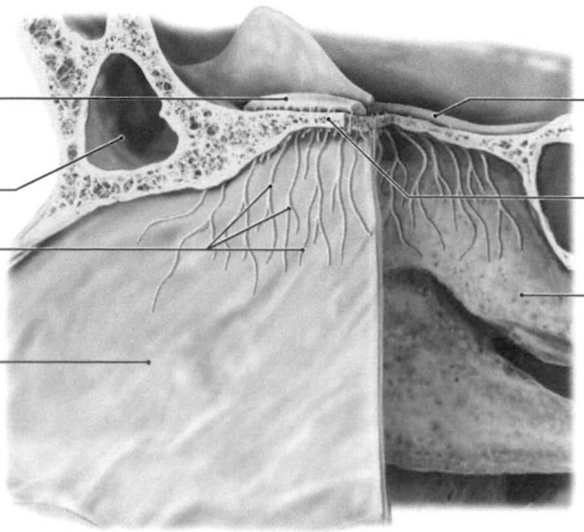

Bulbus olfactorius
Sinus frontalis
Fila olfactoria
Septum nasi
Tractus olfactorius
Lamina cribrosa
Concha nasi superior

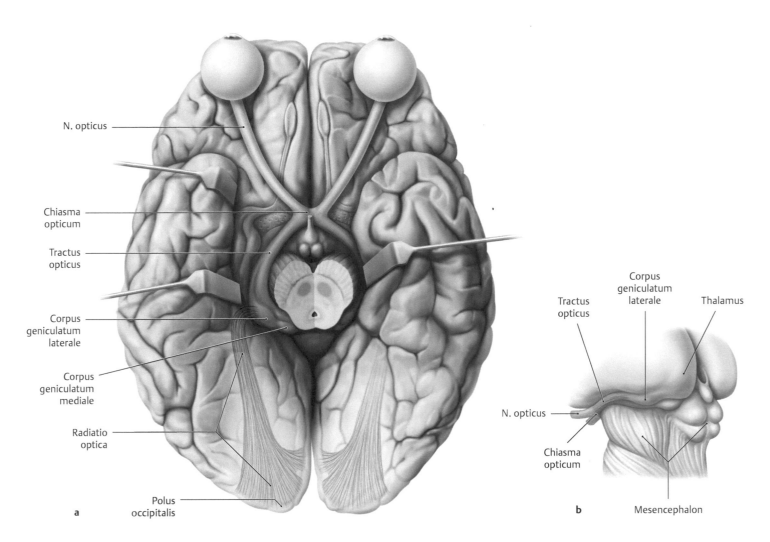

N. opticus

Chiasma
opticum

Tractus
opticus

Corpus
geniculatum
laterale

Corpus
geniculatum
mediale

Radiatio
optica

Polus
occipitalis

a

Corpus
geniculatum
Tractus   laterale   Thalamus
opticus

N. opticus

Chiasma
opticum

b   Mesencephalon

C Eye (oculus), nervus opticus, chiasma opticum, and tractus opticus

a View of the base of the brain, **b** posterolateral view of the left side of the truncus encephali. The termination of the tractus opticus in the corpus geniculatum laterale is shown.

The n. opticus is not a true nerve but an extension of the brain, in this case of the diencephalon. Analogously to the bulbus and tractus olfactorii (see **A**), the n. opticus is sheathed by meninges (removed here) and contains CNS-specific cells (cf. **A**). The n. opticus contains the axons of retinal ganglion cells. These axons terminate mainly in the corpus geniculatum laterale of the diencephalon and in the mesencephalon.

Note: Because the n. opticus is an extension of the brain, the clinician can directly inspect a portion of the brain with an ophthalmoscope. This examination is important in the diagnosis of many neurological diseases (ophthalmoscopy is described on p. 171).

The n. opticus passes from the eyeball (bulbus oculi) through the canalis opticus into the fossa cranii media (see **D**). Many, but not all, retinal cell ganglion axons cross the midline to the contralateral side of the brain in the chiasma opticum (**a**). The tractus opticus extends from the chiasma opticum to the corpus geniculatum laterale (see also **b**).

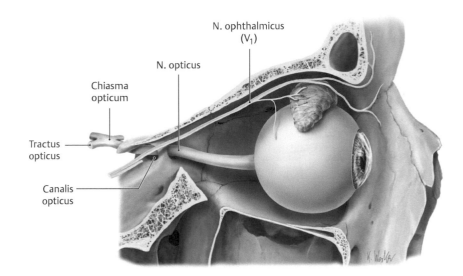

N. ophthalmicus
(V₁)

N. opticus

Chiasma
opticum

Tractus
opticus

Canalis
opticus

D Course of the nervus opticus in the right orbita

Lateral view. The n. opticus extends through the canalis opticus from the orbita into the fossa cranii media. It exits the posterior side of the bulbus oculi within the corpus adiposum orbitae (removed here). The other nn. craniales enter the orbita through the fissura orbitalis superior (only CN V₁ is shown here).

117

4.13 Nervi Craniales of the Extraocular Muscles: Nervus Oculomotorius (CN III), Nervus Trochlearis (CN IV), and Nervus Abducens (CN VI)

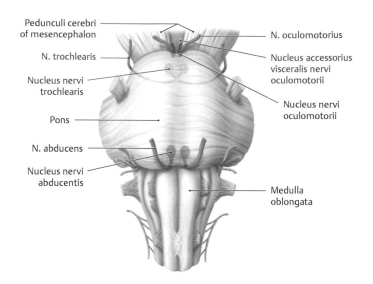

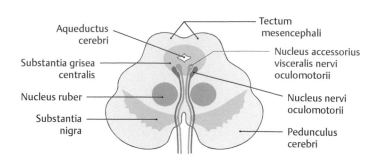

A Emergence of the nerves from the truncus encephali

Anterior view. All three nerves that supply the extraocular muscles emerge from the truncus encephali. The nuclei of the n. oculomotorius and n. trochlearis are located in the midbrain (mesencephalon), while the nucleus of the n. abducens is located in the pons.

Note: Of these three nerves, the n. oculomotorius (CN III) is the only one that contains somatic efferent and visceral efferent fibers and supplies several extraocular muscles (see **C**).

B Overview of the nervus oculomotorius (CN III)

The n. oculomotorius contains *somatic efferent* and *visceral efferent* fibers.

Course: The nerve runs anteriorly from the mesencephalon (midbrain = highest level of the truncus encephali; see pp. 344, 346) and enters the orbita through the fissura orbitalis superior

Nuclei and distribution, *ganglia:*
* *Somatic efferents:* Efferents from a nuclear complex (nucleus nervi oculomotorii) in the midbrain (see **C**) supply the following muscles:
  – M. levator palpebrae superioris (acts on the upper eyelid)
  – Mm. recti superior, medialis, and inferior and m. obliquus inferior (= extraocular muscles, all act on the eyeball).
* *Visceral efferents:* Parasympathetic preganglionic efferents from the nucleus accessorius visceralis nervi oculomotorii (Edinger-Westphal nucleus) synapse with neurons in the ganglion ciliare that innervate the following intraocular muscles:
  – M. sphincter pupillae
  – M. ciliaris

Effects of n. oculomotorius injury:
Oculomotor palsy, severity depending on the extent of the injury.
* Effects of complete oculomotor palsy (paralysis of the extraocular *and* intraocular muscles and m. levator palpebrae):
  – Ptosis (drooping of the lid)
  – Downward and lateral gaze deviation in the affected eye
  – Diplopia (in the absence of complete ptosis)
  – Mydriasis (pupil dilated due to m. sphincter pupillae paralysis)
  – Accommodation difficulties (ciliary paralysis–lens cannot focus).

C Topography of the nucleus nervi oculomotorius

Cross-section through the truncus encephali at the level of the nucleus nervi oculomotorii, superior view.

Note: The visceral efferent, parasympathetic nuclear complex (nucleus accessorius visceralis nervi oculomotorii [Edinger-Westphal nucleus]) can be distinguished from the somatic efferent nuclear complex (nucleus nervi oculomotorii).

D Overview of the nervus trochlearis (CN IV)

The n. trochlearis contains only *somatic efferent* fibers.

Course: The n. trochlearis emerges from the posterior surface of the truncus encephali near the midline, courses anteriorly around the pedunculus cerebri, and enters the orbita through the fissura orbitalis superior.

Special features:
* The n. trochlearis is the only n. cranialis in which all the fibers cross to the opposite side (see **A**). Consequently, lesions of the nucleus or of nerve fibers very close to the nucleus, before they cross the midline, result in n. trochlearis palsy on the side opposite to the lesion (contralateral palsy). A lesion past the site where the nerve crosses the midline leads to n. trochlearis palsy on the same side as the lesion (ipsilateral palsy).
* The n. trochlearis is the only n. cranialis that emerges from the *posterior* side of the truncus encephali.
* It has the longest intracranial course of the three extraocular motor nerves.

Nucleus and distribution: The nucleus of the n. trochlearis is located in the midbrain (mesencephalon). Its efferents supply motor innervation to one extraocular muscle, the m. obliquus superior.

Effects of n. trochlearis injury:
* The affected eye is higher and is also deviated medially because the m. obliquus inferior (responsible for elevation and abduction) becomes dominant due to loss of the m. obliquus superior.
* Diplopia.

E Overview of the nervus abducens (CN VI)

The n. abducens contains only **somatic efferent** fibers.

Course: The nerve follows a long *extradural* path before entering the orbita through the fissura orbitalis superior.

Nucleus and distribution:
* The nucleus of the n. abducens is located in the pons (= midlevel truncus encephali), its fibers emerging at the inferior border of the pons.
* Its efferent fibers supply somatomotor innervation to a single muscle, the m. rectus lateralis.

Effects of n. abducens injury:
* The affected eye is deviated medially.
* Diplopia.

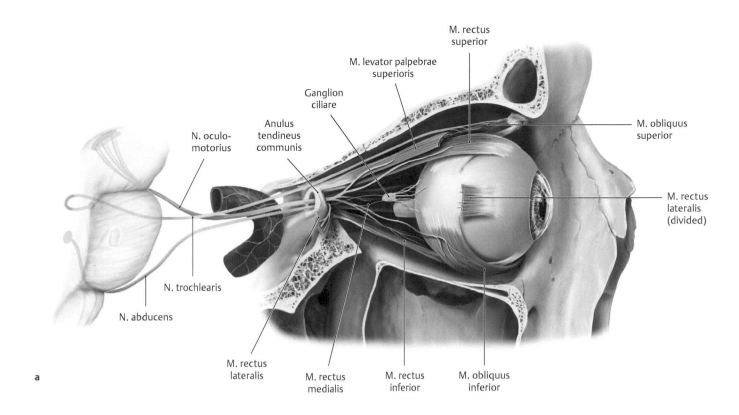

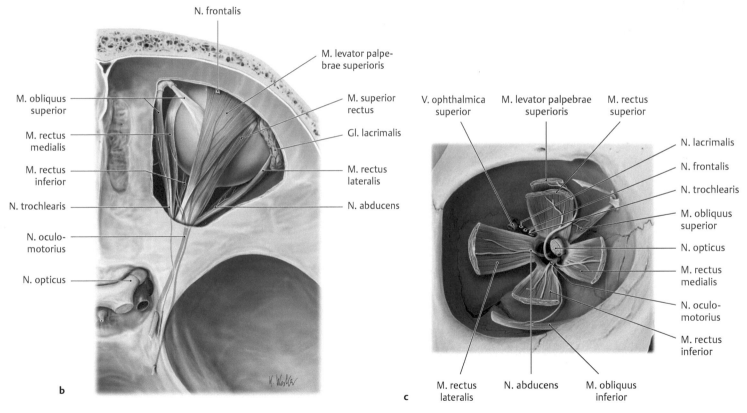

F Course of the nerves supplying the ocular muscles

a Lateral view. Right orbit. **b** Superior view (opened), **c** anterior view. All three nn. craniales extend from the truncus encephali through the fissura orbitalis superior into the orbita. The nn. oculomotorius and abducens pass through the anulus tendineus communis of the extraocular muscles, while the n. trochlearis passes outside the anulus tendineus communis. The *n. abducens* has the longest *extradural* course. Because of this, n. abducens palsy may develop in association with meningitis and subarachnoid hemorrhage. Transient palsy may even occur in cases where lumbar puncture has caused an excessive decrease in CSF pressure, with descent of the truncus encephali exerting traction on the nerve. The *n. oculomotorius* supplies parasympathetic innervation to intraocular muscles (its parasympathetic fibers synapse in the ganglion ciliare) as well as somatic motor innervation to most of the extraocular muscles and the m. levator palpebrae superioris. Oculomotor nerve palsy may affect the parasympathetic fibers exclusively, the somatic motor fibers exclusively, or both at the same time (see **B**). Because the preganglionic parasympathetic fibers for the pupil lie directly beneath the epineurium after emerging from the truncus encephali, they are often the first structures to be affected by pressure due to trauma, tumors, or aneurysms.

4.14 Nervi Craniales: Nervus Trigeminus (CN V), Nuclei and Distribution

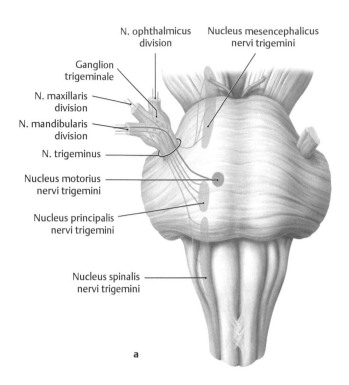

N. ophthalmicus division
Nucleus mesencephalicus nervi trigemini
Ganglion trigeminale
N. maxillaris division
N. mandibularis division
N. trigeminus
Nucleus motorius nervi trigemini
Nucleus principalis nervi trigemini
Nucleus spinalis nervi trigemini

a

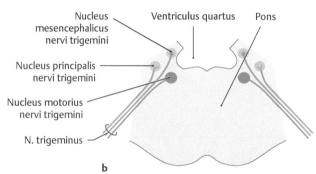

Nucleus mesencephalicus nervi trigemini
Ventriculus quartus
Pons
Nucleus principalis nervi trigemini
Nucleus motorius nervi trigemini
N. trigeminus

b

A   Nuclei and emergence from the pons

a Anterior view. The larger sensory nuclei of the n. trigeminus are distributed along the truncus encephali and extend downward into the medulla spinalis. The *radix sensoria* (major part) of the n. trigeminus forms the bulk of the fibers, while the *radix motoria* (minor part) is formed by fibers arising from the small nucleus motorius nervi trigemini in the pons. They supply motor innervation to the mm. masticatorii (see **B**). The following *somatic afferent* nuclei are distinguished:

- *Nucleus mesencephalicus nervi trigemini:* proprioceptive fibers from the mm. masticatorii. Special feature: the neurons of this nucleus are pseudounipolar ganglion cells that have migrated into the brain.
- *Nucleus principalis nervi trigemini:* chiefly mediates touch.
- *Nucleus spinalis nervi trigemini:* pain and temperature sensation, also touch. A small, circumscribed lesion of the nucleus spinalis nervi trigemini leads to characteristic sensory disturbances in the face (see **D**).

b Cross-section through the pons at the level of emergence of the n. trigeminus, superior view (schematic as the three nuclei are located at different levels).

B   Overview of the nervus trigeminus (CN V)

The n. trigeminus, the sensory nerve of the head, contains mostly *somatic afferent* fibers with a smaller proportion of special *visceral efferent* fibers. Its three major somatic **divisions** have the following **sites of emergence** from the fossa cranii media:

- *N. ophthalmicus division (CN V₁):* enters the orbita through the fissura orbitalis superior.
- *N. maxillaris division (CN V₂):* enters the fossa pterygopalatina through the foramen rotundum.
- *N. mandibularis division (CN V₃):* passes through the foramen ovale to the inferior surface of the basis cranii into the fossa infratemporalis; only division containing motor fibers.

Nuclei and distribution:

- *Special visceral efferent:* Efferent fibers from the nucleus motorius nervi trigemini pass in the n. mandibularis division (CN V₃) to
  - Mm. masticatorii (mm. temporalis, masseter, pterygoidei medialis, and lateralis)
  - Oral floor muscles: m. mylohyoideus and venter anterior musculi digastrici
  - Middle ear muscle: m. tensor tympani
  - Pharyngeal muscle: m. tensor veli palatini
- *Somatic afferent:* The ganglion trigeminale contains pseudounipolar ganglion cells whose central fibers pass to the sensory nuclei of the n. trigeminus (see **Aa**). Their peripheral fibers innervate the facial skin, large portions of the nasopharyngeal mucosa, and the anterior two-thirds of the tongue (somatic sensation, see **C**).
- *"Visceral efferent pathway":* The visceral efferent fibers of some nn. craniales adhere to branches or sub-branches of the n. trigeminus, by which they travel to their destination:
  - The n. lacrimalis (branch of CN V₁) conveys parasympathetic fibers from the n. facialis along the n. zygomaticus (branch of CN V₂) to the gl. lacrimalis.
  - The n. auriculotemporalis (branch of CN V₃) conveys parasympathetic fibers from the n. glossopharyngeus to the gl. parotidea.
  - The n. lingualis (branch of CN V₃) conveys parasympathetic fibers from the chorda tympani of the n. facialis to the gll. submandibularis and sublingualis.
- *"Visceral afferent pathway":* Gustatory fibers from the n. facialis (chorda tympani) travel by the n. lingualis (branch of CN V₃) to supply the anterior two-thirds of the tongue.

Developmentally, the n. trigeminus is the nerve of the arcus pharyngeus primus.

Clinical disorders of the n. trigeminus:
Sensory disturbances and deficits may arise in various conditions:
- Sensory loss due to traumatic nerve lesions.
- Herpes zoster ophthalmicus (involvement of the territory of the first division of the n. trigeminus, including the skin and/or the eye, by the varicella-zoster virus); herpes zoster of the face.

The afferent fibers of the n. trigeminus (like the n. facialis, see p. 124) are involved in the corneal reflex (reflex closure of the eyelid; see **C**, p. 479).

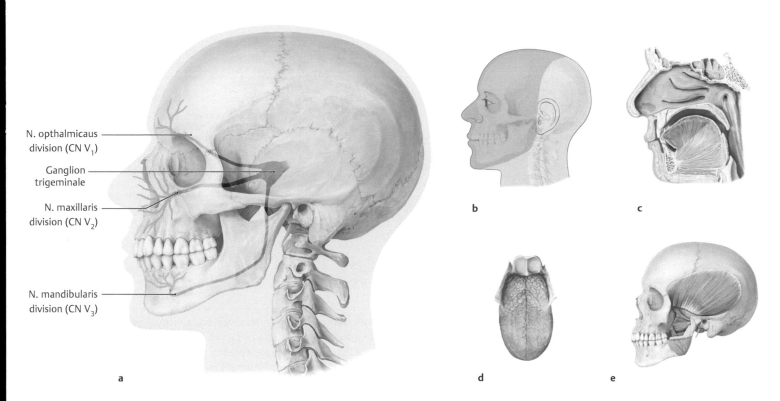

N. opthalmicaus division (CN V₁)

Ganglion trigeminale

N. maxillaris division (CN V₂)

N. mandibularis division (CN V₃)

a

b

c

d

e

C Course and distribution of the nervus trigeminus

a Left lateral view. The three divisions of the n. trigeminus and clinically important terminal branches are shown.

All three divisions of the n. trigeminus supply the skin of the face (**b**) and the mucosa of the pars nasalis pharyngis (**c**). The anterior two-thirds of the tongue (**d**) receives sensory innervation (touch, pain and thermal sensation, but not taste) via the n. lingualis, which is a branch of the n. mandibularis division (CN V₃). The mm. masticatorii are supplied by the radix motoria of the n. trigeminus, whose axons enter the n. mandibularis division (**e**).

Note: The efferent fibers course exclusively in the n. mandibularis division. A peripheral n. trigeminus lesion involving one of its divisions— n. ophthalmicus (CN V₁), n. maxillaris (CN V₂), or n. mandibularis (CN V₃)—may cause loss of somatic sensation (touch, pain, and temperature) in the area innervated by the afferent nerve (see **b**). This contrasts with the more concentric pattern, and more restricted modality, of sensory deficit produced by a central (CNS) lesion involving nucleus spinalis nervi trigemini and pathways (see **D**).

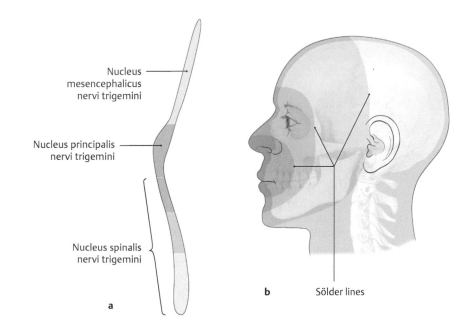

Nucleus mesencephalicus nervi trigemini

Nucleus principalis nervi trigemini

Nucleus spinalis nervi trigemini

a

b   Sölder lines

D Central trigeminal lesion

a Somatotopic organization of the nucleus spinalis nervi trigemini. **b** Facial zones in which sensory deficits (pain and temperature) arise when certain regions of the nucleus spinalis nervi trigemini are destroyed. These zones follow the concentric Sölder lines in the face. Their pattern indicates the corresponding portion of the nucleus spinalis nervi trigemini in which the lesion is located (matching color shades).

4.15 Nervi Craniales: Nervus Trigeminus (CN V), Divisions

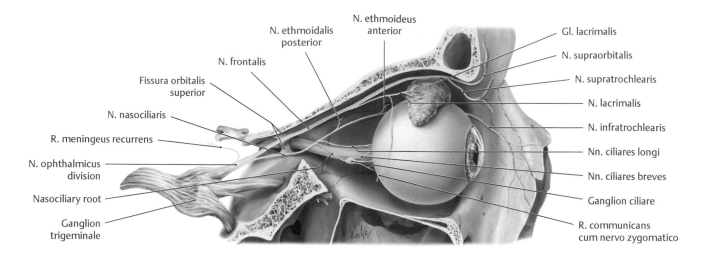

A Branches of the nervus ophthalmicus (= first division of the nervus trigeminus, CN V₁) in the orbital region
Lateral view of the partially opened right orbita. The first small branch arising from the n. ophthalmicus is the r. meningeus recurrens, which supplies sensory innervation to the dura mater. The bulk of the n. ophthalmicus fibers enter the orbita from the fossa cranii media by passing through the *fissura orbitalis superior*. The n. ophthalmicus divides into three branches the names of which indicate their distribution: the **n. lacrimalis, n. frontalis,** and **n. nasociliaris.**

Note: The n. lacrimalis receives postsynaptic, parasympathetic secretomotor fibers from the n. zygomaticus (n. maxillaris division of CN V) via a *ramus communicans* (branch of the n. maxillaris, V₂; see **B**). These fibers travel to the gl. lacrimalis by the n. lacrimalis. Sympathetic fibers accompany the nn. ciliares longi that arise from the n. nasociliaris, traveling in these nerves to the pupilla. The nn. ciliares also contain afferent fibers that mediate the corneal reflex. Sensory fibers from the bulbus oculi course in the radix nasociliaris, passing through the ganglion ciliare to the n. nasociliaris.

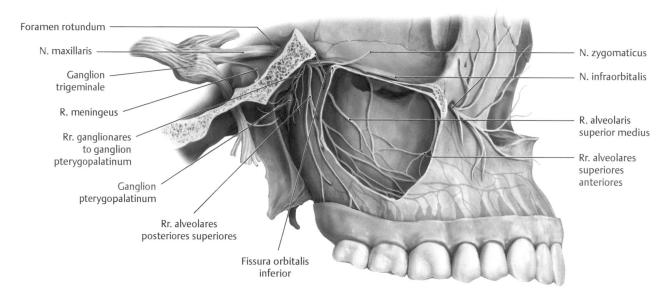

B Branches of the nervus maxillaris (= second division of the nervus trigeminus, CN V₂) in the maxillary region
Lateral view of the partially opened right sinus maxillaris with the arcus zygomaticus removed. After giving off a r. meningeus, the n. maxillaris leaves the fossa cranii media through the foramen rotundum and enters the fossa pterygopalatina, where it divides into the following branches:

- N. zygomaticus
- Rr. ganglionares to the ganglion pterygopalatinum (radix sensoria ganglii pterygopalatini)
- N. infraorbitalis

The **n. zygomaticus** enters the orbita through the *fissura orbitalis inferior*.Its two terminal branches, the r. zygomaticofacialis and r. zygomaticotemporalis (not shown here), supply sensory innervation to the skin

over the arcus zygomaticus and tempora (temple). Parasympathetic, postsynaptic fibers from the ganglion pterygopalatinum are carried to the n. lacrimalis by the ramus communicans (see p. 127). The preganglionic fibers originally arise from the n. facialis. The **n. infraorbitalis** also passes through the fissura orbitalis inferior into the orbita, from which it enters the canalis infraorbitalis. Its fine terminal branches supply the skin between the lower eyelid and upper lip. Its other terminal branches form the *plexus dentalis superior*, which supplies sensory innervation to the maxillary teeth:

- Rr. alveolares superiores anteriores to the dentes incisivi
- R. alveolaris superior medius to the dentes premolares
- Rr. alveolares superiores posteriores to the dentes molares

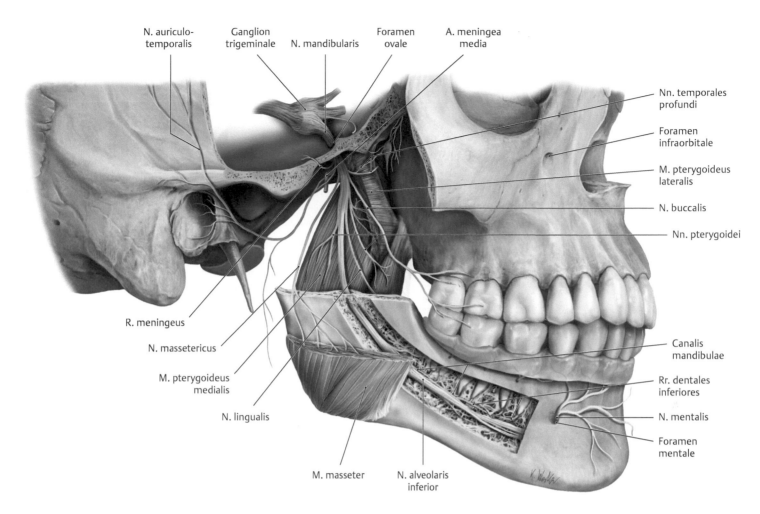

C Branches of the nervus mandibularis (= third division of the nervus trigeminus, CN V₃) in the mandibular region

Right lateral view of the partially opened mandibula with the arcus zygomaticus removed. The mixed afferent-efferent mandibular division leaves the fossa cranii media through the foramen ovale and enters the fossa infratemporalis on the external aspect of the basis cranii. Its r. meningeus re-enters the fossa cranii media to supply sensory innervation to the dura. Its **sensory branches** are as follows:

- N. auriculotemporalis
- N. lingualis
- N. alveolaris inferior (also carries motor fibers, see below)
- N. buccalis

The branches of the *n. auriculotemporalis* supply the temporal skin, the meatus acusticus externa, and the membrana tympanica. The *n. lingualis* supplies sensory fibers to the anterior two-thirds of the tongue, and gustatory fibers from the chorda tympani (n. facialis branch) travel with

it. The *afferent* fibers of the *n. alveolaris inferior* pass through the foramen mandibulae into the canalis mandibulae, where they give off rr. dentales inferiores to the mandibular teeth. The n. mentalis is a terminal branch that supplies the skin of the chin, lower lip, and the body of the mandibula. The *efferent* fibers that branch from the n. alveolaris inferior supply the m. mylohyoideus and the venter anterior of the m. digastricus (not shown). The *n. buccalis* pierces the m. buccinator and supplies sensory innervation to the mucous membrane of the cheek. The pure **motor branches** leave the main nerve trunk just distal to the origin of the r. meningeus. They are:

- N. massetericus (m. masseter)
- Nn. temporales profundi (m. temporalis)
- Nn. pterygoidei (mm. pterygoidei)
- N. musculi tensoris tympani
- N. musculi tensoris veli palatini (not shown)

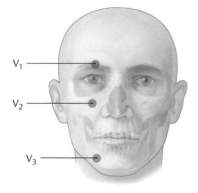

D Clinical assessment of nervus trigeminus function

Each of the three main divisions of the n. trigeminus is tested separately during the physical examination. This is done by pressing on the *nerve exit points* with one finger to test the sensation there (local tenderness to pressure). The typical nerve exit points are as follows:

- For CN V₁: the foramen supraorbitale or incisura supraorbitalis
- For CN V₂: the foramen infraorbitale
- For CN V₃: the foramen mentale

4.16 Nervi Craniales: Nervus Facialis (CN VII), Nuclei and Distribution

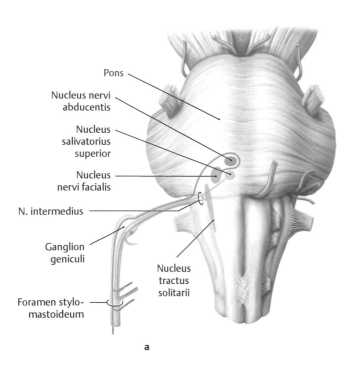

Pons
Nucleus nervi abducentis
Nucleus salivatorius superior
Nucleus nervi facialis
N. intermedius
Ganglion geniculi
Nucleus tractus solitarii
Foramen stylo-mastoideum

a

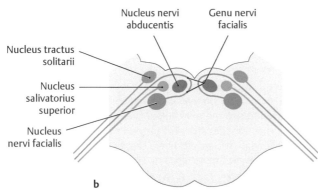

Nucleus nervi abducentis
Genu nervi facialis
Nucleus tractus solitarii
Nucleus salivatorius superior
Nucleus nervi facialis

b

A Nuclei and principal branches of the nervus facialis

a Anterior view of the truncus encephali, showing the site of emergence of the n. facialis from the lower pons. **b** Cross-section through the pons at the level of the genu nervi facialis.

Note: Each of the different fiber types (different sensory modalities) is associated with a particular nucleus.

From the **nucleus nervi facialis**, the *special visceral efferent* axons that innervate the mm. faciei first loop backward around the nucleus nervi abducentis, where they form the genu nervi facialis. They then pass forward and emerge at the lower border of the pons. The **nucleus salivatorius superior** contains *visceromotor*, presynaptic *parasympathetic* neurons. Together with *viscerosensory* (gustatory) fibers from the nucleus tractus solitarii (superior part), they emerge from the pons as the n. intermedius and then are bundled with the *visceromotor* axons from the nucleus nervi facialis to form the n. facialis.

B Overview of the nervus facialis (CN VII)

The n. facialis mainly conveys *special visceral efferent* (branchiogenic) fibers from the nucleus nervi facialis which innervate the skeletal mm. faciei. The other visceral efferent (parasympathetic) fibers from the nucleus salivatorius superior are grouped with the *visceral afferent* (gustatory) fibers from the nucleus tractus solitarii to form the *nervus intermedius* and aggregate with the visceral efferent fibers from the nucleus nervi facialis.

Sites of emergence: The n. facialis emerges in the angulus pontocerebellaris between the pons and oliva. It exits the cavitas cranii through the meatus acusticus internus passing into the pars petrosa of the os temporale, where it divides into its branches:
- The special visceral efferent fibers pass through the *foramen stylomastoideum* to exit the basis cranii to form the plexus intraparotideus (see **C**, exception: n. stapedius).
- The parasympathetic, visceral efferent and visceral afferent fibers, pass through the *fissura petrotympanica* to the basis cranii (see **A**, p. 120). While still in the pars petrosa, the n. facialis gives off the n. petrosus major, n. stapedius, and chorda tympani.

Nuclei and distribution, *ganglia:*
- *Special visceral efferent:* Efferents from the facial nucleus supply the following muscles:
  - Mm. faciei
  - M. stylohyoideus
  - Venter posterior musculi digastrici
  - M. stapedius (n. stapedius)
- *Visceral efferent (parasympathetic):* Parasympathetic presynaptic fibers arising from the nucleus salivatorius superior synapse with neurons in the *ganglion pterygopalatinum* or *ganglion submandibulare*. They innervate the following structures:
  - Gl. lacrimalis
  - Gll. salivatoriae minores of the tunica mucosa cavitatis nasi and of the palata durum and molle
  - Gl. submandibularis
  - Gl. sublingualis
  - Gll. salivatoriae minores on the dorsum of the tongue
- *Special visceral afferent:* Central fibers of pseudounipolar ganglion cells from the ganglion geniculi (corresponds to a spinal ganglion) synapse in the nucleus tractus solitarii. The peripheral processes of these neurons form the *chorda tympani* (gustatory fibers from the anterior two-thirds of the tongue).
- *Somatic afferent neurons:* Some sensory fibers that supply the auricula, the skin of the porus acusticus externus, and the outer surface of the membrana tympanica travel by the n. facialis and *ganglion geniculi* to the nuclei sensorii nervi trigemini. Their precise course is unknown.

Developmentally, the n. facialis is the nerve of the arcus pharyngeus secundus.

Effects of n. facialis injury: A peripheral n. facialis injury is characterized by paralysis of the muscles of expression on the affected side of the face (see **D**). Because the n. facialis conveys various fiber components that leave the main trunk of the nerve at different sites, the clinical presentation of facial paralysis is subject to subtle variations marked by associated disturbances of taste, lacrimation, salivation, etc. (see **B**, p. 126).

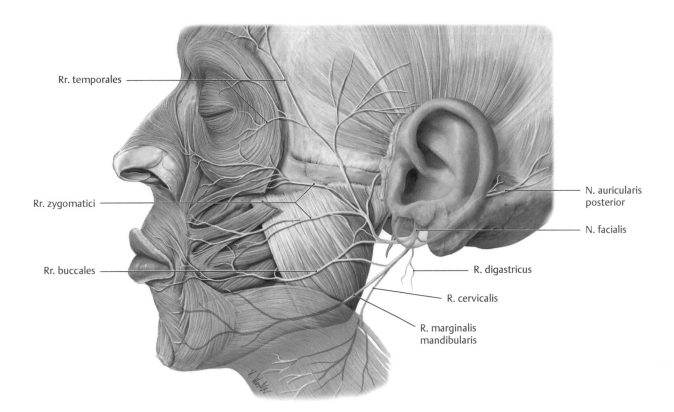

Rr. temporales

Rr. zygomatici

Rr. buccales

N. auricularis posterior

N. facialis

R. digastricus

R. cervicalis

R. marginalis mandibularis

C Nervus facialis branches for the musculi faciei

Note the different fiber types. This unit focuses almost exclusively on the *visceral efferent* (branchiogenic) fibers for the musculi faciei. (The other fiber types are described on p. 126).

The n. stapedius (to the m. stapedius) branches from the n. facialis while still in the pars petrosa ossis temporalis and is mentioned here only because it also contains visceral efferent fibers (its course is shown on p. 126). The first branch that arises from the n. facialis after its emergence from the foramen stylomastoideum is the **n. auricularis posterior;** it supplies *visceral efferent* fibers to the m. auricularis posterior and the venter posterior of the m. occipitofrontalis. It also conveys *somatosensory* fibers from the auris externa, whose pseudounipolar neurons are located in the ganglion geniculi

(see p. 126). After leaving the pars petrosa ossis temporalis, the bulk of the remaining visceral efferent fibers of the n. facialis form the **plexus intraparotideus** in the gl. parotidea, from which successive branches (*rr. temporales, zygomatici, buccales,* and *marginalis mandibularis*) are distributed to the mm. faciei. These n. facialis branches must be protected during the removal of a benign parotid tumor in order to preserve muscle function. Additionally, there are even smaller branches such as the r. digastricus to the venter posterior of the m. digastricus and the r. stylohyoideus to the m. stylohyoideus (not shown). The lowest branch arising from the plexus intraparotideus is the *r. cervicalis.* It joins with the n. transversus cervicalis, an anterior branch of the nervus spinalis C3.

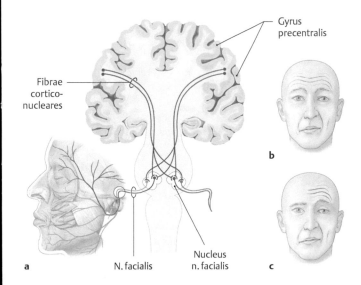

Gyrus precentralis

Fibrae cortico-nucleares

N. facialis

Nucleus n. facialis

a

b

c

D Central and peripheral facial paralysis

a The nucleus nervi facialis contains the cell bodies of lower motor neurons which innervate ipsilateral mm. faciei. The axons (special visceral efferent) of these neurons reach their muscle targets through the n. facialis. These motor neurons are innervated in turn by upper motor

neurons in the primary somatomotor cortex (gyrus precentralis), whose axons enter corticonuclear fiber bundles to reach the nucleus nervi facialis in the truncus encephali.

Note: The nucleus nervi facialis has a "bipartite" structure, its upper part (posterior part) supplying the muscles of the forehead and eyes (rr. temporales) while its lower part (anterior part) supplying the muscles in the lower half of the face. The upper part of the nucleus nervi facialis receives bilateral innervation, the lower part contralateral innervation from cortical (upper) motor neurons.

b Central (supranuclear) paralysis (loss of the upper motor neurons, in this case on the left side) presents clinically with paralysis of the contralateral muscles of facial expression in the lower half of the face, while the contralateral forehead and extraocular muscles remain functional. Thus, the corner of the mouth sags on the right (contralateral) side, but the patient can still wrinkle the forehead and close the eyes on both sides. Speech articulation is impaired.

c Peripheral (infranuclear) paralysis (loss of lower motor neurons, in this case on the right side) is characterized by complete paralysis of the ipsilateral muscles. The patient cannot wrinkle the forehead, the corner of the mouth sags, articulation is impaired, and the eyelid cannot be fully closed. A Bell phenomenon (Bell palsy) is present (the eyeball turns upward and outward, exposing the sclera, when the patient attempts to close the eyelid), and the eyelid closure reflex is abolished. Depending on the site of the lesion, additional deficits may be present such as decreased lacrimation and salivation or loss of taste sensation in the anterior two-thirds of the tongue.

4.17 Nervi Craniales: Nervus Facialis (CN VII), Branches

A Nervus facialis branches in the os temporale

Lateral view of the right os temporale, pars petrosa (petrous bone). The n. facialis, accompanied by the n. vestibulocochlearis (CN VIII, not shown), passes through the meatus acusticus internus (not shown) to enter the pars petrosa. Shortly thereafter it forms the *geniculum* of the n. facialis, which marks the location of the ganglion geniculi. The bulk of the visceral efferent fibers for the muscles of expression pass through the pars petrosa and exit onto the basis cranii at the foramen stylomastoideum (see p. 125). The n. facialis gives off three branches between the ganglion geniculi and foramen stylomastoideum:

- The parasympathetic **n. petrosus major** arises directly at the ganglion geniculi. This nerve leaves the facies anterior partis petrosae at the hiatus canalis nervi petrosi majoris. It continues through the foramen lacerum (not shown), enters the canalis pterygoideus (see **C**), and passes to the ganglion pterygopalatinum.
- The **n. stapedius** passes to the m. stapedius.
- The **chorda tympani** branches from the n. facialis above the foramen stylomastoideum. It contains gustatory fibers as well as presynaptic parasympathetic fibers. It passes through the cavitas tympani and fissura petrotympanica and joins the n. lingualis.

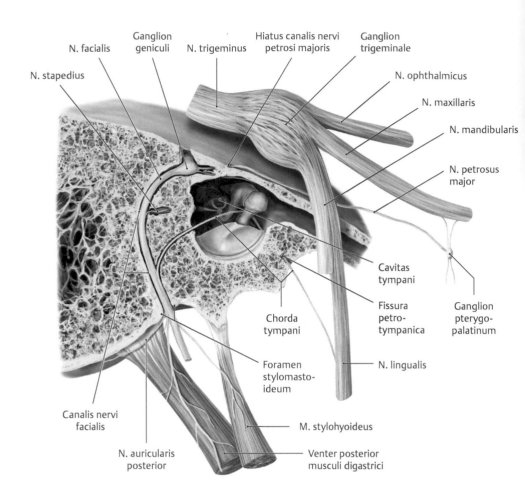

B Branching pattern of the nervus facialis: diagnostic significance in os temporale fractures

The principal signs and symptoms are different depending upon the exact site of the lesion in the course of the n. facialis through the pars petrosa ossis temporalis.

Note: Only the *principal* signs and symptoms associated with a particular lesion site are described here. The more peripheral the site of the nerve injury, the less diverse the signs and symptoms become.

1 A lesion at this level affects the n. facialis in addition to the n. vestibulocochlearis. As a result, peripheral motor facial paralysis is accompanied by hearing loss (deafness) and vestibular dysfunction (dizziness).
2 Peripheral motor facial paralysis is accompanied by disturbances of taste sensation (chorda tympani), lacrimation, and salivation.
3 Motor paralysis is accompanied by disturbances of salivation and taste. Hyperacusis due to paralysis of the m. stapedius has little clinical importance.
4 Peripheral motor paralysis is accompanied by disturbances of taste and salivation.
5 Peripheral motor (facial) paralysis is the only manifestation of a lesion at this level.

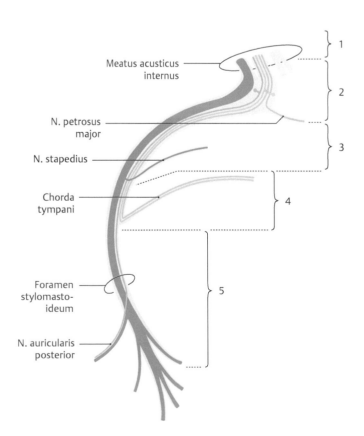

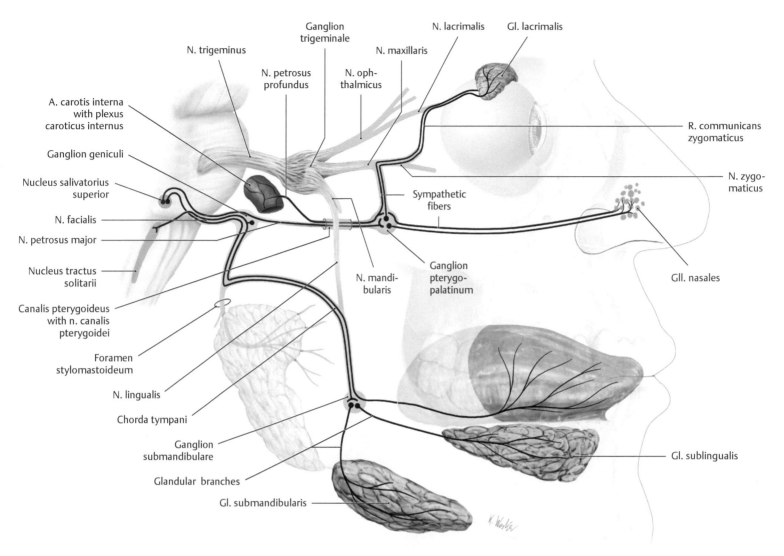

N. trigeminus

Ganglion trigeminale

N. lacrimalis   Gl. lacrimalis

N. petrosus profundus

N. maxillaris

N. oph-thalmicus

A. carotis interna with plexus caroticus internus

R. communicans zygomaticus

Ganglion geniculi

N. zygo-maticus

Nucleus salivatorius superior

Sympathetic fibers

N. facialis

N. petrosus major

Ganglion pterygo-palatinum

Nucleus tractus solitarii

N. mandi-bularis

Gll. nasales

Canalis pterygoideus with n. canalis pterygoidei

Foramen stylomastoideum

N. lingualis

Chorda tympani

Ganglion submandibulare

Gl. sublingualis

Glandular branches

Gl. submandibularis

C Parasympathetic visceral efferents and visceral afferents (gustatory fibers) of the nervus facialis

The presynaptic, parasympathetic, visceral efferent neurons are located in the nucleus salivatorius superior. Their axons enter and leave the pons with the visceral efferent axons as the n. intermedius, then travel with the visceral efferent fibers arising from the nucleus nervi facialis. These preganglionic parasympathetic axons exit the truncus encephali in the n. facialis and branch from it in the n. petrosus major, then mingle with *postganglionic sympathetic axons* (from the ganglion cervicale superius, via the n. petrosus profundus) in the n. canalis pterygoidei. This nerve enters the **ganglion pterygopalatinum,** where the preganglionic parasympathetic motor axons synapse; the sympathetic axons pass through uninterrupted to innervate local blood vessels. The ganglion pterygo-

palatinum supplies the gl. lacrimalis, gll. nasales, and nasal, palatine, and pharyngeal mucosa. Fibers from this ganglion enter the n. maxillaris and travel (via the communicating branch of the n. zygomaticus) with it to innervate the gl. lacrimalis. *Visceral afferent* axons (gustatory fibers) for the anterior two-thirds of the tongue run in the chorda tympani fibers within the n. lingualis. The gustatory fibers originate from pseudounipolar sensory neurons in the **ganglion geniculi,** which corresponds to a spinal sensory (dorsal root) ganglion. The chorda tympani also conveys the presynaptic *parasympathetic visceral efferent fibers* for the gl. submandibularis, gl. sublingualis, and gll. salivariae minores in the anterior two-thirds of the tongue. These fibers also travel with the n. lingualis (CN V_3) and are relayed in the ganglion submandibulare. Glandular branches are then distributed to the respective glands.

D Nerves of the pars petrosa ossis temporalis

N. petrosus major	Branch of CN VII containing preganglionic parasympathetic fibers to the ganglion pterygopalatinum (gl. lacrimalis, gll. nasales)	N. petrosus minor	Branch from CN IX containing preganglionic parasympathetic fibers to the ganglion oticum (gll. parotidea, buccales, and labiales not shown here; see **E**, p. 131)
N. petrosus profundus	Branch from the plexus caroticus internus, containing postganglionic sympathetic fibers; it unites with the n. petrosus minor to form the n. canalis pterygoidei, then continues to the ganglion pterygopalatinum and supplies the same territory as the n. petrosus major (see **C**)		

4.18 Nervi Craniales: Nervus Vestibulocochlearis (CN VIII)

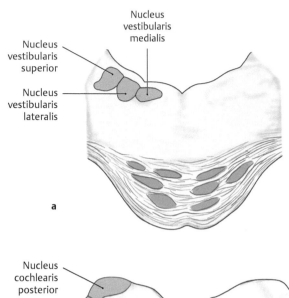

Nucleus vestibularis superior

Nucleus vestibularis medialis

Nucleus vestibularis lateralis

a

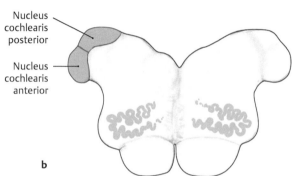

Nucleus cochlearis posterior

Nucleus cochlearis anterior

b

A Nuclei of the nervus vestibulocochlearis (CN VIII)

Cross-sections through the upper medulla oblongata.

a Nuclei vestibulares. Four nuclear complexes are distinguished:

- Nucleus vestibularis superior (of Bechterew)
- Nucleus vestibularis lateralis (of Deiters)
- Nucleus vestibularis medialis (Schwalbe) and
- Nucleus vestibularis inferior (of Roller)

Note: The nucleus vestibularis inferior does not appear in a cross-section at this level (see the location of the cranial nerve nuclei in the brainstem, p. 356).

Most of the axons from the ganglion vestibulare terminate in these four nuclei, but a smaller number pass directly through the pedunculus cerebellaris inferior into the cerebellum (see **Ea**). The nuclei vestibulares appear as eminences on the floor of the rhomboid fossa (see **Eb,** p. 355). Their central connections are shown in **Ea.**

b Nuclei cochleares. Two nuclear complexes are distinguished:

- Nucleus cochlearis anterior
- Nucleus cochlearis posterior

Both nuclei are located lateral and posterior to the nuclei vestibulares (see **Aa,** p. 356). Their central connections are shown in **Eb.**

B Overview of the nervus vestibulocochlearis (CN VIII)

The n. vestibulocochlearis is a *special somatic afferent* (sensory) nerve that consists anatomically and functionally of two components:
- The *n. vestibularis* transmits impulses from the vestibular apparatus.
- The *n. cochlearis* transmits impulses from the auditory apparatus.

These roots are surrounded by a common connective tissue sheath. They pass from the auris interna through the meatus acusticus internus to the angulus pontocerebellaris, where they enter the brain.

Nuclei and distribution, *ganglia:*
- *N. vestibularis:* The *ganglion vestibulare* contains bipolar ganglion cells whose central processes pass to the four nuclei vestibulares on the floor of the fossa rhomboidea of the medulla oblongata. Their peripheral processes begin at the sensory cells of the canales semicirculares, sacculus, and utriculus.
- *N. cochlearis:* The *ganglion spirale* contains bipolar ganglion cells whose central processes pass to the two nuclei cochlearis, which are lateral to the nuclei vestibularis in the fossa rhomboidea. Their peripheral processes begin at the hair cells of the organum spirale.

Every thorough physical examination should include a rapid assessment of both nerve components (hearing and balance tests). A lesion of the n. vestibularis leads to dizziness, while a lesion of the n. cochlearis leads to hearing loss (ranging to deafness).

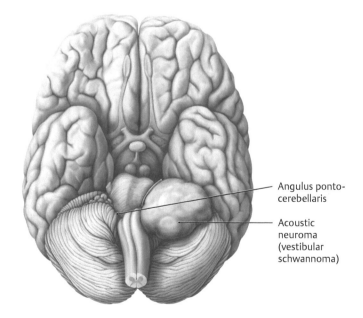

Angulus pontocerebellaris

Acoustic neuroma (vestibular schwannoma)

C Acoustic neuroma in the angulus pontocerebellaris

Acoustic neuromas (more accurately, vestibular schwannomas) are benign tumors of the angulus pontocerebellaris arising from the Schwann cells of the n. vestibularis of CN VIII. As they grow, they compress and displace the adjacent structures and cause slowly progressive hearing loss and gait ataxia. Large tumors can impair the egress of CSF from the ventriculus quartus, causing hydrocephalus and symptomatic intracranial hypertension (vomiting, impairment of consciousness).

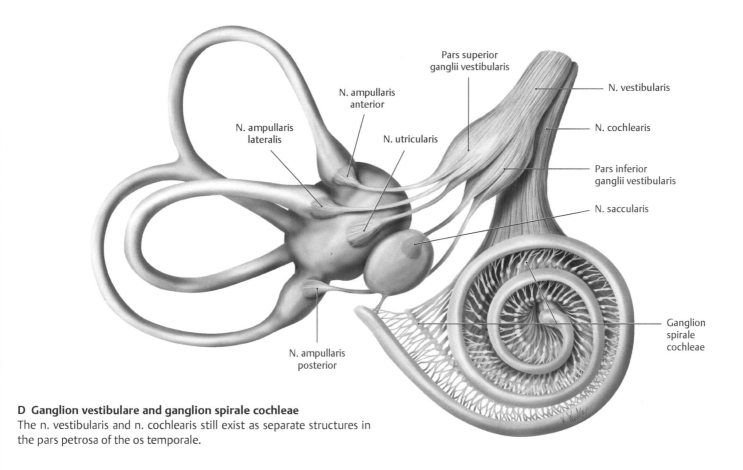

D Ganglion vestibulare and ganglion spirale cochleae
The n. vestibularis and n. cochlearis still exist as separate structures in the pars petrosa of the os temporale.

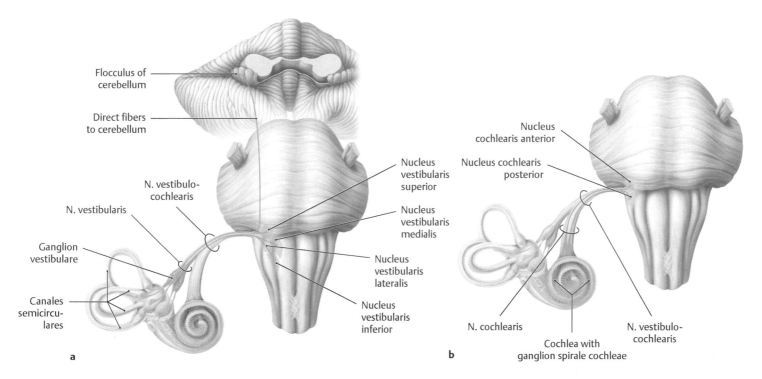

E Nuclei of the nervus vestibulocochlearis in the truncus encephali
Anterior view of the medulla oblongata and pons. The truncus encephali and its connections with the nuclei are shown schematically.

a Vestibular part: The ganglion vestibulare contains bipolar sensory cells whose peripheral processes pass to the canales semicirculares, sacculus, and utriculus. Their axons travel as the n. vestibularis to the four nuclei vestibulares on the floor of the fossa rhomboidea (further connections are shown on p. 486). The vestibular organ processes information concerning orientation in space. An acute lesion of the vestibular organ is manifested clinically by dizziness (vertigo).

b Cochlear part: The ganglion spirale cochleae is a band of nerve cells that follows the course of the bony core of the cochlea. It contains bipolar sensory cells whose peripheral processes pass to the hair cells of the orgnum spirale. Their central processes unite on the floor of the meatus acusticus internus to form the n. cochlearis and are distributed to the two nuclei that are posterior to the nuclei vestibulares. Other connections of the nuclei are shown on p. 484.

4.19 Nervi Craniales: Nervus Glossopharyngeus (CN IX)

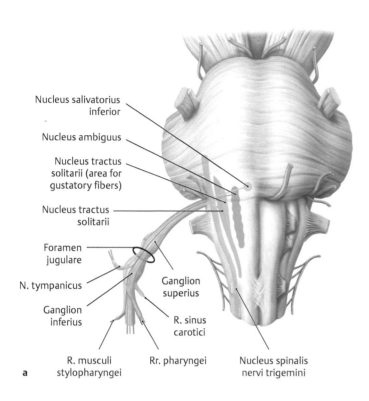

Nucleus salivatorius inferior
Nucleus ambiguus
Nucleus tractus solitarii (area for gustatory fibers)
Nucleus tractus solitarii
Foramen jugulare
N. tympanicus
Ganglion inferius
Ganglion superius
R. sinus carotici
R. musculi stylopharyngei
Rr. pharyngei
Nucleus spinalis nervi trigemini

a

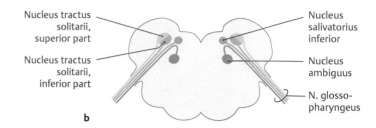

Nucleus tractus solitarii, superior part
Nucleus tractus solitarii, inferior part
Nucleus salivatorius inferior
Nucleus ambiguus
N. glosso-pharyngeus

b

A Nuclei of the nervus glossopharyngeus
a Medulla oblongata, anterior view. **b** Cross-sections through the medulla oblongata at the level of emergence of the n. glossopharyngeus. For clarity, the nuclei of the n. trigeminus are not shown (see **B** for further details on the nuclei).

B Overview of the nervus glossopharyngeus (CN IX)

The n. glossopharyngeus contains *general* and *special visceral efferent fibers* in addition to *visceral afferent* and *somatic afferent fibers*.

Sites of emergence: The n. glossopharyngeus emerges from the medulla oblongata and leaves the cavitas cranii through the foramen jugulare.

Nuclei and distribution, *ganglia:*
- *Special visceral efferent (branchial):* The nucleus ambiguus sends its axons to the constrictor muscles of the pharynx (= pharyngeal branches, join with the nervus vagus to form the plexus pharyngeus) and to the m. stylopharyngeus, m. palatopharyngeus, m. salpingopharyngeus, and m. palatoglossus (see **C**);
- *General visceral efferent (parasympathetic):* The nucleus salivatorius inferior sends parasympathetic presynaptic fibers to the ganglion oticum. Postsynaptic axons from the ganglion oticum are distributed to the gl. parotidea and to the gll. buccales and labiales (see **a** and **E**);
- *Somatic afferent:* Central processes of pseudounipolar sensory ganglion cells located in the *intracranial ganglion superius* or *extracranial ganglion inferius* of the n. glossopharyngeus terminate in the nucleus spinalis nervi trigemini. The peripheral processes of these cells arise from
  - the posterior third of the tongue, palatum molle, pharyngeal mucosa, and tonsillae palatinae (afferent fibers for the gag reflex), see **b** and **c**
  - the mucosa of the cavitas tympani and tuba auditiva (plexus tympanicus), see **d**
  - the skin of the auris externa and porus acusticus externus (blends with the territory supplied by the n. vagus) and the internal surface of the membrana tympanica (part of the plexus tympanicus).
- *Special visceral afferent:* Central processes of pseudounipolar ganglion cells from the ganglion inferius terminate in the superior part of the nucleus tractus solitarii. Their peripheral processes originate in the posterior third of the tongue (gustatory fibers, see **e**).
- *Visceral afferent:* Sensory fibers from the following receptors terminate in the inferior part of the nucleus tractus solitarii:
  - Chemoreceptors in the glomus caroticum
  - Pressure receptors in the sinus caroticus (see **f**).

Developmentally, the n. glossopharyngeus is the nerve of the arcus pharyngis tertius.

Isolated **lesions** of the n. glossopharyngeus are rare. Lesions of this nerve are usually accompanied by lesions of CN X and XI (n. vagus and radix cranialis nervi accessorii) because all three nerves emerge jointly from the foramen jugulare and are all susceptible to injury in basal skull fractures.

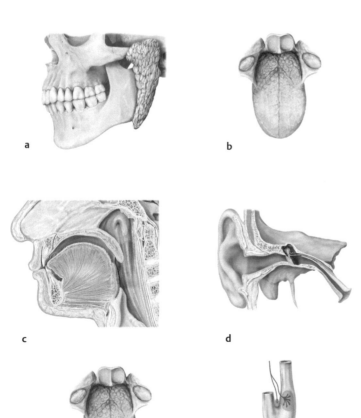

a

b

c

d

e

f

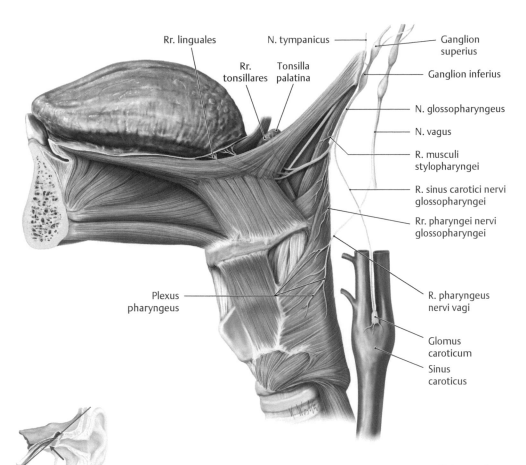

Rr. linguales

N. tympanicus

Ganglion superius

Rr. tonsillares · Tonsilla palatina

Ganglion inferius

N. glossopharyngeus

N. vagus

R. musculi stylopharyngei

R. sinus carotici nervi glossopharyngei

Rr. pharyngei nervi glossopharyngei

Plexus pharyngeus

R. pharyngeus nervi vagi

Glomus caroticum

Sinus caroticus

C Branches of the nervus glossopharyngeus beyond the basis cranii

Left lateral view.

Note the close relationship of the n. glossopharyngeus to the n. vagus (CN X). The sinus caroticus is supplied by both nerves. The most important branches of CN IX seen in the diagram are as follows:

- Rr. pharyngei: three or four branches to the plexus pharyngeus.
- R. musculi stylopharyngei.
- R. sinus carotici: supplies the sinus caroticus and glomus caroticum.
- Rr. tonsillares: to the mucosa of the tonsilla palatina and its surroundings.
- Rr. linguales: somatosensory and gustatory fibers for the posterior third of the tongue.

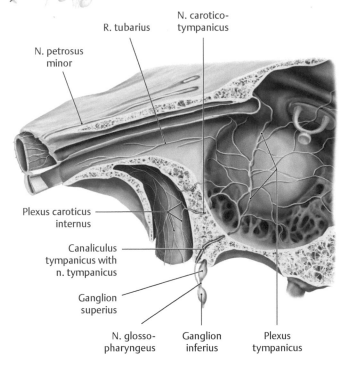

R. tubarius

N. caroticotympanicus

N. petrosus minor

Plexus caroticus internus

Canaliculus tympanicus with n. tympanicus

Ganglion superius

N. glossopharyngeus · Ganglion inferius · Plexus tympanicus

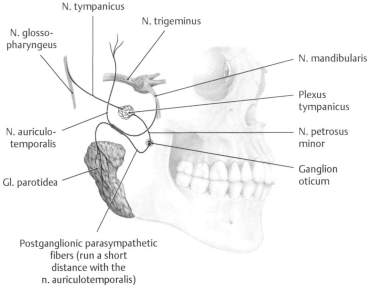

N. tympanicus

N. glossopharyngeus

N. trigeminus

N. mandibularis

Plexus tympanicus

N. auriculotemporalis

N. petrosus minor

Gl. parotidea

Ganglion oticum

Postganglionic parasympathetic fibers (run a short distance with the n. auriculotemporalis)

D Branches of the nervus glossopharyngeus in the cavitas tympani

Left pars petrosa of the ossis temporalis, frontal view. The n. tympanicus, which passes through the canaliculus tympanicus into the cavitas tympani, is the first branch of the n. glossopharyngeus. It contains visceral efferent (presynaptic parasympathetic) fibers for the ganglion oticum and somatic afferent fibers for the cavitas tympani and tuba auditiva. It joins with sympathetic fibers from the plexus caroticus internus (via the n. caroticotympanicus) to form the plexus tympanicus. The parasympathetic fibers travel as the n. petrosus minor to the ganglion oticum (see p. 237), which provides parasympathetic innervation to the gl. parotidea.

E Visceral efferent (parasympathetic) fibers of the nervus glossopharyngeus

The presynaptic parasympathetic fibers from the nucleus salivatorius inferior leave the medulla oblongata with the n. glossopharyngeus and branch off as the n. tympanicus immediately after emerging from the basis cranii. Within the cavitas tympani, the n. tympanicus. bifurcates to form the plexus tympanicus (see **B**, p. 146), which is joined by postganglionic, sympathetic fibers from the plexus caroticus surrounding the a. meningea media (not shown here). The plexus tympanicus gives rise to the n. petrosus minor, which leaves the pars petrosa ossis temporalis through the hiatus canalis nervi petrosi minoris and enters the fossa cranii media. Located below the dura, it passes through the fissura sphenopetrosa to the ganglion oticum. Its fibers enter the n. auriculotemporalis, pass to the n. facialis, and its autonomic fibers are distributed to the gl. parotidea via n. facialis branches.

4.20 Nervi Craniales: Nervus Vagus (CN X)

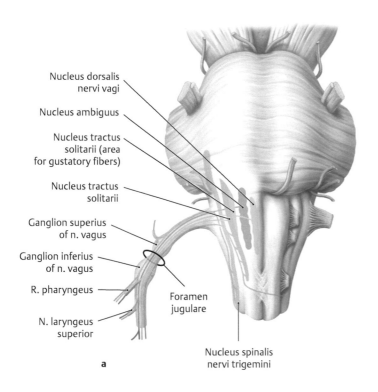

Nucleus dorsalis nervi vagi

Nucleus ambiguus

Nucleus tractus solitarii (area for gustatory fibers)

Nucleus tractus solitarii

Ganglion superius of n. vagus

Ganglion inferius of n. vagus

R. pharyngeus

N. laryngeus superior

Foramen jugulare

Nucleus spinalis nervi trigemini

a

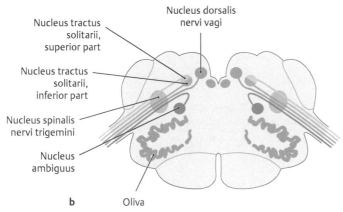

Nucleus tractus solitarii, superior part

Nucleus dorsalis nervi vagi

Nucleus tractus solitarii, inferior part

Nucleus spinalis nervi trigemini

Nucleus ambiguus

b   Oliva

A Nuclei of the nervus vagus

a Medulla oblongata, anterior view showing the site of emergence of the n. vagus.

b Cross-section through the medulla oblongata at the level of the superior olive. Note the various nuclei of the n. vagus and their functions.

The *nucleus ambiguus* contains the *somatic efferent* (branchiogenic) fibers for the nn. laryngei superior and recurrens. It has a somatotopic organization (i.e., the neurons for the n. laryngeus *superior* are above, and those for the n. laryngeus *recurrens* are below). The *nucleus dorsalis nervi vagi* is located on the floor of the fossa rhomboidea and contains presynaptic, parasympathetic visceral efferent neurons. The somatic afferent fibers whose pseudounipolar ganglion cells are located in the ganglion superius (jugular) of the n. vagus terminate in the *nucleus spinalis nervi trigemini*. They use the n. vagus only as a means of conveyance. The central processes of the pseudounipolar ganglion cells from the ganglion inferius (nodose) are gustatory fibers and visceral afferent fibers. They terminate in the *nucleus tractus solitarii*.

B Overview of the nervus vagus (CN X)

The n. vagus contains general and special visceral efferent fibers as well as visceral afferent and somatic afferent fibers. It has the most extensive distribution of all the nn. craniales (n. vagus = "vagabond") and consists of cranial, cervical, thoracic, and abdominal parts. This unit deals mainly with the n. vagus in the head and neck (its thoracic and abdominal parts are described in the volume on the Internal Organs).

Site of emergence: The n. vagus emerges from the medulla oblongata and leaves the cavitas cranii through the foramen jugulare.

Nuclei and distribution, *ganglia:*
- *Special visceral efferent (branchiogenic):* Efferent fibers from the nucleus ambiguus supply the following muscles:
  – Mm. pharyngis (r. pharyngeus, joins with n. glossopharyngeus to form the plexus pharyngeus) and muscles of the palatum molle (levator veli palatini, m. uvulae).
  – All mm. laryngis: The n. laryngeus superior supplies the m. cricothyroideus, while the n. laryngeus recurrens supplies the other mm. laryngis (the origin of the fibers is described on p. 134);
- *General visceral efferent (parasympathetic, see* **Dg**): Parasympathetic presynaptic efferents from the nucleus dorsalis nervi vagi synapse in prevertebral or intramural ganglia with postsynaptic fibers to supply smooth muscle and glands of
  – thoracic viscera and
  – abdominal viscera as far as the flexura coli sinistra (Cannon-Böhm point).
- *Somatic afferent:* Central processes of pseudounipolar ganglion cells located in the ganglion superius (jugular) of the n. vagus terminate in the nucleus spinalis nervi trigemini. The peripheral fibers originate from
  – the dura in the fossa cranii posterior (r. meningeus, see **Df**),
  – the porus acusticus externus (r. auricularis, see **Db**). The r. auricularis is the only cutaneous branch of the n. vagus.
- *Special visceral afferent:* Central processes of pseudounipolar ganglion cells from the ganglion inferius (nodose) terminate in the superior part of the nucleus tractus solitarii. Their peripheral processes supply the gemmae gustatoriae on the epiglottis (see **Dd**).
- *General visceral afferent:* The cell bodies of these afferents are also located in the ganglion inferius. Their central processes terminate in the inferior part of the nucleus tractus solitarii. Their peripheral processes supply the following areas:
  – Mucosa of the lower pharynx at its junction with the esophagus (see **Da**)
  – Laryngeal mucosa above (n. laryngeus superior) and below (n. laryngeus recurrens) the rima glottidis (see **Da**)
  – Pressure receptors in the arcus aortae (see **De**)
  – Chemoreceptors in the glomera aortica (see **De**)
  – Thoracic and abdominal viscera (see **Dg**)

Developmentally, the n. vagus is the nerve of the arcus pharyngei quartus and sextus.

A structure of major **clinical** importance is the *n. laryngeus recurrens*, which supplies visceromotor innervation to the only muscle that abducts the plicae vocales, the m. cricoarytenoideus posterior. Unilateral destruction of this nerve leads to hoarseness, and bilateral destruction leads to respiratory distress (dyspnea).

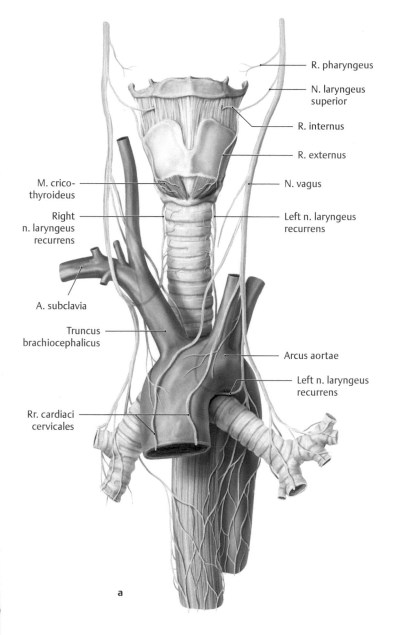

R. pharyngeus

N. laryngeus superior

R. internus

R. externus

N. vagus

M. crico-thyroideus

Right n. laryngeus recurrens

Left n. laryngeus recurrens

A. subclavia

Truncus brachiocephalicus

Arcus aortae

Left n. laryngeus recurrens

Rr. cardiaci cervicales

a

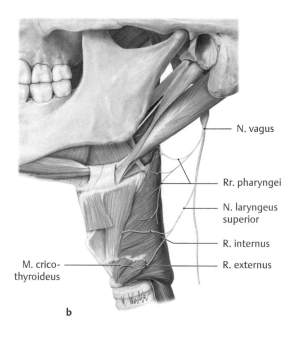

N. vagus

Rr. pharyngei

N. laryngeus superior

R. internus

M. crico-thyroideus

R. externus

b

C Branches of the nervus vagus (CN X) in the neck

a The n.vagus gives off four sets of branches in the neck: r. pharyngeus, the n. laryngeus superior, the n. laryngeus recurrens, and the rr. cardiaci cervicales.

The course of the nn. laryngei recurrentes gives them particular clinical significance. They get damaged as a result of the following:

- Aortic aneurysm, as the left n. laryngeus recurrens winds around the arcus aorticus on the left side
- Lymph node metastases of bronchial carcinoma, as the left n. laryngeus recurrens passes close to the bronchus principalis sinister
- Thyroid operations, as both right and left nn. laryngei recurrentes pass close to the dorsolateral aspects of the gl. thyroidea on either side

In any case, even unilateral damage to a n. laryngeus recurrens leads to hoarseness given that it supplies visceromotor innervation to the only muscle that abducts the plicae vocales, the m. cricoarytenoideus posterior Bilateral nerve damage results in breathing difficulties since the plicae vocales don't open.

b The n. laryngeus superior divides into a r. internus that supplies sensory immervation to the mucosa above the plica vocalis, and a r. externus that is motor to only the m. cricothyroideus.

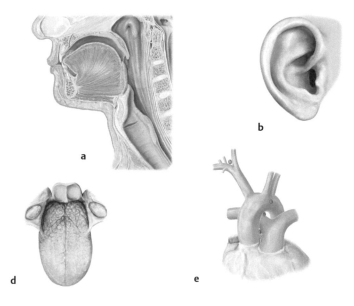

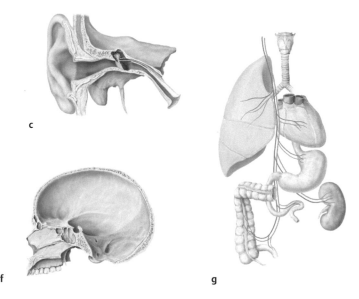

a

b

c

d

e

f

g

D Visceral and sensory distribution of the n. vagus (CN X)

4.21 Nervi Craniales:
Nervus Accessorius (CN XI) and Nervus Hypoglossus (CN XII)

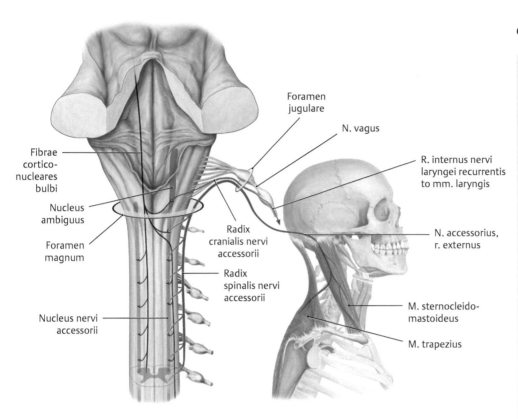

A Nucleus and course of the nervus accessorius
Posterior view of the truncus encephali (with the cerebellum removed). For didactic reasons, the muscles are displayed from the right side (see **C** for further details).

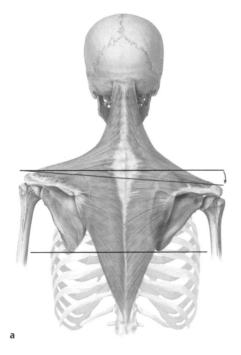

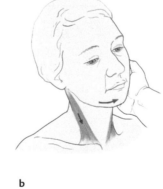

B Lesion of the nervus accessorius (on the right side)
a Posterior view. Paralysis of the m. trapezius causes drooping of the shoulder on the affected side.

b Right anterolateral view. With paralysis of the m. sternocleidomastoideus, it is difficult for the patient to turn the head to the opposite side against a resistance.

C Overview of the nervus accessorius (CN XI)

The n. accessorius is considered by some authors to be an *independent* part of the n. vagus (CN X). It contains both visceral and somatic efferent fibers, and has one radix cranialis and one radix spinalis.

Sites of emergence: The radix spinalis emerges from the medulla spinalis, passes superiorly, and enters the skull through the *foramen magnum*, where it joins with the radix cranialis from the medulla oblongata. Both roots then leave the skull together through the *foramen jugulare*. While still within the foramen jugulare, fibers from the radix cranialis pass to the n. vagus (r. internus). The radix spinalis descends to the nuchal region as the r. externus of the accessory nerve.

Nuclei and distribution:
- *Radix cranialis:* The special visceral efferent fibers of the n. accessorius arise from the caudal part of the *nucleus ambiguus* and form the radix cranialis of the n. accessorius which pass to the n. vagus to be distributed by the n. laryngeus recurrens where they innervate all the mm. laryngis except the m. cricothyroideus.
- *Radix spinalis:* The nucleus nervi accessorii forms a narrow column of cells in the cornu anterius of the medulla spinalis at the level of C2–C5/6. After emerging from the medulla spinalis, its somatic efferent fibers form the r. externus of the n. accessorius, which supplies the trapezius and sternocleidomastoideus.

Effects of n. accessorius injury:
A unilateral lesion results in the following deficits:
- *M. trapezius paralysis:* characterized by drooping of the shoulder and difficulty raising the arm above the horizontal (the m. trapezius supports the m. serratus anterior in elevating the arm past 90°). The part of the accessory nerve that supplies the m. trapezius is vulnerable during operations in the neck (e.g., lymph node biopsies). Since the lower portion of the muscle is also innervated by the C2–4 segments, damage to the n. accessorius does not result in complete loss of muscle control.
- *M. sternocleidomastoideus:* torticollis, damage to the n. accessorius results in flaccid paralysis. With bilateral lesions it is difficult for patients to hold their head in an upright position.

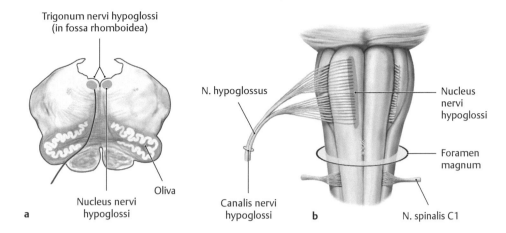

a

Trigonum nervi hypoglossi
(in fossa rhomboidea)

Nucleus nervi
hypoglossi

Oliva

N. hypoglossus

Canalis nervi
hypoglossi

b

Nucleus
nervi
hypoglossi

Foramen
magnum

N. spinalis C1

D Nuclei of the nervus hypoglossus

a Cross-section through the medulla oblongata at the level of the oliva. This section passes through the nucleus nervi hypoglossi. It can be seen that the nucleus lies just beneath the fossa rhomboidea and raises the floor of the fossa to form the trigonum nervi hypoglossi. Because each nucleus is close to the midline, it is common for more extensive lesions to involve the nuclei on both sides, producing the clinical manifestations of a bilateral nuclear lesion.

b Anterior view. The neurons contained in this nuclear column correspond to the alpha motor neurons of the medulla spinalis.

The n. hypoglossus is a purely somatic efferent nerve that supplies the musculature of the tongue.

Nucleus and site of emergence: The nucleus nervi hypoglossi is located in the floor of the fossa rhomboidea. Its somatic efferent fibers emerge from the medulla oblongata, leaving the cavitas cranii through the canalis nervi hypoglossi and descending lateral to the n. vagus. The n. hypoglossus enters the radix linguae above the os hyoideum and distributes its fibers there.

Distribution: The n. hypoglossus supplies all intrinsic and extrinsic muscles of the tongue (except for the m. palatoglossus, CN X). It can be considered a "zeroth" ventral root rather than a true n. cranialis. The ventral fibers of C1 and C2 travel with the n. hypoglossus but leave it again after a short distance to form the radix superior of the ansa cervicalis.

Effects of n. hypoglossus injury:
- Central hypoglossal paralysis (supranuclear): The tongue deviates away from the side of the lesion, since central fibers cross.
- Nuclear or peripheral paralysis: The tongue deviates toward the affected side due to a preponderance of muscular action on the healthy side.

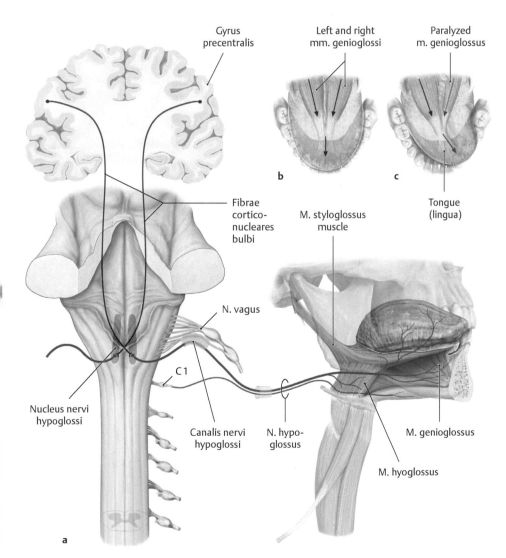

a

Gyrus
precentralis

Fibrae
cortico-
nucleares
bulbi

N. vagus

C1

Nucleus nervi
hypoglossi

Canalis nervi
hypoglossi

N. hypo-
glossus

M. hyoglossus

Left and right
mm. genioglossi

Paralyzed
m. genioglossus

b

c

M. styloglossus
muscle

Tongue
(lingua)

M. genioglossus

F Distribution of the nervus hypoglossus

a Central and peripheral course

b Function of the m. genioglossus

c Deviation of the tongue toward the paralyzed side

The nucleus nervi hypoglossi is innervated (upper motor neurons) by cortical neurons from the contralateral side. With a unilateral *nuclear or peripheral* lesion of the n. hypoglossus, the tongue deviates toward the side of the lesion when protruded because of the relative dominance of the healthy m. genioglossus (**c**). When both nuclei are injured, the tongue cannot be protruded (flaccid paralysis).

4.22 Neurovascular Pathways through the Base of the Skull, Synopsis

Openings between internal surface of basis cranii and other spaces

Fossa cranii anterior

Foramen ethmoidale anterius

- N., a. and v. ethmoidalis anterior

→ *Orbita*

Lamina cribrosa

- Fila olfactoria (I)
- N., a. and v. ethmoidalis anterior

→ *Cavitas nasi*

Fossa cranii media

Canalis opticus

- N. opticus (II)
- A. ophthalmica

→ *Orbita*

Fissura orbitalis superior

① V. ophthalmica superior
② N. ophthalmicus (V_1)
  2a N. lacrimalis
  2b N. frontalis
  2c N. nasociliaris
③ N. abducens (VI)
④ N. oculomotorius (III)
⑤ N. trochlearis (IV)

→ *Orbita*

Hiatus canalis nervi petrosi minoris

- N. petrosus minor (parasympathetic, from IX)
- A. tympanica superior

→ *Hiatus canalis nervi petrosi majoris*

Hiatus canalis nervi petrosi majoris

- N. petrosus major (parasympathetic, from VII)
- V. and a. stylomastoidea

→ *Canalis nervi facialis*

Fossa cranii posterior

Porus and vv. labyrinthi

- A. and vv. labyrinthi
① N. facialis (with n. intermedius) (VII)
② N. vestibulocochlearis (V_3)

→ *Canalis nervi facialis, auris interna*

Openings between internal and external surface of basis cranii

Fossa cranialis media

Foramen rotundum

- N. maxillaris (V_2)

Foramen ovale

- N. mandibularis (V_3)
- A. pterygomeningea
- Plexus venosus foraminis ovalis

Canalis caroticus

- A. carotis interna
- Plexus caroticus internus (sympathetic)
- Plexus venosus caroticus internus

Foramen lacerum

(covered by a. carotis interna)

- N. petrosus profundus
- N. petrosus major (parasympathetic, from VII)

Foramen spinosum

- A. meningea media
- R. meningeus nervi mandibularis (V_3)

Fissura petrosphenoidale

- Lesser petrosal nerve (parasympathetic, from IX)

Fossa cranii posterior

Foramen jugulare

① N. glossopharyngeus (IX)
② N. vagus (X)
③ Sinus petrosus inferior
④ N. accessorius (XI)
⑤ A. meningea posterior
⑥ V. jugularis interna

Foramen magnum

See right-hand side

Canalis nervi hypoglossi

- N. hypoglossus (XII)
- Plexus venosus canalis nervi hypoglossi

Canalis condylaris

- V. emissaria condylaris (inconstant)

Foramen mastoideum

- V. emissaria mastoidea
- R. mastoideus arteriae occipitalis

Labels on illustration: Fossa cranii anterior; Fossa cranii media; Fossa cranii posterior; 2a, 2b, 2c; ① ② ③ ④ ⑤ ⑥

Openings between external and surfaces of basis cranii

Foramen rotundum

(not visible here, since located in fossa cranii media)

- N. maxillaris (V_2)

Foramen ovale

- N. mandibularis (V_3)
- A. pterygomeningea
- Plexus venosus foraminis ovalis

Foramen spinosum

- A. meningea media
- R. meningeus nervi mandibularis (V_3)

Fissura sphenopetrosa

- N. petrosus minor
  (parasympathetic, from IX)

Foramen lacerum

- N. petrosus profundus (sympathetic)
- N. petrosus major
  (parasymphathetic, from VII)

Canalis caroticus

- A. carotis interna
- Plexus caroticus internus
  (sympathetic)
- Plexus venosus caroticus internus

Canalis nervi hypoglossi

- N. hypoglossus (XII)
- Plexus venosus canalis nervi hypoglossi

Foramen magnum

① A. spinalis anterior
② Aa. vertebrales
③ Medulla spinalis
④ Radix spinalis nervi accessorii (XI)
⑤ A. spinalis posterior
⑥ V. spinalis posterior

Canalis condylaris

- V. emissaria condylaris (inconstant)

Foramen jugulare

① N. glossopharyngeus (IX)
② N. vagus (X)
③ Sinus petrosus inferior
④ A. meningea posterior
⑤ N. accessorius
⑥ V. jugularis interna

Foramen mastoideum

- V. emissaria mastoidea
- R. mastoideus arteriae occipitalis

Openings between internal surface of basis cranii and other spaces

Fossa incisiva with foramen incisivum

- N. nasopalatinus (from V_2)
- A. sphenopalatina

→ *Cavitas nasi*

Foramen palatinum majus

- N. palatinus major
- A. palatina major

→ *Fossa pterygopalatina*

Foramen palatinum minus

- Nn. palatini minores
- Aa. palatinae minores

→ *Fossa pterygopalatina*

Fossa pterygoidea

- N. petrosus major
  (parasympathetic, from VII)
- N. petrosus profundus (sympathetic)
- A. and v. canalis pterygoidei

→ *Fossa pterygopalatina*

Fissura petrotympanica

- A. tympanica anterior
- Chorda tympani
  (parasympathetic and taste, from VII)

→ *Cavitas tympani*

Canaliculus tympanicus

- N. tympanicus
  (parasympathetic and sensory, from IX)
- A. tympanica inferior

→ *Cavitas tympani*

Foramen stylomastoideum

- N. facialis (VII)
- A. and v. stylomastoidea

→ *Canalis nervi facialis*

A Exit points of neurovascular structures through the basis cranii

Left side Internal surface of cranial base (Basis cranii interna); right side external surface of cranial base.

(symp. = sympathetic, parasymp. = parasympathetic)

4.23 Overview of the Nervous System in the Neck and the Distribution of Spinal Nerve Branches

A Overview of the nervous system in the neck

The following structures of the peripheral nervous system are present in the neck: nn. spinales, nn. craniales, and nerves of the autonomic nervous system. The table below reviews the most important structures, following the sequence in which they are discussed in the next sections.

The nn. spinales that supply the neck arise from the C1–C4 segments of the cervical medulla spinalis. The nn. spinales divide into rr. posteriores (dorsales) and rr. anteriores (ventrales):

- The rr. posteriores of the nn. spinales arising from the C1–C3 medulla spinalis segments (n. suboccipitalis, n. occipitalis major, n. occipitalis tertius) supply motor innervation to the intrinsic nuchal muscles and sensory innervation to the C2 and C3 dermatomes on the back of the neck and occiput (see **B**).
- The rr. anteriores of the nn. spinales arising from C1–C4 medulla spinalis segments supply motor innervation to the deep neck muscles (short, direct branches from the rr. anteriores) and finally unite in the neck to form the plexus cervicalis (see **C**). This plexus supplies the skin and musculature of the anterior and lateral neck (all but the nuchal region).

The neck contains the following nn. craniales, which arise from the truncus encephali:

- N. glossopharyngeus (CN IX)
- N. vagus (CN X)
- N. accessorius (CN XI)
- N. hypoglossus (CN XII)

These nerves supply motor and sensory innervation to the pharynx and larynx (CN IX and X) and motor innervation to the mm. trapezius and sternocleidomastoideus (CN XI), lingual muscles (CN XII), and floor of the mouth.

The **truncus sympathicus** is part of the autonomic nervous system, consisting of a nerve trunk with three ganglia that extends along the columna vertebralis on each side. The postganglionic fibers follow the aa. carotides to their territories in the head and neck region.

Another part of the autonomic nervous system, the **parasympathetic system**, is represented in the neck by the n. vagus.

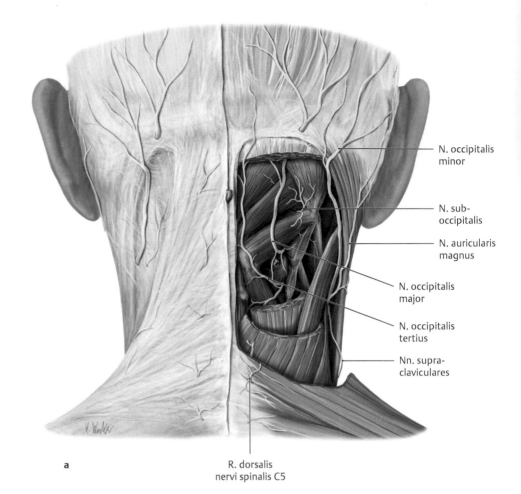

N. occipitalis minor

N. sub-occipitalis

N. auricularis magnus

N. occipitalis major

N. occipitalis tertius

Nn. supra-claviculares

a

R. dorsalis nervi spinalis C5

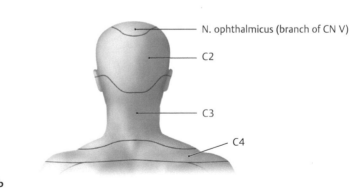

N. ophthalmicus (branch of CN V)

C2

C3

C4

b

B Motor and sensory innervation of the nuchal region

Posterior view. **a** N. spinalis branches in the nuchal region. **b** Segmental distribution.

The nuchal region receives most of its motor and sensory innervation from rr. *posteriores* of the cervical spinal nerves arising from the C1–C3 cord segments:

- N. suboccipitalis (C1)
- N. occipitalis major (C2)
- N. occipitalis tertius (C3)

Note their subcutaneous course on the left side (**a**). The following nerves are derived from rr. *anteriores* of the cervical spinal nerves and enter the nuchal region from the lateral side:

- N. occipitalis minor
- N. auricularis magnus

Note: The r. dorsalis of the first cervical spinal nerve (the n. suboccipitalis) is purely motor (see **a**), and consequently there is no C1 dermatome.

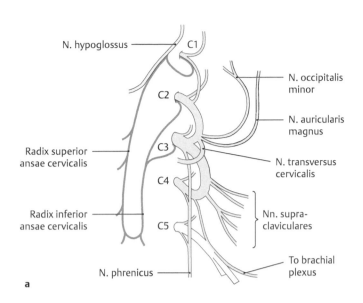

a

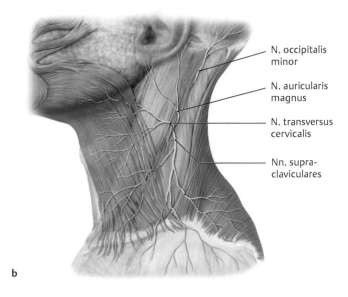

b

C Motor and sensory innervation of the anterior and lateral neck

The anterolateral portions of the neck, unlike the nuchal region and occiput, are supplied entirely by rr. *anteriores* of the C1–C4 cervical spinal nerves. These rami distribute short branches to the deep neck muscles (see **c**). They also give off branches that form the plexus cervicalis, which consists of a sensory part and a motor part supplying the skin and muscles of the neck.

a Branching pattern of the plexus cervicalis (viewed from the left side). The motor fibers from C1–C3 form the ansa cervicalis*, which innervates the mm. infrahyoidei (see **c**). The fibers from C1 course briefly with the n. hypoglossus, without exchanging fibers with it, before they separate to form the *radix superior* of the ansa cervicalis, which supplies the mm. omohyoideus, sternothyroideus and sternohyoideus. Only the fibers for the mm. thyrohyoideus and geniohyoideus continue to course with the n. hypoglossus. Other fibers from C2 unite with the fibers from C3 to form the *radix inferior* of the ansa cervicalis. The bulk of the fibers from C4 descend in the n. phrenicus to the diaphragma (see **D**).

b Sensory innervation of the anterior and lateral neck (viewed from the left side). Erb's point is located approximately at the midposterior border of the m. sternocleidomastoideus, and is the site where the following nerves of the plexus cervicalis emerge to supply sensory innervation to the skin of the anterior and lateral neck (the *sensory part* of the plexus cervicalis):

- N. occipitalis minor
- N. auricularis magnus with its rr. anterior and posterior
- N. transversus cervicalis
- Nn. supraclaviculares

These nerves course along the surface of the fascia the entire distance (including the pars descendens musculi trapezii, shown here without its fascia for greater clarity). The only muscle they perforate is the platysma, which lacks a fascia.

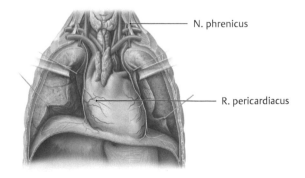

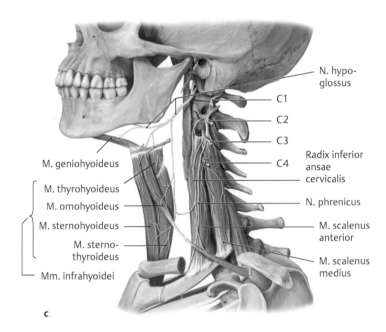

c

c Motor innervation of the anterior and lateral neck. Most of the anterior and lateral neck muscles are supplied by rr. ventrales of the nn. spinales. Their motor fibers either pass directly as short fibers from the rr. ventrales to the deep neck muscles or combine to form the *motor root* of the plexus cervicales.

* The ansa cervicalis (profunda) is the loop of nerves in the plexus cervicalis shown here. This is distinct from the ansa cervicalis superficialis, which represents an anastomosis between the n. transversus colli and the r. cervicalis nervi facialis (see p. 241).

D Nervus phrenicus

Anterior view. The n. phrenicus arises from the C3, 4, and 5 anterior roots ("C3, 4 and 5 keep the diaphragm alive"), with the major contribution from C4. It descends through the cervical region in front of the m. scalenus anterior, behind the m. sternocleidomastoideus, through the apertura thoracis superior to the diaphragma, which it provides with motor innervation. Although this is an unusual anatomical relation between nerve origin and target location in the adult, the embryonic diaphragma develops from a precursor (the septum transversum) at the cervical level, and carries its innervation with it as it migrates inferiorly. If the C4 segment of the medulla spinalis (the main root of the n. phrenicus) sustains bilateral injury in an accident, the victim will usually die at the scene from asphyxiation brought on by paralysis of the diaphragma.

4.24 Nervi Craniales and Autonomic Nervous System in the Neck

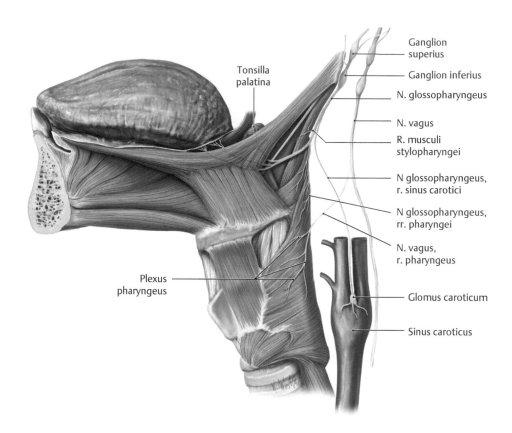

A Nervus glossopharyngeus
Left lateral view. The n. glossopharyngeus (CN IX) carries the motor fibers for the m. stylopharyngeus as well as sensory fibers for the pharyngeal mucosa, the tonsillae palatinae, and the posterior third of the tongue including the gustatory fibers. It sends small branches to anastomose with both the truncus sympathicus and the n. vagus. It also sends nerve fibers (r. sinus carotici) to the bifurcatio carotidis, which contains specialized collections of cells that are important in autonomic control of the circulatory system. Mechanoreceptors in the sinus caroticus sense blood pressure, and chemoreceptors in the glomus caroticum monitor blood pH and carbon dioxide and oxygen levels. This information is relayed by the n. glossopharyngeus to the centers regulating breathing and heart rate in the truncus encephali.

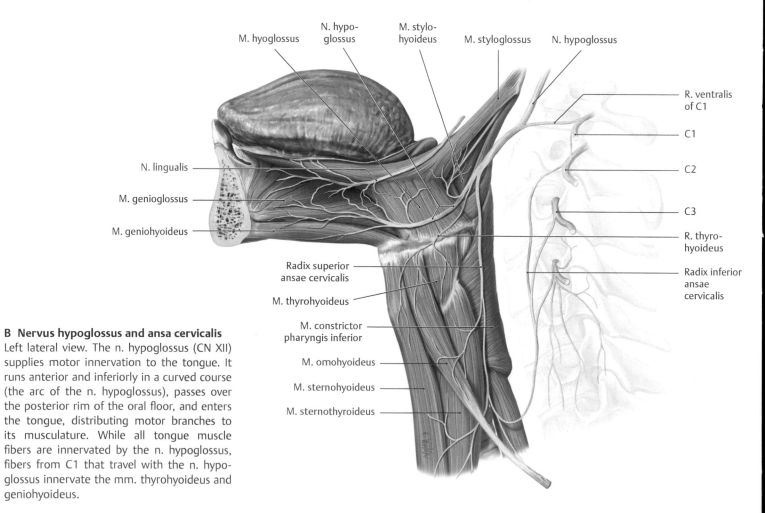

B Nervus hypoglossus and ansa cervicalis
Left lateral view. The n. hypoglossus (CN XII) supplies motor innervation to the tongue. It runs anterior and inferiorly in a curved course (the arc of the n. hypoglossus), passes over the posterior rim of the oral floor, and enters the tongue, distributing motor branches to its musculature. While all tongue muscle fibers are innervated by the n. hypoglossus, fibers from C1 that travel with the n. hypoglossus innervate the mm. thyrohyoideus and geniohyoideus.

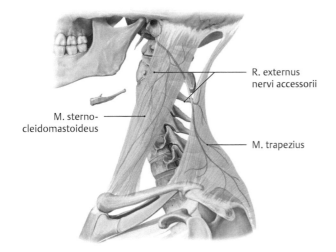

R. externus nervi accessorii

M. sternocleidomastoideus

M. trapezius

C Nervus accessorius in the neck

Left lateral view. The n. accessorius (CN XI) is purely motor. Some of its fibers enter the m. sternocleidomastoideus from behind while others continue on to the m. trapezius. A deep (prescalene) lymph node biopsy may injure the n. accessorius in the neck. Damage to the fibers supplying the m. trapezius results in lateral rotation of the scapula and some shoulder drop. Damage to the fibers supplying the m. sternocleidomastoideus leads to weakness in turning the head to the opposite side.

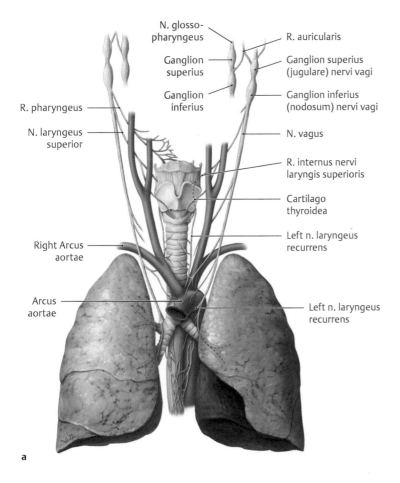

N. glossopharyngeus

R. auricularis

Ganglion superius

Ganglion superius (jugulare) nervi vagi

Ganglion inferius

Ganglion inferius (nodosum) nervi vagi

R. pharyngeus

N. vagus

N. laryngeus superior

R. internus nervi laryngis superioris

Cartilago thyroidea

Left n. laryngeus recurrens

Right Arcus aortae

Arcus aortae

Left n. laryngeus recurrens

a

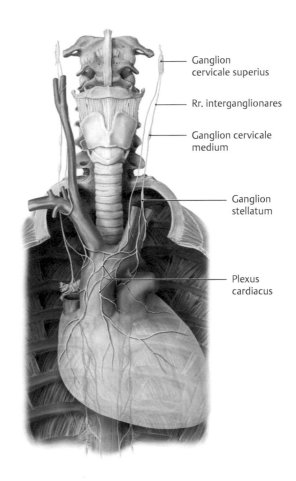

Ganglion cervicale superius

Rr. interganglionares

Ganglion cervicale medium

Ganglion stellatum

Plexus cardiacus

b

D Nervus vagus in the neck and the cervical truncus sympathicus

a Anterior view. The n. vagus (CN X) conveys the fibers of the cranial portion of the parasympathetic nervous system (part of the autonomic nervous system) that supply the neck, thorax, and parts of the cavitas abdominis. It passes down the neck in the vagina carotica (see topographical anatomy, p. 242), giving off only a few branches in the head and neck:

- The r. auricularis, a somatic afferent branch that supplies the back surface of the ear and the porus acusticus externus
- The r. pharyngeus, special visceral efferent fibers for supplying muscles of the pharynx and palatum molle
- The n. laryngeus superior, a mixed nerve with sensory and special visceral efferent fibers, that innervate the mm. cricothyroidei and the mucosa surrounding them

- The n. laryngeus recurrens, which supplies the skeletal mm. laryngis and the mucosa surrounding them (see p. 208). The n. laryngeus recurrens winds around the a. subclavia on the right side and the arcus aortae on the left side.

b Anterior view. The paravertebral chain of sympathetic ganglia terminates in the cervical region at the ganglion cervicale superius, approximately 2 cm below the base of the skull. Postganglionic fibers from this ganglion follow both the aa. carotis interna and externa to provide sympathetic innervation to the entire cranial vasculature, to the iris, and to glands and mucosa in the head. The lowest of the ganglia cervicalia in the paravertebral chain is often fused with the first thoracic sympathetic ganglion to form the ganglion stellatum.

5.1 Ear (Auris): Overview and Supply to the External Ear (Auris Externa)

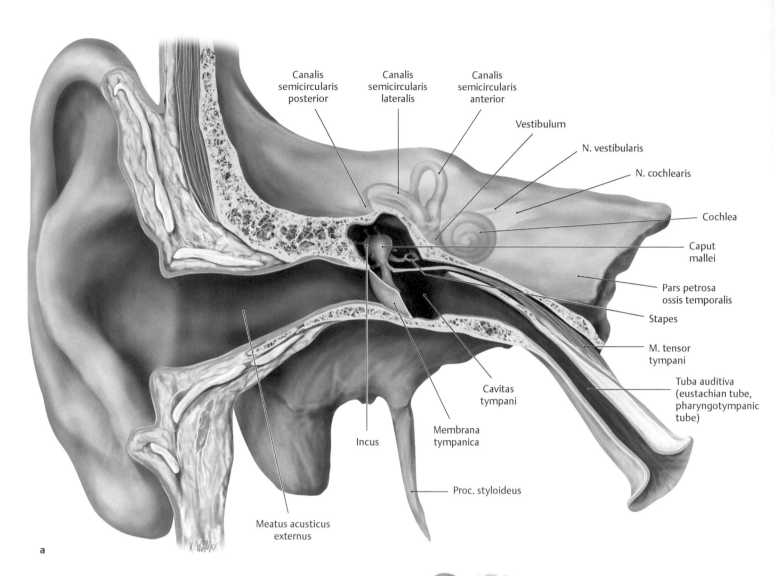

- Canalis semicircularis posterior
- Canalis semicircularis lateralis
- Canalis semicircularis anterior
- Vestibulum
- N. vestibularis
- N. cochlearis
- Cochlea
- Caput mallei
- Pars petrosa ossis temporalis
- Stapes
- M. tensor tympani
- Tuba auditiva (eustachian tube, pharyngotympanic tube)
- Cavitas tympani
- Membrana tympanica
- Incus
- Proc. styloideus
- Meatus acusticus externus

a

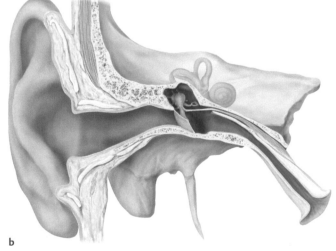

b

A Auditory and vestibular apparatus in situ

a Coronal section through the right ear, anterior view. **b** Main parts of the auditory apparatus: auris externa (yellow), auris media (blue), and auris interna (green).

The auditory and vestibular apparatus are located deep in the pars petrosa of the os temporale (petrous bone). The **auditory apparatus** consists of the auris externa, auris media, and auris interna (see **b**). Sound waves are captured by the auris *externa* (auricula, see **B**) and travel through the meatus acusticus externus to the membrana tympanica, which marks the lateral boundary of the auris *media*. The sound waves set the membrana tympanica into motion, and these mechanical vibrations are transmitted by the chain of ossicula auditoria in the auris media to the oval window (fenestra vestibuli), which leads into the auris *interna* (see p. 146). The ossicular chain induces vibrations in the membrane covering the fenestra vestibuli, and these in turn cause a fluid column in the auris interna to vibrate, setting receptor cells in motion (see p. 153). The transformation of sound waves into electrical impulses takes place in the auris interna, which is the actual organ of hearing. The auris externa and auris media, on the other hand, constitute the *sound conduction apparatus*. The organ of balance is the **vestibular apparatus**, which is also located in the auditory apparatus and

will be described after the units that deal with the auditory apparatus. It contains the *canales semicirculares* for the perception of angular acceleration (rotational head movements) and the *sacculus* and *utriculus* for the perception of linear acceleration. Diseases of the vestibular apparatus produce dizziness (vertigo).

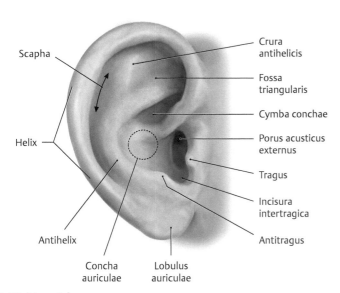

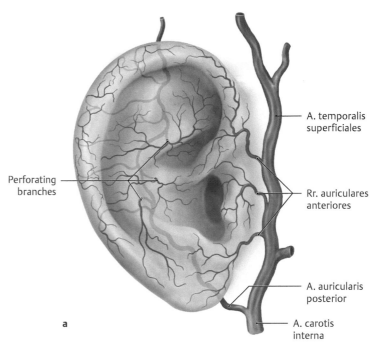

B Right auricle
The auricle of the ear encloses a cartilaginous framework (cartilago auriculae) that forms a funnel-shaped receptor for acoustic vibrations.

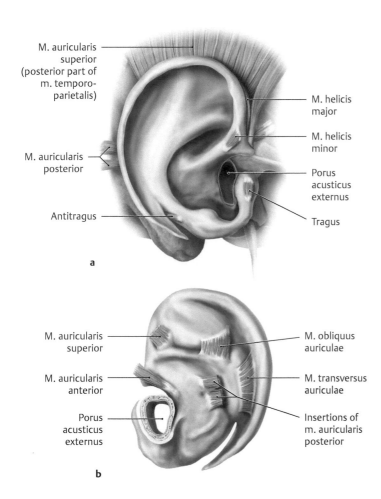

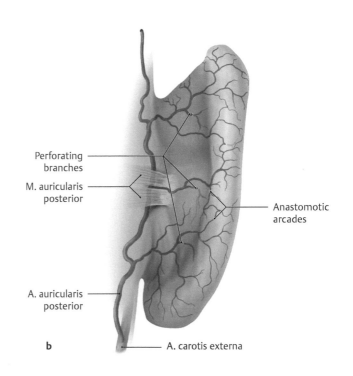

C Cartilage and muscles of the auricle
a Lateral view of the external surface. **b** Medial view of the posterior surface of the right ear.
The skin (removed here) is closely applied to the elastic cartilago auriculae (shown in light blue). The muscles of the ear are classified as mm. faciei and, like the other members of this group, are supplied by the n. facialis. Prominent in other mammals, the mm. auriculares are vestigial in humans, with no significant function.

D Arterial supply of the right auricle
Lateral view (**a**) and posterior view (**b**).
The proximal and medial portions of the laterally directed anterior surface of the ear are supplied by the rr. auriculares anteriores, which arise from the a. temporalis superficialis (see p. 101). The other parts of the ear are supplied by branches of the a. auricularis posterior, which arises from the a. carotis externa. These vessels are linked by extensive anastomoses, so operations on the auris externa are unlikely to compromise the auricular blood supply. The copious blood flow through the auricula contributes to temperature regulation: dilation of the vessels helps dissipate heat through the skin. The lack of insulating fat predisposes the ear to frostbite, which is particularly common in the upper third of the auricula. The lymphatic drainage and innervation of the auricula are covered in the next unit.

143

5.2 External Ear: Auricula, Auditory Canal (Meatus Acusticus Externus), and Tympanic Membrane (Membrana Tympanica)

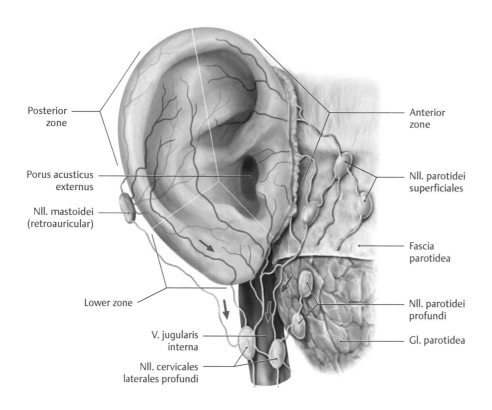

Posterior zone

Porus acusticus externus

Nll. mastoidei (retroauricular)

Lower zone

V. jugularis interna

Nll. cervicales laterales profundi

Anterior zone

Nll. parotidei superficiales

Fascia parotidea

Nll. parotidei profundi

Gl. parotidea

A Auricula and meatus acusticus externus: lymphatic drainage and regional groups of nodi lymphoidei
Right ear, oblique lateral view. The cartilaginous framework and blood supply of the ear were described in the previous unit. The lymphatic drainage of the ear is divided into three zones, all of which drain directly or indirectly into the nodi lymphoidei cervicales laterales profundi along the v. jugularis interna. The lower zone drains directly into the nodi lymphoidei cervicales laterales profundi. The anterior zone first drains into the nodi parotidei superficiales, the posterior zone into the nodi mastoidei.

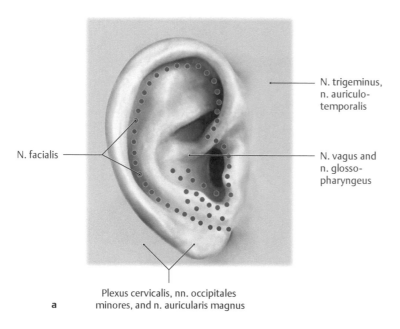

N. facialis

N. trigeminus, n. auriculo-temporalis

N. vagus and n. glosso-pharyngeus

Plexus cervicalis, nn. occipitales minores, and n. auricularis magnus

a

N. trigeminus, n. auriculo-temporalis

N. vagus and n. glosso-pharyngeus

N. facialis

Plexus cervicalis, nn. occipitales minores, and n. auricularis magnus

b

B Sensory innervation of the auricle
Right ear, lateral view (**a**) and posterior view (**b**). The auricular region has a complex nerve supply because, developmentally, it is located at the boundary between nn. craniales (pharyngeal arch nerves) and branches of the plexus cervicalis. Four nn. craniales contribute to the innervation of the auricula:

- N. trigeminus (CN V),
- N. facialis (CN VII; the skin area that receives sensory innervation from the n. facialis is not precisely known)
- N. glossopharyngeus (CN IX) and n. vagus (CN X)

Two branches of the **plexus cervicalis** are involved:

- N. occipitalis minor (C_2)
- N. auricularis magnus (C_2, C_3)

Note: Because the n. vagus (see pp. 132 and 141) contributes to the innervation of the meatus acusticus externus (r. auricularis, see below), mechanical cleaning of the meatus acusticus (by inserting an aural speculum or by irrigating the ear) may evoke coughing and nausea. The r. auricularis of the n. vagus passes through the canaliculus mastoideus and through a space between the proc. mastoideus and the pars tympanica ossis temporalis (fissura tympanomastoidea, see p. 29) to the auris externa and porus acusticus externus. The meatus acusticus receives sensory fibers from the n. glossopharyngeus through its r. communicans cum ramo auriculare nervi vagi.

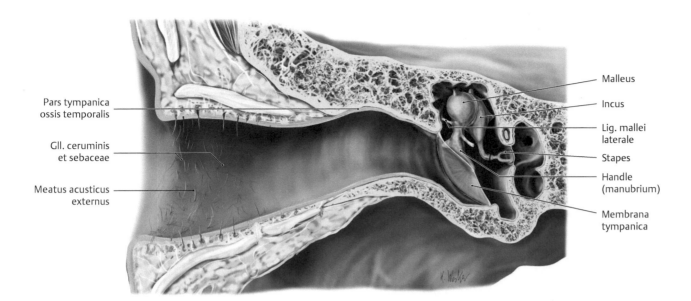

Pars tympanica ossis temporalis

Gll. ceruminis et sebaceae

Meatus acusticus externus

Malleus

Incus

Lig. mallei laterale

Stapes

Handle (manubrium)

Membrana tympanica

C Meatus acusticus externus, membrana tympanica, and cavitas tympani

Right ear, coronal section, anterior view. The membrana tympanica (eardrum, see **E**) separates the meatus acusticus internus from the cavitas tympani, which is part of the auris media (see p. 146). The meatus acusticus externus is an S-shaped tunnel (see **D**) that is approximately 3 cm long with an average diameter of 0.6 cm. The outer third of the ear canal is cartilaginous. The inner two-thirds of the canal are osseous, the wall being formed by the pars tympanica of the os temporale. The cartilaginous part in particular bears numerous sebaceous and cerumen glands beneath the keratinized stratified squamous epithelium. The glandula ceruminis produce a watery secretion that combines with the sebum and sloughed epithelial cells to form a protective barrier (cerumen, "earwax") that screens out foreign bodies and keeps the epithelium from drying out. If the cerumen absorbs water (e.g., water in the ear canal after swimming), it may obstruct the meatus acusticus (cerumen impaction), temporarily causing a partial loss of hearing.

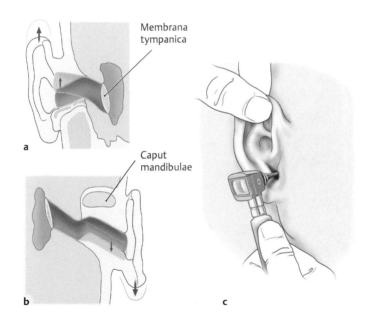

Membrana tympanica

Caput mandibulae

a

b

c

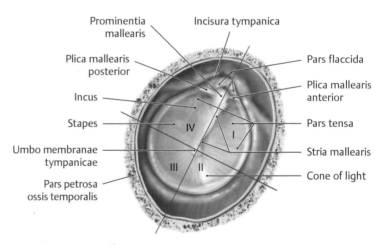

Prominentia mallearis

Incisura tympanica

Plica mallearis posterior

Incus

Stapes

Umbo membranae tympanicae

Pars petrosa ossis temporalis

Pars flaccida

Plica mallearis anterior

Pars tensa

Stria mallearis

Cone of light

D Curvature of the meatus acusticus externus

Right ear, anterior view (**a**) and transverse section (**b**).
The meatus acusticus externus is most curved in its cartilaginous portion. It is important for the clinician to know how the meatus acusticus is curved. When the membrana tympanica is inspected with an otoscope, the auricula should be pulled backward and upward in order to straighten the cartilaginous part of the meatus acusticus so that the speculum of the otoscope can be introduced (**c**).
Note the proximity of the cartilaginous anterior wall of the meatus acusticus externus to the art. temporomandibularis. This allows the examiner to palpate movements of the caput mandibulae by inserting the small finger into the outer part of the meatus acusticus.

E Tympanic membrane

Right membrana tympanica, lateral view. The healthy membrana tympanica has a pearly gray color and an oval shape with an average surface area of approximately 75 mm². It consists of a lax portion, the *pars flaccida* (Shrapnell membrane), and a larger taut portion, the *pars tensa*, which is drawn inward at its center to form the umbo ("navel") membranae tympanicae. The umbo marks the lower tip of the handle (manubrium) of the malleus, which is attached to the membrana tympanica all along its length. It is visible through the pars tensa as a light-colored streak (stria mallearis). The membrana tympanica is divided into four quadrants in a clockwise direction: anterosuperior (I), anteroinferior (II), posteroinferior (III), posterosuperior (IV). The boundary lines of the quadrants are the stria mallearis and a line intersecting it perpendicularly at the umbo. The quadrants of the membrana tympanica are clinically important because they are used in describing the location of lesions. The function of the membrana tympanica is reviewed on pp. 142 and 148. A triangular area of reflected light can be seen in the anteroinferior quadrant of a normal membrana tympanica. The location of this "cone of light" is helpful in evaluating the tension of the membrana tympanica.

5.3 Middle Ear (Auris Media): Tympanic Cavity (Cavitas Tympani) and Pharyngotympanic Tube (Tuba Auditiva)

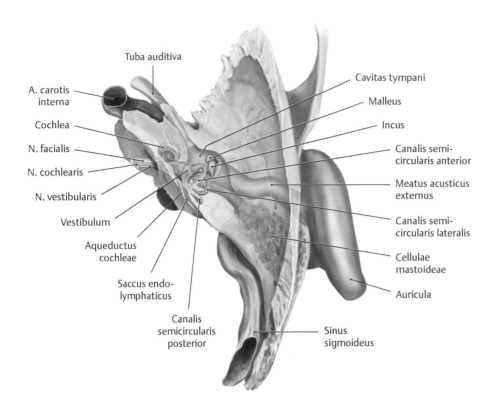

Tuba auditiva

A. carotis interna

Cochlea

N. facialis

N. cochlearis

N. vestibularis

Vestibulum

Aqueductus cochleae

Saccus endo-lymphaticus

Canalis semicircularis posterior

Cavitas tympani

Malleus

Incus

Canalis semi-circularis anterior

Meatus acusticus externus

Canalis semi-circularis lateralis

Cellulae mastoideae

Auricula

Sinus sigmoideus

A The auris media and associated structures

Right pars petrosa ossis temporalis, superior view. The auris media (light blue) is located within the pars petrosa ossis temporalis between the auris externa (yellow) and auris interna (green). The cavitas tympani of the auris media contains the chain of ossicula auditoria, of which the malleus (hammer) and incus (anvil) are visible here. The cavitas tympani communicates anteriorly with the pharynx via the tuba auditiva, and it communicates posteriorly with the cellulae mastoideae. Infections can spread from the pharynx to the cellulae mastoideae by this route (see **C**).

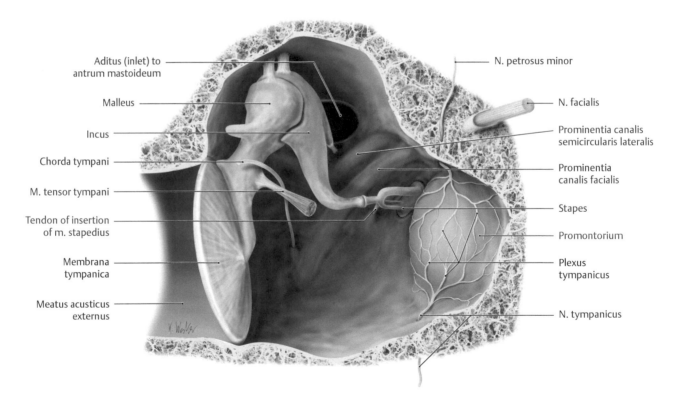

Aditus (inlet) to antrum mastoideum

Malleus

Incus

Chorda tympani

M. tensor tympani

Tendon of insertion of m. stapedius

Membrana tympanica

Meatus acusticus externus

N. petrosus minor

N. facialis

Prominentia canalis semicircularis lateralis

Prominentia canalis facialis

Stapes

Promontorium

Plexus tympanicus

N. tympanicus

B Walls of the cavitas tympani

Anterior view with the anterior wall removed. The cavitas tympani is a slightly oblique space that is bounded by six walls:

- Lateral wall (paries membranaceus): boundary with the auris externa; formed largely by the membrana tympanica.
- Medial wall (paries labyrinthicus): boundary with the auris interna; formed largely by the promontorium, or the bony eminence, overlying the basal turn of the cochlea.

- Inferior wall (paries jugularis): forms the floor of the cavitas tympani and borders on the bulbus superior venae jugularis.
- Posterior wall (paries mastoideus): borders on the cellulae of the proc. mastoideus, communicating with the cells through the aditus (inlet) of the antrum mastoideum.
- Superior wall (paries tegmentalis): forms the roof of the cavitas tympani.
- Anterior wall (paries caroticus, removed here): includes the opening to the tuba auditiva and borders on the canalis caroticus.

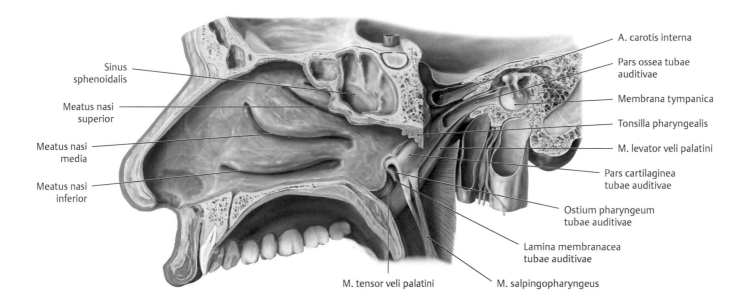

C Cavitas tympani: clinically important anatomical relationships
Oblique sagittal section showing the medial wall of the cavitas tympani (cf. **B**). The anatomical relationships of the cavitas tympani are particularly important in treating chronic suppurative otitis media. During this inflammation of the auris media, pathogenic bacteria may spread upward to adjacent regions. For example, bacteria may spread upward through the paries tegmentalis of the cavitas tympani into the fossa cranii media (inciting meningitis or a cerebral abscess, especially of the lobus temporalis); they may invade the cellulae mastoideae (mastoiditis) or sinus sigmoideus (sinus thrombosis); they may pass through the air cells of the apex partis petrosae ossis temporalis and enter the CSF space, causing abducent paralysis, n. trigeminus irritation, or visual disturbances (Gradenigo syndrome); or they may invade the canalis nervi facialis, resulting in facial paralysis.

D Tuba auditiva
Medial view of the right half of the head. The tuba auditiva (auditory tube) creates an open channel between the auris media and pharynx. One-third of the tube is bony and two-thirds are cartilaginous. The pars ossea of the tube is located in the pars petrosa ossis temporalis, and the pars cartilaginea continues onward to the pharynx, where it expands into a funnel-shaped orifice. As it expands, it forms a hook (hamulus) which is attached to a membranous part (lamina membranacea) that enlarges toward the pharynx. The tuba auditiva also opens during swallowing. Air passing through the tube serves to equalize the air pressure on the two sides of the membrana tympanica. This equalization is essential for maintaining normal membrana tympanica mobility, which, in turn, is necessary for normal hearing. The tuba auditiva is opened by the muscles of the palatum molle (mm. tensor veli palatini and levator veli palatini) and by the m. salpingopharyngeus, which is part of the m. constrictor pharyngis superior. The fibers of the m. tensor veli palatini arising from the lamina membranacea of the tuba auditiva are of special significance: When the m. tensor veli palatini tenses the palatum molle during swallowing, its fibers attached to the lamina membranacea simultaneously open the tuba auditiva. The tuba auditiva is lined with ciliated respiratory epithelium whose cilia beat toward the pharynx, thus inhibiting the passage of microorganisms into the auris media. If this nonspecific protective mechanism fails, bacteria may migrate up the tuba auditiva and incite a purulent auris media infection (cf. C).

5.4 Middle Ear: Auditory Ossicles (Ossicula Auditoria) and Tympanic Cavity (Cavitas Tympani)

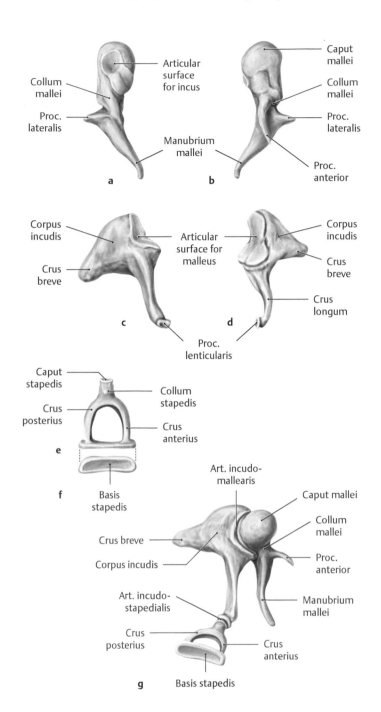

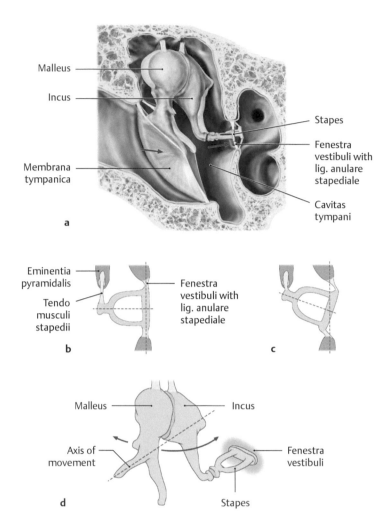

A Ossicula auditoria

The ossicula auditoria of the left ear. The ossicular chain consists of three small bones in the auris media (chain function is described in **B**). It establishes an articular connection from the membrana tympani to the fenestra vestibuli and consists of the following bones:

- Malleus ("hammer")
- Incus ("anvil")
- Stapes ("stirrup")

a, b Malleus: posterior view and anterior view
c, d Incus: medial view and anterolateral view
e, f Stapes: superior view and medial view
g Medial view of the ossicular chain

Note the articulations between the malleus and incus (art. incudomallearis) and between the incus and stapes (art. incudostapedialis).

B Function of the ossicular chain

Anterior view.

a Sound waves (periodic pressure fluctuations in the air) set the membrana tympanica into vibration. The ossicular chain transmits the vibrations of the membrana tympanica (and thus the sound waves) to the fenestra vestibuli, which in turn communicates them to an aqueous medium, the perilympha. While sound waves encounter very little resistance in air, they encounter considerably higher impedance when they reach the fluid interface of the inner ear (perilympha). The sound waves must therefore be amplified ("impedance matching"). The difference in surface area between the membrana tympanica and fenestra vestibuli increases the sound pressure by a factor of 17, and this is augmented by the 1.3-fold mechanical advantage of the lever action of the ossicular chain. Thus, in passing from the membrana tympanica to the auris interna, the sound pressure is amplified by a factor of 22. If the ossicular chain fails to transform the sound pressure between the membrana tympanica and basis stapedis (footplate), the patient will experience conductive hearing loss of magnitude approximately 20 dB.

b, c Sound waves impinging on the membrana tympanica induce motion in the ossicular chain, causing a tilting movement of the stapes (**b** normal position, **c** tilted position). The lig. anulare of the stapes forms a mobile connection between the borders of the foramen ovale and the stapes. The movements of the basis stapedis then induce corresponding waves in the fluid column in the inner ear.

d The movements of the ossicular chain are essentially rocking movements (the dashed line indicates the axis of the movements, the arrows indicate their direction). Two muscles affect the mobility of the ossicular chain: the m. tensor tympani and the m. stapedius (see **C**).

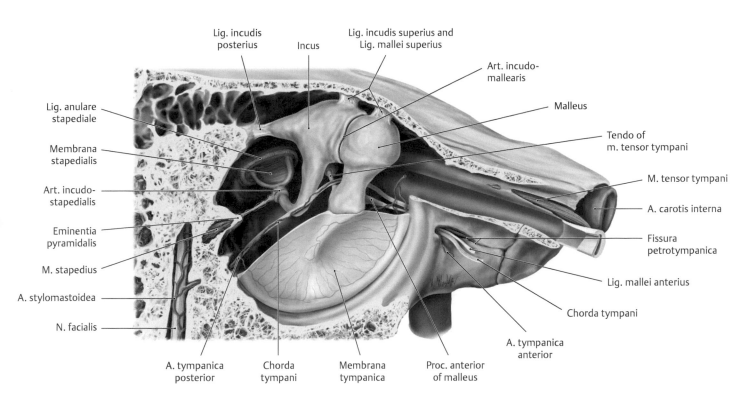

Lig. incudis posterius
Incus
Lig. incudis superius and Lig. mallei superius
Art. incudo-mallearis
Malleus
Tendo of m. tensor tympani
M. tensor tympani
A. carotis interna
Fissura petrotympanica
Lig. mallei anterius
Chorda tympani
A. tympanica anterior

Lig. anulare stapediale
Membrana stapedialis
Art. incudo-stapedialis
Eminentia pyramidalis
M. stapedius
A. stylomastoidea
N. facialis

A. tympanica posterior
Chorda tympani
Membrana tympanica
Proc. anterior of malleus

C Ossicular chain in the cavitas tympani
Lateral view of the right ear. The joints and their stabilizing ligaments can be seen. The two muscles of the middle ear—the m. stapedius and m. tensor tympani—can also be identified. The *m. stapedius* (innervated by the n. stapedius branch of the n. facialis) inserts on the stapes. When it contracts, it stiffens the sound conduction apparatus and decreases sound transmission to the auris media. This filtering function is believed to be particularly important at high sound frequencies ("high-pass filter"). When sound is transmitted into the auris media through a probe placed in the meatus acusticus externus, one can measure the action of the m. stapedius (stapedius reflex test) by measuring the change in acoustic impedance (i.e., the amplification of the sound waves). Contraction of the *m. tensor tympani* (Innervation: n. musculi tensoris tympani, V3) stiffens the membrana tympanica, thereby reducing the transmission of sound. Both muscles undergo a reflex contraction in response to loud acoustic stimuli.

Note: The chorda tympani, which contains gustatory fibers for the anterior two-thirds of the tongue, passes through the middle ear without a bony covering (making it susceptible to injury during otological surgery).

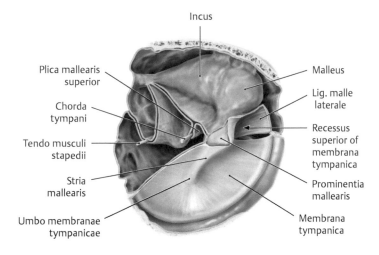

Incus
Plica mallearis superior
Chorda tympani
Tendo musculi stapedii
Stria mallearis
Umbo membranae tympanicae

Malleus
Lig. malle laterale
Recessus superior of membrana tympanica
Prominentia mallearis
Membrana tympanica

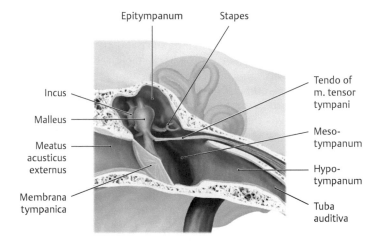

Epitympanum
Stapes
Incus
Malleus
Meatus acusticus externus
Membrana tympanica

Tendo of m. tensor tympani
Meso-tympanum
Hypo-tympanum
Tuba auditiva

D Tunica mucosa cavitatis tympani
Posterolateral view with the membrana tympanica partially removed. The cavitas tympani and the structures it contains (ossicular chain, tendons, nerves) are covered with mucosa that is raised into folds and deepened into depressions conforming to the covered surfaces. The epithelium consists mainly of a simple squamous type, with areas of ciliated columnar cells and goblet cells. Because the cavitas tympani communicates directly with the respiratory tract through the tuba auditiva, it can also be interpreted as a specialized sinus paranasalis. Like the sinuses, it is susceptible to frequent infections (otitis media).

E Clinically important levels of the cavitas tympani
The cavitas tympani is divided into three levels in relation to the membrana tympanica:

• The epitympanum (recessus epitympanicus, attic) above the membrana tympanica
• The mesotympanum medial to the membrana tympanica
• The hypotympanum (hypotympanic recess) below the membrana tympanica

The epitympanum communicates with the cellulae mastoideae, and the hypotympanum communicates with the tuba auditiva.

5.5   Inner Ear (Auris Interna): Overview

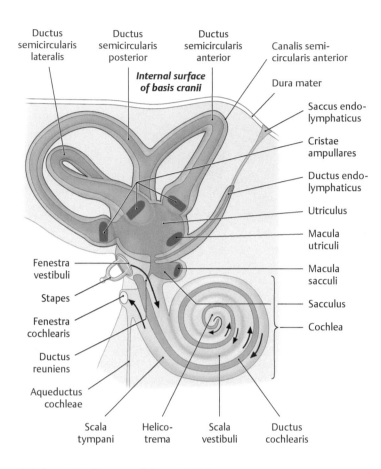

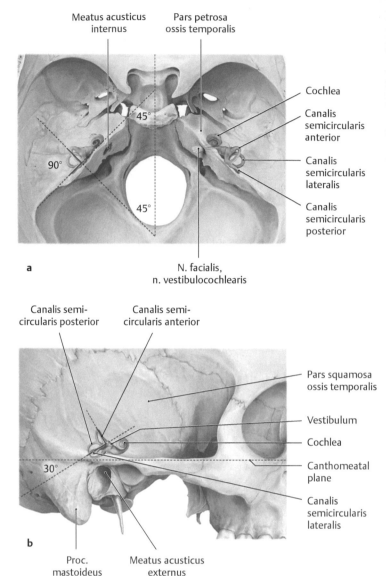

a   Superior view of the pars petrosa ossis temporalis.

b   Right lateral

a   N. facialis, n. vestibulocochlearis

A Schematic diagram of the auris interna

The inner ear is embedded within the pars petrosa of the os temporale (see **B**) and contains the auditory and vestibular apparatus for hearing and balance (see p. 146 ff). It comprises a *labyrinthus membranaceus* contained within a similarly shaped *labyrinthus osseus*. The **auditory apparatus** consists of the labyrinthus cochlearis with the membranous *ductus cochlearis*. The membranous duct and its bony shell make up the *cochlea*, which contains the sensory epithelium of the auditory apparatus (organum spirale, or *organ of Corti*). The **vestibular apparatus** includes the labyrinthus vestibularis with three *canales semicirculares* (ductus semicirculares), a *sacculus*, and an *utriculus*, each of which contains sensory epithelium. While each of the membranous ductus semicirculares is encased in its own bony shell (canalis semicircularis), the utriculus and sacculus are contained in a common bony capsule, the *vestibulum*. The cavity of the *labyrinthus osseus* is filled with perilympha (*spatium perilymphaticum*, beige), whose composition reflects its being an ultrafiltrate of blood. The spatium perilymphaticum is connected to the spatium subarachnoideum by the aqueductus cochleae (= perilymphatic duct). It ends at the external basis cranii medial to the fossa jugularis. The *labyrinthus membranaceus* "floats" in the labyrinthus osseus, being loosely attached to it by connective-tissue fibers. It is filled with endolympha (*spatium endolymphaticum*, blue-green), whose ionic composition corresponds to that of intracellular fluid. The spatia endolymphatica of the auditory and vestibular apparatus communicate with each other through the *ductus reuniens* and are connected by the *ductus endolymphaticus* to the saccus endolymphaticus, an epidural sac at the looks like inner surface of the pars petrosa ossis temporalis between meatus acusticus internus and sulcus sinus sigmoidei in which the endolympha is absorbed.

B Projection of the auris interna onto the bony skull

a Superior view of the pars petrosa ossis temporalis. **b** Right lateral view of the pars squamosa ossis temporalis.

The apex of the cochlea is directed anteriorly and laterally—not upward as might be intuitively expected. The bony canales semicirculares are oriented at an approximately 45° angle to the cardinal body planes (coronal, transverse, and sagittal). It is important to know this arrangement when interpreting thin-slice CT scans of the pars petrosa.

Note: The location of the canales semicirculares is of clinical importance in thermal function tests of the vestibular apparatus. The canalis semicircularis lateralis (horizontal) is directed 30° forward and upward (see b). If the head of the supine patient is elevated by 30°, the canalis semicircularis lateralis will assume a vertical alignment. Since warm fluids tend to rise, irrigating the meatus acusticus externus with warm (44° C) or cool (30° C) water (relative to the normal body temperature) can induce a thermal current in the endolympha of the canalis semicircularis, causing the patient to manifest vestibular nystagmus (jerky eye movements, vestibulo-ocular reflex). Because head movements always stimulate both vestibular apparatuses, caloric testing is the only method of *separately* testing the function of each vestibular apparatus (important in the diagnosis of unexplained vertigo).

Ductus semi-circularis anterior
N. ampullaris anterior
Pars superior ganglii vestibularis
N. vestibulo-cochlearis, n. vestibularis
N. facialis
Aqueductus vestibuli
Pars inferior ganglii vestibularis
Dura mater
R. communicans cochlearis
Saccus endo-lymphaticus
N. intermedius
N. ampullaris lateralis
N. vestibulo-cochlearis, n. cochlearis
Crus membranacea commune
N. saccularis
N. utricularis
N. ampullaris posterior
Ductus semicircularis lateralis
Modiolus cochleae
Ductus semicircularis posterior
Ganglion spirale cochleae
Ampulla membrana-cea posterior
Fenestra vestibuli
Fenestra cochleae

C Innervation of the labyrinthus membranaceus
Right ear, anterior view. **Afferent impulses** from the receptor organs of the utriculus, sacculus, and canales semicirculares (i.e., the **vestibular apparatus**) are first relayed by dendritic (peripheral) processes to the two-part *ganglion vestibulare* (partes superior and inferior), which contains the cell bodies of the afferent neurons (bipolar ganglion cells). Their central processes form the *n. vestibularis* part of the *n. vestibulocochlearis* through the meatus acusticus internus and the angulus pontocerebellaris to the truncus encephali.

Afferent impulses from the receptor organs of the cochlea (i.e., the **auditory apparatus**) are first transmitted by dendritic (peripheral) processes to the *ganglion spirale cochleae*, which contains the cell bodies of the bipolar ganglion cells. They are located in the central bony core of the cochlea (modiolus cochleae). Their central processes form the *n. cochlearis* part of the *n. vestibulocochlearis*.
Note also the section of the n. facialis with its parasympathetic fibers (n. intermedius) within the meatus acusticus internus (see D).

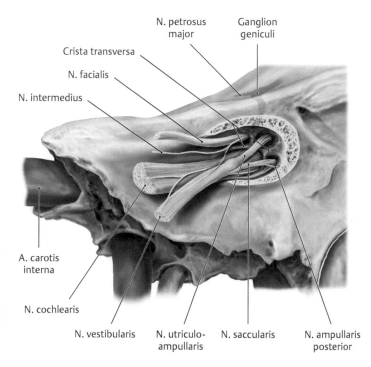

N. petrosus major
Ganglion geniculi
Crista transversa
N. facialis
N. intermedius
A. carotis interna
N. cochlearis
N. vestibularis
N. utriculo-ampullaris
N. saccularis
N. ampullaris posterior

D Passage of nervi craniales through the right meatus acusticus internus
Posterior oblique view of the fundus of the internal acoustic meatus. The approximately 1 cm long internal auditory canal begins at the internal acoustic meatus on the posterior wall of the petrous bone. It contains

- the n. vestibulocochlearis with its n. cochlearis and n. vestibularis parts,
- the markedly thinner n. facialis with its parasympathetic fibers (n. intermedius), and
- the a. and v. labyrinthi (not shown).

Given the close proximity of the n. vestibulocochlearis and n. facialis in the bony canal, a tumor of the n. vestibulocochlearis (*acoustic neuroma*) may exert pressure on the n. facialis, leading to peripheral facial paralysis (see also p. 125). Acoustic neuroma is a benign tumor that originates from the Schwann cells of vestibular fibers, and so it would be more accurate to call it a *vestibular schwannoma* (see also p. 128). Tumor growth always begins in the meatus acusticus internus; as the tumor enlarges it may grow into the angulus pontocerebellaris. Acute, unilateral auris interna dysfunction with hearing loss (sudden sensorineural hearing loss), often accompanied by tinnitus, typically reflects an underlying vascular disturbance (vasospasm of the a. labyrinthi causing decreased blood flow).

5.6   Ear: Auditory Apparatus

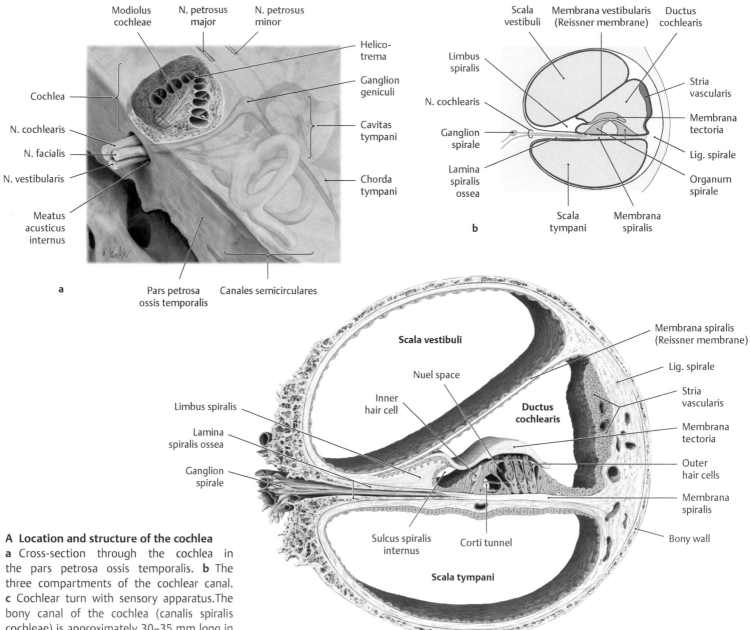

Modiolus cochleae
N. petrosus major
N. petrosus minor
Helico-trema
Ganglion geniculi
Cochlea
Cavitas tympani
N. cochlearis
N. facialis
N. vestibularis
Chorda tympani
Meatus acusticus internus
a
Pars petrosa ossis temporalis
Canales semicirculares

Scala vestibuli
Membrana vestibularis (Reissner membrane)
Ductus cochlearis
Limbus spiralis
Stria vascularis
N. cochlearis
Membrana tectoria
Ganglion spirale
Lig. spirale
Lamina spiralis ossea
Organum spirale
Scala tympani
Membrana spiralis
b

Scala vestibuli
Nuel space
Membrana spiralis (Reissner membrane)
Inner hair cell
Lig. spirale
Limbus spiralis
Stria vascularis
Ductus cochlearis
Lamina spiralis ossea
Membrana tectoria
Ganglion spirale
Outer hair cells
Membrana spiralis
Sulcus spiralis internus
Corti tunnel
Bony wall
Scala tympani
c

A Location and structure of the cochlea

a Cross-section through the cochlea in the pars petrosa ossis temporalis. **b** The three compartments of the cochlear canal. **c** Cochlear turn with sensory apparatus. The bony canal of the cochlea (canalis spiralis cochleae) is approximately 30–35 mm long in the adult. It makes 2½ turns around its bony axis, the *modiolus cochleae*, which is permeated by branched cavities and contains the ganglion spirale cochleae (cell bodies of the afferent neurons). The base of the cochlea is directed toward the imeatus acusticus internus (**a**). A cross-section through the canalis spiralis cochleae displays three membranous compartments arranged in three levels (**b**). The upper and lower compartments, the *scala vestibuli* and *scala tympani*, each contain peri-lympha, while the middle level, the *ductus cochlearis* (scala media), contains endolympha. The spatia perilymphatica are interconnected at the apex by the *helicotrema*, while the spatium endolymphaticum ends blindly at the apex. The ductus cochlearis, which is triangular in cross-section, is separated from the scala vestibuli by the *membrana vestibularis* (*Reissner membrane*) and from the scala tympani by the *membrana spiralis*. The membrana spiralis

represents a bony projection of the modiolus cochleae (*lamina spiralis ossea*) and widens steadily from the basis cochleae to the apex. High frequencies (up to 20,000 Hz) are perceived by the narrow portions of the membrana spiralis while low frequencies (down to about 200 Hz) are perceived by its broader portions (*tonotopic organization*). The membrana spiralis and lamina spiralis ossea form the floor of the ductus cochlearis, upon which the actual organ of hearing, the organum spirale (organ of Corti), is located. This organ consists of a system of sensory cells and supporting cells covered by an acellular gelatinous flap, the *membrana tectoria*. The sensory cells (inner and outer hair cells) are the receptors of the organ of Corti (**c**). These cells bear approximately 50–100 stereocilia, and on their apical surface synapse on their basal side with

the endings of afferent and efferent neurons. They have the ability to transform mechanical energy into electrochemical potentials (see below). A magnified cross-sectional view of a cochlear turn (**c**) also reveals the *stria vascularis*, a layer of vascularized epithelium in which the endolympha is formed. This endolympha fills the labyrinthus membranaceus (appearing here as the ductus cochlearis, which is part of the labyrinth). The organ of Corti is located on the membrana spiralis. It transforms the energy of the acoustic traveling wave into electrical impulses, which are then carried to the brain by the n. cochlearis. The principal cell of signal transduction is the inner hair cell. The function of the membrana spiralis is to transmit acoustic waves to the inner hair cell, which transforms them into impulses that are received and relayed by the cochlear ganglion.

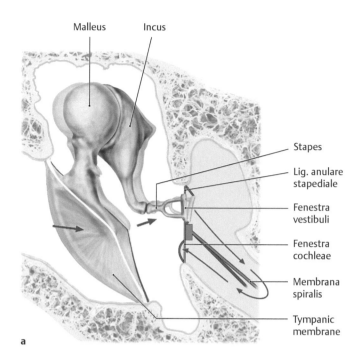

a

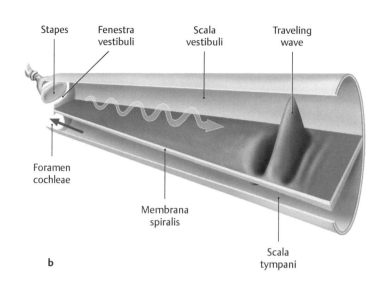

b

B Sound conduction during hearing

a Sound conduction from the auris media to the auris interna: Sound waves in the air deflect the membrana tympanica, whose vibrations are conducted by the ossicular chain to the fenestra vestibularis. The sound pressure induces motion of the oval window membrane, whose vibrations are in turn, transmitted through the perilymph to the membrana spiralis of the auris interna (see **b**). The fenestra cochleae equalizes pressures between the auris media and internum.

b Formation of a traveling wave in the cochlea: The sound wave begins at the oval window and travels up the scala vestibuli to the apex of the cochlea ("traveling wave"). The amplitude of the traveling wave gradually increases as a function of the sound frequency and reaches a maximum value at particular sites (shown greatly exaggerated in the drawing). These are the sites where the receptors of the organum spirale are stimulated and signal transduction occurs. To understand this process, one must first grasp the structure of the organum spirale (the actual organ of hearing), which is depicted in **C**.

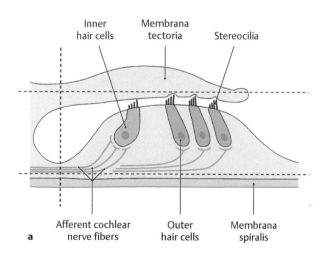

a

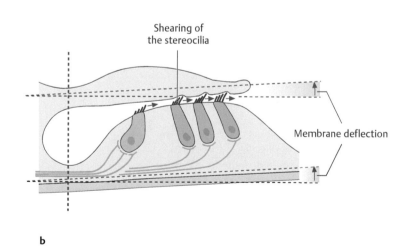

b

C Organum spirale at rest (a) and deflected by a traveling wave (b)
The traveling wave is generated by vibrations of the fenestra vestibuli membrane (cf. **Bb**). At each site that is associated with a particular sound frequency, the traveling wave causes a maximum deflection of the membrana spiralis and in turn of the membrana tectoria, setting up shearing movements between the two membranes. These shearing movements cause the stereocilia on the outer hair cells to bend. In response, the hair cells actively change their length, thereby increasing the local amplitude of the traveling wave. This additionally bends the stereocilia of the *inner* hair cells, stimulating the release of glutamate at their basal pole. The release of this substance generates an excitatory potential on the afferent nerve fibers, which is transmitted to the brain.

5.7 Inner Ear: Vestibular Apparatus

A Structure of the vestibular apparatus

The vestibular apparatus is the organ of balance. It consists of the membranous ductus semicirculares, which contain sensory ridges (cristae ampullares) in their dilated portions (ampullae), and of the sacculus and utriculus with their macular organs (their location in the pars petrosa ossis temporalis is shown in B, p. 144). The sensory organs in the ductus semicirculares respond to angular acceleration while the macular organs, which have an approximately vertical and horizontal orientation, respond to horizontal (macula utriculi) and vertical (macula sacculi) linear acceleration, as well as to gravitational forces.

B Structure of the ampulla and crista ampullaris

Cross-section through the ampulla of a canalis semicircularis. Each canal has a bulbous expansion at one end (ampulla) that is traversed by a connective tissue ridge with sensory epithelium (crista ampullaris). Extending above the crista ampullaris is a gelatinous cupula ampullaris, which is attached to the roof of the ampulla. Each of the sensory cells of the crista ampullaris (approximately 7000 in all) exhibits one long kinocilium and approximately 80 shorter stereocilia on their apical pole, which project into the cupula. When the head is rotated in the plane of a particular canalis semicircularis, the inertial lag of the endolympha acauses a deflection of the cupula, which in turn causes a bowing of the stereocilia. The sensory cells are either depolarized (excitation) or hyperpolarized (inhibition), depending on the direction of ciliary displacement (see details in **E**).

C Structure of the utricular and saccular maculae

The maculae are thickened oval areas in the epithelial lining of the utriculus and sacculus, each averaging 2 mm in diameter and containing arrays of sensory and supporting cells. Like the sensory cells of the crista ampullaris, those of the macular organs bear specialized stereocilia, which project into an otolithic membrane (membrana statoconiorum). The latter consists of a gelatinous layer, similar to the cupula ampullaris, but it has calcium carbonate crystals or otoliths (*statoconia*) embedded in its surface. With their high specific gravity, these crystals exert traction on the gelatinous mass in response to linear acceleration, and this induces shearing movements of the cilia. The sensory cells are either depolarized or hyperpolarized by the movement, depending on the orientation of the cilia. There are two distinct categories of vestibular hair cells (type I and type II); type I cells (light red) are goblet-shaped.

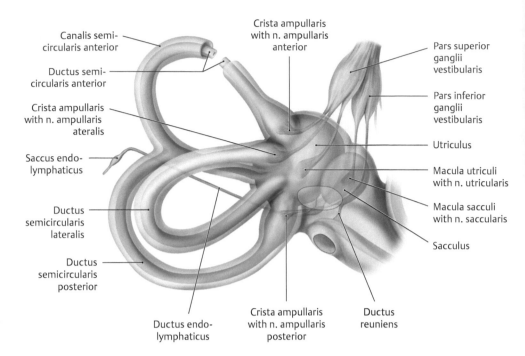

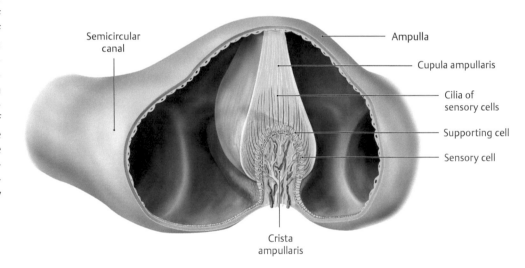

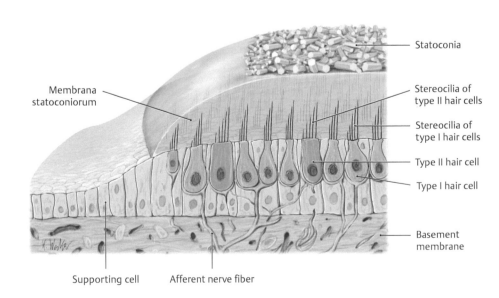

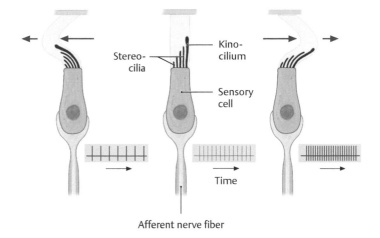

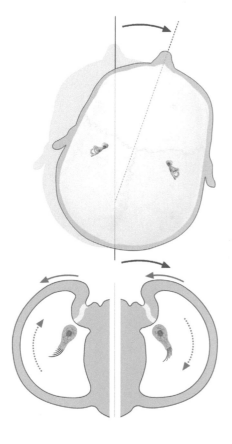

D Stimulus transduction in the vestibular sensory cells

Each of the sensory cells of the maculae and cristae ampullares bears on its apical surface one long kinocilium and approximately 80 stereocilia of graduated lengths, forming an array that resembles a pipe organ. This arrangement results in a polar differentiation of the sensory cells. The cilia are straight while in a resting state. When the stereocilia are deflected toward the kinocilium, the sensory cell depolarizes and the frequency of action potentials (discharge rate of impulses) is increased (right side of diagram). When the stereocilia are deflected away from the kinocilium, the cell hyperpolarizes and the discharge rate is decreased (left side of diagram). This mechanism regulates the release of the transmitter glutamate at the basal pole of the sensory cell, thereby controlling the activation of the afferent nerve fiber (depolarization stimulates glutamate release, and hyperpolarization inhibits it). In this way the brain receives information on the magnitude and direction of movements and changes of position.

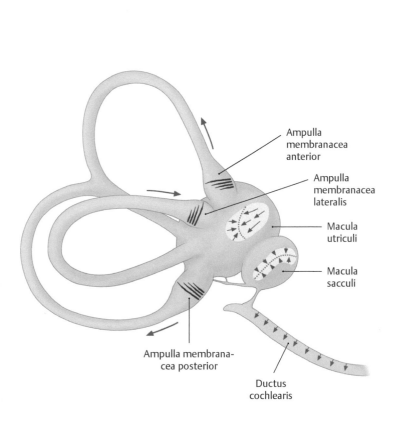

E Specialized orientations of the stereocilia in the vestibular apparatus (cristae ampullares and maculae)

Because the stimulation of the sensory cells by deflection of the stereocilia *away from* or *toward* the kinocilium is what initiates signal transduction, the spatial orientation of the cilia must be specialized to ensure that every position in space and every movement of the head stimulates or inhibits certain receptors. The ciliary arrangement shown here ensures that every direction in space will correlate with the maximum sensitivity of a particular receptor field. The arrows indicate the polarity of the cilia (i.e., each of the arrowheads points in the direction of the kinocilium in that particular field).

Note that the sensory cells show an opposite, reciprocal arrangement in the sensory fields of the utriculus and sacculus.

F Interaction of contralateral canales semicirculares during head rotation

When the head rotates to the right (red arrow), the endolympha flows to the left because of its inertial mass (solid blue arrow, taking the head as the reference point). Owing to the alignment of the stereocilia, the left and right ductus semicirculares are stimulated in opposite fashion. On the right side, the stereocilia are deflected toward the kinocilium (dotted arrow; the discharge rate increases). On the left side, the stereocilia are deflected away from the kinocilium (dotted arrow; the discharge rate decreases). This arrangement heightens the sensitivity to stimuli by increasing the stimulus contrast between the two sides. The difference between the decreased firing rate on one side and the increased firing rate on the other side enhances the perception of the kinetic stimulus.

5.8 Ear: Blood Supply

A Origin of the principal arteries of the cavitas tympani

Except for the aa. caroticotympanicae, which arise from the pars petrosa of the a. carotis interna, all of the vessels that supply blood to the cavitas tympani arise from the a. carotis externa. The vessels have many anastomoses with one another and reach the ossicula auditoria, for example, through folds of mucosa. The ossicula are also traversed by intraosseous vessels.

Artery	Origin	Distribution
Aa. caroticotympanicae	A. carotis interna	Tuba auditiva and paries caroticus of the cavitas tympani
A. stylomastoidea	A. auricularis posterior	Paries mastoideus of the cavitas tympani, cellulae mastoideae, m. stapedius, stapes
A. tympanica inferior	A. pharyngea ascendens	Paries jugularis of the cavitas tympani, promontorium
A. auricularis profunda	A. maxillaris	Membrana tympanica, paries jugularis of the cavitas tympani
A. tympanica posterior	A. stylomastoidea (alternatively: a. auricularis posterior, see **Ab**, p. 98)	Chorda tympani, membrana tympanica, malleus
A. tympanica superior	A. meningea media	M. tensor tympani, paries tegmentalis of the cavitas tympani, stapes
A. tympanica anterior	A. maxillaris	Membrana tympanica, antrum mastoideum, malleus, incus

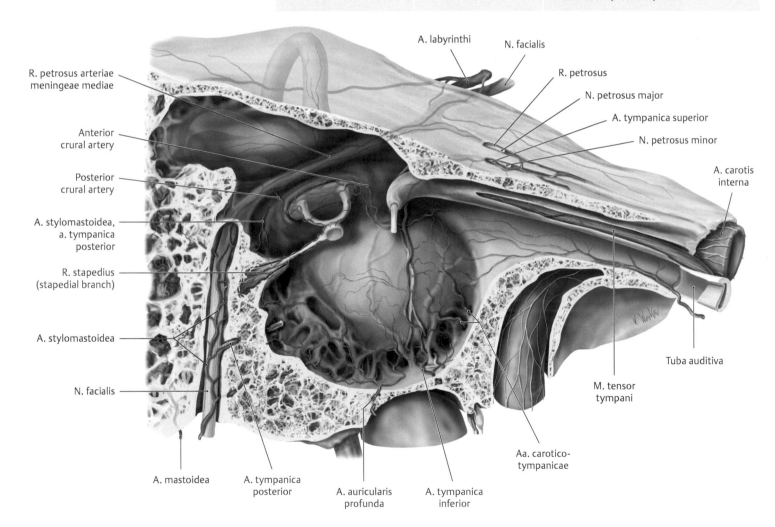

B Arteries of the cavitas tympani and cellulae mastoideae

Pars petrosa of the right os temporale, lateral oblique view. The malleus, incus, portions of the chorda tympani, and the a. tympanica anterior have been removed.

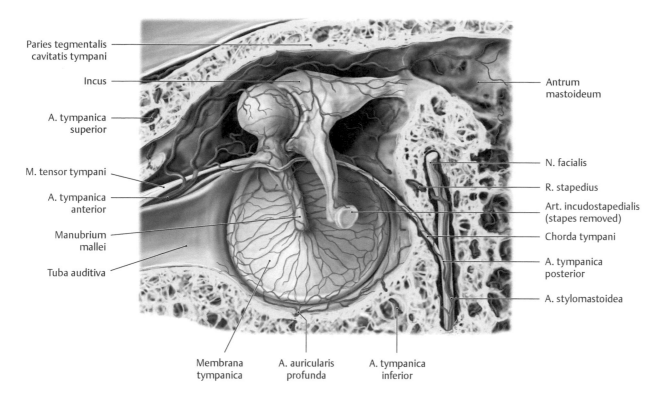

Paries tegmentalis cavitatis tympani

Incus

A. tympanica superior

M. tensor tympani

A. tympanica anterior

Manubrium mallei

Tuba auditiva

Antrum mastoideum

N. facialis

R. stapedius

Art. incudostapedialis (stapes removed)

Chorda tympani

A. tympanica posterior

A. stylomastoidea

Membrana tympanica

A. auricularis profunda

A. tympanica inferior

C Vascular supply of the ossicular chain and membrana tympanica
Medial view of the right membrana tympanica. This region receives most of its blood supply from the a. tympanica anterior. With inflammation of the membrana tympanica, the arteries may become so dilated that their course in the membrana tympanica can be seen, as illustrated here.

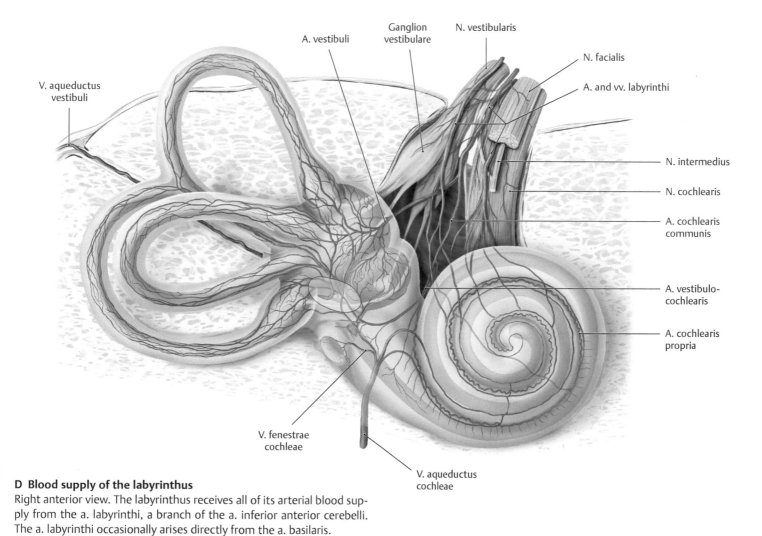

V. aqueductus vestibuli

A. vestibuli

Ganglion vestibulare

N. vestibularis

N. facialis

A. and vv. labyrinthi

N. intermedius

N. cochlearis

A. cochlearis communis

A. vestibulo-cochlearis

A. cochlearis propria

V. fenestrae cochleae

V. aqueductus cochleae

D Blood supply of the labyrinthus
Right anterior view. The labyrinthus receives all of its arterial blood supply from the a. labyrinthi, a branch of the a. inferior anterior cerebelli. The a. labyrinthi occasionally arises directly from the a. basilaris.

157

5.9 Eye: Orbital Region, Eyelids, and Conjunctiva

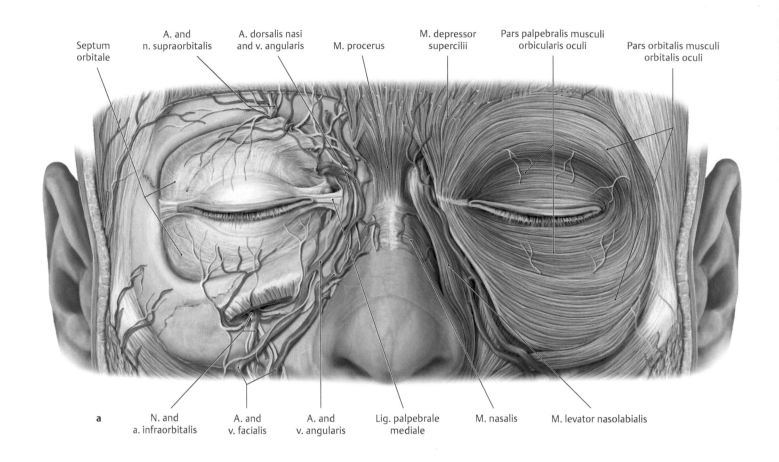

Septum orbitale — A. and n. supraorbitalis — A. dorsalis nasi and v. angularis — M. procerus — M. depressor supercilii — Pars palpebralis musculi orbicularis oculi — Pars orbitalis musculi orbitalis oculi

N. and a. infraorbitalis — A. and v. facialis — A. and v. angularis — Lig. palpebrale mediale — M. nasalis — M. levator nasolabialis

a

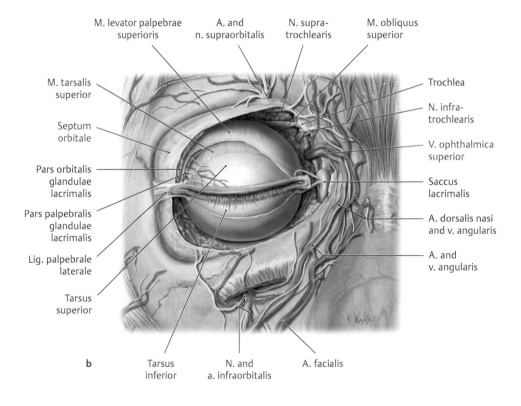

M. levator palpebrae superioris — A. and n. supraorbitalis — N. supra-trochlearis — M. obliquus superior

M. tarsalis superior

Septum orbitale

Pars orbitalis glandulae lacrimalis

Pars palpebralis glandulae lacrimalis

Lig. palpebrale laterale

Tarsus superior

Trochlea

N. infra-trochlearis

V. ophthalmica superior

Saccus lacrimalis

A. dorsalis nasi and v. angularis

A. and v. angularis

b — Tarsus inferior — N. and a. infraorbitalis — A. facialis

A Superficial and deep neurovascular structures of the orbital region

Right eye, anterior view.

a Superficial layer. The septum orbitale on the right side has been exposed by removal of the m. orbicularis oculi. **b** Deep layer. Anterior orbital structures have been exposed by partial removal of the septum orbitale.

The regions supplied by the a. carotis *interna* (a. supraorbitalis) and a. carotis *externa* (a. infraorbitalis, a. facialis) meet in this region. The anastomosis between the v. angularis (extracranial) and vv. ophthalmicae superiores (intracranial) creates a portal of entry by which microorganisms may reach the sinus cavernosus (risk of sinus thrombosis, meningitis); therefore it is sometimes necessary to ligate this anastomosis in the orbital region, in patients with extensive infections of the external facial region (see p. 227).

Note the passage of the nn. supra and infraorbitalis (branches of CN V_1 and CN V_2) through the foramina of the same name. The sensory function of these two n. trigeminus divisions can be tested at these nerve exit points.

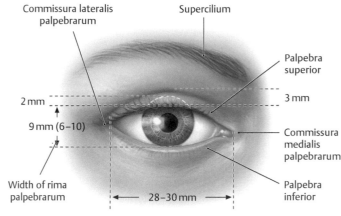

B Surface anatomy of the eye

Right eye, anterior view. The measurements indicate the width of the normal palpebral fissure (rima palpebrarum). It is important to know these measurements because there are a number of diseases in which they are altered. For example, the rima palpebrarum may be widened in peripheral facial paralysis or narrowed in ptosis (drooping of the eyelid) due to oculomotor palsy.

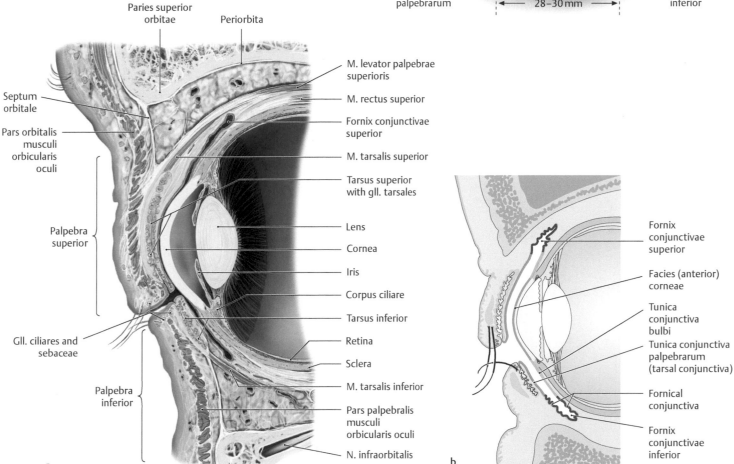

C Structure of the palpebrae and tunica conjunctiva

a Sagittal section through the anterior cavitas orbitalis. **b** Anatomy of the tunica conjunctiva.

The palpebra consists clinically of an outer and an inner layer with the following components:

- Outer layer: palpebral skin, gll. sudoriferae, gll. ciliares (modified sweat glands, Moll glands), gll. sebaceae (Zeis glands), and two skeletal muscles, the m. orbicularis oculi and m. levator palpebrae (palpebra superior only), innervated by the n. facialis and the n. oculomotorius, respectively.
- Inner layer: the tarsus (fibrous connective tissue plate), the mm. tarsales superior and inferior (of Müller; smooth muscle innervated by sympathetic fibers), the tunica conjunctiva palpebrarum, and the gll. tarsales (Meibomian glands).

Regular blinking (20–30 times per minute) keeps the eyes from drying out by evenly distributing the lacrimal fluid and glandular secretions (see p. 161). Mechanical irritants (e.g., grains of sand) evoke the blink reflex, which also serves to protect the cornea and **tunica conjunctiva**. The conjunctiva (tunica conjunctiva) is a vascularized, thin, serous mucous membrane that is subdivided into the *tunica conjunctiva palpebrarum* (see above), *fornical conjunctiva*, and *tunica conjunctiva bulbi*. The tunica conjunctiva bulbi borders directly on the corneal surface and combines with it to form the **saccus conjunctivalis**, whose functions include

- facilitating ocular movements,
- enabling painless motion of the tunica conjunctiva palpebralis and tunica conjunctiva bulbi relative to each other (lubricated by lacrimal fluid), and
- protecting against infectious pathogens (collections of lymphocytes along the fornices).

The fornices conjunctivae superior and inferior are the sites where the conjunctiva is reflected from the upper and lower eyelid, respectively, onto the eyeball. They are convenient sites for the instillation of ophthalmic medications. *Inflammation of the conjunctiva* is common and causes a dilation of the conjunctival vessels resulting in "pink eye." Conversely, a deficiency of red blood cells (anemia) may lessen the prominence of vascular markings in the conjunctiva. This is why the conjunctiva should be routinely inspected in every clinical examination.

5.10 Eye: Lacrimal Apparatus (Apparatus Lacrimalis)

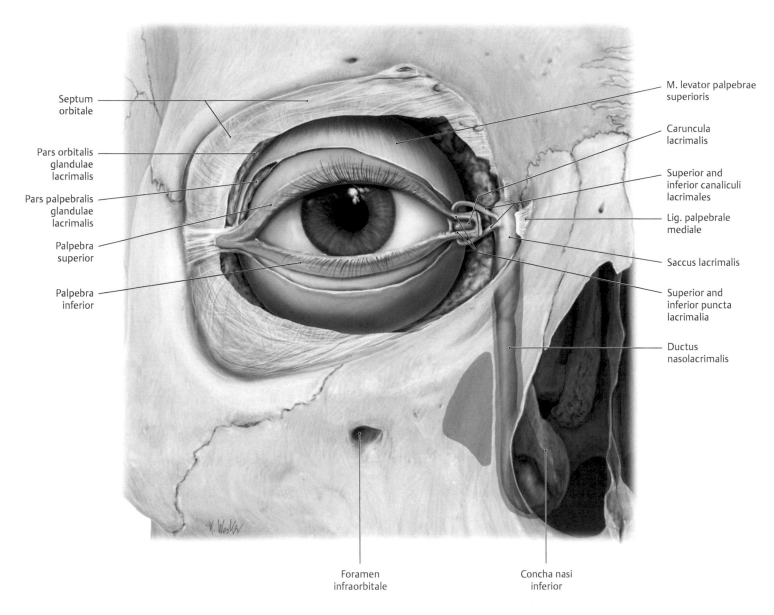

Septum orbitale

Pars orbitalis glandulae lacrimalis

Pars palpebralis glandulae lacrimalis

Palpebra superior

Palpebra inferior

M. levator palpebrae superioris

Caruncula lacrimalis

Superior and inferior canaliculi lacrimales

Lig. palpebrale mediale

Saccus lacrimalis

Superior and inferior puncta lacrimalia

Ductus nasolacrimalis

Foramen infraorbitale

Concha nasi inferior

A Apparatus lacrimalis

Right eye, anterior view. The septum orbitale has been partially removed, and the tendon of insertion of the m. levator palpebrae superioris has been divided. The hazelnut-sized **gl. lacrimalis** is located in the fossa glandulae lacrimalis of the os frontale and produces most of the lacrimal fluid. Smaller *gll. lacrimales accessoriae* (Krause or Wolfring glands) are also present. The tendon of m. levator palpebrae superioris subdivides the gl. lacrimalis, which normally is not visible or palpable, into a *pars orbitalis* (two-thirds of gland) and a *pars palpebralis* (one-third). The sympathetic fibers innervating the gl. lacrimalis originate from the ganglion cervicale superius and travel along arteries to reach the gl. lacrimalis. The parasympathetic innervation of the gl. lacrimalis is complex (see p. 127). The function of the **apparatus lacrimalis** can be understood by tracing the flow of lacrimal fluid obliquely downward from upper right to lower left. From the superior and inferior *puncta lacrimalia*, the lacrimal fluid enters the superior and inferior *canaliculi lacrimales*, which direct the fluid into the saccus lacrimalis. Finally it drains through the *ductus nasolacrimalis* to an outlet below the concha nasi inferior. "Watery eyes" are a typical cold symptom caused by obstruction of the inferior opening of the ductus nasolacrimalis.

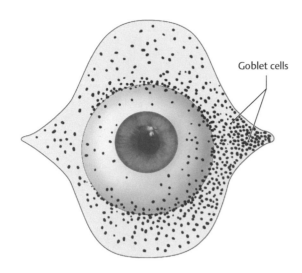

Goblet cells

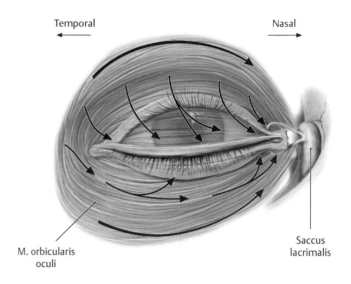

Temporal

Nasal

M. orbicularis
oculi

Saccus
lacrimalis

B Distribution of goblet cells in the tunica conjunctiva
(after Calabria and Rolando)

Goblet cells are mucous-secreting cells with an epithelial covering. Their secretions (mucins) are an important constituent of the lacrimal fluid (see **C**). Besides the goblet cells, mucins are also secreted by the main gl. lacrimalis.

D Mechanical propulsion of the lacrimal fluid

During closure of the palpebrae, contraction of the m. orbicularis oculi proceeds in a temporalto-nasal direction. The successive contraction of these muscle fibers propels the lacrimal fluid toward the lacrimal passages.

Note: Facial paralysis prevents closure of the palpebrae, causing the eye to dry out.

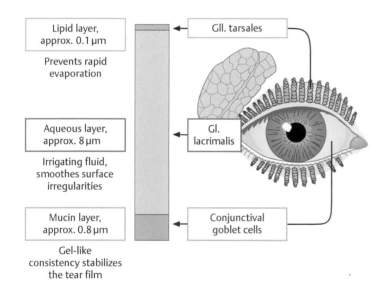

Lipid layer,
approx. 0.1 μm

Prevents rapid
evaporation

Aqueous layer,
approx. 8 μm

Irrigating fluid,
smoothes surface
irregularities

Mucin layer,
approx. 0.8 μm

Gel-like
consistency stabilizes
the tear film

Gll. tarsales

Gl.
lacrimalis

Conjunctival
goblet cells

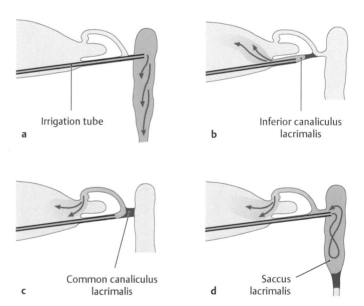

Irrigation tube

a

Inferior canaliculus
lacrimalis

b

Common canaliculus
lacrimalis

c

Saccus
lacrimalis

d

C Structure of the tear film (after Lang)

The tear film is a complex fluid with several morphologically distinct layers, whose components are produced by individual glands. The outer lipid layer, produced by the gll. tarsales, protects the aqueous middle layer of the tear film from evaporating.

E Obstructions to lacrimal drainage (after Lang)

Sites of obstruction in the lacrimal drainage system can be located by irrigating the system with a special fluid. To make this determination, the examiner must be familiar with the anatomy of the lacrimal apparatus and the normal drainage pathways for lacrimal fluid (see **A**).

a No obstruction to lacrimal drainage (cf. A).

b, c Stenosis in the inferior or common canaliculus lacrimalis. The stenosis causes a damming back of lacrimal fluid behind the obstructed site. In b the fluid refluxes through the inferior canaliculus lacrimalis, and in c it flows through the superior canaliculus lacrimalis.

d Stenosis below the level of the saccus lacrimalis (postlacrimal sac stenosis). When the entire saccus lacrimalis has filled with fluid, the fluid begins to reflux into the superior canaliculus lacrimalis. In such cases, the lacrimal fluid often has a purulent, gelatinous appearance.

161

5.11 Eyeball (Bulbus Oculi)

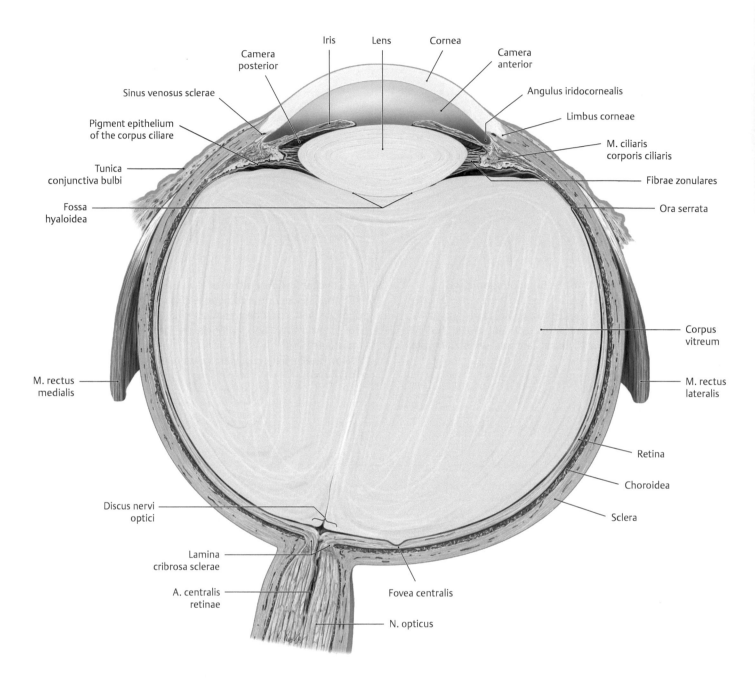

A Transverse section through the bulbus oculi

Right eye, superior view. Most of the bulbus oculi is composed of three concentric layers (from outside to inside): the sclera, choroidea, and retina.

The anterior portion of the bulbus oculi has a different structure, however. The **outer coat** of the eye in this region is formed by the **cornea** (anterior portion of the **tunica fibrosa bulbi**). As the "window of the eye," it bulges forward while covering the structures behind it. At the limbus corneae, the cornea is continuous with the less convex **sclera**, which is the posterior portion of the tunica fibrosa bulbi. It is a firm layer of connective tissue that gives attachment to the tendons of all the extraocular muscles. Anteriorly, the sclera in the angulus iridocornealis of the camera anterior forms the reticulum trabeculare (see p. 161), which is connected to the sinus venosus sclerae. On the posterior side of the bulbus oculi, the axons of the n. opticus pierce the lamina cribrosa sclerae. Beneath the sclera is the **tunica vasculosa bulbi**, also called the **uveal tract**. It consists of three parts in the anterior portion of the eye: the iris, corpus ciliare, and choroidea, the latter

being distributed over the entire bulbus oculi. The iris shields the eye from excessive light (see p. 167) and covers the lens. Its root is continuous with the corpus ciliare, which contains the m. ciliaris for visual accommodation (alters the refractive power of the lens, see p. 165). The epithelium of the corpus ciliare produces the humor aquosus. The *corpus ciliare* is continuous at the ora serrata with the middle layer of the eye, the **choroidea**. The choroidea is the most highly vascularized region in the body and serves to regulate the temperature of the eye and to supply blood to the outer layers of the retina. The **tunica interna bulbi** is the **retina**, which includes an inner layer of photosensitive cells (the sensory retina, stratum nervosum) and an outer layer of retinal pigment epithelium (stratum pigmentosum). The latter is continued forward as the pigment epithelium of the corpus ciliare and the epithelium of the iris. The *fovea centralis* is a depressed area in the central retina that is approximately 4 mm temporal to the discus nervi optici. Incident light is normally focused onto the fovea centralis, which is the site of greatest visual acuity. The interior of the bulbus oculi is occupied by the **humor vitreus (corpus vitreum**, see **C**).

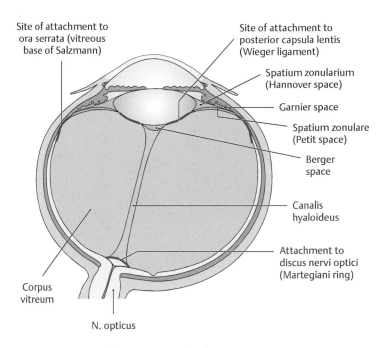

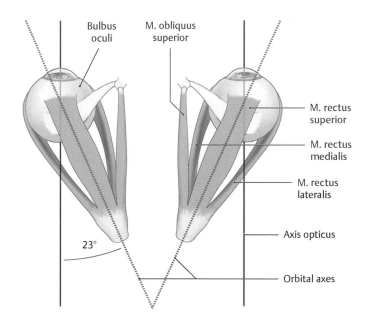

B Reference lines and points on the eye

The line marking the greatest circumference of the bulbus oculi is the *equator*. Lines perpendicular to the equator are called *meridians*.

C Corpus vitreum (humor vitreus) (after Lang)

Right eye, transverse section viewed from above. Sites where the corpus vitreum is attached to other ocular structures are shown in red, and adjacent spaces are shown in green. The corpus vitreum stabilizes the eyeball and protects against retinal detachment. Devoid of nerves and vessels, it consists of 98% water and 2% hyaluronic acid and collagen. The canalis hyaloideus is an embryological remnant of the a. hyaloidea. For the treatment of some diseases, the corpus vitreum may be surgically removed (vitrectomy) and the resulting cavity filled with physiological saline solution.

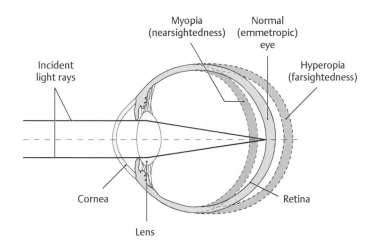

D Light refraction in a normal (emmetropic) eye and in myopia and hyperopia

Parallel rays from a distant light source are normally refracted by the cornea and lens to a focal point on the retinal surface.

- Shortsightedness (myopia, red): bulbus oculi is too short, the light is focused in front of the retina.
- Farsightedness (hyperopia, blue): the bulbus oculi is too long, the light is focused behind the retina

In addition to the ocular anomalies discussed here, myopia and hyperopia can also be the result of other rare causes such as refractive anomalies.

E Axis opticus and orbital axis

Superior view of both eyes showing the m. recti medialis, lateralis and superior and the m. obliquus superior. The axis opticus deviates from the orbital axis by 23°. Because of this disparity, the point of maximum visual acuity, the fovea centralis, is lateral to the "blind spot" of the discus nervi optici (see **A**).

5.12 Eye: Lens and Cornea

A Overview: Position of the lens and cornea in the bulbus oculi

Histological section through the cornea, lens, and suspensory apparatus of the lens. The normal lens is clear and transparent and is only 4 mm thick. It is suspended in the fossa hyaloidea of the corpus vitreum (see p. 156). The lens is attached by rows of fibrils (fibrae zonulares) to the m. ciliaris, whose contractions alter the shape and focal length of the lens (the structure of the corpus ciliare is shown in **B**). The lens is a dynamic structure that can change its shape in response to visual requirements (see **Cb**). The camera anterior of the eye is situated in front of the lens, and the camera posterior is located between the iris and the anterior epithelium lentis (see p. 160). The lens, like the corpus vitreum, is devoid of nerves and blood vessels and is composed of elongated epithelial cells—the fibrae lentis.

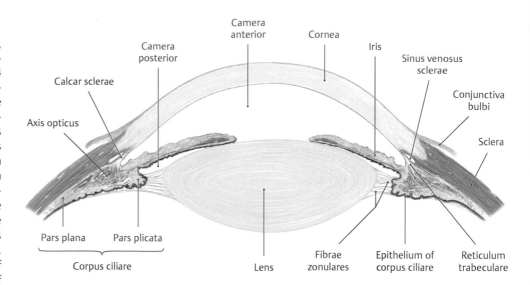

B The lens and corpus ciliare

Posterior view. The curvature of the lens is regulated by the muscle fibers of the annular corpus ciliare (see **Cb**). The *corpus ciliare* lies between the ora serrata and the root of the iris and consists of a relatively flat part (pars plana) and a part that is raised into folds (pars plicata). The latter part is ridged by approximately 70–80 radially oriented procc. ciliares, which surround the lens like a halo when viewed from behind. The procc. ciliares contain large capillaries, and their epithelium secretes the humor aquosus (see p. 167). Very fine *fibrae zonulares* extend from the lamina basalis of the procc. ciliares to the equator of the lens. These fibers and the spaces between them constitute the suspensory apparatus of the lens, called the *zonule*. Most of the corpus

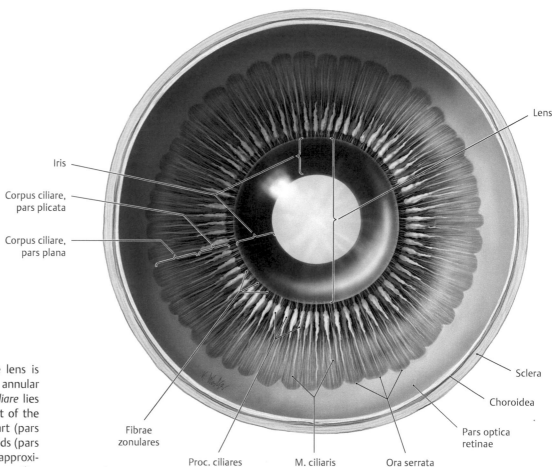

ciliare is occupied by the m. ciliaris, a smooth muscle composed of fibrae meridionales, radiales, and circulares. It arises mainly from the calcar sclerae (a reinforcing ring of sclera just below the sinus venosus sclerae), and it attaches to structures including the lamina basalis of the choroid and the inner surface of the sclera. When the m. ciliaris contracts, it pulls the choroidea forward and relaxes the fibrae zonulares. As these fibers become lax, the intrinsic resilience of the lens causes it to assume the more convex relaxed shape that is necessary for near vision (see **Cb**). This is the basic mechanism of visual accommodation.

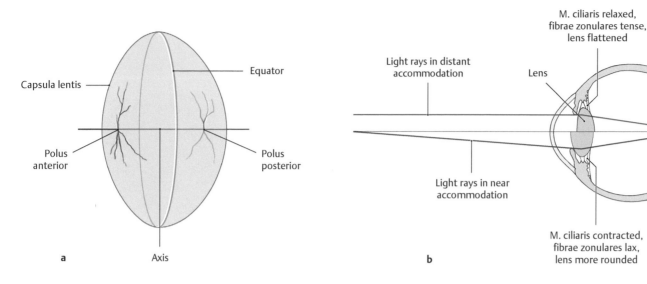

C Reference lines and dynamics of the lens

a Principal reference lines of the lens: The lens has a *polus anterior* and *polus posterior*, an *axis* passing between the poles, and an equator. The lens has a biconvex shape with a greater radius of curvature posteriorly (16 mm) than anteriorly (10 mm). Its function is to transmit light rays and make fine adjustments in refraction. Its refractive power ranges from 10 to 20 diopters, depending on the state of accommodation. The cornea has a considerably higher refractive power of 43 diopters.

b Light refraction and dynamics of the lens:
- Upper half of diagram: fine adjustment of the eye for far vision. Parallel light rays arrive from a distant source, and the lens is flattened.
- Lower half of diagram: For near vision (accommodation to objects less than 5 m from the eye), the lens assumes a more rounded shape (see **B**). This is effected by contraction of the m. ciliaris (parasympathetic innervation from the n. oculomotorius), causing the fibrae zonulares to relax and allowing the lens to assume a more rounded shape because of its intrinsic resilience.

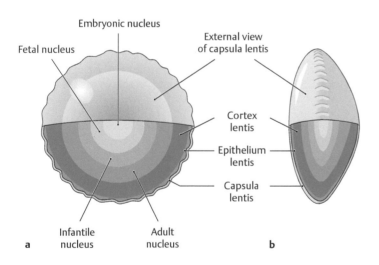

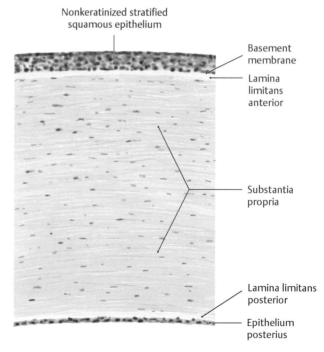

D Growth of the lens and zones of discontinuity (after Lang)

a Anterior view, **b** lateral view.

The lens continues to grow throughout life, doing so in a manner opposite to that of other epithelial structures, i.e., the youngest cells are at the surface of the lens while the oldest cells are deeper. Due to the constant proliferation of epithelial cells, which are all firmly incorporated in the capsula lentis, the tissue of the lens becomes increasingly dense with age. A slit-lamp examination will demonstrate zones of varying cell density (zones of discontinuity). The zone of highest cell density, the *embryonic nucleus*, is at the center of the lens. With further growth, it becomes surrounded by the *fetal nucleus*. The *infantile nucleus* develops after birth, and finally the *adult nucleus* begins to form during the third decade of life. These zones are the basis for the morphological classification of cataracts, a structural alteration in the lens, causing opacity, that is more or less normal in old age (present in 10% of all 80-year-olds).

E Structure of the cornea

The cornea is covered externally by nonkeratinized stratified squamous epithelium whose basal membrane borders on the lamina limitans anterior (Bowman membrane). The stroma (substantia propria) makes up approximately 90% of the corneal thickness and is bounded on its deep surface by the lamina limitans posterior (Descemet membrane). Beneath is a single layer of corneal endothelium (endothelium of anterior chamber, epithelium posterius). The cornea does have a nerve supply (for corneal reflexes) but it is not vascularized and therefore has an immunologically privileged status: normally, a corneal transplant can be performed without fear of a host rejection response.

5.13 Eye: Iris and Ocular Chambers

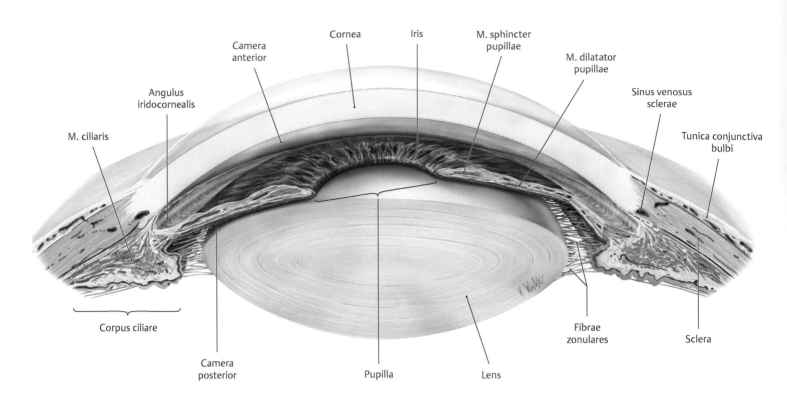

A Location of the iris and the camerae anterior and posterior
Transverse section through the segmentum anterius of the eye, superior view. The iris, the choroidea, and the corpus ciliare at the periphery of the iris are part of the uveal tract. In the iris, the pigments are formed that determine eye color (see **D**). The iris is an optical diaphragm with a central aperture, the pupilla, placed in front of the lens. The pupilla is 1–8 mm in diameter; it constricts on contraction of the m. sphincter pupillae (*parasympathetic* innervation via the n. oculomotorius and ganglion ciliare) and dilates on contraction of the m. dilatator pupillae (*sympathetic* innervation from the ganglion cervicale superius via the plexus caroticus internus). Together, the iris and lens separate the camera anterior of the eye from the camera posterior. The camera posterior behind the iris is bounded posteriorly by the corpus vitreum, centrally by the lens, and laterally by the corpus ciliare. The camera anterior is bounded anteriorly by the cornea and posteriorly by the iris and lens.

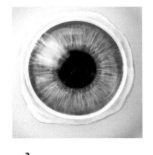
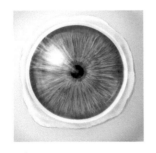
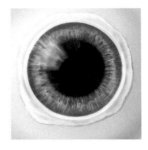

a   b   c

B Pupil size
a Normal pupil size, **b** maximum constriction (miosis), **c** maximum dilation (mydriasis). The regulation of pupil size is aided by the two intraocular muscles, the m. sphincter pupillae and m. dilatator pupillae (see **D**). The m. sphincter pupillae, which receives parasympathetic innervation, narrows the pupil while the m. dilatator pupillae, which receives sympathetic innervation, enlarges the pupil. Pupil size is normally adjusted in response to incident light and serves mainly to optimize visual acuity. Normally, the pupillae are circular in shape and equal in size (3–5 mm). Various influences (listed in C) may cause the pupil size to vary over a range from 1.5 mm (miosis) to 8 mm (mydriasis). The condition of unequal pupil size is called anisocoria. Mild anisocoria is physiological in some indivuals. Pupillary reflexes such as convergence and the consensual light response are described on p. 480.

C Causes of miosis and mydriasis
(after Füeßl and Middecke)

Miosis (Bb)	Mydriasis (Bc)
Light	Darkness
Sleep, fatigue	Pain, excitement
Miotics (parasympathomimetics, e.g. pilocarpine and sympatholytics)	Mydriatics (parasympatholytics, e.g. atropine and sympathomimetics, e.g. adrenaline)
Horner syndrome (including ptosis and a narrow rima palpebrarum)	Oculomotor palsy
Morphine abuse	Migraine, glaucoma
Pontine lesion, meningitis	Mesencephalic lesion
Anesthesia	Cocaine

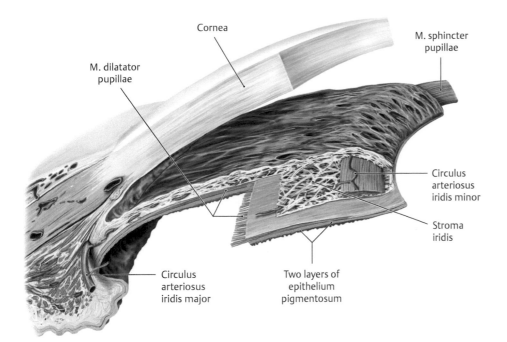

Cornea

M. sphincter pupillae

M. dilatator pupillae

Circulus arteriosus iridis minor

Stroma iridis

Circulus arteriosus iridis major

Two layers of epithelium pigmentosum

D Structure of the iris

The basic structural framework of the iris is the vascularized stroma iridis, which is bounded on its deep surface by two layers of epithelium pigmentosum. The loose, collagen-containing stroma iridis contains outer and inner vascular circles (circuli arteriosi iridis major and minor), which are interconnected by small anastomotic arteries. The m. sphincter pupillae is an annular muscle located in the stroma bordering the pupil. The radially disposed m. dilatator is not located in the stroma iridis; rather it is composed of numerous myofibrils in the iris epithelium (myoepithelium). The stroma iridis is permeated by pigmented connective tissue cells (melanocytes). When heavily pigmented, these melanocytes of the anterior border zone of the stroma render the iris brown or "black." Otherwise, the characteristics of the underlying stroma iridis and epithelium determine eye color, in a manner that is not fully understood.

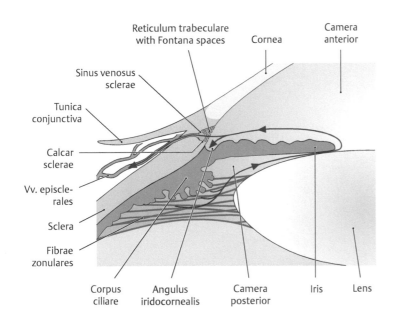

Reticulum trabeculare with Fontana spaces

Cornea

Camera anterior

Sinus venosus sclerae

Tunica conjunctiva

Calcar sclerae

Vv. episclerales

Sclera

Fibrae zonulares

Corpus ciliare

Angulus iridocornealis

Camera posterior

Iris

Lens

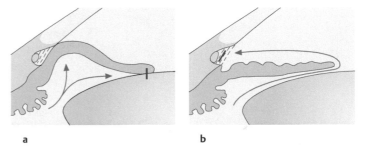

a

b

F Obstruction of aqueous drainage and glaucoma

The normal intraocular pressure in adults (15 mm Hg) is necessary for a functioning optical system, partly because it maintains a smooth curvature of the corneal surface and helps keep the photoreceptor cells in contact with the stratum pigmentosum. When *glaucoma* is present (see **D**, p. 159), the intraocular pressure is elevated and the n. opticus becomes constricted at the lamina cribrosa sclerae, where it emerges from the bulbus oculi through the sclera. This constriction of the n. opticus eventually leads to blindness. The elevated pressure is caused by an obstruction that hampers the normal drainage of humor aquosus, which can no longer overcome the pupillary or trabecular resistance (see **E**). One of two conditions may develop:

- *Acute or angle-closure glaucoma* (**a**), in which the angulus iridocornealis is obstructed by iris tissue. The humor aquosus cannot drain into the camera anterior and pushes portions of the iris upward, blocking the angulus iridocornealis.
- *Chronic or open-angle glaucoma* (**b**), in which the angulus iridocornealis is open but drainage through the reticulum trabeculare is impaired (the red bar marks the location of each type of obstruction).

By far the most common form (approximately 90% of all glaucomas) is primary chronic open-angle glaucoma (**b**), which becomes more prevalent after 40 years of age. The primary goal of treatment is to improve the drainage of humor aquosus (e.g., with parasympathomimetics that induce sustained contraction of the m. ciliaris and m. sphincter pupillae) or decrease its production.

E Normal drainage of humor aquosus

The humor aquosus (approximately 0.3 mL per eye) is an important determinant of the intraocular pressure (see **F**). It is produced by the nonpigmented ciliary epithelium of the procc. ciliares in the camera *posterior* (approximately 0.15 mL/hour) and passes through the pupil into the camera *anterior* of the eye. The humor aquosus seeps through the spaces of the reticulum trabeculare (Fontana spaces) in the angulus iridocornealis and enters the canal of Schlemm (sinus venosus sclerae), through which it drains to the vv. episclerales. The draining humor aquosus flows toward the angulus iridocornealis along a pressure gradient (intraocular pressure = 15 mm Hg, pressure in the vv. episclerales = 9 mm Hg) and must surmount a physiological resistance at two sites:

- the *pupillary resistance* (between the iris and lens) and
- the *trabecular resistance* (narrow spaces in the reticulum trabeculare).

Approximately 85% of the humor aquosus flows through the reticulum trabeculare into the sinus venosus sclerae. Only 15% drains through the uveoscleral vascular system into the vv. vorticosae (uveoscleral drainage route).

5.14 Eye: Retina

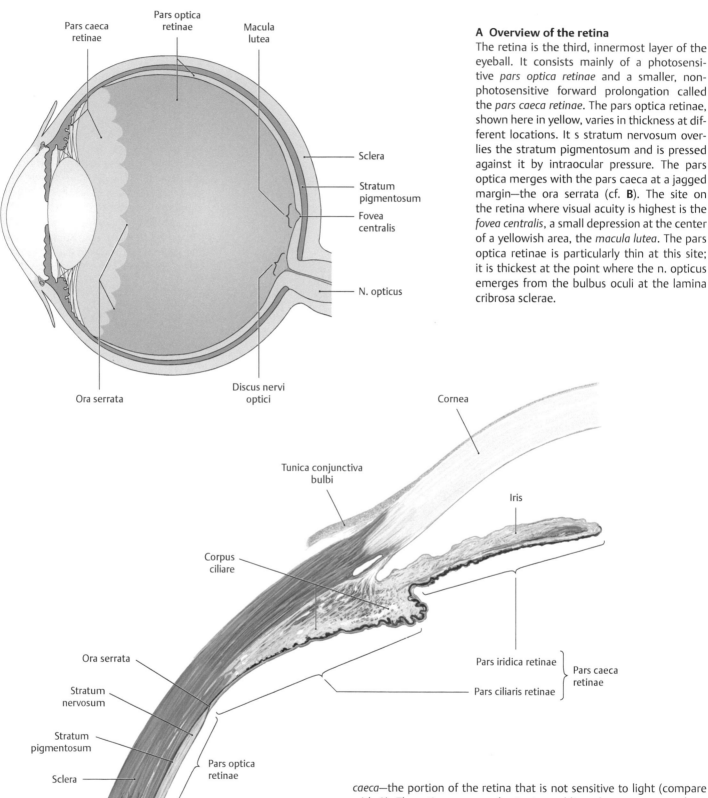

Pars caeca retinae

Pars optica retinae

Macula lutea

Pars caeca retinae

Sclera

Stratum pigmentosum

Fovea centralis

N. opticus

Ora serrata

Discus nervi optici

Cornea

Tunica conjunctiva bulbi

Iris

Corpus ciliare

Ora serrata

Stratum nervosum

Stratum pigmentosum

Sclera

Pars optica retinae

Pars iridica retinae

Pars ciliaris retinae

Pars caeca retinae

A Overview of the retina
The retina is the third, innermost layer of the eyeball. It consists mainly of a photosensitive *pars optica retinae* and a smaller, nonphotosensitive forward prolongation called the *pars caeca retinae*. The pars optica retinae, shown here in yellow, varies in thickness at different locations. It s stratum nervosum overlies the stratum pigmentosum and is pressed against it by intraocular pressure. The pars optica merges with the pars caeca at a jagged margin—the ora serrata (cf. **B**). The site on the retina where visual acuity is highest is the *fovea centralis*, a small depression at the center of a yellowish area, the *macula lutea*. The pars optica retinae is particularly thin at this site; it is thickest at the point where the n. opticus emerges from the bulbus oculi at the lamina cribrosa sclerae.

B Parts of the retina
The posterior surface of the iris bears a double layer of pigment epithelium, the pars *iridica* retinae. Just peripheral to it is the pars *ciliaris* retinae, also formed by a double layer of epithelium (one of which is pigmented) and covering the posterior surface of the corpus ciliare. The partes iridica and ciliaris retinae together constitute the *retina*

caeca—the portion of the retina that is not sensitive to light (compare with **A**). The retina caeca ends at a jagged line, the ora serrata, where the light-sensitive *pars optica* of the retina begins. Consistent with the development of the retina from the embryonic cupula optica, two layers can be distinguished within the pars optica:

• An outer layer nearer the sclera: the *stratum pigmentosum*, consisting of a single layer of pigmented retinal epithelium (cf. **Ca**).
• An inner layer nearer the corpus vitreum: the *stratum nervosum*, comprising a system of receptor cells, interneurons, and ganglion cells (see **Cb**).

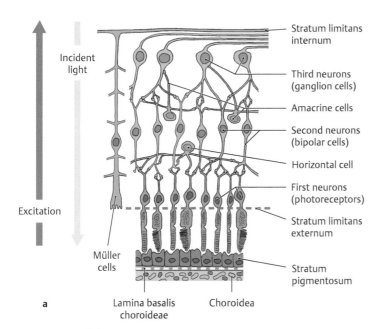

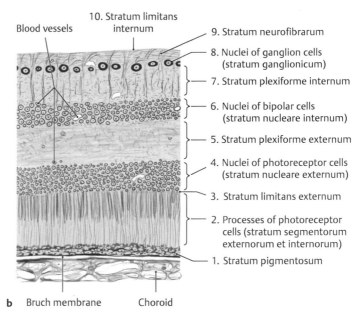

C Structure of the retina

a Schematic diagram of the first three neurons in the visual pathway and their connections. **b** The ten anatomical layers of the retina. Light must pass through all the inner layers of the retina (the layers nearest the corpus vitreum) before reaching the photosensitive elements of the photoreceptors. The direction of transmission of sensory information, however, is inward, opposite to the direction of the incoming light. The first three neurons of the visual pathway are located within the retina. Starting with the outermost neuron, they are as follows (**a**):

- First neuron: Photoreceptor cells (rods and cones) are light-sensitive sensory cells that transform light stimuli into electrochemical signals. The two types of *photoreceptors* are rods and cones, named for the shape of their receptor segment. The retina contains 100–125 million rods, which are responsible for twilight and night vision, but only about 6–7 million cones. Different cones are specialized for the perception of red, green, and blue.
- Second neuron: bipolar cells that receive impulses from the photoreceptors and relay them to the ganglion cells.
- Third neuron: retinal ganglion cells whose axons converge at the discus nervi opticis to form the n. opticus and reach the corpus geniculatum laterale and colliculus superior.

In addition to these largely "vertical" connections, there are also horizontal cells and amacrine cells that function as *interneurons* to establish lateral connections. In this way the impulses transmitted by the receptor cells are processed and organized while still within the retina (signal convergence). The retinal *Müller cells* are glial cells that span the stratum nervosum radially from the stratum limitans internum to stratum limitans externum and create a supporting framework for the neurons. External to these cells is the *stratum pigmentosum*, whose basement membrane is attached to the lamina basalis choroideae (contains elastic fibers and collagen fibrils) and mediates the exchange of substances between the adjacent choroidea (choriocapillaris) and the photoreceptor cells.

Note: The outer segments of the photoreceptors are in contact with the stratum pigmentosum but are not attached to it. The intraocular pressure alone pushes the stratum nervosum against the stratum pigmentosum. This explains why the stratum nervosum may become separated from the stratum pigmentosum (retinal detachment; untreated, leads to blindness). Traditionally, a histological section of the retina consists of ten layers (**b**) that are formed by elements of the three neurons (e.g., nuclei or cellular processes) that occupy a consistent level within any given layer.

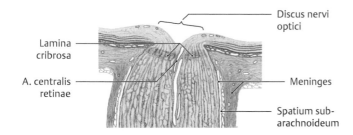

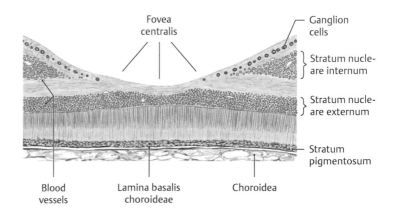

D Discus nervi optici ("blind spot") and lamina cribrosa sclerae

The unmyelinated axons of the retinal ganglion cells (approximately 1 million axons per eye) pass to a collecting point at the polus posterior of the eye, the discus nervi optici. There they unite to form the n. opticus and leave the retina through numerous perforations in the sclera (lamina cribrosa sclerae). In the n. opticus, these axons are myelinated by oligodendrocytes.

Note the a. centralis retinae entering the eye at this location (see p. 171) and the coverings of the n. opticus. Because the n. opticus is a forward prolongation of the diencephalon, it has all the coverings of the brain (dura mater, arachnoidea mater, and pia mater). It is surrounded by a spatium subarachnoideum that contains liquor cerebrospinalis and communicates with the spatia subarachnoidea of the brain and medulla spinalis.

E Macula lutea and fovea centralis

Temporal to the discus nervi optici is the macula lutea. At its center is a funnel-shaped depression approximately 1.5 mm in diameter, the fovea centralis, which is the site of maximum visual acuity. At this site the inner retinal layers are heaped toward the margin of the depression, so that the cells of the photoreceptors (just cones, no rods) are directly exposed to the incident light. This arrangement significantly reduces scattering of the light rays.

169

5.15 Eye: Blood Supply

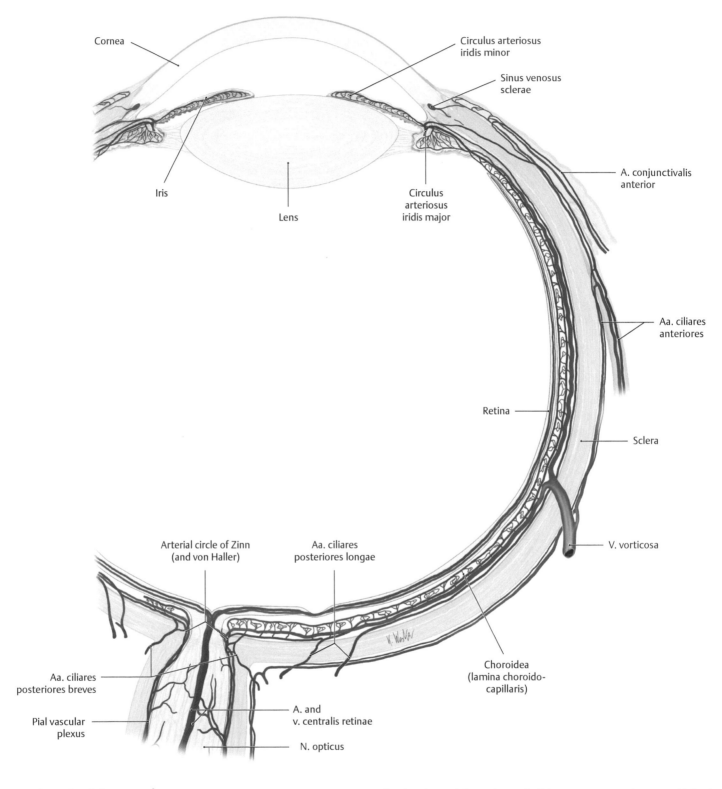

A Blood supply of the eye

Horizontal section through the right eye at the level of the n. opticus, viewed from above. All of the arteries that supply the eye arise from the *a. ophthalmica*, a terminal branch of the a. carotis interna (see p. 103). Its ocular branches are as follows:

- A. centralis retinae to the retina (see **B**)
- Aa. ciliares posteriores breves to the choroidea
- Aa. ciliares posteriores longae to the corpus ciliare and iris, where they supply the circuli arteriosi iridis major and minor (see **D**, p. 167)
- Aa. ciliares anteriores, which arise from the vessels of the mm. recti of the eye and anastomose with the posterior ciliary vessels

Blood is drained from the eyeball by 4 to 8 vv. vorticosae, which pierce the sclera behind the equator and open into the v. opththalmica superior or inferior.

B Arterial blood supply of the n. opticus and discus nervi optici

Lateral view. The a. centralis retinae, the first branch of the a. ophthalmica, enters the n. opticus from below approximately 1 cm behind the bulbus oculi and courses with it to the retina while giving off multiple small branches. The a. ciliaris posterior also gives off several small branches that supply the n. opticus. The discus nervi optici receives its arterial blood supply from an arterial ring (circle of Zinn and von Haller) formed by anastomoses among the side branches of the aa. ciliares posteriores breves and a. centralis retinae.

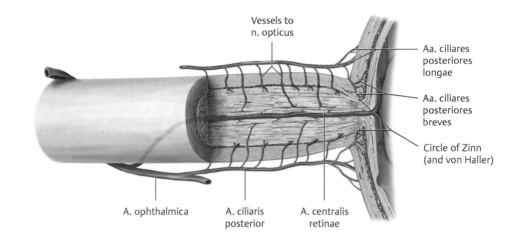

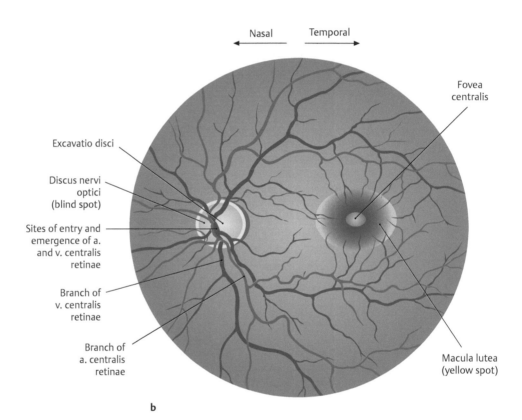

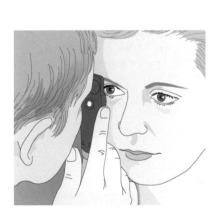

C Ophthalmoscopic examination of the optic fundus

a Examination technique (direct ophthalmoscopy). **b** Normal appearance of the optic fundus.

In direct ophthalmoscopy, the following structures of the optic fundus can be directly evaluated at approximately 16x magnification:

- The condition of the retina
- The blood vessels (particularly the a. centralis retinae)
- The discus nervi optici (where the n. opticus emerges from the bulbus oculi)
- The macula lutea and fovea centralis

Because the retina is transparent, the color of the optic fundus is determined chiefly by the stratum pigmentosum and the blood vessels of the choroidea. It is uniformly pale red in light-skinned persons and is considerably browner in dark-skinned persons. Abnormal detachment of the retina is usually associated with a loss of retinal transparency, and the retina assumes a yellowish-white color. The a. and v. centralis retinae can be distinguished from each other by their color and caliber: arteries have a brighter red color and a smaller caliber than the veins. This provides a means for the early detection of vascular changes (e.g., stenosis, wall thickening, microaneurysms), such as those occurring in diabetes mellitus (diabetic retinopathy) or hypertension. The discus nervi optici normally has sharp margins, a yellow-orange color, and a central depression, the excavatio disci. The disk is subject to changes in pathological conditions such as elevated intracranial pressure (papilledema with ill-defined disk margins). On examination of the *macula lutea*, which is 3–4 mm temporal to the discus nervi optici, it can be seen that numerous branches of the a. centralis retinae radiate toward the macula but do not reach its center, the fovea centralis (the fovea receives its blood supply from the choroidea). A common age-related disease of the macula lutea is macular degeneration, which may gradually lead to blindness.

5.16 Orbita: Extraocular Muscles (Musculi Externi Bulbi Oculi)

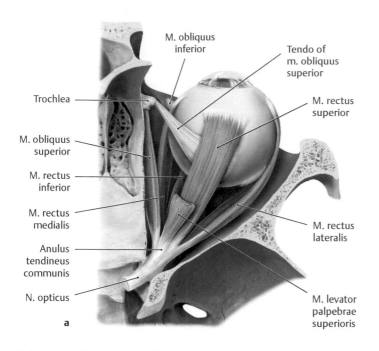

a

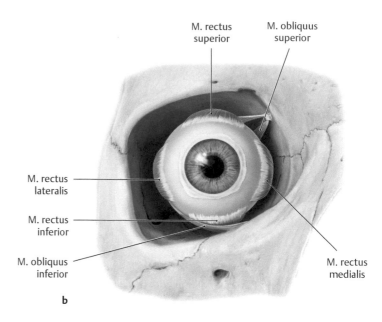

b

A Location of the extraocular muscles (extrinsic eye muscles)
Right eye, superior view (**a**) and anterior view (**b**).
The bulbus oculi is moved in the orbita by four mm. recti (superior, inferior, medial, and lateral) and two mm. obliqui (superior and inferior); innervation and direction of movements are shown in **B** and **D**. Except for the m. obliquus inferior (origin on the medial margin of the orbita), all of the mm. externi bulbi oculi arise from the anulus tendineus around the optic canal (common tendinous ring). All of the extraocular muscles insert on the sclera. The tendon of insertion of the m. obliquus superior first passes through a tendinous loop (trochlea) attached to the

superomedial margo orbitae, which redirects it posteriorly at an acute angle to its insertion on the temporal aspect of the superior surface of the bulbus oculi. The functional competence of all six extraocular muscles and their coordinated interaction are essential in directing both eyes toward the visual target. It is the task of the brain to process the two perceived retinal images in a way that provides binocular visual perception. If the coordinated actions of these muscles are impaired, due, for example, to the paralysis of one eye muscle (see **E**), the patient will perceive a double image (diplopia), i.e., the visual axis of one eye will deviate from its normal position.

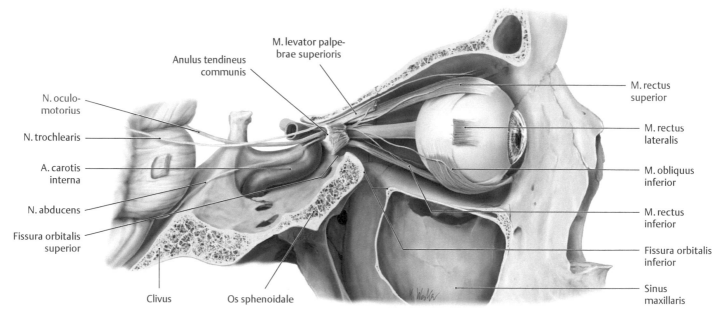

B Innervation of the extraocular muscles
Right eye, lateral view with the temporal wall of the orbit removed. Except for the m. obliquus superior (n. trochlearis) and m. rectus lateralis (n. abducens), the ocular muscles (m. rectus superior, m. rectus medialis, m. rectus inferior, and m. obliquus inferior) are supplied by the n. oculomotorius. Its r. superior supplies the m. rectus superior and the m. levator palpebrae superioris, which is not one of the

mm. externi bulbi oculi. Its r. inferior supplies the m. rectus inferior, m. rectus medialis, and m. obliquus inferior.
After emerging from the brainstem, nervi craniales III, IV, and VI first pass through the sinus cavernosus (or its lateral wall, see **A**, p. 170), where they are in close proximity to the a. carotis interna. From there they traverse the fissura orbitalis superior (see **B**, p. 170) to enter the orbit and supply their respective muscles.

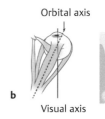

Horizontal axis (elevation, depression)

Sagittal axis (internal and external rotation)

Orbital axis

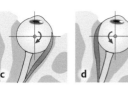

a

b

Visual axis

Longitudinal axis (abduction, adduction)

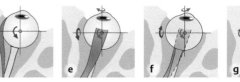 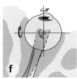 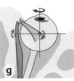 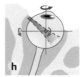

c d e f g h

	Muscle	Primary action	Secondary action	Innervation
Mm. externi bulbi oculi horizontales	• M. rectus lateralis • M. rectus medialis	• Abduction • Adduction	• None • None	• N. abducens (VI) • N. oculomotorius (III), r. inferior
Mm. externi bulbi oculi verticales recti	• M. rectus inferior • M. rectus superior	• Depression • Elevation	External rotation and adduction • Internal rotation and adduction	• N. oculomotorius (III), r. inferior • N. oculomotorius (III), r. superior
Mm. externi bulbi oculi verticales obliqui	• Inferior oblique • Superior oblique	• External rotation (excycloduction) • Internal rotation (incycloduction)	• Elevation and abduction • Depression and abduction	N. oculomotorius (III), r. inferior • N. trochlearis (IV)

C Ocular axes; function and innervation of the mm. externi bulbi oculi
Right eye. Except for **a**, superior view. Longitudinal axis is visible only as a point in **b–h**.
a and **b** Eye movements occur around three perpendicular axes. In primary position, the eye is turned slightly inward, i.e., the orbital axis is not identical to the visual axis or, respectively, the visual axis is externally rotated about 23°. To evaluate the mobility of individual ocular muscles, the eye must be brought into a specific cardinal direction of gaze (see **E**).
c–h The six mm. externi bulbi oculi are thus considered in pairs. See table. The two **mm. externi bulbi oculi verticales recti** are the most important elevators and depressors over their entire range of eye motion. These primary actions are more pronounced in abduction than in adduction (direction of pull of the muscle corresponds to the orbital axis, see **b**). The two muscles also have secondary actions: The m. rectus superior internally

rotates the eye (incycloduction), the m. rectus inferior externally rotates it (excycloduction). Both also have a slight adductive effect. Note that both secondary actions are strongest in maximum adduction and decrease as the eye moves through the primary position toward abduction.
Mm. externi bulbi oculi verticales obliqui: The main action of the m. obliquus superior is incycloduction, which can be expected to be strongest in abduction. The most important secondary action is depression. In contrast to incycloduction, it is strongest in adduction. The main action of the m. obliquus inferior is excycloduction, whereas its most important secondary action is elevation. As with the m. obliquus superior, the muscle's main action is strongest in abduction and its secondary action is strongest in adduction. Both mm. externi bulbi oculi verticales obliqui also have a slight abductive effect.

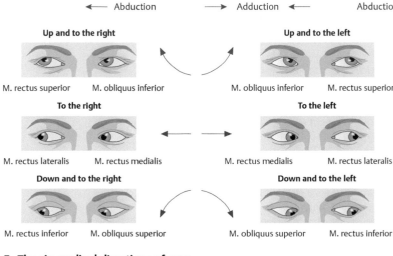

M. obliquus inferior   M. rectus superior   M. obliquus inferior
Elevation   Internal rotation
M. obliquus inferior   M. rectus medialis   M. rectus lateralis
Depression   External rotation
M. obliquus inferior   M. rectus inferior   M. obliquus superior
← Abduction   → Adduction ←   Abduction →

D Primary action of the mm. externi bulbi oculi on the bulbus oculi in primary position
In primary position (looking straight ahead) the maximum combined effect of all mm. externi bulbi oculi, i.e., all primary and secondary actions are performed, yet none of them to the full extent (red arrows; linear effect, black arrows: rotational effect).

Up and to the right
M. rectus superior   M. obliquus inferior
To the right
M. rectus lateralis   M. rectus medialis
Down and to the right
M. rectus inferior   M. obliquus superior

Up and to the left
M. obliquus inferior   M. rectus superior
To the left
M. rectus medialis   M. rectus lateralis
Down and to the left
M. obliquus superior   M. rectus inferior

E The six cardinal directions of gaze
(schematic diagram after Hering)
Displayed here are the directions of gaze in which the function of individual ocular muscles is evaluation or which are most heavily affected when a primary ocular muscle is paralyzed (increasing condition of double vision). Note: The rotational effect cannot be identified without additional methods of testing.

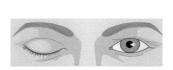 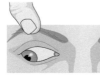

F Oculomotor palsy
Complete oculomotor palsy involves the failure of both the mm. externi bulbi oculi (superior, inferior, medial rectus and the inferior oblique; see **C**) as well as the mm. interni bulbi oculi: m. ciliaris and m. sphincter pupillae and the mm. levatores palpebrarum, which also receive their parasympathetic supply from the n. oculomotorius. The result is impaired bulbar motility and pupil motor function: The affected eye is depressed and externally rotated, the pupilla is dilated (mydriasis due to failure of the m. sphincter pupillae). Loss of near-field accommodation (failure of the m. ciliaris) occurs, and the palpebra is more or less closed (ptosis) due to failure of the m. levator palpebrae superioris. In complete ptosis as shown here, the patient does not have diplopia because only one eye is functional. Intrinsic and extraocular oculomotor palsies, in which only the intrinsic or only the mm. externi bulbi oculi are paralyzed, are discussed on p. 118.

5.17 Orbita: Subdivisions and Neurovascular Structures

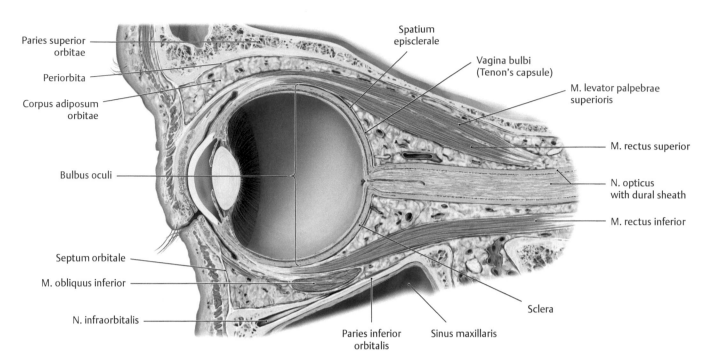

Paries superior orbitae
Periorbita
Corpus adiposum orbitae
Bulbus oculi
Septum orbitale
M. obliquus inferior
N. infraorbitalis
Spatium episclerale
Vagina bulbi (Tenon's capsule)
M. levator palpebrae superioris
M. rectus superior
N. opticus with dural sheath
M. rectus inferior
Sclera
Paries inferior orbitalis
Sinus maxillaris

A Subdivision of the orbita into upper, middle, and lower levels
Sagittal section through the right orbita viewed from the medial side. The orbit is lined by periosteum (periorbita) and contains the following structures, which are embedded within the corpus adiposum orbitae: bulbus oculi, n. opticus, gl. lacrimalis (not visible in this plane of section), musculi externi bulbi oculi, and the neurovascular structures that supply them. The corpus adiposum orbitae is bounded anteriorly by the septum orbitale and toward the bulbus oculi by a mobile sheath of con-

nective tissue (vagina bulbi, Tenon's capsule). The narrow space between the vagina bulbi and sclera is called the spatium episclerale. Topographically, the orbit is divided into three levels with the following boundaries:

• *Upper level:* between paries superior orbitae and the m. rectus superior
• *Middle level:* between m. rectus superior and m. rectus inferior
• *Lower level:* between m. rectus inferior and paries inferior orbitae

The contents of the different levels are listed in **B**.

B The three orbital levels and their main contents
The gl. lacrimalis is the dominant structure in the upper level, whereas the bulbus oculi is the landmark in the middle level. (The sites of entry of neurovascular structures into the orbita are described on p. 36.)

Level	Contents	Source/associated structures
Upper level	• N. lacrimalis	• Branch of n. ophthalmicus (CN V_1)
	• A. lacrimalis	• Branch of a. ophthalmica (from a. carotis interna)
	• V. lacrimalis	• Passes to v. ophthalmica superior
	• N. frontalis	• Branch of n. ophthalmicus (CN V_1)
	• N. supraorbitalis and n. supratrochlearis	• Terminal branches of n. frontalis
	• A. supraorbitalis	• Terminal branch of a. ophthalmica
	• V. supraorbitalis	• Unites with vv. supratrochleares to form v. angularis
	• N. trochlearis	• Nucleus of n. trochlearis in mesencephalon
	• N. infratrochlearis	• R. nervi nasociliaris (r. rami nervi ophthalmici [V^1])"
Middle level	• A. ophthalmica	• Branch of a. carotis interna
	• A. centralis retinae	• Branch of a. ophthalmica
	• Aa. ciliares posteriores	• Branches of a. ophthalmica
	• N. nasociliaris	• Branch of n. ophthalmicus (CN V_1)
	• N. abducens	• Nucleus nervi abducentis in pons
	• R. superior nervi oculomotorii	• Nucleus nervi oculomotorii in mesencephalon
	• N. opticus	• Retina (retinal ganglion cells)
	• Nn. ciliares breves	• Postsynaptic autonomic fibers to the bulbus oculi
	• Ganglion ciliare	• Parasympathetic ganglion for m. ciliaris and m. sphincter pupillae
	• Radix parasympathica ganglii ciliaris	• Presynaptic autonomic fibers of n. oculomotorius
	• Sympathetic root	• Postsynaptic fibers from the ganglion cervicale superius
	• N. nasociliaris	• Sensory fibers from bulbus oculi through ganglion ciliare to n. nasociliaris
	• V. ophthalmica superior	• Passes into sinus cavernosus
Lower level	• R. inferior nervi oculomotorii	• Nucleus nervi oculomotorii in mesencephalon
	• V. ophthalmica inferior	• Passes into sinus cavernosus
	• N. infraorbitalis	• Branch of n. maxillaris (CN V_2)
	• A. infraorbitalis	• Terminal branch of a. maxillaris (a. carotis externa)

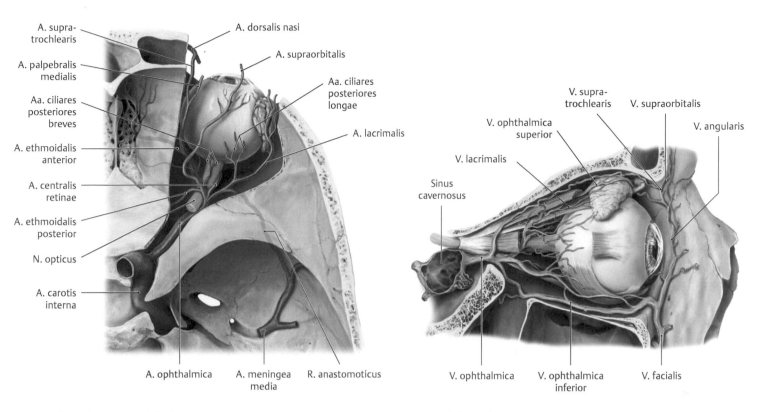

C Branches of arteria ophthalmica

Right orbit, superior view after opening of the canalis opticus and paries superior orbitae. The a. ophthalmica is a branch of the a. carotis interna. It runs below the n. opticus through the canalis opticus into the orbita and supplies the intraorbital structures including the bulbus oculi.

D Veins of the orbita

Right orbit, lateral view with the paries lateralis orbitae removed and the sinus maxillaris opened. The veins of the orbita communicate with the veins of the superficial and deep facial region and with the sinus cavernosus in the fossa cranii media (potential spread of infectious pathogens).

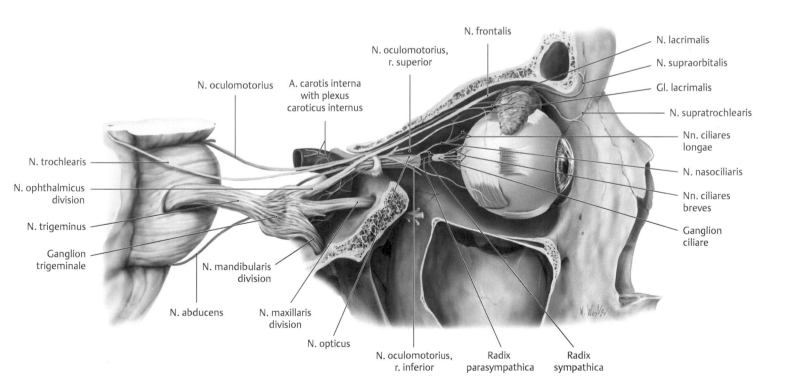

E Innervation of the orbit

Right orbita, lateral view with the temporal bony wall removed. The orbit receives motor, sensory and autonomic innervation from four nn. craniales: the n. oculomotorius (CN III), the n. trochlearis (CN IV), the n. abducens (CN VI), and the n. ophthalmicus division of the n. trigeminus (CN V1). The n. oculomotorius also conveys presynaptic parasympathetic fibers to the ganglion ciliare. Postsynaptic sympathetic fibers pass into the orbita by way of the plexus caroticus internus and plexus ophthalmicus.

5.18 Orbita: Topographical Anatomy

A Topography of the right orbita: contents of the upper level

Superior view.

a The paries superior orbitae osseus has been removed and the periorbita partially cut away. Dissection of the contents of the orbita with careful removal of the corpus adiposum orbitae.

b The periorbita of the entire paries superior orbitae and the corpus adiposum orbitae have been completely removed.

Note in **a** the course of the n. frontalis on the m. levator palpebrae superioris. The n. frontalis is the first nerve that one sees after opening the periorbita from a superior approach.

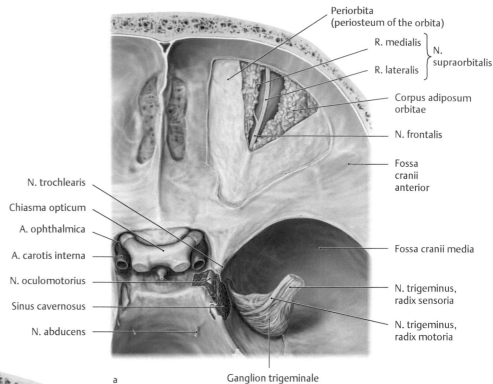

Periorbita (periosteum of the orbita)

R. medialis ⎫ N.
R. lateralis ⎬ supraorbitalis

Corpus adiposum orbitae

N. frontalis

Fossa cranii anterior

Fossa cranii media

N. trigeminus, radix sensoria

N. trigeminus, radix motoria

Ganglion trigeminale

N. trochlearis
Chiasma opticum
A. ophthalmica
A. carotis interna
N. oculomotorius
Sinus cavernosus
N. abducens

a

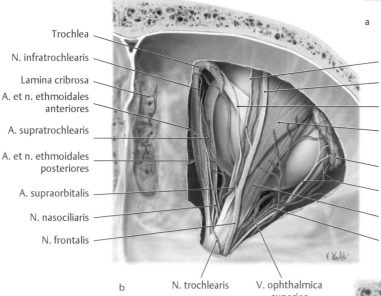

Trochlea
N. infratrochlearis
Lamina cribrosa
A. et n. ethmoidales anteriores
A. supratrochlearis
A. et n. ethmoidales posteriores
A. supraorbitalis
N. nasociliaris
N. frontalis

R. medialis ⎫ N. supraorbitalis
R. lateralis ⎭
N. supratrochlearis
M. levator palpebrae superioris
Gl. lacrimalis
A. et n. lacrimales
M. rectus superior
N. abducens

b   N. trochlearis   V. ophthalmica superior

B Topography of the right orbita: contents of the middle level

Superior view. The m. levator palpebrae superioris and the m. rectus superior have been divided and reflected posteriorly, and all fatty tissue has been removed to better expose the n. opticus.

Note: The ganglion ciliare is approximately 2 mm in diameter and lies lateral to the n. opticus approximately 2 cm behind the bulbus oculi. The parasympathetic innervation for the mm. interni bulbi oculi (mm. ciliaris et sphincter pupillae) is relayed through the ganglion ciliare where they synapse. The postsynaptic sympathetic fibers for the m. dilator pupillae, from the ganglion cervicale superius, also pass through this ganglion.

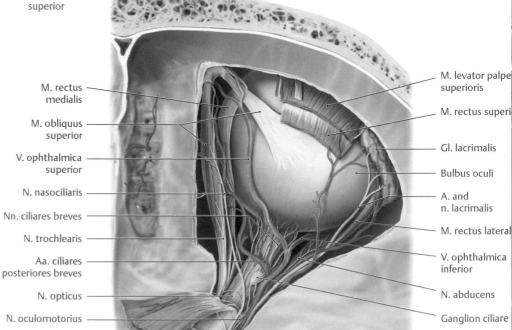

M. rectus medialis
M. obliquus superior
V. ophthalmica superior
N. nasociliaris
Nn. ciliares breves
N. trochlearis
Aa. ciliares posteriores breves
N. opticus
N. oculomotorius

M. levator palpebrae superioris
M. rectus superior
Gl. lacrimalis
Bulbus oculi
A. and n. lacrimalis
M. rectus lateralis
V. ophthalmica inferior
N. abducens
Ganglion ciliare

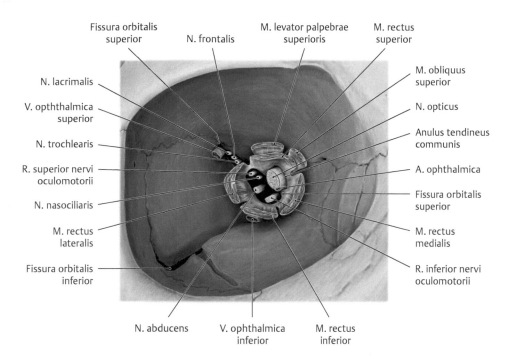

Fissura orbitalis superior
N. frontalis
M. levator palpebrae superioris
M. rectus superior

N. lacrimalis
M. obliquus superior
V. opththalmica superior
N. opticus
N. trochlearis
Anulus tendineus communis
R. superior nervi oculomotorii
A. ophthalmica
N. nasociliaris
Fissura orbitalis superior
M. rectus lateralis
M. rectus medialis
Fissura orbitalis inferior
R. inferior nervi oculomotorii

N. abducens
V. ophthalmica inferior
M. rectus inferior

C Topography of the right orbita: contents of the upper level
Superior view. The paries superior osseus orbitae, the periorbita, and the corpus adiposum orbitae have been removed.

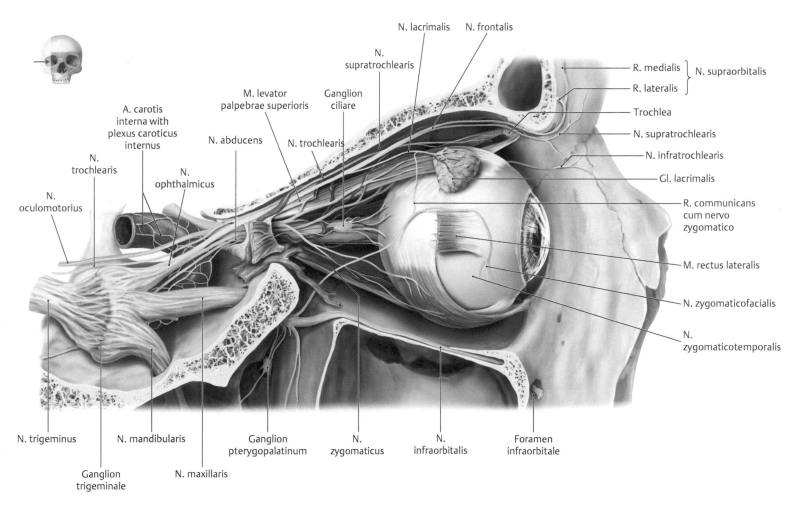

N. lacrimalis
N. frontalis
N. supratrochlearis
M. levator palpebrae superioris
Ganglion ciliare
A. carotis interna with plexus caroticus internus
N. abducens
N. trochlearis
R. medialis
N. supraorbitalis
R. lateralis
Trochlea
N. supratrochlearis
N. infratrochlearis
Gl. lacrimalis
N. trochlearis
N. ophthalmicus
N. oculomotorius
R. communicans cum nervo zygomatico
M. rectus lateralis
N. zygomaticofacialis
N. zygomaticotemporalis
N. trigeminus
N. mandibularis
Ganglion pterygopalatinum
N. zygomaticus
N. infraorbitalis
Foramen infraorbitale
Ganglion trigeminale
N. maxillaris

D Right orbita
Lateral view.
The following structures have been removed: paries lateralis orbitae as far as the fissura orbitalis inferior (see navigator), lateral portions of the paries superior orbitae as well as corpus adiposum orbitae and the anterior two-thirds of the m. levator palpebrae superioris. The m. rectus lateralis has been divided. The entire orbital contents can now be easily dissected, especially the ganglion ciliare and the r. communicans

cum nervo zygomatico (parasympathetic fibers from the ganglion pterygopalatinum for the gl. lacrimalis). If one also removes the ala major ossis sphenoidalis, one will also see the ganglion trigeminale and the opened sinus cavernosus.
Note that the removed facies orbitalis of the os zygomaticum contains the points of entry of the rr. zygomaticofacialis et zygomaticotemporalis, the rr. terminales sensorii nervi zygomatici supplying the skin over the os zygomaticum and tempora.

5.19 Topography of the Sinus Cavernosus

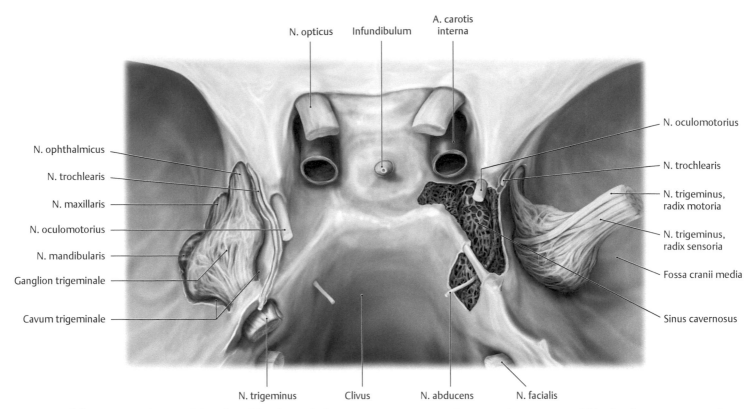

A Course of the nn. craniales supplying the orbita through the cavernous sinus

Sella turcica with partially opened sinus cavernosus on the right side, superior view. The two ganglia trigeminalia are exposed. The right ganglion has also been retracted laterally (thus opening the trigeminal cave) to demonstrate the open sinus cavernosus with the pars cavernosa arteriae carotidis internae coursing within it.

Note the n. abducens which also courses within the sinus cavernosus immediately adjacent to the a. carotis interna. All the other nerves coursing here (nn. oculomotorius, trochlearis, et trigeminus) course in a rostral or inferior direction in the lateral wall of the dura mater of the sinus

cavernosus. An a. carotis aneurysm within the sinus cavernosus therefore most often affects the n. abducens, and often that nerve alone. The expanding aneurysm compresses the nerve, causing loss of function. Therefore, one should always consider an a. carotis aneurysm as a possible cause of a sudden isolated n. abducens palsy (see **D**). In contrast, an isolated *n. trochlearis* palsy is very rare. The *n. trochlearis* tends to be affected *secondarily*, for example in the setting of sinus cavernosus thrombosis, which then affects all nerves passing through the sinus cavernosus, often including the first two rr. nervi trigemini.

B Coronal section through the sinus cavernosus at the level of the hypophysis

Rostral view.

Note the structures coursing within the lateral wall and within the sinus cavernosus.

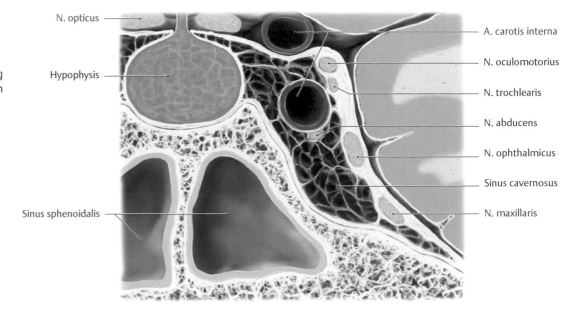

C Topography of the extradural course of the n. abducens on the clivus and in the opened left sinus cavernosus.

Left view.

Note the long extradural course of the n. abducens. This begins as it exits from the dura mater in the superior third of the clivus (before which its subarachnoid segment lies at the cisterna pontocerebellaris) over the "abducent bridge" (deep to the lig. petrosphenoidale through the canalis petrosphenoidalis) at the level of tip of the margo superior partis petrosae (passing from the fossa cranii posterior to the fossa cranii media). It continues through the sinus cavernosus immediately adjacent to the a. carotis interna, finally entering the orbita through the fissura orbitalis superior.

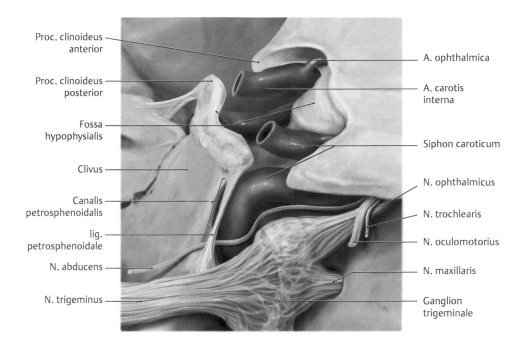

Proc. clinoideus anterior — Proc. clinoideus posterior — Fossa hypophysialis — Clivus — Canalis petrosphenoidalis — lig. petrosphenoidale — N. abducens — N. trigeminus

A. ophthalmica — A. carotis interna — Siphon caroticum — N. ophthalmicus — N. trochlearis — N. oculomotorius — N. maxillaris — Ganglion trigeminale

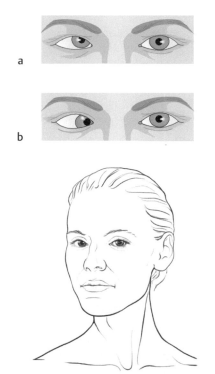

a

b

c

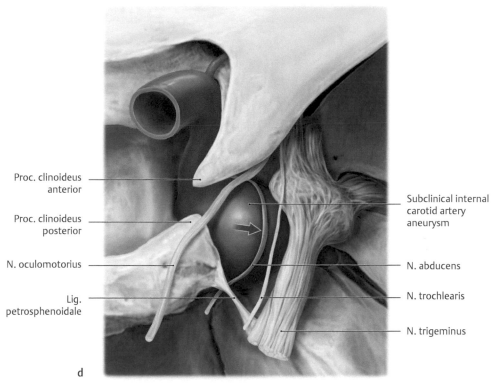

Proc. clinoideus anterior — Proc. clinoideus posterior — N. oculomotorius — Lig. petrosphenoidale

Subclinical internal carotid artery aneurysm — N. abducens — N. trochlearis — N. trigeminus

d

D Trochlear and n. abducens palsies

a Right n. trochlearis palsy; **b** right n. abducens palsy (patient looking straight ahead in each case); **c** compensatory head posture in right n. abducens palsy; **d** subclinical internal carotid artery aneurysm within the sinus cavernosus compressing the n. abducens.

Ophthalmoplegia can result from a lesion in the nucleus, along the course of the respective cranial nerve, or within the ocular muscle itself (see p. 173). Sequelae include an abnormal gaze of the affected eye that varies according to the muscle involved and the occurrence of diplopia, which the patient attempts to avoid with a compensatory head posture. For example, loss of the n. abducens (at 47% of all cases,

n. abducens palsies are the most common peripheral neurogenic disturbance of ocular motility) causes the affected eye to deviate medially even in primary position due to the isolated loss of the m. rectus lateralis (esotropia). The disturbing diploplia induces a compensatory head posture (**c**), that is a head posture in which diplopia does not occur or is greatly reduced. The patient turns the head laterally toward the side of the affected muscle (a position in which the paretic muscle has no effect anyway). A. carotis interna aneurysms within the sinus cavernosus can lie in a supraclinoid or infraclinoid position, whereby the infraclinoid aneurysms (**d**) in particular exhibit a slowly progressive mass effect leading to isolated compression of the n. abducens.

5.20 Nose: Overview

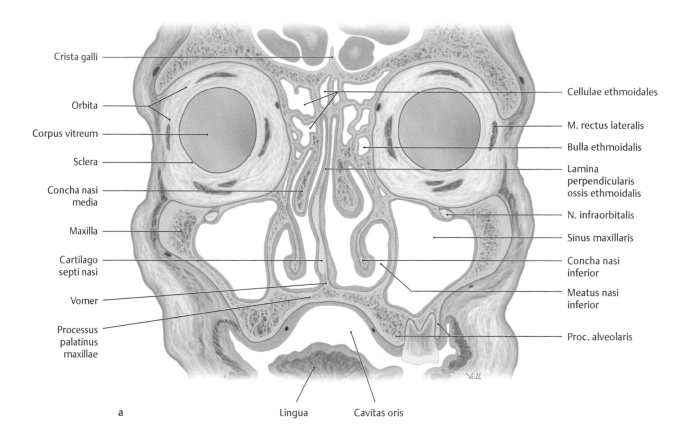

Crista galli
Orbita
Corpus vitreum
Sclera
Concha nasi media
Maxilla
Cartilago septi nasi
Vomer
Processus palatinus maxillae

Cellulae ethmoidales
M. rectus lateralis
Bulla ethmoidalis
Lamina perpendicularis ossis ethmoidalis
N. infraorbitalis
Sinus maxillaris
Concha nasi inferior
Meatus nasi inferior
Proc. alveolaris

a   Lingua Cavitas oris

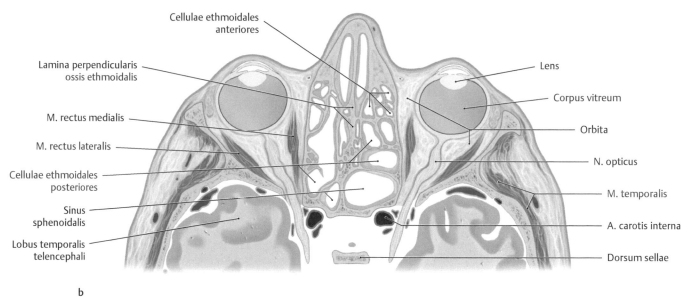

Cellulae ethmoidales anteriores
Lamina perpendicularis ossis ethmoidalis
M. rectus medialis
M. rectus lateralis
Cellulae ethmoidales posteriores
Sinus sphenoidalis
Lobus temporalis telencephali

Lens
Corpus vitreum
Orbita
N. opticus
M. temporalis
A. carotis interna
Dorsum sellae

b

A Overview of the nose and sinus paranasales

a Coronal section, anterior view. **b** Transverse section, superior view. The reader is assumed to be familiar with the bony anatomy of the cavitas nasi (especially the openings of the various passages below the conchae nasi, see p. 42 f). The cavitates nasi and sinus paranasales are arranged in pairs. The left and right cavitates nasi are separated by the septum nasi and have an approximately triangular shape. Below the base of the triangle is the cavitas oris. The following paired sinus paranasales are shown in the drawings:

- Cellulae ethmoidales (ethmoid sinus*)
- Sinus maxillaris
- Sinus sphenoidalis

The interior of each sinus is lined with ciliated pseudostratified columnar epithelium with goblet cells (respiratory epithelium) (see p. 184).

*The term "ethmoid sinus" has been dropped from the latest anatomical nomenclature, although it is still widely used by medical practitioners.

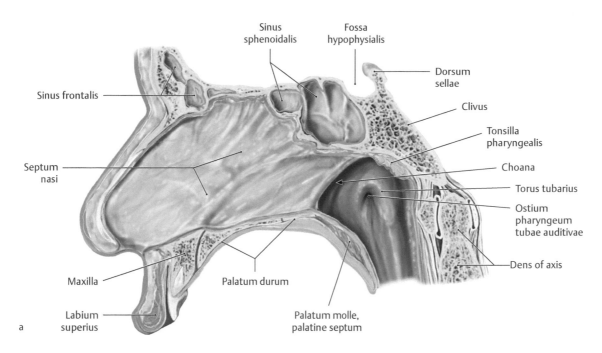

a Tunica mucosa of the septum nasi, parasagittal section viewed from the left side.

Labels (clockwise): Sinus sphenoidalis · Fossa hypophysialis · Dorsum sellae · Clivus · Tonsilla pharyngealis · Choana · Torus tubarius · Ostium pharyngeum tubae auditivae · Dens of axis · Palatum molle, palatine septum · Palatum durum · Labium superius · Maxilla · Septum nasi · Sinus frontalis

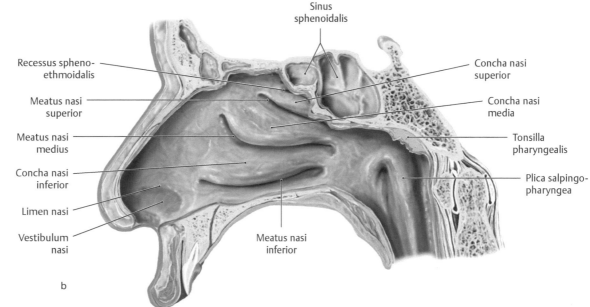

b Tunica mucosa of the right lateral nasal wall, viewed from the left side.

Labels: Sinus sphenoidalis · Recessus spheno-ethmoidalis · Meatus nasi superior · Meatus nasi medius · Concha nasi inferior · Limen nasi · Vestibulum nasi · Meatus nasi inferior · Concha nasi superior · Concha nasi media · Tonsilla pharyngealis · Plica salpingopharyngea

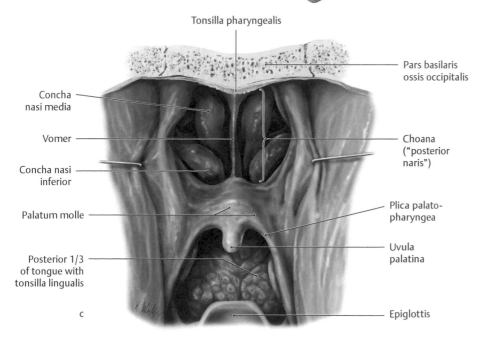

c Posterior view through the choanae into the cavitas nasi.

Labels: Tonsilla pharyngealis · Concha nasi media · Vomer · Concha nasi inferior · Palatum molle · Posterior 1/3 of tongue with tonsilla lingualis · Pars basilaris ossis occipitalis · Choana ("posterior naris") · Plica palatopharyngea · Uvula palatina · Epiglottis

B Mucosa of the nasal cavity

a Tunica mucosa of the septum nasi, parasagittal section viewed from the left side. **b** Tunica mucosa of the right lateral nasal wall, viewed from the left side. **c** Posterior view through the choanae into the cavitas nasi.

While the medial wall of the cavitas nasi is smooth, its lateral wall is raised into folds by the three conchae (conchae nasi superior, media, and inferior). These increase the surface area of the cavitas nasi, enabling it to warm and humidify the inspired air more efficiently (cf. p. 184). A section of the right sinus sphenoidalis is shown in **b**. The choanae (**c**) are the posterior openings by which the cavitas nasi communicates with the pars nasalis pharyngis. Note the close proximity of the choanae to the tuba auditiva and tonsilla pharyngealis (see p. 197).

181

5.21 Nasal Cavity (Cavitas Nasi): Neurovascular Supply

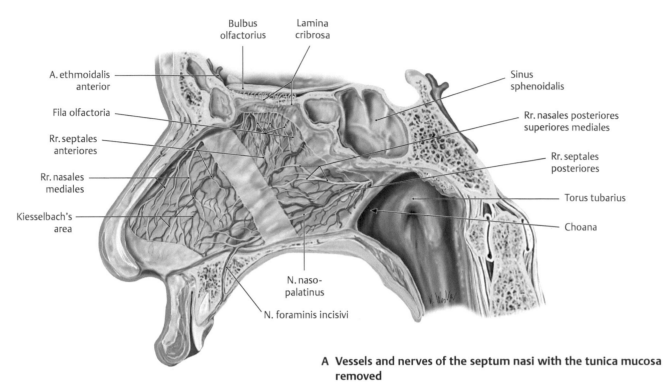

A Vessels and nerves of the septum nasi with the tunica mucosa removed

Parasagittal section, viewed from the left side. The arterial supply of the septum nasi is of particular clinical interest in the diagnosis and treatment of nosebleed (see **C**).

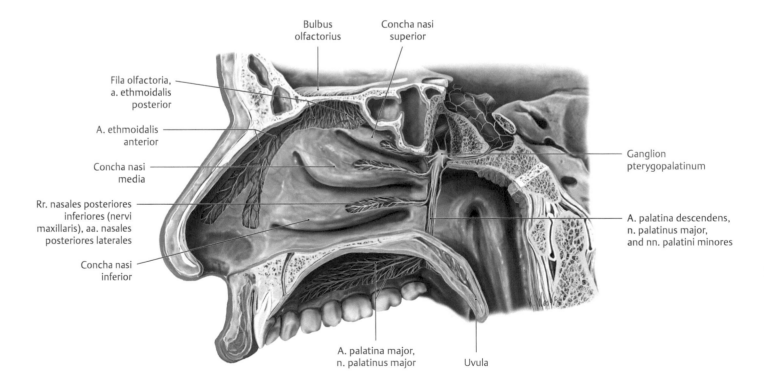

B Vessels and nerves of the right lateral nasal wall

Left lateral view. The ganglion pterygopalatinum, an important relay in the parasympathetic nervous system (see pp. 127 and 239), has been exposed here by partial resection of the os sphenoidale. The nerve fibers arising from it pass to the small gll. nasales of the conchae nasi, entering the conchae from the posterior side with the blood vessels. At the level of the concha nasi superior, the fila olfactoria pass through the lamina cribrosa (ossis ethmoidalis) to the pars **olfactoria tunicae mucosae nasi**. The nasal wall is supplied from above by the two aa. ethmoidales, which arise from the a. ophthalmica. It is supplied from behind by the aa. nasales posteriores laterales, which arise from the a. sphenopalatina.

The figures below depict the functional groups of arteries and nerves supplying the cavitas nasi. As in a dissection, the septum is displayed first, followed by the lateral wall.

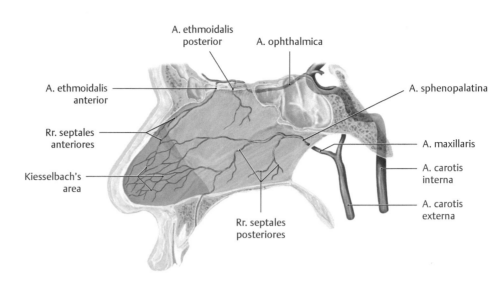

C Arteries of the septum nasi
Left lateral view. The vessels of the septum nasi arise from branches of the aa. carotides externa and interna. The anterior part of the septum contains a highly vascularized area called Kiesselbach's area (indicated by color shading), which is supplied by vessels from both major arteries. This area is the most common site of significant nosebleed.

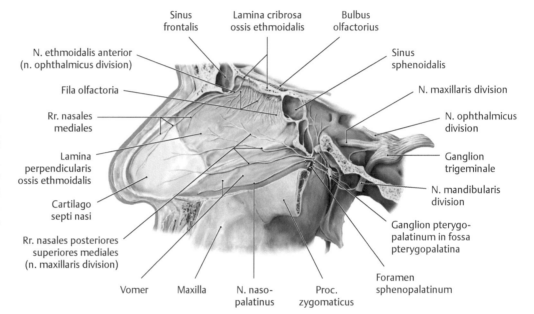

D Nerves of the septum nasi
Left lateral view. The septum nasi receives its sensory innervation from branches of the n. trigeminus (CN V). The anterosuperior part of the septum is supplied by branches of the n. ophthalmicus division (CN V_1), and the rest by branches of the n. ophthalmicus division (CN V_2). Bundles of fila olfactoria (CN I) arise from receptors in the pars olfactoria tunicae mucosae nasi.

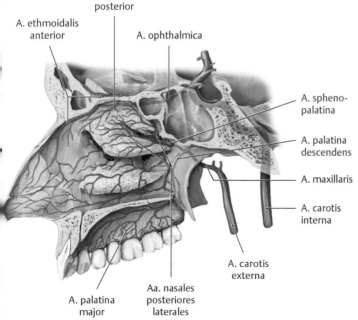

E Arteries of the right lateral nasal wall
Left lateral view.
Note the vascular supply from the branches of the a. carotis interna (from above) and the a. carotis externa (from behind).

F Nerves of the right lateral nasal wall
Left lateral view. The lateral nasal wall derives its sensory innervation from branches of the n. ophthalmicus division (CN V_1) and the n. maxillaris division (CN V_2) of the n. trigeminus. Receptor neurons in the pars olfactoria tunicae mucosae nasi send their axons in the n. olfactorius (CN I) to the bulbus olfactorius.

5.22 Nose and Paranasal Sinuses (Sinus Paranasales): Histology and Clinical Anatomy

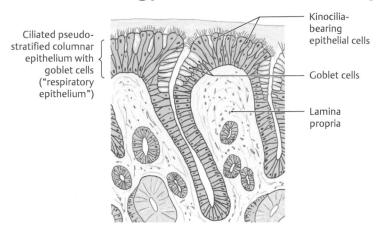

Ciliated pseudo-stratified columnar epithelium with goblet cells ("respiratory epithelium")

Kinocilia-bearing epithelial cells

Goblet cells

Lamina propria

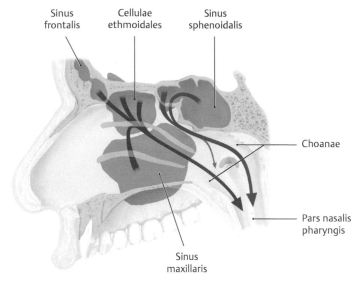

Sinus frontalis — Cellulae ethmoidales — Sinus sphenoidalis

Choanae

Pars nasalis pharyngis

Sinus maxillaris

A Histology of the nasal tunica mucosa

The surface of the respiratory epithelium of the nasal tunica mucosa consists of kinocilia-bearing cells and goblet cells, the latter secreting their mucus into a watery film on the epithelial surface. Serous and sero-mucous glands are embedded in the lamina propria and also release secretions into the superficial fluid film. The directional fluid flow produced by the cilia (see **C** and **D**) is an important component of the nonspecific immune response. If coordinated beating of the cilia is impaired, the patient will suffer chronic recurring infections of the respiratory tract.

B Normal drainage of secretions from the sinus paranasales

Left lateral view. The beating cilia propel the mucous blanket over the cilia (see **D**) and through the choana into the pars nasalis pharyngis, where it is swallowed.

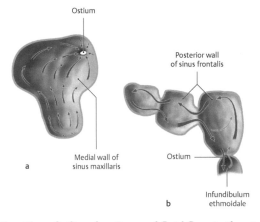

Ostium

Posterior wall of sinus frontalis

Medial wall of sinus maxillaris

Ostium

Infundibulum ethmoidale

a   b

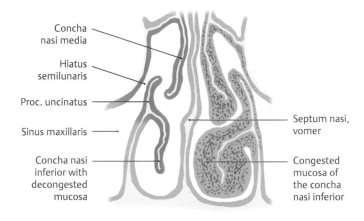

Concha nasi media

Hiatus semilunaris

Proc. uncinatus

Sinus maxillaris

Septum nasi, vomer

Concha nasi inferior with decongested mucosa

Congested mucosa of the concha nasi inferior

C Direction of ciliary beating and fluid flow in the right maxillary sinus and frontal sinus

Schematic coronal sections of the right sinus maxillaris (**a**) and sinus frontalis (**b**), anterior view. The location of the sinuses is shown in **C**.
Beating of the cilia produces a flow of fluid in the sinus paranasales that is always directed toward the sinus ostium. This clears the sinus of particles and microorganisms that are trapped in the mucous layer. If the ostium is obstructed due to swelling of the mucosa, inflammation may develop in the affected sinus (*sinusitis*). This occurs most commonly in the ostiomeatal unit of the sinus maxillaris—ethmoid ostium (see p. 30 f) (after Stammberger and Hanke).

D Functional states of the mucosa in the nasal cavity

Coronal section, anterior view.
The function of the tunica mucosa cavitatis nasi is to warm and humidify the inspired air. This is accomplished by an increase of blood flow through the tunica mucosa (see pp. 101 and 103), placing it in a congested (swollen) state. The mucous membranes are not simultaneously congested on both sides, however, but undergo a normal cycle of congestion and decongestion that lasts approximately 6 hours (the right side is decongested in the drawing). Examination of the cavitas nasi can be facilitated by first administering a decongestant to shrink the tunica mucosa, roughly as it appears here on the left side.

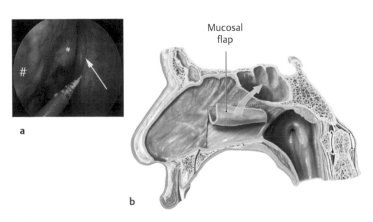

Mucosal flap

a

b

E Sparing the pars olfactoria tunicae mucosae nasi in operations on the sphenoid sinus

a Endoscopic image of the pars olfactoria tunicae mucosae nasi (from: Harvey R. et al. The Olfactory Strip and Its Preservation in Endoscopic Pituitary Surgery Maintains Smell and Sinonasal Function in: Neurol Surg B 2015; 76(06): 464–470; for the angle of vision with the endoscope see **F**)

b Lateral nasal wall. Left view. The pars olfactoria is the lighter (less perfused) region (arrow; *concha nasi suprema; # concha nasi media in **a**). This region should be spared in operations on the sinus sphenoidalis. The mucosal region deep to the pars olfactoria can be grafted as a mucosal flap.

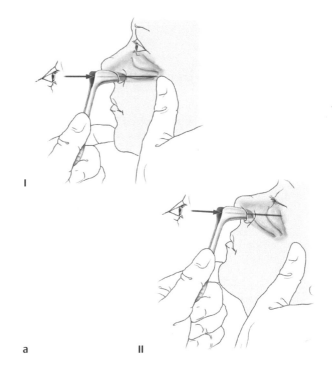

a

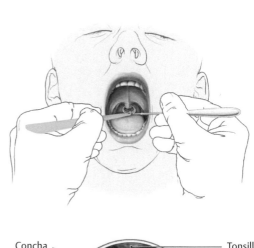

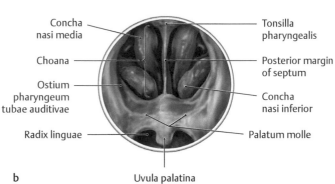

Concha nasi media

Choana

Ostium pharyngeum tubae auditivae

Radix linguae

Tonsilla pharyngealis

Posterior margin of septum

Concha nasi inferior

Palatum molle

b Uvula palatina

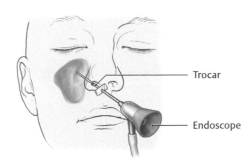

— Trocar

— Endoscope

F Endoscopy of the sinus maxillaris
Anterior view. The sinus maxillaris is not accessible to direct inspection and must therefore be examined with an endoscope. To enter the sinus maxillaris, the examiner pierces the thin bony wall below the concha nasi inferior with a trocar and advances the endoscope through the opening. The scope can then be angled and rotated to inspect all of the mucosal surfaces.

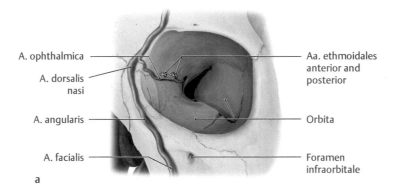

A. ophthalmica

A. dorsalis nasi

A. angularis

A. facialis

Aa. ethmoidales anterior and posterior

Orbita

Foramen infraorbitale

a

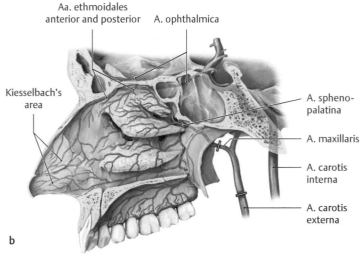

Aa. ethmoidales anterior and posterior   A. ophthalmica

Kiesselbach's area

A. spheno-palatina

A. maxillaris

A. carotis interna

A. carotis externa

b

G Anterior and posterior rhinoscopy
a **Anterior rhinoscopy** is a procedure for inspection of the cavitas nasi. Two different positions (I, II) are used to ensure that all of the anterior cavitas nasi is examined.
b In posterior rhinoscopy, the choanae and tonsilla pharyngealis are accessible to clinical examination. The rhinoscope can be angled and rotated to demonstrate the structures shown in the composite image. Today the rhinoscope is frequently replaced by an endoscope.

H Sites of arterial ligation for the treatment of severe nosebleed
If a severe nosebleed cannot be controlled with ordinary intranasal packing, it may be necessary to ligate relatively large arterial vessels. The following arteries may be ligated:

• In the case of anterior nasal bleeding, the aa. ethmoidales anterior and posterior (**a**)
• In the case of posterior nasal bleeding, the a. sphenopalatina or the a. maxillaris (**b**)
• In very severe cases, the a. carotis externa (**b**)

185

5.23 Oral Cavity (Cavitas Oris): Overview

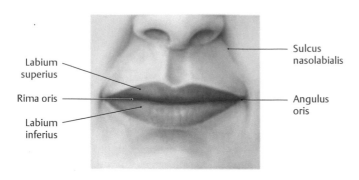

A Lips (labia oris) and labial creases
Anterior view. The upper and lower lips (labia superius and inferius) meet at the angulus oris. The rima oris opens into the cavitas oris. Changes in the lips noted on visual inspection may yield important diagnostic clues: Blue lips (cyanosis) suggest a disease of the heart, lung, or both, while deep sulci nasolabiales may reflect chronic diseases of the digestive tract.

B Cavitas oris
Anterior view. The arcus dentales with the processus alveolaris maxillae and pars alveolaris mandibulae subdivide the cavitas oris into several parts (see also **C**):

- Vestibulum oris: the part of the cavitas oris bounded on one side by the dentes and on the other side by the labia oris or buccae
- Cavitas oris propria: the cavity of the mouth in the strict sense (within the arcus dentales, bounded posteriorly by the arcus palatoglossus)
- Fauces: the throat (boundary with the pharynx: arcus palatopharyngeus)

The fauces communicate with the pharynx through the isthmus faucium. The cavitas oris is lined with nonkeratinized, stratified squamous epithelium which is moistened by secretions from the gll. salivariae (see p. 211). Squamous cell carcinomas of the cavitas oris are particularly common in smokers and heavy drinkers.

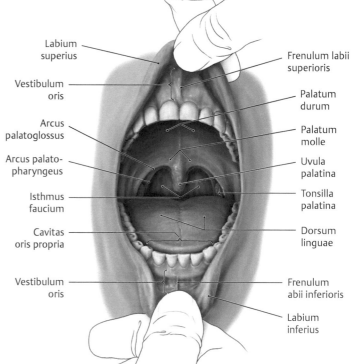

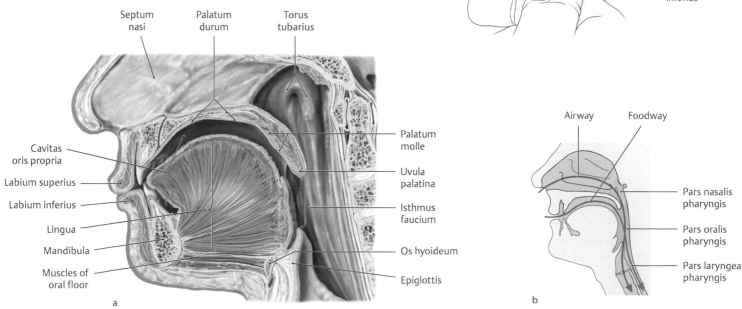

C Organization and boundaries of the cavitas oris
Midsagittal section, left lateral view. The muscles of the oral floor and the adjacent tongue (lingua) together constitute the inferior boundary of the cavitas oris propria. The roof of the cavitas oris is formed by the palatum durum in its anterior two-thirds and by the palatum molle (velum) in its posterior third (see **F**). The uvula palatina hangs from the palatum molle between the cavitas oris and pharynx. The keratinized stratified squamous epithelium of the skin blends with the nonkeratinized stratified squamous epithelium of the cavitas oris at the vermilion border of the lip. The cavitas oris is located below the cavitas nasi and anterior to the pharynx. The midportion of the pharynx, called the pars oralis pharyngis, is the area in which the airway and foodway intersect (**b**).

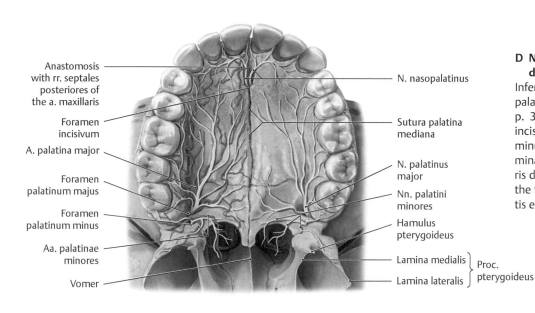

Anastomosis with rr. septales posteriores of the a. maxillaris

Foramen incisivum

A. palatina major

Foramen palatinum majus

Foramen palatinum minus

Aa. palatinae minores

Vomer

N. nasopalatinus

Sutura palatina mediana

N. palatinus major

Nn. palatini minores

Hamulus pterygoideus

Lamina medialis ⎱ Proc.
Lamina lateralis ⎰ pterygoideus

D Neurovascular structures of the palatum durum

Inferior view. The arteries and nerves of the palatum durum (skeletal anatomy is shown on p. 38) pass downward through the foramen incisivum and the foramina palatina majus and minus into the cavitas oris. The nerves are terminal branches of the n. trigeminus n. maxillaris division (CN V$_2$), and the arteries arise from the territory of the a. maxillaris off the a. carotis externa (neither are shown here).

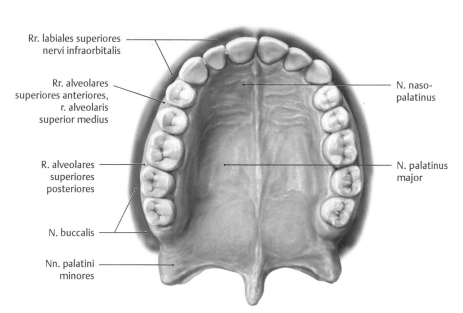

Rr. labiales superiores nervi infraorbitalis

Rr. alveolares superiores anteriores, r. alveolaris superior medius

R. alveolares superiores posteriores

N. buccalis

Nn. palatini minores

N. nasopalatinus

N. palatinus major

E Sensory innervation of the palatal tunica mucosa, labium superius, buccae, and gingiva

Inferior view.

Note that the region shown in the drawing receives sensory innervation from different branches of the n. trigeminus (n. buccalis from the n. mandibularis division (CN V$_3$, all other branches are from the n. maxillaris division, CN V$_2$).

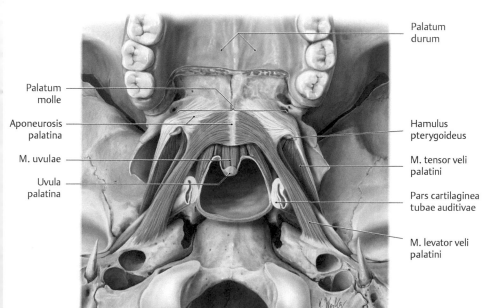

Palatum molle

Aponeurosis palatina

M. uvulae

Uvula palatina

Palatum durum

Hamulus pterygoideus

M. tensor veli palatini

Pars cartilaginea tubae auditivae

M. levator veli palatini

F Muscles of the palatum molle

Inferior view. The palatum molle forms the posterior boundary of the cavitas oris, separating it from the pars oralis pharyngis. The muscles are attached at the midline to the aponeurosis palatina, which forms the connective tissue foundation of the palatum molle. The m. tensor veli palatini, m. levator veli palatini, and m. uvulae can be identified in this dissection. While the m. tensor veli palatini tightens the palatum molle, simultaneously opening the inlet to the tuba auditiva, the m. levator veli palatini raises the palatum molle to a horizontal position. Both of these muscles, but not the m. uvulae, also contribute structurally to the lateral pharyngeal wall.

5.24 Tongue (Lingua): Muscles and Mucosa

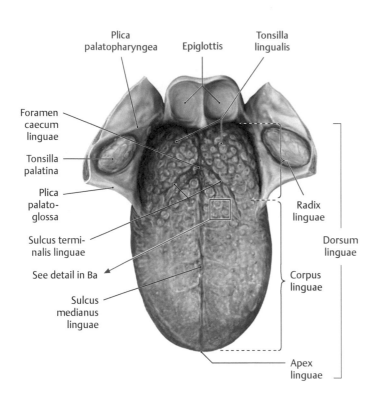

Plica palatopharyngea · Epiglottis · Tonsilla lingualis

Foramen caecum linguae

Tonsilla palatina

Plica palato-glossa

Sulcus termi-nalis linguae

See detail in Ba

Sulcus medianus linguae

Radix linguae

Dorsum linguae

Corpus linguae

Apex linguae

A Surface anatomy of the lingual mucosa

Superior view. While the motor properties of the tongue are functionally important during mastication, swallowing, and speaking, its equally important sensory functions include taste and fine tactile discrimination. The tongue is endowed with a very powerful muscular body (see **Ca**). The upper surface (dorsum linguae) of the tongue is covered by a highly specialized mucosal coat and consists, from front to back, of an apex (tip), corpus linguae (body), and radix linguae (root).

The V-shaped furrow on the dorsal surface (the sulcus terminalis) further divides the tongue into an anterior (oral, presulcal) part and a posterior (pharyngeal, postsulcal) part. The pars anterior comprises the anterior two-thirds of the tongue, and the pars posterior comprises the posterior third. At the tip of the "V" is the foramen caecum linguae (vestige of embryological migration of the gl. thyroidea). This subdivision is a result of embryological development and explains why each part has a different nerve supply (see p. 191). The tunica mucosa of the pars anterior is composed of numerous papillae (see B), and the connective tissue between the mucosal surface and musculature contains many gll. salivariae minores. The physician should be familiar with them because they may give rise to tumors (usually malignant).

The gemmae gustatoriae are bordered by serous glands (see **Bb–e**) that are known also as von *Ebner glands*; they produce a watery secretion that keeps the taste buds clean.

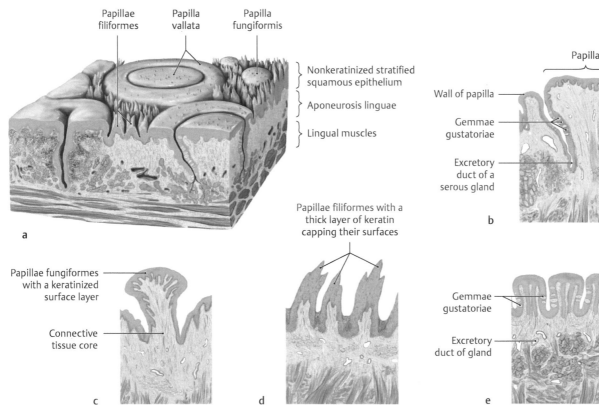

Papillae filiformes · Papilla vallata · Papilla fungiformis

Nonkeratinized stratified squamous epithelium

Aponeurosis linguae

Lingual muscles

a

Papillae fungiformes with a keratinized surface layer

Connective tissue core

c

Papillae filiformes with a thick layer of keratin capping their surfaces

d

Papilla

Sulcus

Wall of papilla

Gemmae gustatoriae

Excretory duct of a serous gland

Serous glands (von Ebner glands)

b

Gemmae gustatoriae

Excretory duct of gland

Papillae foliatae

Serous gland

e

B The papillae of the tongue

a Sectional block diagram of the lingual papillae. **b–e** Types of papillae. The papillae are divided into four morphologically distinct types:

b Papillae vallatae: encircled by a depression and containing abundant gemmae gustatoriae on their lateral surfaces

c Papillae fungiformes: mushroom-shaped, located at the sides of the tongue (they exhibit mechanical receptors, thermal receptors, and gemmae gustatoriae)

d Papillae filiformes: rasplike papillae with a thick cap of keratin that are sensitive to tactile stimulie Papilla

e foliatae: located on the posterior sides of the tongue, containing numerous gemmae gustatoriae

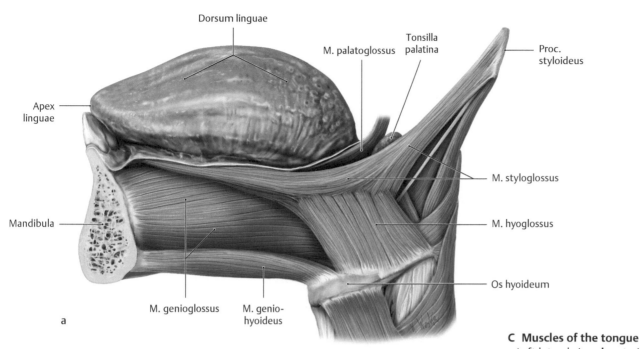

a

Dorsum linguae

M. palatoglossus

Tonsilla palatina

Proc. styloideus

Apex linguae

M. styloglossus

Mandibula

M. hyoglossus

Os hyoideum

M. genioglossus

M. genio-hyoideus

C Muscles of the tongue

a Left lateral view, **b** anterior view of a coronal section.

There are two sets of lingual muscles: extrinsic and intrinsic. The extrinsic muscles are attached to specific bony sites outside the tongue, while the intrinsic muscles have no attachments to skeletal structures. The extrinsic lingual muscles include the

- m. genioglossus,
- m. hyoglossus,
- m. palatoglossus,
- m. styloglossus.

The *intrinsic* lingual muscles include the

- m. longitudinalis superior,
- m. longitudinalis inferior,
- m. transversus linguae,
- m. verticalis linguae.

The extrinsic muscles move the tongue as a whole, while the intrinsic muscles alter its shape. All of the genuine mm. linguae mentioned here are innervated by the n. hypoglossus (CN XII). Although the m. palatoglossus (see **a**) acts on the tongue, it is in fact a muscle of the palatum molle vel fauces, belonging to the mm. palati mollis et faucium and not to the mm. linguae. Accordingly, it is still supplied by the n. glossopharyngeus.

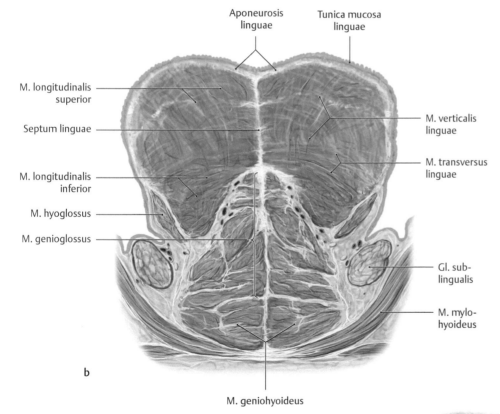

Aponeurosis linguae

Tunica mucosa linguae

M. longitudinalis superior

M. verticalis linguae

Septum linguae

M. transversus linguae

M. longitudinalis inferior

M. hyoglossus

M. genioglossus

Gl. sub-lingualis

M. mylo-hyoideus

b

M. geniohyoideus

D Unilateral nervus hypoglossus palsy

Active protrusion of the tongue with an intact n. hypoglossus (**a**) and with a unilateral n. hypoglossus lesion (**b**).

When the n. hypoglossus is damaged on one side, the m. genioglossus muscle is paralyzed on the affected side. As a result, the healthy (innervated) m. genioglossus on the opposite side dominates the tongue across the midline toward the affected side. When the tongue is protruded, it deviates toward the paralyzed side.

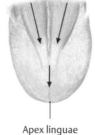

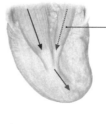

Paralyzed m. genioglossus on affected side

a   Apex linguae

b

5.25 Tongue: Neurovascular Structures and Lymphatic Drainage

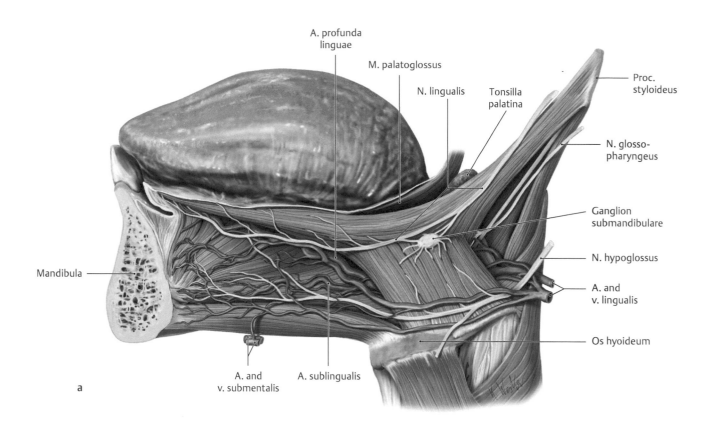

A. profunda linguae

M. palatoglossus

N. lingualis

Tonsilla palatina

Proc. styloideus

N. glosso-pharyngeus

Ganglion submandibulare

N. hypoglossus

A. and v. lingualis

Os hyoideum

Mandibula

A. and v. submentalis

A. sublingualis

a

A Nerves and vessels of the tongue

a Left lateral view, **b** view of the inferior surface of the tongue.

The tongue is supplied by the *a. lingualis* (from the a. carotis externa), which divides into its terminal branches, the a. carotis externa and the a. sublingualis. The v. lingualis usually runs parallel to the artery and drains into the *v. jugularis interna*. The tunica mucosa linguae receives its somatosensory innervation (sensitivity to thermal and tactile stimuli) from the *n. lingualis*, which is a branch of the n. trigeminus n. mandibularis division (CN V_3). The n. lingualis transmits fibers from the chorda tympani of the n. facialis (CN VII), among them the afferent taste fibers for the pars anterior (anterior two-thirds) of the tongue. The chorda tympani also contains presynaptic, parasympathetic visceromotor axons which synapse in the ganglion submandibulare, whose neurons in turn innervate the gll. submandibulares and gll. sublinguales (see p. 127 for further details). The m. palatoglossus receives its somatosensory innervation from the n. glossopharyngeus (CN IX). The remaining tongue muscles are innervated by the n. hypoglossus (CN XII).

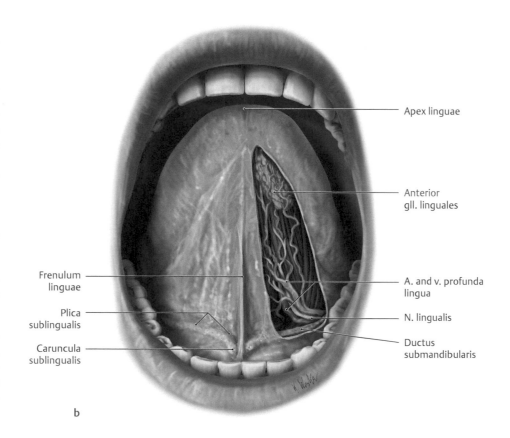

Apex linguae

Anterior gll. linguales

Frenulum linguae

A. and v. profunda lingua

Plica sublingualis

N. lingualis

Caruncula sublingualis

Ductus submandibularis

b

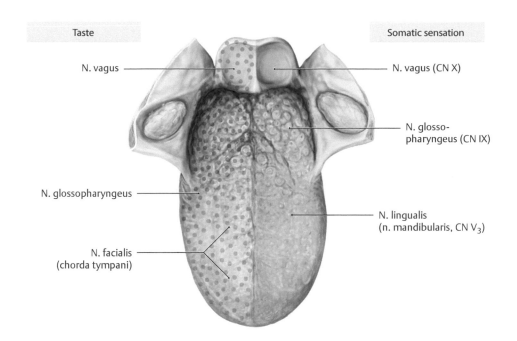

Taste | Somatic sensation

N. vagus — — N. vagus (CN X)

— N. glosso-pharyngeus (CN IX)

N. glossopharyngeus —

— N. lingualis (n. mandibularis, CN V$_3$)

N. facialis (chorda tympani)

B Somatosensory innervation (left side) and taste innervation (right side) of the tongue

Anterior view. The tongue receives its somatosensory innervation (e.g., touch, pain, thermal sensation) from three cranial nerve branches:

- N. lingualis (branch of n. mandibularis CN V$_3$),
- N. glossopharyngeus (CN IX)
- N. vagus (CN X)

Three nn. craniales also convey the taste fibers: CN VII (n. facialis, chorda tympani), CN IX (n. glossopharyngeus), and CN X (n. vagus). Thus, a disturbance of taste sensation involving the anterior two-thirds of the tongue indicates the presence of a n. facialis lesion, whereas a disturbance of tactile, pain, or thermal sensation indicates a n. trigeminus lesion (see also pp. 121 and 127).

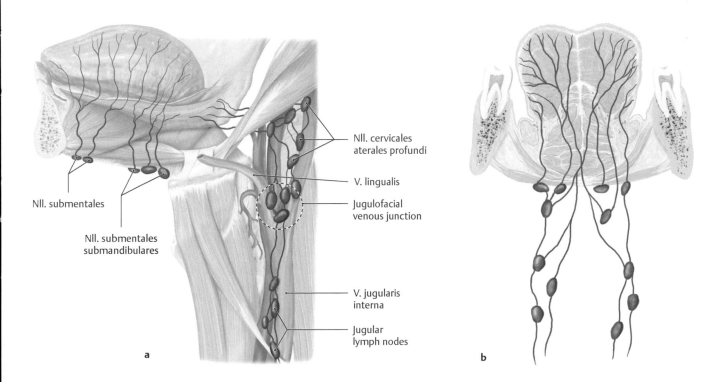

Nll. cervicales aterales profundi

V. lingualis

Nll. submentales

Jugulofacial venous junction

Nll. submentales submandibulares

V. jugularis interna

Jugular lymph nodes

a

b

C Lymphatic drainage of the tongue and oral floor

Left lateral view (**a**) and anterior view (**b**).

The lymphatic drainage of the tongue and oral floor is mediated by submental and submandibular groups of lymph nodes that ultimately drain into the lymph nodes along the v. jugularis interna (**a**, jugular lymph nodes). Because the lymph nodes receive drainage from both the ipsilateral and contralateral sides (**b**), tumor cells may become widely disseminated in this region (for example, metastatic squamous cell carcinoma, especially on the lateral border of the tongue, frequently metastasizes to the opposite side).

191

5.26 Topography of the Cavitas Oris Aperta

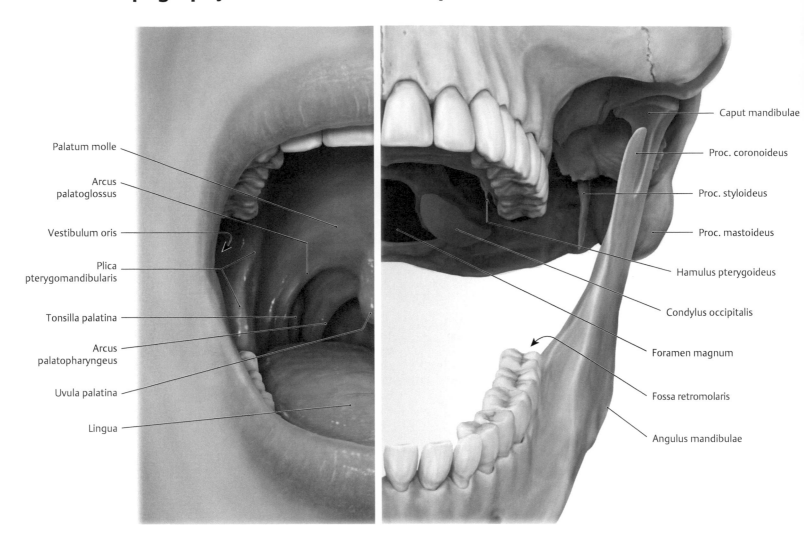

Palatum molle

Arcus palatoglossus

Vestibulum oris

Plica pterygomandibularis

Tonsilla palatina

Arcus palatopharyngeus

Uvula palatina

Lingua

Caput mandibulae

Proc. coronoideus

Proc. styloideus

Proc. mastoideus

Hamulus pterygoideus

Condylus occipitalis

Foramen magnum

Fossa retromolaris

Angulus mandibulae

A   Mucosal structures versus bony architecture of the upper and lower jaw

Anterior view with the mouth fully open.

The comparison shows where which **bony structures (b)** lie under the **tunica mucosa oris (a)**. Here one is looking past the isthmus faucium at the posterior wall of the pharynx. Anterior to the margo lateralis faucium, i.e., anterior to the arcus palatopharyngeus, arcus palatoglossus, and tonsilla palatina between them, there is a readily visible mucosal fold on both sides that extends in a arcus medialis. This is the plica pterygomandibularis. This thick ridge defines the margo posterior vestibuli oris. It extends from the fossa retromolaris of the lower jaw (posterior to the last molar and part of the trigonum retromolare, see p. 48) in the direction of the palatum durum to the hamulus pterygoideus. The base of the plica pterygomandibularis is a well-defined tendinous strip (raphe pterygomandibularis) between fossa et hamulus. Inserting into it are both the m. constrictor pharyngis superior (pars buccopharyngea) and m. buccinator, occasionally referred to as the "trumpeter's muscle." It represents an important landmark for administering a nerve block of the n. alveolaris inferior (see **B, b**). A fully open cavitas oris is practically never seen in an **anatomy lab** as the donor cadavers are usually fixed with the mouth shut so that the tongue more or less completely fills

the cavitas oris. There are also often only a few teeth or even none. The oral cavity is usually dissected in half a head divided by a median sagittal section. The anatomy student never sees the entire, fully open cavitas oris. Yet in **clinical reality**, inspection of the open cavitas oris and the anulus lymphoideus pharyngis (lips, tunica mucosa oris, tongue, tonsillae palatinae, and pharynx as well as teeth and gums) is an integral part of the even the most cursory physical examination. This is because the cavitas oris reflects habits (such as whether a person smokes), indicates the extent of personal care (condition of the teeth), and shows signs of disorders of internal organs (such as atrophic glossitis or "bald tongue," atrophy of the papillae in iron-deficiency anemia or Crohn's disease) and of the cavitas oris itself. Thus, every irregularity (leukoplakia, nodes, ulceration, etc.) in the mucosa should be evaluated as a suspected malignancy. In addition to inspection, palpation plays an important role, as one can obtain information about the consistency and extent of irregularities and changes in coloration within the oral mucosa. Findings in the paries inferior cavitatis oris or the cheek region are palpated with both hands from inside and outside the cavitas oris (see p. 211). Finally, familiarity with the topography of the open cavitas oris is an important requirement for properly administering local anesthesia, for example in dental procedures.

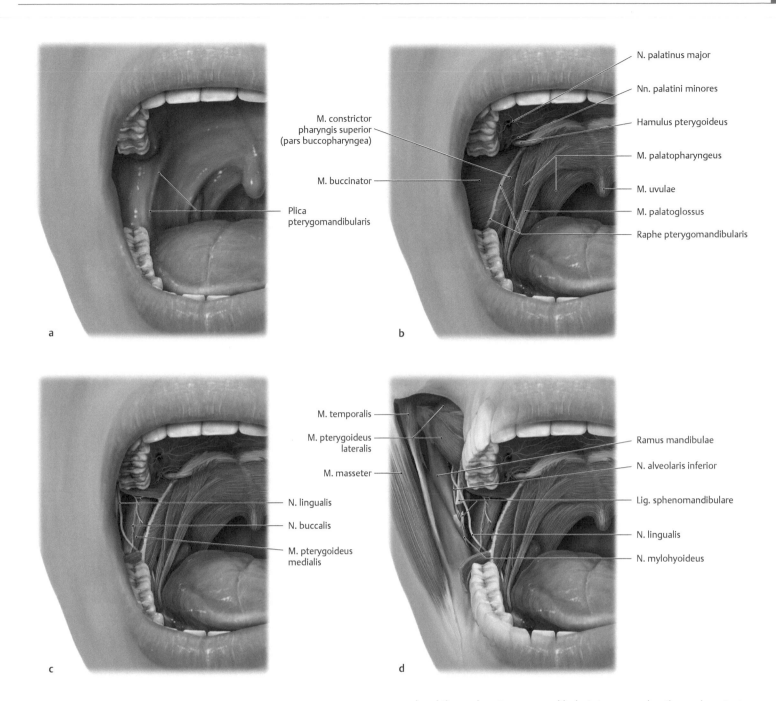

M. constrictor
pharyngis superior
(pars buccopharyngea)

M. buccinator

Plica
pterygomandibularis

N. palatinus major

Nn. palatini minores

Hamulus pterygoideus

M. palatopharyngeus

M. uvulae

M. palatoglossus

Raphe pterygomandibularis

M. temporalis

M. pterygoideus
lateralis

M. masseter

N. lingualis

N. buccalis

M. pterygoideus
medialis

Ramus mandibulae

N. alveolaris inferior

Lig. sphenomandibulare

N. lingualis

N. mylohyoideus

a

b

c

d

**B Course of the n. alveolaris inferior, n. lingualis, and n. mylohyoideus in the region of the regio medialis rami mandibulae
(spatium pterygomandibularis)**

a–d Anterolateral views of various layers of the lower jaw. In these
views, the neurovascular structures, muscles, and plica pterygomandibularis lie in different positions relative to one another than they do in
the anterior view (see **A**). As one invariably approaches the most frequently anesthetized nerve, the n. alveolaris inferior, from the contralateral premolar region, this lateral view is extremely important for
orientation. The lower jaw is in focus here as that is where not only the
n. alveolaris inferior courses, but also the n. lingualis and n. mylohyoideus. These latter structures can be easily injured if the wrong approach
is chosen. The various layers also convey an impression of the size of the
spatium pterygomandibulare.
a View of the tunica mucosa oris in the region of the plica pterygomandibularis dextra; **b** the tunica mucosa oris has been completely remo

ved and the raphe pterygomandibularis is exposed; **c** the m. buccinator
has been cut away or reflected, exposing the m. pterygoideus medialis
and the spatium pterygomandibulare, through which the n. alveolaris
inferior as well as the nn. lingualis et mylohyoideus course; **d** the skin of
the cheek has been cut away, revealing the lig. sphenomandibulare. It
courses on the medial aspect of the ramus mandibulae from the spina
ossis sphenoidalis to the lingula (foraminis) mandibulae and covers the
n. alveolaris inferior immediately before its point of entry into the foramen mandibulae. With the pars distalis ligamenti cut away, one can see
the bifurcatio nervi mylohyoidei at the level of the lingula mandibulae.
Note: Injuries to the n. lingualis can occur in the setting of facial trauma
as well as in dental procedures (for example surgical removal of wisdom
teeth or administration of an n. alveolaris inferior block).

193

5.27 Oral Floor

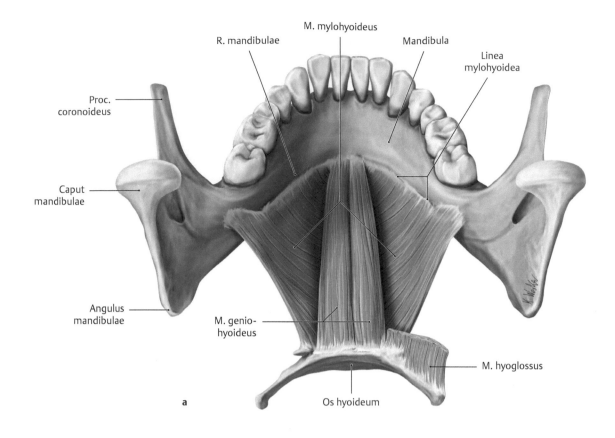

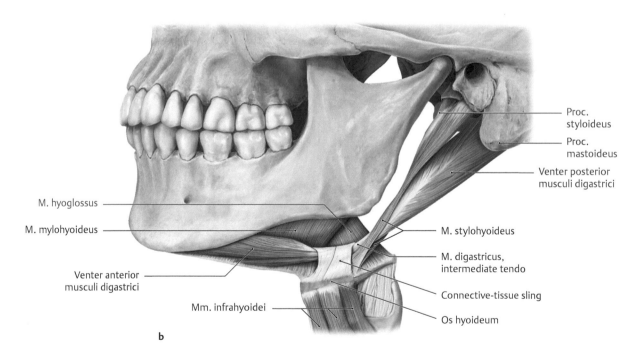

A Muscles of the oral floor

Superior view (**a**) and left lateral view (**b**).

The oral floor is formed by a muscular sheet that stretches between the two rami of the mandibula. This sheet consists of four muscles, all of which are located above the os hyoideum and are thus collectively known as the mm. suprahyoidei:

1. M. mylohyoideus: The muscle fibers from each side fuse in a median raphe (covered superiorly by the m. geniohyoideus).

2. M. geniohyoideus: strengthens the central portion of the oral floor.
3. M. digastricus: The venter anterior of the m. digastricus is located in the oral floor region; its venter posterior arises from the processus mastoideus.
4. M. stylohyoideus: arises from the proc. styloideus. Its tendon is perforated by the intermediate tendon of the m. digastricus.

All four muscles participate in active opening of the mouth. They also elevate the os hyoideum and move it forward during swallowing.

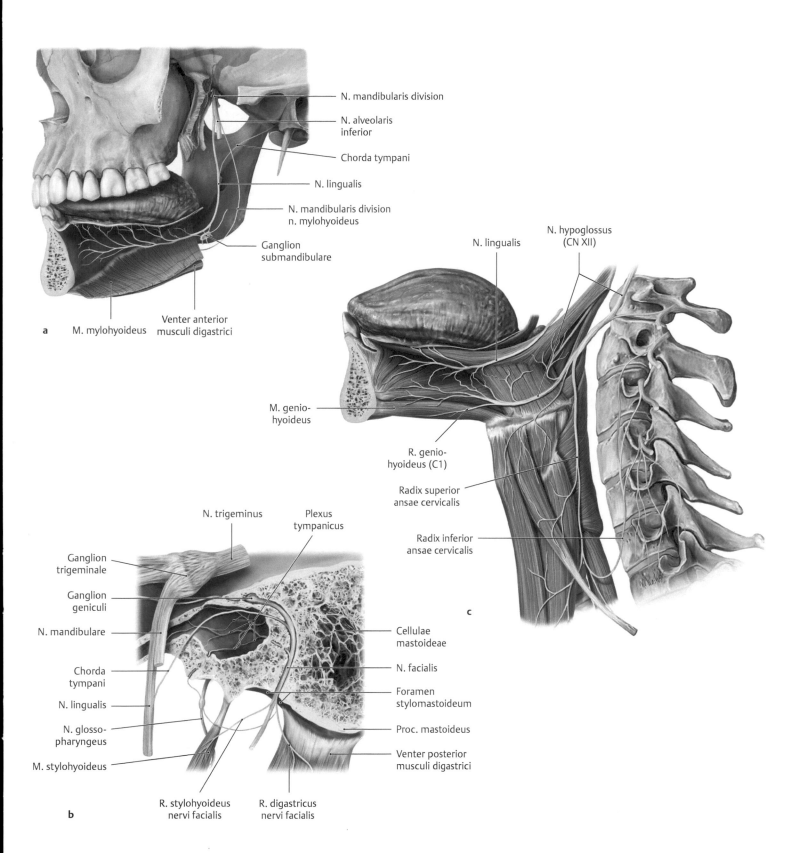

B Innervation of the oral floor muscles
a Left lateral view (right half of the mandibula viewed from the medial side). **b** Sagittal section through the right pars petrosa ossis temporalis at the level of the proc. mastoideus and cellulae mastoideae, viewed from the medial side. **c** Left lateral view.
The muscles of the oral floor have a complex nerve supply due to different arcus pharyngeus derivations, with contributions from three different nerves:

a The derivatives of the arcus pharyngeus primus (m. mylohyoideus, venter anterior of the m. digastricus) are supplied by the n. mylohyoideus, a branch of the n. mandibularis division (CN V₃).
b The derivatives of the arcus pharyngeus secundus (venter posterior of the m. digastricus, m. stylohyoideus) are supplied by the n. facialis.
c The m. geniohyoideus (and the m. thyrohyoideus) are supplied by the ramus anterior of n. spinalis C1, which travels with the n. hypoglossus.

5.28 Oral Cavity: Pharynx and Tonsils (Tonsillae)

A Waldeyer's ring

Posterior view of the opened pharynx. All the components of the anulus lymphoideus pharyngis (Waldeyer's ring) can be seen in this view. The anulus lymphoideus pharyngis is composed of immunocompetent lymphatic tissue (tonsillae and lymph follicles). The tonsillae are "immunological sentinels" surrounding the passageways from the cavitas oris and cavitas nasi to the pharynx. The lymph follicles are distributed over all of the epithelium, showing marked regional variations. the anulus lymphoideus pharyngis consists of the following structures:

- The unpaired tonsilla pharyngealis on the roof of the pharynx
- The paired tonsillae palatinae
- The tonsilla lingualis
- The paired tubal tonsils (tonsillae tubariae), which may be thought of as lateral extensions of the tonsilla pharyngealis
- The paired lateral bands.

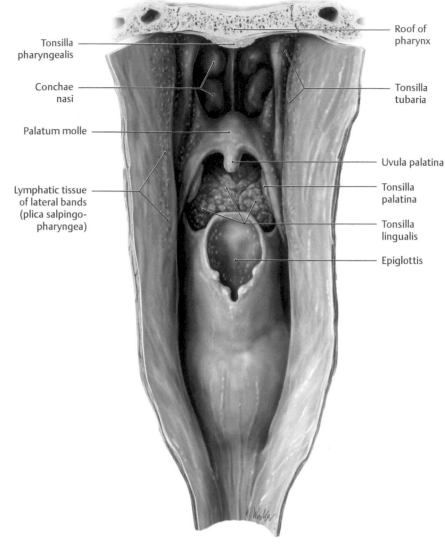

B Tonsillae palatinae: location and abnormal enlargement
Anterior view of the oral cavity.

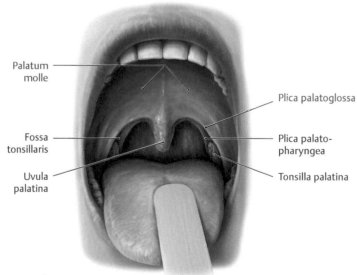

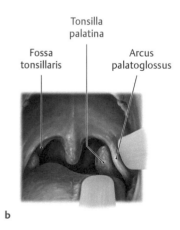

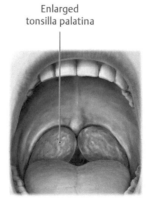

a The tonsillae palatinae occupy a shallow recess on each side, the fossa tonsillaris, which is located between the anterior and posterior pillars (arci palatoglossus and palatopharyngeus).

b and c The tonsilla palatina is examined clinically by placing a tongue depressor on the anterior pillar and displacing the tonsilla from its fossa while a second instrument depresses the tongue. Severe enlargement of the tonsilla palatina (due to viral or bacterial infection, as in tonsillitis) may significantly narrow the outlet of the cavitas oris, causing difficulty in swallowing (dysphagia).

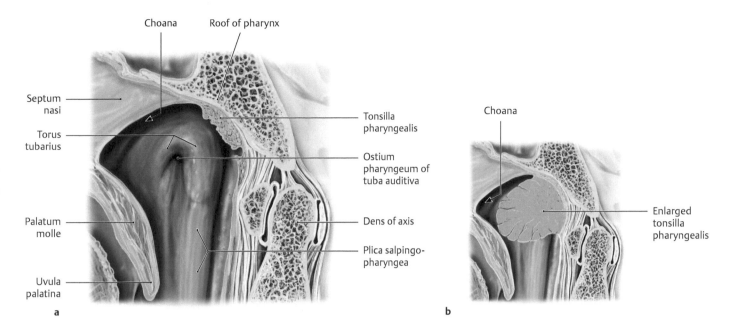

| Choana | Roof of pharynx | | Choana |
| a | | | b |

C Tonsilla pharyngealis: location and abnormal enlargement
Sagittal section through the roof of the pharynx.

a Located on the roof of the pharynx, the unpaired tonsilla pharyngealis can be examined by means of posterior rhinoscopy (see p. 177). It is particularly well developed in (small) children and begins to regress at 6 or 7 years of age.

b An enlarged tonsilla pharyngealis is very common in preschool-age children. (Chronic recurrent nasopharyngeal infections at this age often evoke a heightened immune response in the lymphatic tissue, causing "adenoids" or "polyps.") The enlarged tonsilla pharyngealis blocks the choanae, obstructing the nasal airway and forcing the child to breathe through the mouth. Since the mouth is then constantly open during respiration at rest, an experienced examiner can quickly diagnose the adenoidal condition by visual inspection.

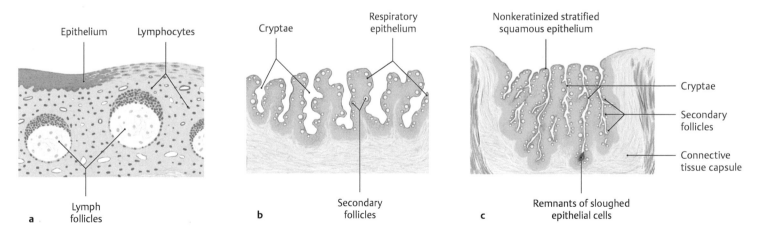

D Histology of the lymphatic tissue of the cavitas oris and pharynx
Due to the close anatomical relationship between the epithelium and lymphatic tissue, the lymphatic tissue of the anulus lymphoideus pharyngis is also des ignated lymphoepithelial tissue.

a Lymphoepithelial tissue. Lymphatic tissue, both organized and diffusely distributed, is found in the lamina propria of all mucous membranes and is known as mucosa-associated lymphatic tissue (MALT). The epithelium acquires a looser texture, with abundant lymphocytes and macrophages. Besides the well-defined tonsillae, smaller collections of lymph follicles may be found in the lateral bands (plicae

salpingopharyngeae). They extend almost vertically from the lateral wall to the posterior wall of the pars oralis and pars nasalis pharyngis.
b Structure of the tonsilla pharyngealis. The mucosal surface of the tonsilla pharyngealis is raised into ridges that greatly increase its surface area. The ridges and intervening cryptae are lined by ciliated respiratory epithelium.
c Structure of the tonsilla palatina. The surface area of the tonsilla palatina is increased by deep depressions (cryptae) in the mucosal surface (creating an active surface area as large as 300 cm²). The mucosa is covered by nonkeratinized stratified squamous epithelium.

5.29 Pharynx: Muscles

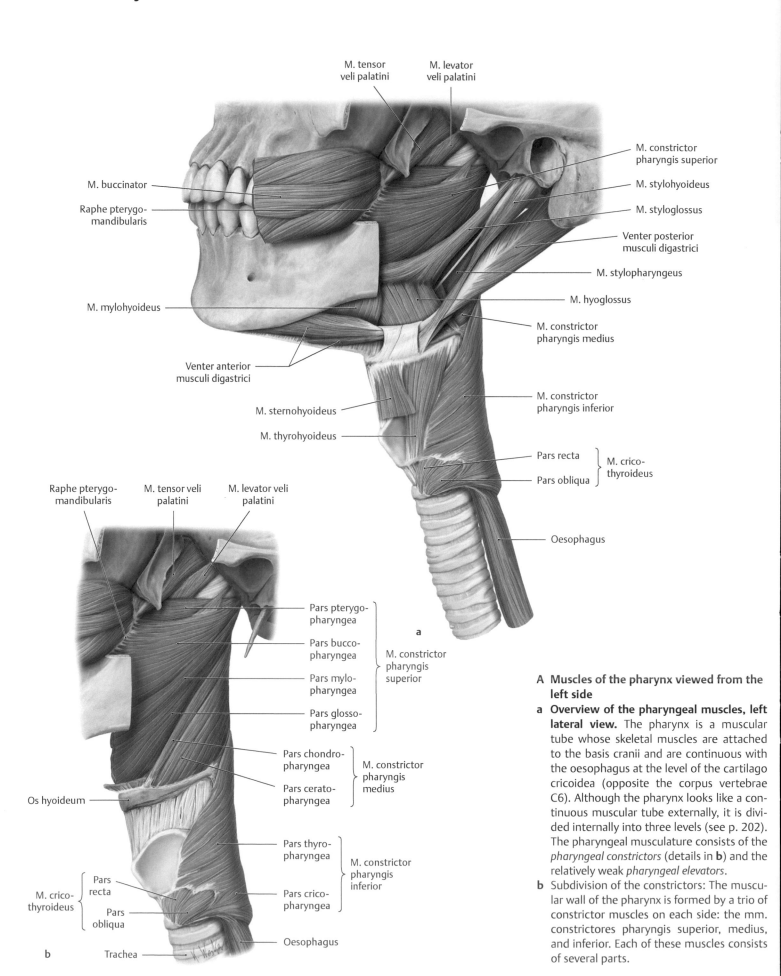

M. tensor veli palatini

M. levator veli palatini

M. constrictor pharyngis superior

M. buccinator

Raphe pterygo-mandibularis

M. stylohyoideus

M. styloglossus

Venter posterior musculi digastrici

M. stylopharyngeus

M. mylohyoideus

M. hyoglossus

M. constrictor pharyngis medius

Venter anterior musculi digastrici

M. constrictor pharyngis inferior

M. sternohyoideus

M. thyrohyoideus

Pars recta
Pars obliqua } M. crico-thyroideus

Oesophagus

a

Raphe pterygo-mandibularis

M. tensor veli palatini

M. levator veli palatini

Pars pterygo-pharyngea
Pars bucco-pharyngea
Pars mylo-pharyngea
Pars glosso-pharyngea } M. constrictor pharyngis superior

Pars chondro-pharyngea
Pars cerato-pharyngea } M. constrictor pharyngis medius

Os hyoideum

Pars thyro-pharyngea
Pars crico-pharyngea } M. constrictor pharyngis inferior

M. crico-thyroideus { Pars recta
Pars obliqua

b

Trachea

Oesophagus

A Muscles of the pharynx viewed from the left side

a Overview of the pharyngeal muscles, left lateral view. The pharynx is a muscular tube whose skeletal muscles are attached to the basis cranii and are continuous with the oesophagus at the level of the cartilago cricoidea (opposite the corpus vertebrae C6). Although the pharynx looks like a continuous muscular tube externally, it is divided internally into three levels (see p. 202). The pharyngeal musculature consists of the *pharyngeal constrictors* (details in **b**) and the relatively weak *pharyngeal elevators*.

b Subdivision of the constrictors: The muscular wall of the pharynx is formed by a trio of constrictor muscles on each side: the mm. constrictores pharyngis superior, medius, and inferior. Each of these muscles consists of several parts.

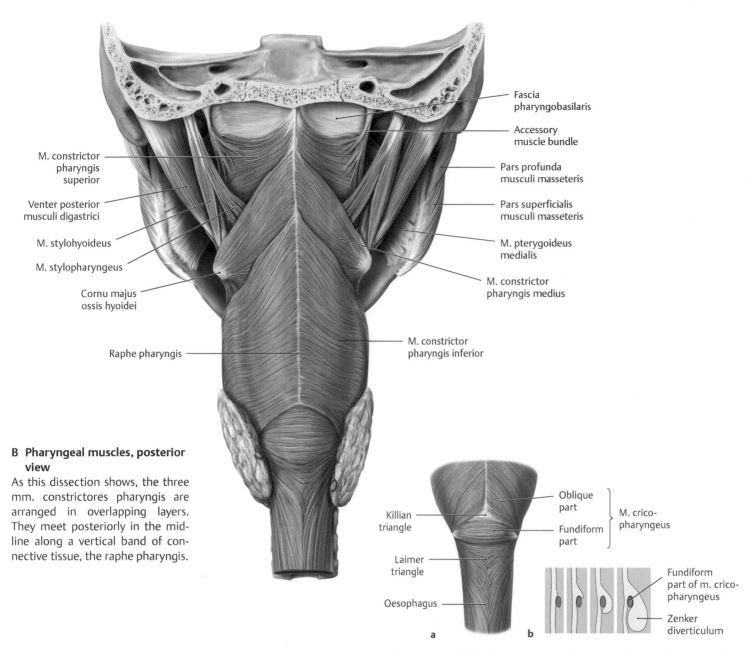

M. constrictor
pharyngis
superior

Venter posterior
musculi digastrici

M. stylohyoideus

M. stylopharyngeus

Cornu majus
ossis hyoidei

Raphe pharyngis

Fascia
pharyngobasilaris

Accessory
muscle bundle

Pars profunda
musculi masseteris

Pars superficialis
musculi masseteris

M. pterygoideus
medialis

M. constrictor
pharyngis medius

M. constrictor
pharyngis inferior

B Pharyngeal muscles, posterior view

As this dissection shows, the three mm. constrictores pharyngis are arranged in overlapping layers. They meet posteriorly in the midline along a vertical band of connective tissue, the raphe pharyngis.

Killian
triangle

Laimer
triangle

Oesophagus

Oblique
part

Fundiform
part

M. crico-
pharyngeus

Fundiform
part of m. crico-
pharyngeus

Zenker
diverticulum

a   b

D Junction of the pharyngeal and esophageal musculature and the development of Zenker diverticula

a Posterior view, **b** left lateral view.

The pars cricopharyngea of the m. constrictor pharyngis inferior is further subdivided into an oblique part and a fundiform part. Between these two parts is an area of muscular weakness known as the Killian triangle. At the inferior border of the fundiform part, the muscle fibers form a V-shaped area called the Laimer triangle. The weak spot at the Killian triangle may allow the tunica mucosa of the pars laryngea pharyngis to bulge outward through the fundiform part of the m. cricopharyngeus (**b**). *Note:* Killian's triangle and Laimer's triangle are often used synonymously.

This can result in a *Zenker diverticulum*, a sac-like protrusion in which food residues may collect and gradually expand the sac (with risk of obstructing the esophageal lumen by extrinsic pressure from the diverticulum). The diagnosis is suggested by the regurgitation of trapped food residues. Zenker diverticula are most common in middle-aged and elderly individuals. In elderly patients, who can undergo surgeries only to a limited extent, the fundiform part of the m. constrictor pharyngis inferior is cut endoscopically.

Note: Because a Zenker diverticulum is located at the junction of the pars laryngea pharyngis with the oesophagus, it is known also as a pharyngoesophageal diverticulum (the term "esophageal diverticulum," while common, is incorrect).

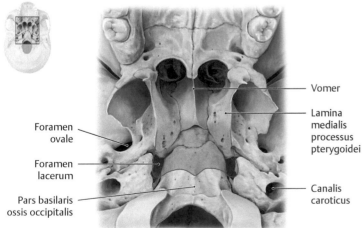

Foramen
ovale

Foramen
lacerum

Pars basilaris
ossis occipitalis

Vomer

Lamina
medialis
processus
pterygoidei

Canalis
caroticus

C Fascia pharyngobasilaris at the basis cranii

Inferior view. The pharyngeal muscles originate from the basis cranii with a dense connective tissue membrane, the fascia pharyngobasilaris. Their insertion is projected onto the basis cranii and marked as a red line. The U-shaped area surrounded by fascia and muscles is part of the bony roof of the pharynx (light red).

199

5.30 Pharynx: Surface Anatomy of the Mucosa and Its Connections with the Skull Base

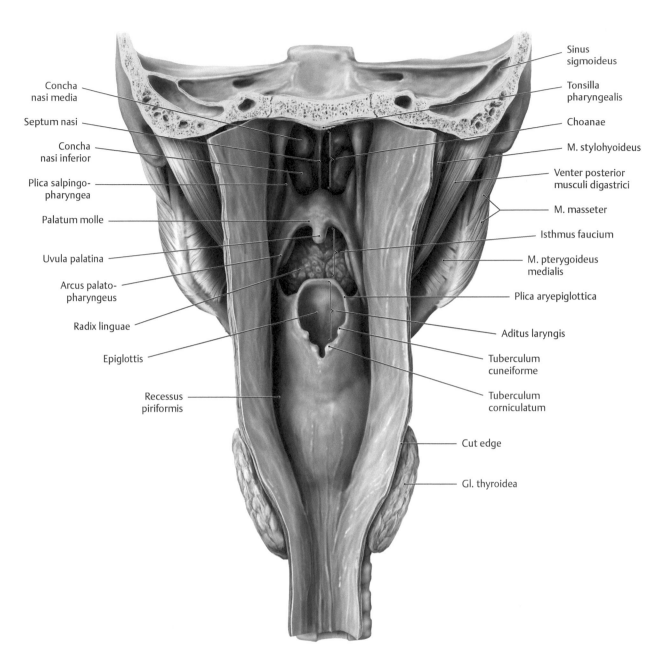

Concha nasi media
Septum nasi
Concha nasi inferior
Plica salpingo-pharyngea
Palatum molle
Uvula palatina
Arcus palato-pharyngeus
Radix linguae
Epiglottis
Recessus piriformis

Sinus sigmoideus
Tonsilla pharyngealis
Choanae
M. stylohyoideus
Venter posterior musculi digastrici
M. masseter
Isthmus faucium
M. pterygoideus medialis
Plica aryepiglottica
Aditus laryngis
Tuberculum cuneiforme
Tuberculum corniculatum
Cut edge
Gl. thyroidea

A Surface anatomy of the pharyngeal mucosa

Posterior view. The muscular posterior wall of the pharynx is opened along its midline.

The anterior part of the pharyngeal wall is interrupted by three openings:

- To the cavitas nasi (choanae)

- To the cavitas oris (isthmus faucium)
- To the laryngeal inlet (aditus laryngis)

The pharynx is divided accordingly into a pars nasalis, pars oralis, and pars laryngea pharyngis (see p. 202).

B Posterior rhinoscopy

The pars nasalis pharyngis can be visually inspected by posterior rhinoscopy.

a Technique of holding the tongue blade and mirror. The angulation of the mirror is continually adjusted to permit complete inspection of the pars nasalis pharyngis (see **b**).

b Composite posterior rhinoscopic image acquired at various mirror angles. The ostium pharyngeum of the tuba auditiva and tonsilla pharyngealis can be identified (see p. 196).

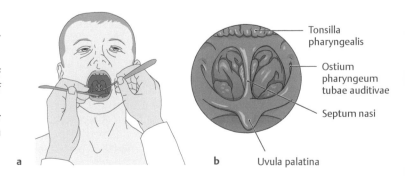

Tonsilla pharyngealis
Ostium pharyngeum tubae auditivae
Septum nasi

a

b Uvula palatina

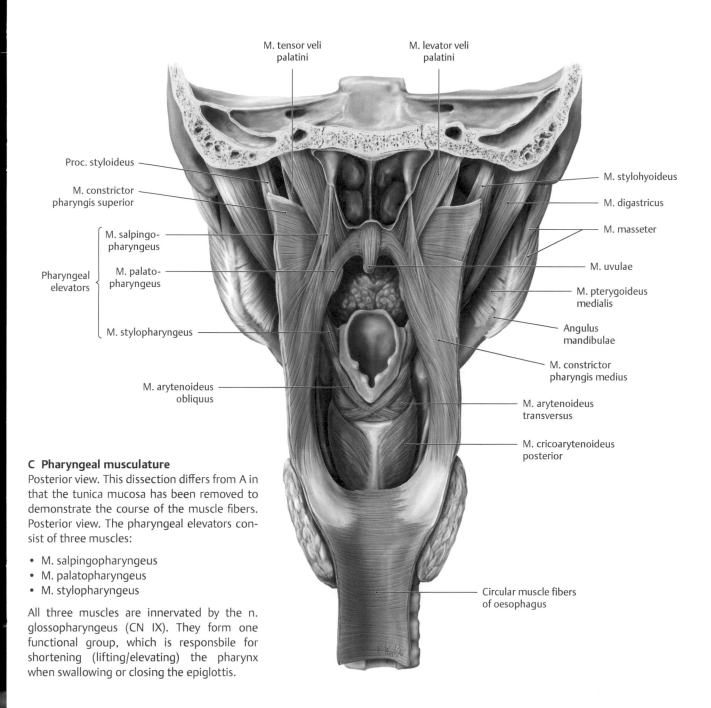

M. tensor veli palatini

M. levator veli palatini

Proc. styloideus

M. constrictor pharyngis superior

Pharyngeal elevators
- M. salpingo-pharyngeus
- M. palato-pharyngeus
- M. stylopharyngeus

M. arytenoideus obliquus

M. stylohyoideus

M. digastricus

M. masseter

M. uvulae

M. pterygoideus medialis

Angulus mandibulae

M. constrictor pharyngis medius

M. arytenoideus transversus

M. cricoarytenoideus posterior

Circular muscle fibers of oesophagus

C Pharyngeal musculature

Posterior view. This dissection differs from A in that the tunica mucosa has been removed to demonstrate the course of the muscle fibers. Posterior view. The pharyngeal elevators consist of three muscles:

- M. salpingopharyngeus
- M. palatopharyngeus
- M. stylopharyngeus

All three muscles are innervated by the n. glossopharyngeus (CN IX). They form one functional group, which is responsbile for shortening (lifting/elevating) the pharynx when swallowing or closing the epiglottis.

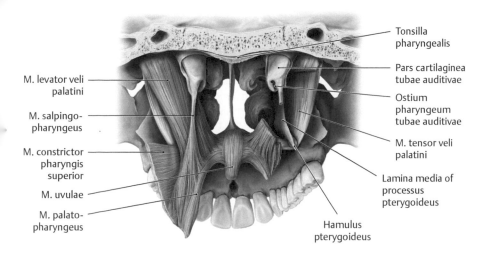

M. levator veli palatini

M. salpingo-pharyngeus

M. constrictor pharyngis superior

M. uvulae

M. palato-pharyngeus

Tonsilla pharyngealis

Pars cartilaginea tubae auditivae

Ostium pharyngeum tubae auditivae

M. tensor veli palatini

Lamina media of processus pterygoideus

Hamulus pterygoideus

D Muscles of the palatum molle and tuba auditiva

Posterior view. The os sphenoidale has been sectioned posterior to the choanal opening in the coronal plane, and the following muscles have been resected on the right side: m. levator veli palatini, m. salpingopharyngeus, m. palatopharyngeus, and m. constrictor pharyngis superior. These muscles are part of the pharynx (space between the palatum molle, arcus palatoglossus and palatopharyngeus, and dorsum linguae) that forms the posterior boundary of the cavitas oris.

5.31 Pharynx: Topographical Anatomy and Innervation

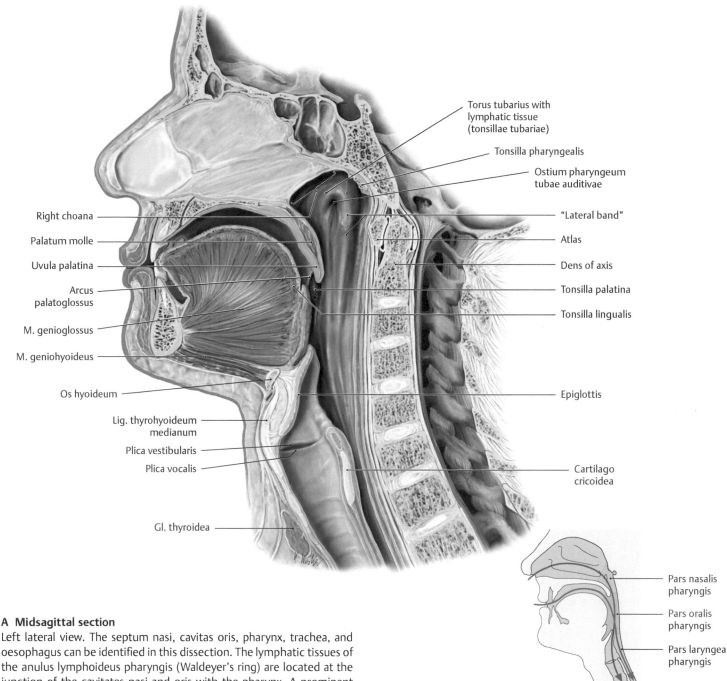

A Midsagittal section

Left lateral view. The septum nasi, cavitas oris, pharynx, trachea, and oesophagus can be identified in this dissection. The lymphatic tissues of the anulus lymphoideus pharyngis (Waldeyer's ring) are located at the junction of the cavitates nasi and oris with the pharynx. A prominent part of this defensive ring is the array of tonsillae that play an important role in the early recognition of pathogenic microorganisms and the initiation of an immune response (more complex infections spread to the spatium peripharyngeum, see p. 204). This array consists of the single tonsilla pharyngealis (on the roof of the pharynx), the paired tonsillae palatinae (between the plicae faucium), and the paired tonsillae linguae (at the radix linguae). Additional masses of lymphatic tissue are located around the ostium pharyngeum of each tuba auditiva (tonsillae tubariae) and are continued inferiorly as the "lateral bands."

The tuba auditiva connects the pharynx with the cavitas tympani and serves to equalize the air pressure in the auris media. Swelling around the ostium pharyngeum tubae auditivae (tonsillae tubariae), which may occur even with a mild inflammation, may occlude the orifice and prevent pressure equalization in the auris media. This restricts the mobility of the tympanic membrane, causing a mild degree of hearing loss. Enlargement of the tonsilla pharyngealis (e. g., polyps in small children) may also obstruct the lumen of the tuba auditiva.

B Levels of the cavitas pharyngis

Left lateral view. The cavitas pharyngis is divided into the pars nasalis pharyngis, pars oralis pharyngis, and pars laryngea pharyngis. The upper airway and lower foodway intersect in the pars oralis pharyngis. The following synonyms for the three pharyngeal levels are in common use:

Upper level:	Pars nasalis pharyngis	Nasopharynx	Epipharynx
Middle level:	Pars oralis pharyngis	Oropharynx	Mesopharynx
Lower level:	Pars laryngea pharyngis	Laryngopharynx	Hypopharynx

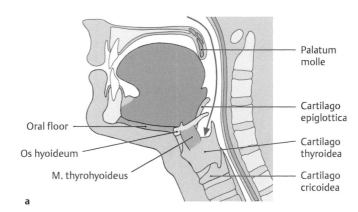

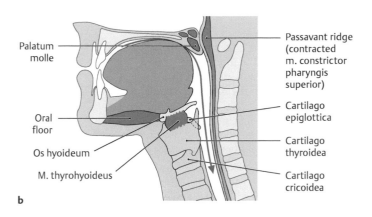

C Anatomy of swallowing

As part of the airway, the larynx in the adult is located at the inlet to the digestive tract (**a**). During swallowing (**b**), therefore, the airway must be briefly occluded to keep food from entering the trachea. The act of swallowing consists of three phases:

1. Voluntary initiation of swallowing
2. Reflex closure of the airway
3. Reflex transport of the food bolus down the pharynx and oesophagus

During the second phase of swallowing, the oral floor muscles (mm. mylohyoideus and digastricus) and the mm. thyrohyoideus elevate the larynx and the epiglottis covers the aditus laryngis, sealing off the lower airway. Meanwhile the palatum molle is tightened, elevated, and apposed to the posterior pharyngeal wall, sealing off the upper airway.

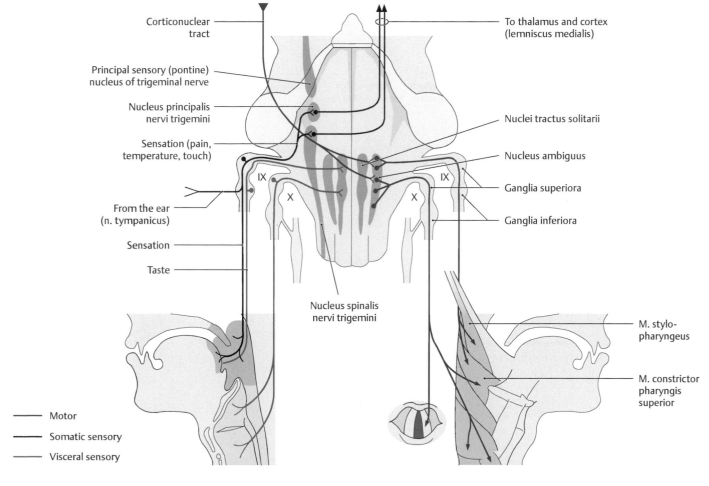

D Nervus vagus and nervus glossopharyngeus: their peripheral distribution and nuclei in truncus encephali (after Duus)

Posterior view. Both the n. glossopharyngeus (CN IX) and the n. vagus (CN X) originate from nuclei in the truncus encephali. In this simplified schematic, motor pathways are depicted on the right and sensory pathways on the left.

Note that both nerves contribute to the sensory and motor supply of the pharynx. Together they form the plexus pharyngeus.

5.32 Pharynx: The Parapharyngeal Space and Its Clinical Significance

A Parapharyngeal space

Horizontal section, at the level of dens axis and fossa tonsillaris (after Töndury). The spatium peripharyngeum is an area of connective tissue, which extends from the basis cranii to the mediastinum. Topographically, it is divided into a spatium lateropharyngeum (parapharyngeum) (①+②) on either side of the pharynx and a *spatium retropharyngeum* (③) posterior to the pharynx. The border separating the two is the septum sagittale made of connective tissue that extends between the lamina prevertebralis fasciae cervicalis and the posterior pharyngeal wall.

- The unpaired **spatium retropharyngeum** is a thin gap between the posterior wall of the pharynx and the lamina prevertebralis fasciae cervicalis which covers the prevertebral neck muscles. The space includes branches of the a. pharyngea ascendens and veins of the plexus pharyngeus.
- The paired **spatia lateropharyngea** contain loose connective tissue and are divided by the stylopharyngeal aponeurosis (the common connective tissue sheath of muscles which arise from the processus styloideus) into an anterior part (prestyloid) and posterior part (*retrostyloid*).

  - ① *Anterior part:* communicates with the fossa retromandibularis and contains all the structures which run from the fossa infratemporalis to the face (e.g., m. pterygoideus medialis, n. alveolaris inferior, n. lingualis, n. auriculotemporalis, ganglion oticum, as well as the a. maxillaris and its branches).

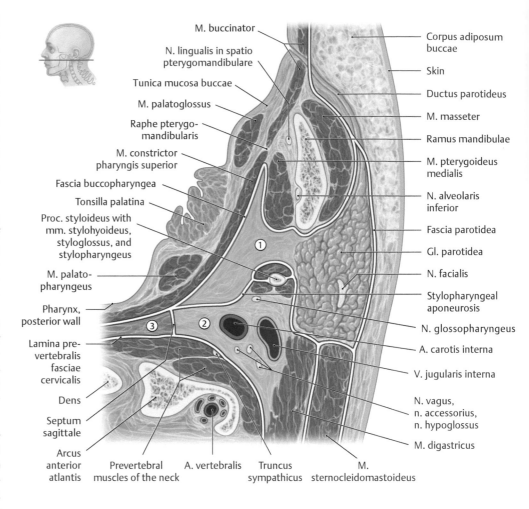

  - ② Posterior part: includes the a. carotis interna, v. jugularis interna, nn. craniales IX-XII as well as the truncus sympathicus, which runs below or along the lamina prevetrebralis fasciae cervicalis.

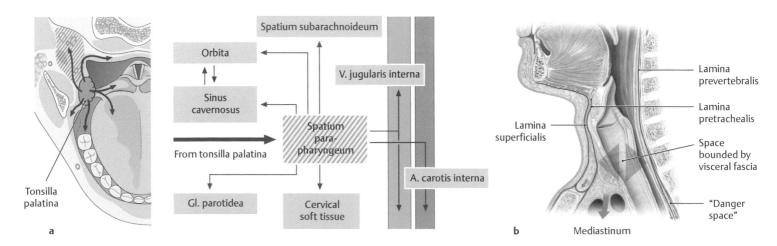

B Clinical significance of the spatium parapharyngeum
(after Becker, Naumann, and Pfaltz)

a Bacteria and inflammatory cells in the tonsilla palatina can infiltrate into the spatium parapharyngeum from where they can spread

- into the v. jugularis interna—risk of sepsis
- into the spatium subarachnoideum—risk of meningitis

b Additional complications include sinking abscesses (the inflammation spreads between the superficial and medial layers of the fascia cervicalis or along the vagina carotica into the mediastinum causing mediastinitis). From the "danger space" (a cleft-like divided space of the lamina prevertebralis) infections can directly reach the posterior mediastinum. By administering modern antibiotics early and broadly, these complications now rarely occur.

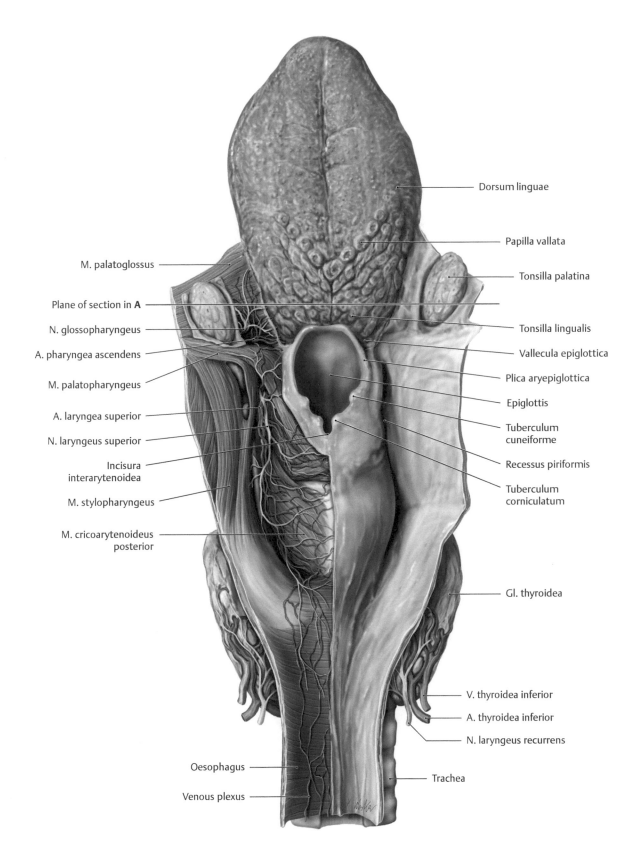

Dorsum linguae

Papilla vallata

Tonsilla palatina

Tonsilla lingualis

Vallecula epiglottica

Plica aryepiglottica

Epiglottis

Tuberculum cuneiforme

Recessus piriformis

Tuberculum corniculatum

Gl. thyroidea

V. thyroidea inferior

A. thyroidea inferior

N. laryngeus recurrens

Trachea

M. palatoglossus

Plane of section in **A**

N. glossopharyngeus

A. pharyngea ascendens

M. palatopharyngeus

A. laryngea superior

N. laryngeus superior

Incisura interarytenoidea

M. stylopharyngeus

M. cricoarytenoideus posterior

Oesophagus

Venous plexus

C Neurovascular structures of the spatium peripharyngeum
(after Platzer)

Posterior view of a specimen composed of the tongue, larynx, esophagus, and thyroid gland, as it would be resected at autopsy for pathologic evaluation of the neck. This dissection clearly demonstrates the branching pattern of the neurovascular structures that occupy the plane between the pharyngeal muscles. The large neck pathways and their organ-supplying vessels and nerves (see p. 230 f.) are embedded in an area of connective tissue, the peripharyngeal space (cf. **A**). This allows for their mobility during neck movement. The bifurcation of the pathways in the layer between the pharyngeal muscles is clearly identifiable. The rr. tonsillares arise from the ascending a. palatina as shown here but occasionally directly from the a. facialis as well.

Note the vascular supply to the palatine tonsil and its proximity to the neurovascular bundle, which creates a risk of hemorrhage during tonsillectomy.

5.33 Pharynx:
Neurovascular Structures in the Parapharyngeal Space (Superficial Layer)

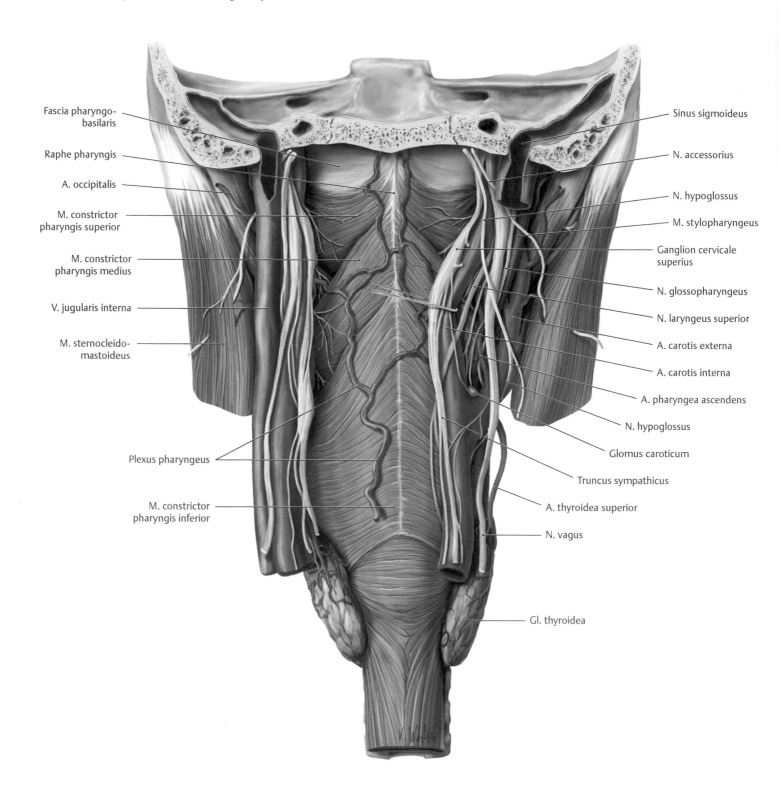

Fascia pharyngo-basilaris

Raphe pharyngis

A. occipitalis

M. constrictor pharyngis superior

M. constrictor pharyngis medius

V. jugularis interna

M. sternocleido-mastoideus

Plexus pharyngeus

M. constrictor pharyngis inferior

Sinus sigmoideus

N. accessorius

N. hypoglossus

M. stylopharyngeus

Ganglion cervicale superius

N. glossopharyngeus

N. laryngeus superior

A. carotis externa

A. carotis interna

A. pharyngea ascendens

N. hypoglossus

Glomus caroticum

Truncus sympathicus

A. thyroidea superior

N. vagus

Gl. thyroidea

A Spatium parapharyngeum, posterior view
The columna vertebralis and all structures posterior to it have been completely removed to display the posterior wall of the pharynx from the posterior aspect. The neurovascular structures on the left side are intact, while the right v. jugularis interna has been removed to demonstrate neurovascular structures lying anterior to the vein. After passing through the base of the skull, the a. carotis interna, n. vagus, and truncus sympathicus are shifted medially to the spatium lateropharyngeum. Note the exposed glomus caroticum, which is innervated by the n. vagus and truncus sympathicus.

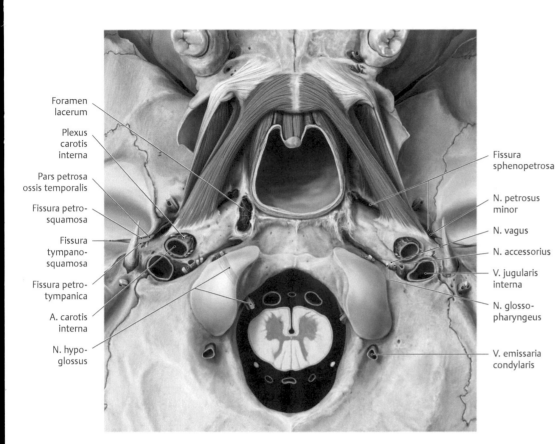

Foramen lacerum
Plexus carotis interna
Pars petrosa ossis temporalis
Fissura petrosquamosa
Fissura tympanosquamosa
Fissura petrotympanica
A. carotis interna
N. hypoglossus

Fissura sphenopetrosa
N. petrosus minor
N. vagus
N. accessorius
V. jugularis interna
N. glossopharyngeus
V. emissaria condylaris

B Neurovascular structures in the spatium peripharyngeum: points of emergence from the basis cranii

The neurovascular structures use the following openings:

- **Fissura petrotympanica (Glaserian fissure)**
  - Chorda tympani
- **Fissura tympanosquamosa**
- **Fissura sphenopetrosa;** its wide extension forms the foramen lacerum
  - N. petrosus minor
- **Foramen lacerum**
  - N. petrosus major
- **Foramen jugulare**
  - V. jugularis interna
  - N. glossopharyngeus (CN IX)
  - N. vagus (CN X)
  - N. accessorius (CN XI)
- **Canalis nervi hypoglossi**
  - N. hypoglossus (CN XII)
- **Canalis condylaris**
  - V. emissaria condylaris
- **Canalis caroticus**
  - A. carotis interna, Plexus caroticus internus

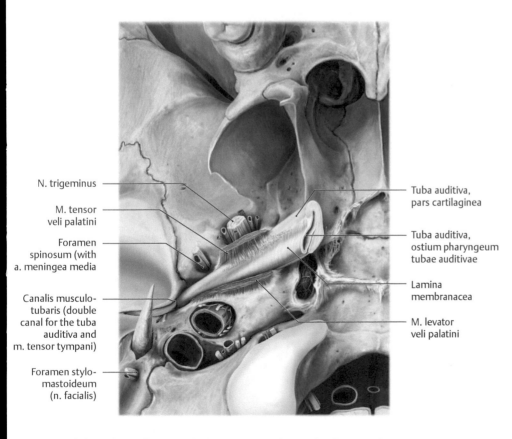

N. trigeminus
M. tensor veli palatini
Foramen spinosum (with a. meningea media
Canalis musculotubaris (double canal for the tuba auditiva and m. tensor tympani)
Foramen stylomastoideum (n. facialis)

Tuba auditiva, pars cartilaginea
Tuba auditiva, ostium pharyngeum tubae auditivae
Lamina membranacea
M. levator veli palatini

C Course of the tuba auditiva at the basis cranii

Detail of B. Directly below the basis cranii, in the cranial aspect of the spatium lateropharyngeum lies the **pars cartilaginea** of the tuba auditiva. When projected onto the basis cranii,

it lies in the fissura sphenopetrosa, an extension of the fissura petrosquamosa (the exit point of the n. petrosus minor, see **B**).

Medially, the fissura sphenopetrosa widens toward the *foramen lacerum* (exit point of the n. petrosus major), which is covered by

fibrocartilagious tissue. The pars cartilaginea of the tuba auditiva begins at the funnel-shaped opening (opening of the tuba auditiva) lateral to the superior margin of the pharyngeal wall close to the choanae and runs obliquely in a lateral-posterior direction (at a 45° angle to the mid-sagittal plane). The pars cartilaginea tubae auditivae creates a channel which is open at its lateral and inferior margin - where the tubal mucosa is located. In cross-section it appears hook-shaped. The lateral wall is composed of connective tissue and forms the lamina membranacea.

The **pars ossea** of the tuba auditiva represents around one-third of the tuba auditiva entire length and runs together with the m. tensor tympani in the canali musculotubarius to the cavitas tympani. Its opening is located between the canalis caroticus and the foramen spinosum (at the level of the fissura petrosquamosa). The narrowest part of the tuba auditiva (the isthmus tubae auditivae) is between the partes cartilaginea and ossea. For functions of the mm. levator and tensor veli palatini see p. 147.

207

5.34 Pharynx: Neurovascular Structures in the Parapharyngeal Space (Deep Layer)

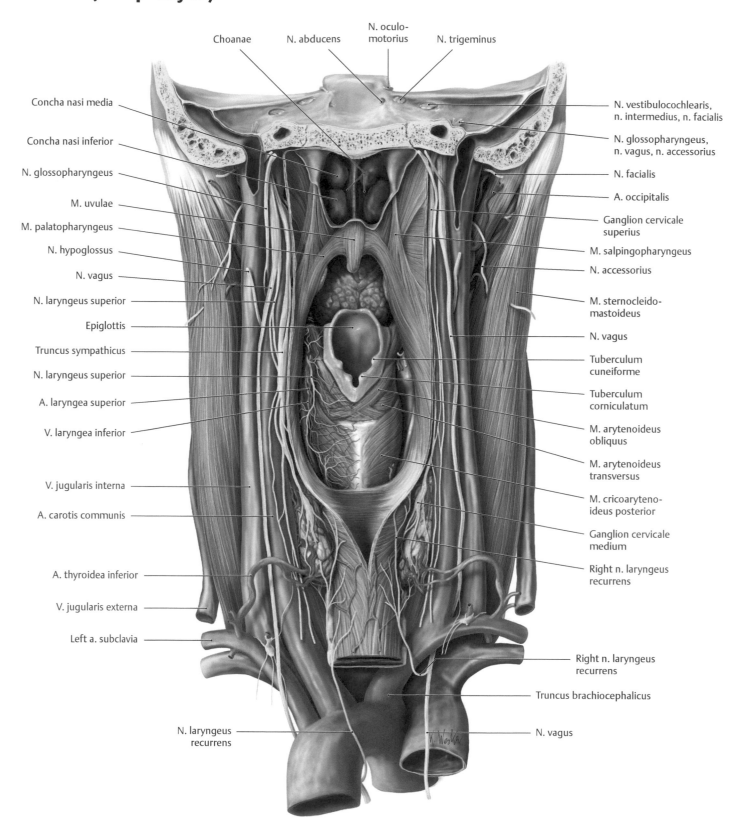

Choanae N. abducens N. oculo-motorius N. trigeminus

Concha nasi media

Concha nasi inferior

N. glossopharyngeus

M. uvulae

M. palatopharyngeus

N. hypoglossus

N. vagus

N. laryngeus superior

Epiglottis

Truncus sympathicus

N. laryngeus superior

A. laryngea superior

V. laryngea inferior

V. jugularis interna

A. carotis communis

A. thyroidea inferior

V. jugularis externa

Left a. subclavia

N. laryngeus recurrens

N. vestibulocochlearis, n. intermedius, n. facialis

N. glossopharyngeus, n. vagus, n. accessorius

N. facialis

A. occipitalis

Ganglion cervicale superius

M. salpingopharyngeus

N. accessorius

M. sternocleido-mastoideus

N. vagus

Tuberculum cuneiforme

Tuberculum corniculatum

M. arytenoideus obliquus

M. arytenoideus transversus

M. cricoaryteno-ideus posterior

Ganglion cervicale medium

Right n. laryngeus recurrens

Right n. laryngeus recurrens

Truncus brachiocephalicus

N. vagus

A Spatium parapharyngeum
Posterior view. The neurovascular structures in the spatium parapharyngeum are fully displayed from the fossa cranii posterior to the apertura thoracis superior. Also, the posterior wall of the pharynx has been longitudinally incised and spread open to demonstrate the cavitas pharyngis from the choanae down to the oesophagus.

Note: The major neurovascular structures in the neck course along the pharynx in a tightly clustered configuration. Stab injuries that perforate the lumen (from accidentally ingested bones, for example) may lead to inflammation of the spatium parapharyngeum, causing significant damage (see p. 204). Even minor injuries may incite a purulent bacterial inflammation that spreads rapidly within this connective tissue space (cellulitis).

Rr. pharyngeales of
a. pharyngea ascendens

R. pharyngeus of
a. palatina descendens

Rr. tonsillares of
nn. palatini minores

Tonsilla palatina

M. palatoglossus

R. tonsillaris of
a. palatina ascendens

Rr. tonsillares of
n. glossopharyngeus

Rr. dorsales linguae
of a. lingualis

N. glossopharyngeus

B Vascular and nerve supply of the tonsilla palatina (after Tillmann)
Median sagittal section, medial view. The tonsilla palatina lies between the arcus palatoglossus and palatopharyngeus. For a better illustration of its pathways, the tonsil has been detached from the tonsillar bed and tilted cranially. The pathways originate from, or extend to, the spatium peripharyngeum.

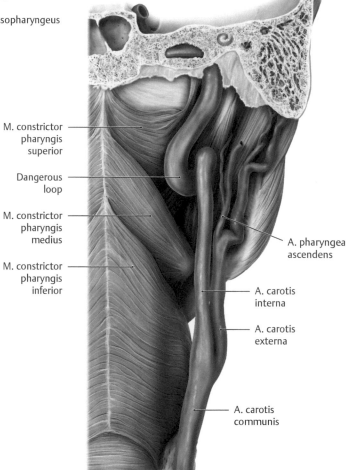

M. constrictor
pharyngis
superior

Dangerous
loop

M. constrictor
pharyngis
medius

M. constrictor
pharyngis
inferior

A. pharyngea
ascendens

A. carotis
interna

A. carotis
externa

A. carotis
communis

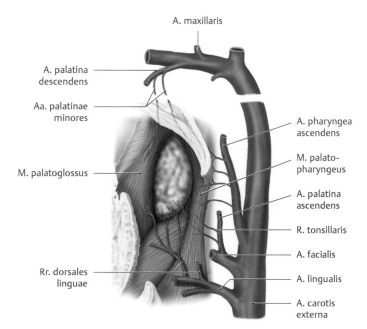

A. maxillaris

A. palatina
descendens

Aa. palatinae
minores

A. pharyngea
ascendens

M. palato-
pharyngeus

M. palatoglossus

A. palatina
ascendens

R. tonsillaris

A. facialis

Rr. dorsales
linguae

A. lingualis

A. carotis
externa

C Arterial supply of the tonsilla palatina (after Tillmann)
During tonsillectomies, branches of those arteries must be cauterized or ligated to prevent them from bleeding.

D Dangerous loop of the arteria carotis interna
(based on a specimen, which is part of the anatomical collection of the University in Kiel)
Dorsal view. A siphon-shaped loop of the a. carotis on the mm. constrictores pharyngis in the area around the tonsillar bed can be found in approximately 5% of the population. Damaging this loop during a tonsillectomy is dangerous and can result in severe arterial bleeding.

5.35 Salivary Glands (Glandulae Salivariae)

A Glandulae salivariae majores

Lateral view (**a**) and superior view (**b**).
Three large, paired sets of glands are distinguished:

1. Gll. parotideae
2. Gll. submandibulares
3. Gll. sublinguales

The gl. parotidea is a purely serous gland (watery secretions). The gl. submandibularis is a mixed seromucous gland, and the gl. sublingualis is a predominantly mucous-secreting (mucoserous) gland. The glands produce approximately 0.5–2 liters of saliva per day. Their excretory ducts open into the oral cavity. The excretory duct of the gl. parotidea (the ductus parotideus) crosses over the m. masseter, pierces the m. buccinator, and opens in the oral vestibule opposite the second upper molar. The excretory duct of the gl. submandibularis (ductus submandibularis) opens on the sublingual papilla behind the lower incisor teeth. The gl. sublingualis has many smaller excretory ducts that open on the plica sublingualis, or into the ductus submandibularis. The saliva keeps the oral mucosa moist, and it contains the starch-splitting enzyme amylase and the bactericidal enzyme lysozyme. The presynaptic *parasympathetic* fibers (not shown here) for autonomic control of the salivary glands arise from the superior and inferior salivatory nuclei and are distributed to the glands in various nerves (see pp. 124, 127, and 130), where they synapse with clusters of local ganglion cells, or in the ganglion submandibulare. *Sympathetic* fibers are distributed to the ducts along vascular pathways. The long winding duct of the gl. submandibularis has a tendency to become obstructed by salivary stones.

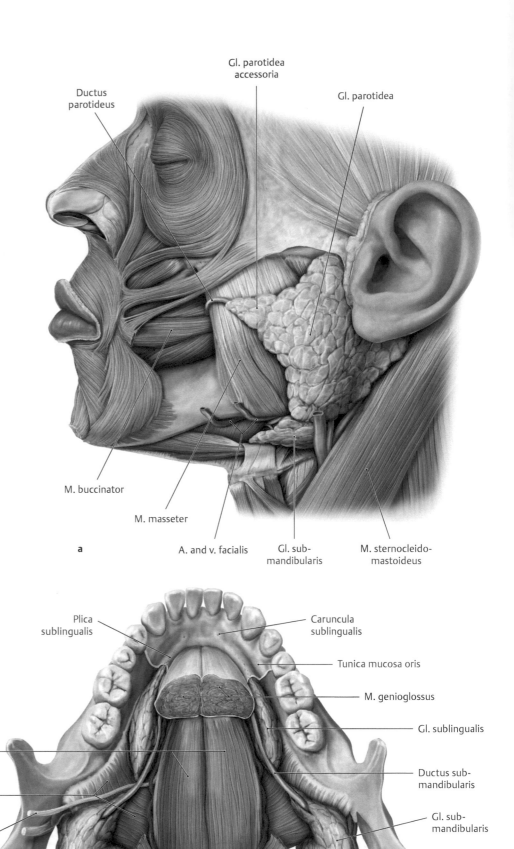

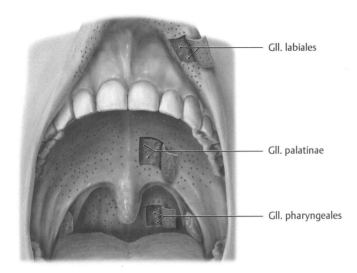

Gll. labiales

Gll. palatinae

Gll. pharyngeales

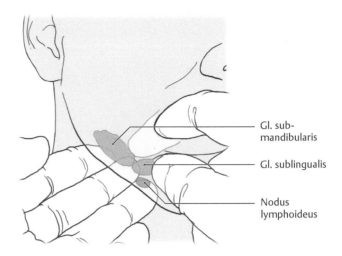

Gl. sub-
mandibularis

Gl. sublingualis

Nodus
lymphoideus

B Glandulae salivariae minores
In addition to the three major paired glands, 700–1000 minor gland-salso secrete saliva into the cavitas oris. They produce only 5–8% of the total output but this amount keeps the mouth moist when the gll. salivariae majores secrete only during mastication.
Note: Tumors originating in the gll. salivariae minores are more often malignant than those originating in the gll. salivariae majores. This is another reason for the clinical significance of these glands.

C Bimanual examination of the glandulae salivariae
The two gll. salivariae of the mandibula, the gl. submandibularis and gl. sublingualis, and the adjacent nodi lymphoidei are grouped around the mobile oral floor, and so they must be palpated against resistance. This is done with bimanual examination.

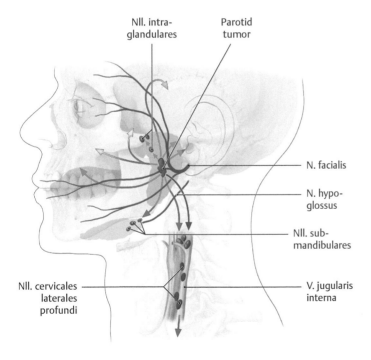

Nll. intra-
glandulares

Parotid
tumor

N. facialis

N. hypo-
glossus

Nll. sub-
mandibulares

Nll. cervicales
laterales
profundi

V. jugularis
interna

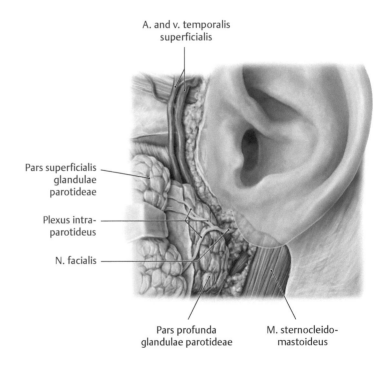

A. and v. temporalis
superficialis

Pars superficialis
glandulae
parotideae

Plexus intra-
parotideus

N. facialis

Pars profunda
glandulae parotideae

M. sternocleido-
mastoideus

D Spread of malignant parotid tumors along anatomical pathways
Malignant tumors of the gl. parotidea may directly invade surrounding structures (open arrows); they may also spread via regional nodi lymphoidei (solid arrows), or spread systemically (metastasize) through the vascular system.

E Intraglandular course of the nervus facialis in the glandula parotidea
The n. facialis divides into branches within the gl. parotidea (the plexus intraparotideus separates the gland into a pars superficialis and pars profunda) and is vulnerable during the surgical removal of parotid tumors. To preserve the n. facialis during parotidectomy, it is first necessary to locate and identify the facial nerve trunk. The best landmark for locating the nerve trunk is the tip of the cartilago meatus acustici.

5.36 Larynx: Location, Shape, and Laryngeal Cartilages

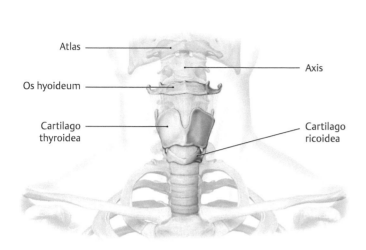

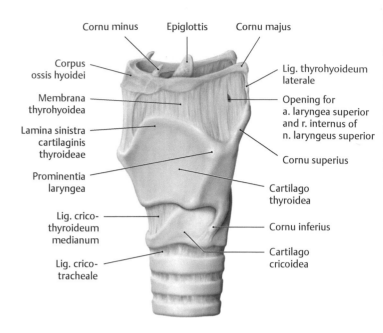

A Location of the larynx in the neck

Anterior view. In the adult male, when the head is upright and the larynx is centered in the neck:

- The os hyoideum is at the level of the C3 vertebra.
- The superior border of the cartilago thyroidea is at the C 4 level.
- The laryngotracheal junction is at the C6–C7 level.

These structures are located approximately one-half vertebra higher in women and children. The upper part of the larynx (the cartilago thyroidea, see **B**) is especially prominent in the male, forming the prominentia laryngea or "Adam's apple."

B General features of the larynx

Left anterior oblique view. The following cartilaginous structures of the larynx can be identified in this view:

- Epiglottis (see **D**)
- Thyroid thyroidea (see **E**)
- Cricoid cricoidea (see **F**)

These cartilages are connected to one another and to the trachea and os hyoideum by elastic ligaments, which allow some degree of laryngeal motion during swallowing (see p. 193). The cartilagines arytenoideae and cartilago corniculata are not visible in this view (see **G**).

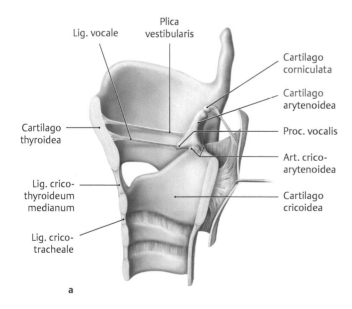

a

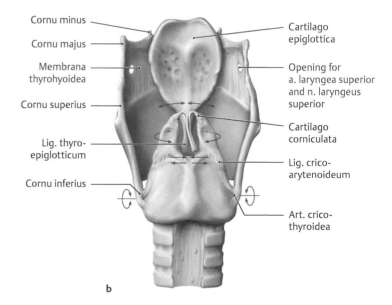

b

C Laryngeal cartilages and ligaments

a Sagittal section, viewed from the left medial aspect. The cartilago thyroidea encloses most of the laryngeal cartilages, its inferior part articulating with the cartilago cricoidea (art cricothyroidea).

b Posterior view. Arrows indicate the directions of movement in the various joints. The cartilago thyroidea can tilt relative to the cartilago

cricoidea in the art. cricothyroidea. The base of the cartilago arytenoidea on each side can translate or rotate relative to the upper edge of the cartilago cricoidea at the art. cricoarytenoidea. The arytenoid cartilages move during phonation.

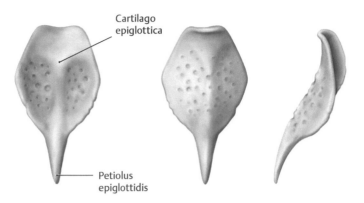

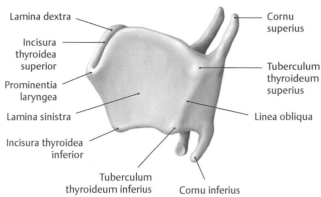

D Cartilago epiglottica
Laryngeal, lingual, and left lateral views. The internal skeleton of the epiglottis is composed of elastic cartilage shown here (the cartilago epiglottica). This cartilage enables the epiglottis to return spontaneously to its initial position at the end of swallowing (when muscular traction is lost). If the epiglottis is removed as part of a tumor resection, the patient must go through an arduous process of learning how to swallow effectively without an epiglottis, avoiding aspiration of ingested material into the trachea.

E Cartilago thyroidea
Left oblique view. This hyaline cartilage consists of two quadrilateral plates, the laminae dextra and sinsitra, which are joined in the midline to form a keel-shaped projection. At the upper end of this junction is the prominentia laryngea, called the "Adam's apple" in the male. The posterior ends of the laminae are prolonged to form the cornua superius and inferius, which serve as anchors for ligaments (see **B**).

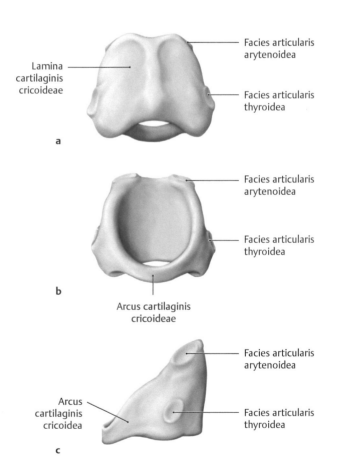

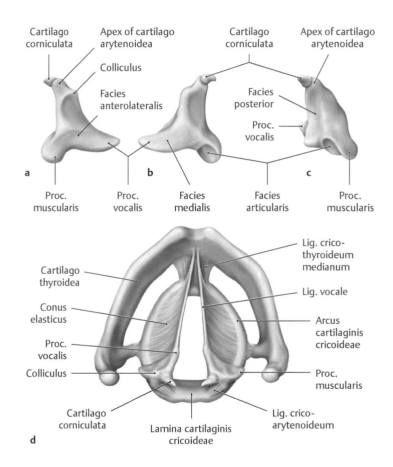

F Cricoid cartilage
Posterior view (**a**), anterior view (**b**), left lateral view (**c**). This hyaline cartilage is shaped like a signet ring. It consists posteriorly of an expanded cartilaginous plate, the lamina cartilaginis cricoideae. The upper end of the plate bears an articular facet for the cartilago arytenoidea, and the lower end bears a facet for the cartilago thyroidea. The inferior border of the cartilago cricoidea is connected to the highest cartilago trachealis by the lig. cricotracheale (see **B** and **C**).

G Cartilago arytenoidea and cartilago corniculata
Right cartilages, viewed from the lateral (**a**), medial (**b**), posterior (**c**), and superior (**d**) aspects. The function of the cartilago arytenoidea ("arytenoid" literally means "ladle-shaped") is to alter the position of the plicae vocales during phonation (see p. 207). The pyramid-shaped, hyaline cartilago arytenoidea has three surfaces (facies anterolateralis, medialis, and posterior), a base with two processes (procc. vocalis and muscularis), and an apex. The apex articulates with the tiny cartilago corniculata, which is composed of elastic fibrocartilage.

213

5.37 Larynx: Internal Features and Neurovascular Structures

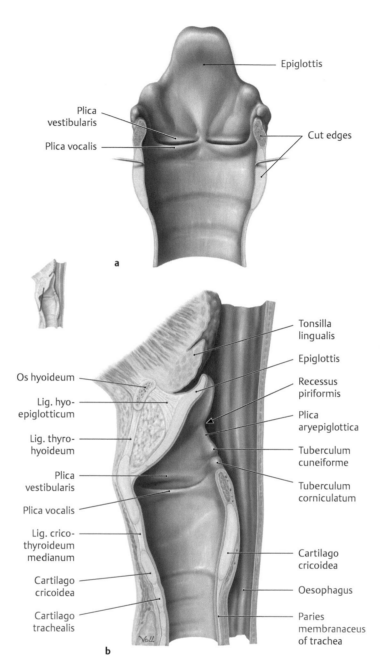

a

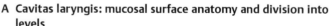

b

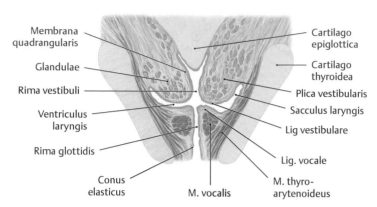

B Plicae vestibulares and plicae vocales

The plicae vestibulares ("false vocal cords") are clearly displayed in this coronal section. They contain the lig. vestibulare, which is the free inferior end of the membrana quadrangularis. The fissure between the plicae vestibulares is the rima vestibuli. Below the plicae vestibulares are the plicae vocales (also called the true vocal folds), which contain the lig. vocale and the m. vocalis. The fissure between the plicae vocales is the rima glottidis (glottis), which is narrower than the rima vestibuli.
Note: The loose connective tissue of the aditus laryngeus may become markedly swollen in response to an insect bite or inflammatory process, obstructing the rima vestibuli. This laryngeal edema (often incorrectly called "glottic edema") presents clinically with dyspnea and a risk of asphyxiation.

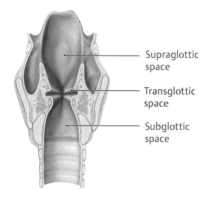

A Cavitas laryngis: mucosal surface anatomy and division into levels

a **Posterior view.** The muscular tube of the pharynx and oesophagus has been incised posteriorly and spread open (cut edges). Mucous membrane completely lines the interior of the larynx and, except at the plicae vocales, is loosely applied to its underlying tissue (creating the potential for laryngeal edema, see **B**). The plicae aryepiglotticae are located on each side of the cavitas laryngis between the cartilagines arytenoideae and epiglottis, and lateral to those folds are pear-shaped mucosal fossae, the recessus piriformes.
Note: These recesses have an important role in food transport. The airway and foodway intersect in this region, and the recessus piriformes channel food past the larynx and into the oesophagus. The epiglottis seals off the aditus laryngis during swallowing (see p. 203).

b **Midsagittal section viewed from the left side.** The cavitas laryngis can be divided into three levels or spaces to aid in describing the precise location of a laryngeal lesion (cf. **C**).

C Clinical classification of the major laryngeal regions and their borders

Posterior view. The larynx is divided into three levels from above downward to aid in describing the precise location of abnormalities. These three levels are also important in terms of lymphatic drainage.

Levels of the larynx	Extent
Level I: supraglottic space (Vestibulum laryngis)	From the aditus laryngis to the plicae vestibulares
Level II: transglottic space (intermediate laryngeal cavity)	From the plicae vestibulares across the ventriculus laryngis (lateral evagination of mucosa) to the plicae vocales
Level III: subglottic space (infraglottic cavity)	From the plicae vocales to the inferior margin of the cartilago cricoidea

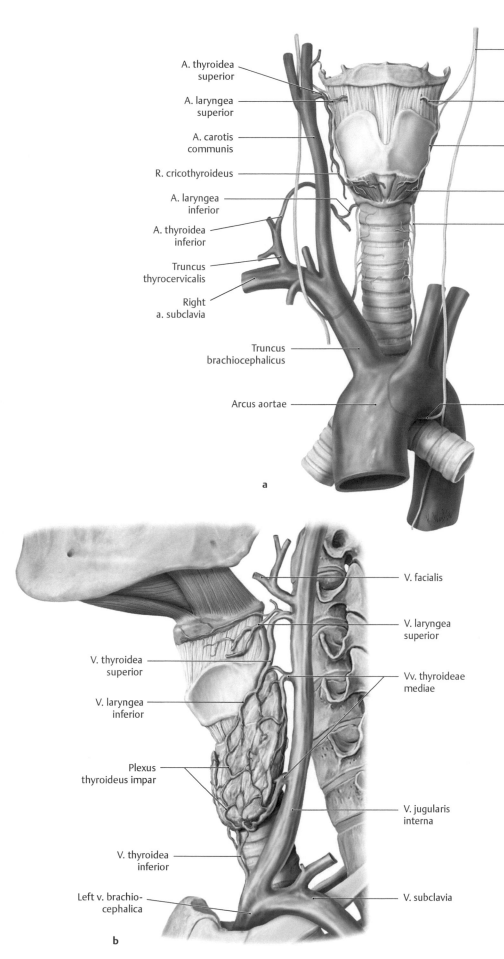

A. thyroidea superior

A. laryngea superior

A. carotis communis

R. cricothyroideus

A. laryngea inferior

A. thyroidea inferior

Truncus thyrocervicalis

Right a. subclavia

Truncus brachiocephalicus

Arcus aortae

N. vagus

R. internus nervi laryngei superioris

R. externus nervi laryngei superioris

M. cricothyroideus

Left n. laryngeus recurrens (terminal branch which used to be called inferior laryngeal nerve)

Left n. laryngeus recurrens

a

V. facialis

V. laryngea superior

V. thyroidea superior

Vv. thyroideae mediae

V. laryngea inferior

Plexus thyroideus impar

V. jugularis interna

V. thyroidea inferior

Left v. brachio-cephalica

V. subclavia

b

D Blood supply and innervation

a Arterial and nerve supply. Anterior view. The larynx derives its *blood supply* from two major arteries: (1) the a. laryngea superior from the a. thyroidea superior branch of the a. carotis externa and (2) the a. laryngea inferior from the a. laryngea inferior off the a. subclavia. Thus the arterial supply of the larynx is analogous to that of the gl. thyroidea. Responsible for the innervation are the nn. laryngei superior and recurrens (both from the n. vagus, see p. 141).

Note: Owing to the close proximity of the nerves and arteries, a left-sided aortic aneurysm may cause left n. laryngeus recurrens palsy resulting in hoarseness (the pathophysiology is explored more fully on p. 219).

b Venous drainage. Left lateral view. The v. laryngea superior drains into the v. thyroidea superior, which terminates at the v. jugularis interna. The v. laryngea inferior drains into the plexus thyroideus impar, which usually drains into the left v. brachiocephalica via the v. thyroidea inferior.

215

5.38   Larynx: Muscles

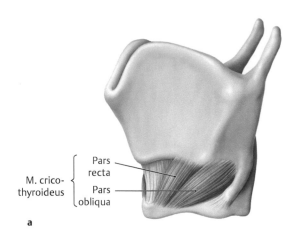

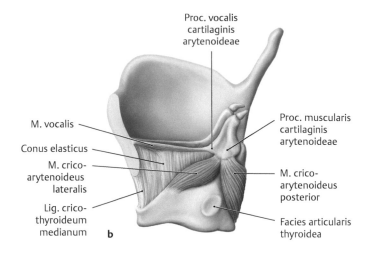

a   Left lateral oblique view

b   Left lateral view with the left half of the cartilago thyroidea removed

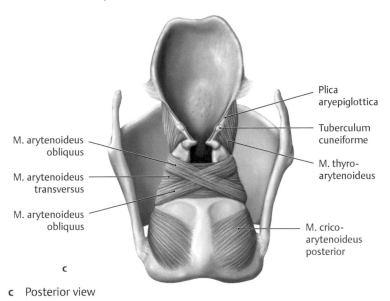

c   Posterior view

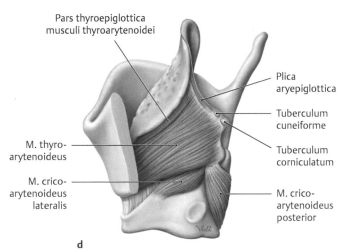

d   Left lateral view, left half of the cartilago thyroidea has been removed almost completely for better exposure of the epiglottis and m. thyroarytenoideus, external part*

A Mm. laryngis

a Extrinsic mm. laryngis. The m. cricothyroideus (or anterior cricothyroid) is the only laryngeal muscle that attaches to the external surface of the larynx. Contraction of the m. cricothyroideus tilts the cartilago cricoidea posteriorly, acting with the m. vocalis (see **b**) to increase tension on the plicae vocales. The *m. cricothyroideus* is the only muscle innervated by the r. externus of the n. laryngeus superior.

b–d Intrinsic mm. laryngis (the mm. cricoarytenoidei posterior and lateralis and the m. thyroarytenoideus). These muscles insert on the cartilago arytenoidea and can alter the position of the plicae vocales. Contraction of the *m. cricoarytenoideus posterior* rotates the cartilago arytenoidea outward and slightly to the side; thus it is the only laryngeal muscle that abducts the plicae vocales. The *m. cricoarytenoideus lateralis* adducts the plicae. It opens the intercartilaginous portion (part of glottis located between the cartilagines arytenoideae) and closes the intermembranous portion (part of the glottis located between the cartilago thyroidea and the tip of the proc. vocalis, see **B**) which brings the tips of the procc. vocales close to each other. Because this mechanism initiates speech production, this intrinsic laryngeal muscle is also called the muscle of phonation. Besides the m. vocalis, the *mm. arytenoideus transversus* and *thyroarytenoideus* produce *complete* closure of the rima glottidis (see **c**).

Note: All intrinsic mm. laryngis receive their motor innervation via the n. laryngeus recurrens. Unilateral loss of the n. laryngeus recurrens (e.g., on the left side due to nodal metastases from a hilar bronchial carcinoma) leads to ipsilateral palsy of the m. cricoarytenoideus posterior. This prevents complete abduction of the plicae vocales, resulting in hoarseness. Bilateral loss of the n. laryngeus recurrens (e.g., due to thyroid surgery) leads to dominance of the muscles that close the rima glottidis, causing adduction of the plicae vocales with a risk of asphyxiation, but speech is not completely lost (see p. 132).

The muscles described here move the laryngeal cartilages relative to one another and affect the tension and/or position of the plicae vocales. The muscles that move the larynx as a whole (mm. infra- and suprahyoidei as well as m. constrictor pharyngis inferior) are described on p. 84.

---

* In older nomenclature, the pars thyroepiglottica of the m. thyroarytenoideus was called the thyroepiglottic m. and the band of muscle fibers below the plica aryepiglottica was the aryepiglottic m.

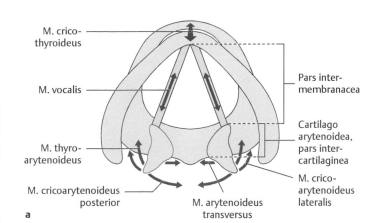

M. crico-thyroideus

M. vocalis

M. thyro-arytenoideus

M. cricoarytenoideus posterior

M. arytenoideus transversus

Pars inter-membranacea

Cartilago arytenoidea, pars inter-cartilaginea

M. crico-arytenoideus lateralis

a

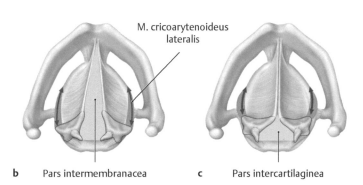

M. cricoarytenoideus lateralis

b Pars intermembranacea

c Pars intercartilaginea

B Mm. laryngis and their actions (arrows indicate directions of pull)

M. cricoarytenoideus posterior	Abduct the vocal folds (open the rima glottidis)
M. cricoarytenoideus lateralis (see **b** and **c**)	Adduct the vocal folds (close the rima glottidis)
M. arytenoideus transversus, m. thyroarytenoideus	Adduct the vocal folds (close the rima glottidis)
M. cricothyroideus, m. vocalis	Tighten the vocal folds

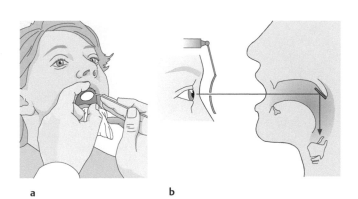

a   **b**

C Indirect laryngoscopy

a From the perspective of the examiner: The larynx—without anesthesia—can only be viewed indirectly with the aid of a mirror (laryngoscope, alternatively endoscope) (cf. **Da**). The examiner holds the patient's tongue while introducing the mirror with the other hand.

b Optical path in laryngoscopy: The mirror directs the light—from the uvula palatina—in a caudal direction to the larynx (findings see **D**).

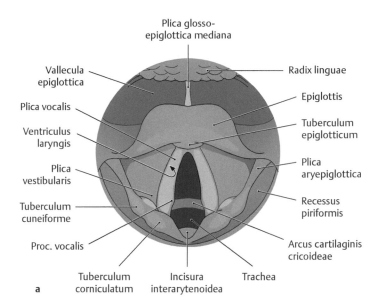

Plica glosso-epiglottica mediana

Vallecula epiglottica

Plica vocalis

Ventriculus laryngis

Plica vestibularis

Tuberculum cuneiforme

Proc. vocalis

Radix linguae

Epiglottis

Tuberculum epiglotticum

Plica aryepiglottica

Recessus piriformis

Arcus cartilaginis cricoideae

Tuberculum corniculatum   Incisura interarytenoidea   Trachea

a

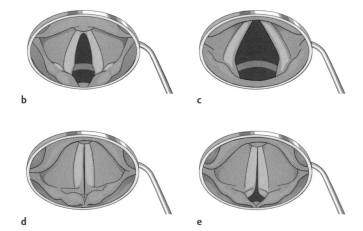

b   **c**

d   **e**

D Mirror image seen by laryngoscopy
(after Berghaus, Rettinger, and Böhme)

a The **mirror image** is a virtual image that shows an anatomically correct portrayal of the left and right side: The right plica vocalis appears on the right side of the mirror image. However, anatomically anterior and posterior structures appear at the top or at the bottom of the image: that is radix linguae, valleculae epiglotticae or epiglottis (all anterior) at the top, the incisura interarytenoidea (posterior) at the bottom. The plicae vocales appear as smooth-edged bands. Unlike the surrounding mucosa, the plicae vocales do not have blood vessels and are thus markedly lighter in color. The glottis is evaluated in both the respiratory (open) and phonation (closed) positions by having the patient alternately breathe and sing "hiii." The evaluation is based on pathoanatomical (redness, swelling, ulceration) as well as functional changes (e.g., abnormal plica vocalis position).

b–e Physiological findings: *Respiratory positions:* opening of the rima glottidis during normal (**b**) and vigorous respiration (**c**). Phonation position with the plicae vocales completely adducted (**d**). During whispered speech, the plicae vocales are slightly abducted in their posterior third (**e**).

5.39 Larynx: Topographical and Clinical Anatomy

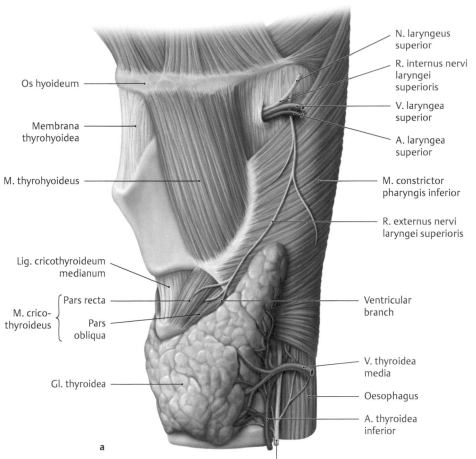

Os hyoideum

Membrana thyrohyoidea

M. thyrohyoideus

Lig. cricothyroideum medianum

M. crico-thyroideus { Pars recta / Pars obliqua

Gl. thyroidea

N. laryngeus superior

R. internus nervi laryngei superioris

V. laryngea superior

A. laryngea superior

M. constrictor pharyngis inferior

R. externus nervi laryngei superioris

Ventricular branch

V. thyroidea media

Oesophagus

A. thyroidea inferior

N. laryngeus recurrens

a

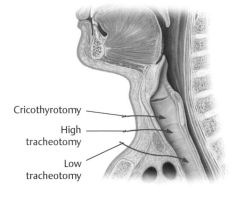

Cricothyrotomy

High tracheotomy

Low tracheotomy

B Approaches to the larynx and trachea
Midsagittal section, left lateral view. When an acute edematous obstruction of the larynx (e. g., due to an allergic reaction) poses an acute risk of asphyxiation, the following surgical approaches are available for creating an emergency airway:

- Division of the median cricothyroid ligament (cricothyrotomy)
- Incision of the trachea (tracheotomy) at a level just below the cricoid cartilage (high tracheostomy) or just superior to the jugular notch (low tracheostomy).

A Topographical anatomy of the larynx: blood supply and innervation
Left lateral view. **a** Superficial layer, **b** deep layer. The m. cricothyroideus and lamina sinistra cartilaginis thyroideae have been removed, and the pharyngeal tunica mucosa has been mobilized and retracted. Arteries and veins enter the larynx mainly from the posterior side. *Note*: The motor branch (r. externus) of the n. laryngeus superior supplies the m. crico-thyroideus, and its sensory branch (r. internus) supplies the laryngeal tunica mucosa down to the level of the plicae vocales. The n. laryngeus recurrens, supplies motor innervation to all other (intrinsic) larynx muscles as well as sensory innervation to the laryngeal tunica mucosa below the plicae vocales.
The r. externus of the n. laryngeus superior gives off an endolaryngeal branch, the ventricular branch. It runs in a cranial direction along the interior surface of the larynx and ends at the level of the plicae vestibulares. It probably innervates the ventricular m. but is not yet included in the *Terminologia Anatomica*.

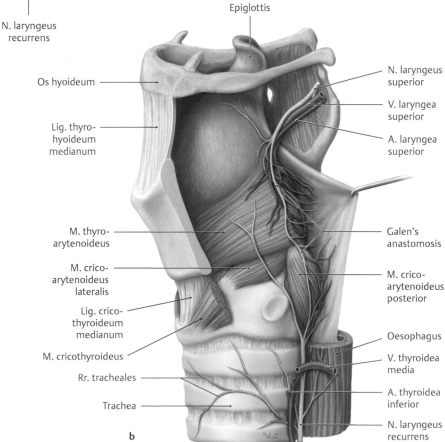

Os hyoideum

Lig. thyro-hyoideum medianum

M. thyro-arytenoideus

M. crico-arytenoideus lateralis

Lig. crico-thyroideum medianum

M. cricothyroideus

Rr. tracheales

Trachea

Epiglottis

N. laryngeus superior

V. laryngea superior

A. laryngea superior

Galen's anastomosis

M. crico-arytenoideus posterior

Oesophagus

V. thyroidea media

A. thyroidea inferior

N. laryngeus recurrens

b

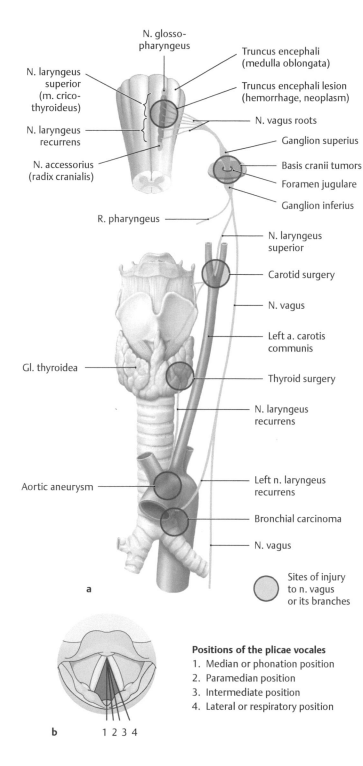

Positions of the plicae vocales
1. Median or phonation position
2. Paramedian position
3. Intermediate position
4. Lateral or respiratory position

b   1 2 3 4

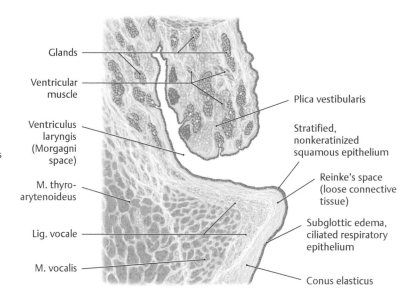

D Structure of the plica vocalis

Schematic coronal histologic section, posterior view. Subjected to severe mechanical stress, the plicae vocales are covered by nonkeratinized stratified squamous epithelium (degenerative changes may lead to squamous cell carcinoma). Respiratory (ciliated) epithelium is located in the adjacent subglottic space. The tunica mucosa sits on loose connective tissue. Chronic irritation from smoking may cause chronic edema in Reinke's space which can result in a hoarse voice ("smoker's voice").

Particularly at the base of the plicae vestibulares, but also occasionally at the fold itself, exist bands of skeletal muscle, referred to as the ventricular muscle. The official nomenclature does not list this muscle any longer, yet several authors have described it. Functionally, every voice pathologist is familiar with it, because the plicae vestibulares contract with the help of this muscle.

C Vagus nerve and the position of the vocal folds

The motor fibers of the n. vagus innervate the mm. pharyngis and laryngis. They originate in the truncus encephali in the nucleus ambiguus, the cell groups of which are arranged in somatic order: Between the fibers of the n. glossopharyngeus (cranial origin) and n. accessorius (caudal origin) lie the original neurons of the nn. laryngeus superior and recurrens as well as the motor fibers for the muscles of the palatum molle and pharynx. Central or high peripheral vagal lesions lead to pharyngeal or laryngeal muscle palsy and thereby influence the positions of the plicae vocales:

- *Central lesions in the truncus encephali or highe* involving the nucleus ambiguus (e. g., caused by a tumor or hemorrhage) → an intermediate or paramedian position of the vocal fold on the affected side (see **b**).
- *Peripheral lesions of the n. vagus* have variable effects, depending on the site of the lesion:

- Basis cranii lesions at the level of the foramen jugulare (e.g., caused by a nasopharyngeal tumor) → an intermediate or paramedian position of the affected plica vocalis due to a flaccid paralysis of all intrinsic and extrinsic mm. laryngis (see **b**) → inability to close the glottis with severe hoarseness. Sensation is lost in the larynx on the affected side.
- N. laryngeus superior in the midcervical region (e.g., as a complication of carotid surgery) → hypotonicity of the m. cricothyroideus → mild hoarseness with a weak voice, especially at higher frequencies. Sensation is lost above the plica vocalis.
- N. laryngeus recurrens in the lower neck (e.g., lesion caused by thyroid surgery, bronchial carcinoma, or an aortic aneurysm) → paralysis of all intrinsic mm. laryngis on the affected side → a median or paramedian position of the plica vocalis, mild hoarseness, poor tonal control, rapid voice fatigue, no dyspnea. Sensation is lost below the plica vocalis.

Note: Bilateral lesions usually worsen the symptoms; e.g., n. laryngeus recurrens palsy results in the plica vocalis being in the paramedian position, significant dyspnea and inspiratory stridor (necessitating tracheotomy in acute cases, see **B**). In addition to motor deficits, sensation is lost at various sites in the laryngeal tunica mucosa depending on the location of the lesion (see **Ab**). Moreover, n. vagus lesions lead to diminished gag reflexes, swallowing difficulty, foreign-body sensation, coughing and hypernasal speech (deficient closure of the oronasal cavity); usually drooping of the palatum molle on the affected side (dysfunction of the m. levator veli palatini) and deviation of the uvula palatina to the unaffected side.

5.40 Endotracheal Intubation

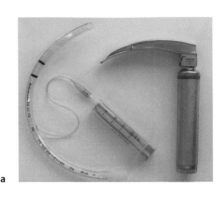

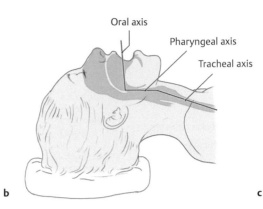

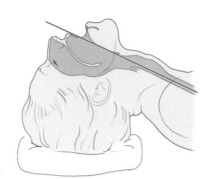

Oral axis
Pharyngeal axis
Tracheal axis

a

b

c

A Equipment and positioning of the head for endotracheal intubation

a Endotracheal (ET) tube with an inflatable cuff (left) and laryngoscope with handle and curved spatula (right).
b, c Unfavorable and optimal positioning of the head for endotracheal intubation.

Endotracheal intubation, inserting a tube into the trachea of a patient, is the safest way to keep the airways clear to allow for effective ventilation. Depending on access there are four ways to achieve endotracheal intubation:

- orotracheal = via the mouth (gold standard),
- nasotracheal = via the nose (performed if orotracheal intubation is not possible), and
- pertracheal = intubation through tracheostomy (used for long-term ventilation), and

- cricothyrotomy (used only in an emergencies when there is the threat of impending suffocation).

Endotracheal intubation requires the use of a laryngoscope and an ET tube (**a**). The tubes are available in different sizes (10–22 cm) and diameters (2.5–8 mm). They have a circular cross piece that has a proximal connector for a ventilation hose and a beveled distal end. An inflatable cuff on the ET ensures that the trachea is hermetically sealed (see **Cb**). With orotracheal intubation, the oral, pharyngeal, and tracheal axes should lie in a straight line (the "sniffing position," see **c**). This facilitates direct visualization of the laryngeal inlet (see **B**) and shortens the distance between the teeth and glottis in young adults (13–16 cm).

Note: In patients with suspected cervical spine injury, manipulation of the head position without maintaining the stability of the cervical spine is contraindicated.

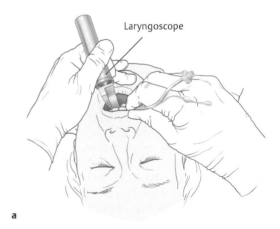

Laryngoscope

a

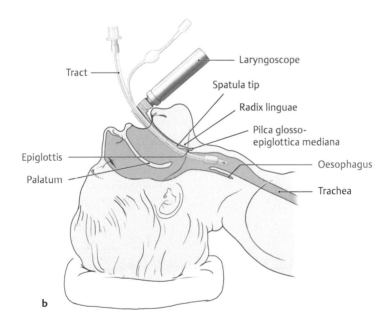

Laryngoscope
Spatula tip
Radix linguae
Pilca glosso-epiglottica mediana
Oesophagus
Trachea
Tract
Epiglottis
Palatum

b

B Placement of the laryngoscope and the endotracheal tube (ET)

a Handling and placement of the laryngoscope from the perspective of the physician. **b** Placement of the ET tube.

To place the ET tube, the physician stands at the head of the patient and introduces the spatula of the laryngoscope into the patient's mouth. The spatula is then used to push the patient's tongue to the left to get a clear view of the larynx.

Under direct visualization, the spatula tip is then advanced until its lies in the vallecula.

Note: If the spatula is introduced too deep, its tip reaches behind the epiglottis, and orientation is difficult.

The physician then pulls the spatula in the direction of the floor of mouth without using the upper teeth as a fulcrum. This elevates the epiglottis and the base of the tongue such that the physician now has an unobstructed view of the laryngeal inlet (see **Ca**). The physician then pushes

the ET tube through the rima glottis into the trachea (see **b**). Placement under laryngoscopic control ensures that the ET tube is placed in the trachea and does not accidentally enter the esophagus.

Note: The ET tube has markings in centimeter increments that serve as an orientation aid to the physician. The distance from the upper teeth to the center of the trachea in the adult is about 22 cm and in newborns is about 11 cm. Distances greater than these might be an indicator that the tube is inserted too deeply and is in the right main bronchus.

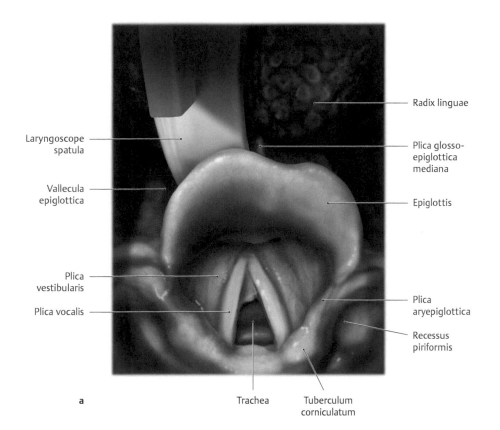

Radix linguae

Laryngoscope spatula

Plica glosso-epiglottica mediana

Vallecula epiglottica

Epiglottis

Plica vestibularis

Plica vocalis

Plica aryepiglottica

Recessus piriformis

a

Trachea

Tuberculum corniculatum

C View of the laryngeal inlet and location of the endotracheal tube after intubation
a Laryngoscopic view of larynx, epiglottis, and median glossoepiglottic fold. **b** Median sagittal section viewed from the right of an ET tube in situ with its cuff inflated.

a Shows the entrance to the trachea after placement of the laryngoscope (cf. **Ba**). **b** Depicts the ET tube in situ in the trachea. The inflatable cuff seals the trachea in all directions and eliminates leakage during ventilation and prevents aspiration of foreign bodies, mucus, or gastric juice.

To check if the ET tube has been placed correctly, the physician looks at the patient's chest to evaluate if chest movement is symmetrical, he auscultates for equal breath sounds over both lung fields and the absence of breath sounds over the stomach. Further indicators that the ET tube is placed correctly include vapor condensation on the inside of the ET tube with exhalation and measurement of end-tidal carbon dioxide. If there is any doubt as to the positioning of the tube, it should be removed.

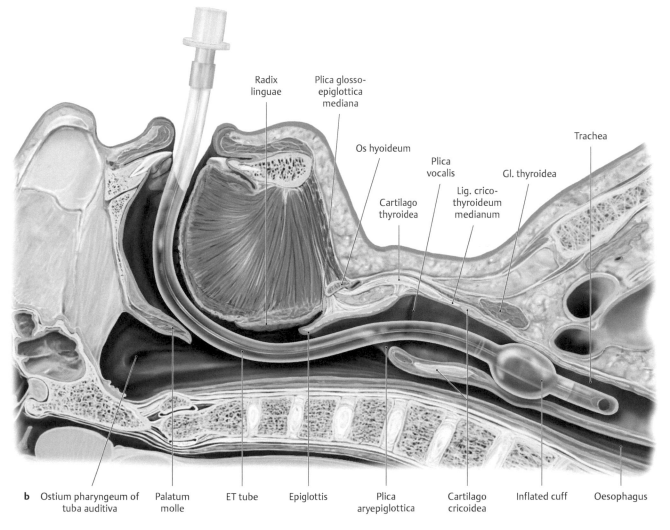

Radix linguae

Plica glosso-epiglottica mediana

Os hyoideum

Plica vocalis

Trachea

Cartilago thyroidea

Lig. crico-thyroideum medianum

Gl. thyroidea

b Ostium pharyngeum of tuba auditiva

Palatum molle

ET tube

Epiglottis

Plica aryepiglottica

Cartilago cricoidea

Inflated cuff

Oesophagus

221

5.41 Thyroid Gland (Glandula Thyroidea) and Parathyroid Glands (Glandulae Parathyroideae)

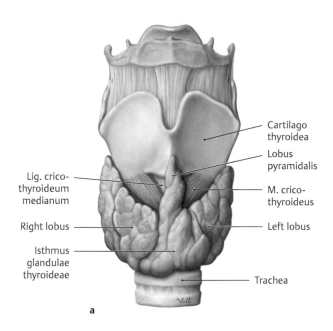

a

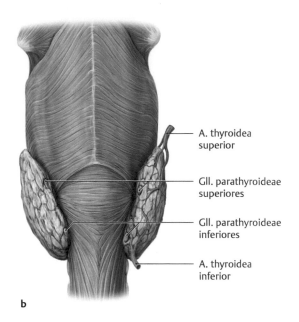

b

A Glandula thyroidea and glandulae parathyroideae

a Gl. thyroidea, anterior view. The gl. thyroidea consists of two laterally situated lobi and a central narrowing or isthmus. In place of the isthmus glandulae thyroideae there is often a lobus pyramidalis, whose apex points cranially to the embryonic origin of the gl. thyroidea at the base of the tongue (see p.11).

b Gl. thyroidea and gll. parathyroideae, posterior view.
The gll. parathyroideae may show considerable variation in their number (generally four) and location.

Note: Because the parathyroid glands are usually contained within the capsule of the thyroid gland, there is a considerable risk of removing them during thyroid surgery (see **B**).

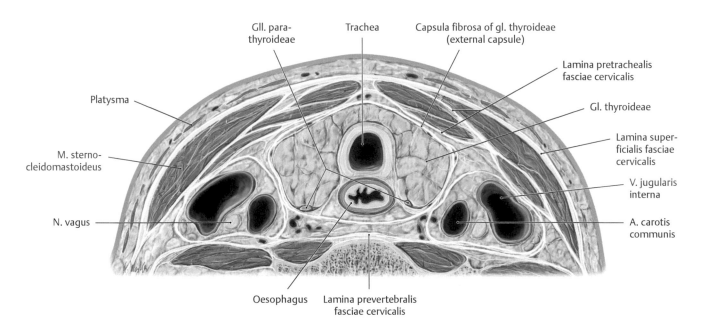

B Relationship of the glandula thyroidea to the trachea and neurovascular structures

Transverse section through the neck at the level of T1 superior view. The gl. thyroidea partially surrounds the trachea and is bordered posterolaterally by the neurovascular bundle within the vagina carotica. When the gl. thyroidea is pathologically enlarged (e.g., due to iodine-deficiency goiter), it may gradually compress and narrow the tracheal lumen, causing respiratory distress.

Note the arrangement of the fasciae: The gl. thyroidea is surrounded by a capsula fibrosa composed of an internal and external layer. The delicate internal layer (*internal capsule*, not shown here) directly invests the gl. thyroidea and is fused with its glandular parenchyma. Vascularized fibrous slips extend from the internal capsule into the substance of the gland, subdividing it into lobules. The internal capsule is covered by the tough *external capsule*, which is part of the lamina pretrachealis of the fascia cervicalis. This capsule invests the gl. thyroidea and gll. parathyroideae and is also called the "surgical capsule" because it must be opened to gain surgical access to the gl. thyroidea. Between the external and internal capsules is a potential space that is traversed by vascular branches and is occupied by the gll. parathyroideae.

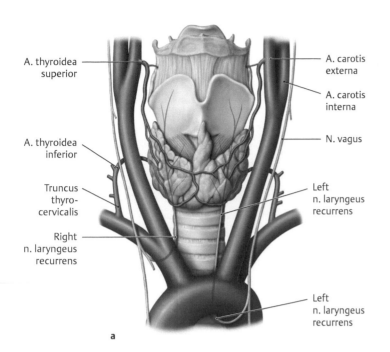

A. thyroidea superior
A. carotis externa
A. carotis interna
A. thyroidea inferior
N. vagus
Truncus thyro-cervicalis
Left n. laryngeus recurrens
Right n. laryngeus recurrens
Left n. laryngeus recurrens

a

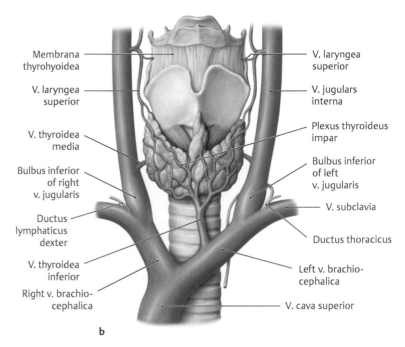

Membrana thyrohyoidea
V. laryngea superior
V. laryngea superior
V. jugulars interna
V. thyroidea media
Plexus thyroideus impar
Bulbus inferior of right v. jugularis
Bulbus inferior of left v. jugularis
Ductus lymphaticus dexter
V. subclavia
Ductus thoracicus
V. thyroidea inferior
Right v. brachio-cephalica
Left v. brachio-cephalica
V. cava superior

b

C Blood supply and innervation of the glandula thyroidea
Anterior view.

a Arterial supply: The gl. thyroidea derives most of its arterial blood supply from the a. thyroidea superior (the first branch of the a. carotis externa), which runs forward and downward to supply the gland. It is supplied from below by the a. thyroidea inferior, which branches from the truncus thyrocervicalis (see p. 214). All of these arteries, which course on the right and left sides of the organ, must be ligated during surgical removal of the gl. thyroidea.
Note: Operations on the gl. thyroidea carry a risk of injury to the n. laryngeus recurrens, which is closely related to the posterior surface of the gland. Because it supplies important laryngeal muscles, unilateral injury to the nerve will cause postoperative hoarseness while bilateral injury may additionally result in dyspnea (difficulty in breathing). Prior to thyroid surgery, therefore, an otolaryngologist should confirm the integrity of the nerve supply to the mm. laryngis and exclude any preexisting nerve lesion.

b Venous drainage: The gl. thyroidea is drained anteroinferiorly by a well-developed *plexus thyroideus impar*, which usually drains through the v. thyroidea inferior to the left v. brachiocephalica. Blood from the gl. thyroidea also drains to the v. jugularis interna via the vv. thyroideae superior and mediae.

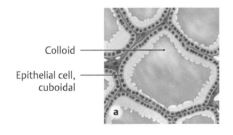

Colloid
Epithelial cell, cuboidal

a

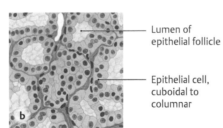

Lumen of epithelial follicle
Epithelial cell, cuboidal to columnar

b

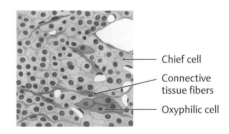

Chief cell
Connective tissue fibers
Oxyphilic cell

D Histology of the glandula thyroidea
The gl. thyroidea absorbs iodide from the blood and uses it to make the thyroid hormones, thyroxine (T4, tetraiodothyronine) and triiodothyronine (T3). These hormones are stored at extracellular sites in the gland, bound to protein, and when needed they are mobilized from the thyroid follicles and secreted into the bloodstream. A special feature of the gl. thyroidea is the appearance of its epithelium, which varies depending on whether it is storing hormones or releasing them into the blood. The epithelial cells are low cuboidal in shape when in their resting or "storage state" (**a**), but they are columnar in shape when in their active or "secretory state" (**b**). The epithelial morphology thus indicates the current functional state of the cells. Iodine deficiency causes an enlargement of the colloidal follicular lumen, which eventually results in a gross increase in the size of the gl. thyroidea (goiter). With prolonged iodine deficiency there is a reduction in body metabolism, and concomitant lethargy, fatigue, and mental depression. Conversely, hyperactivity of the gl. thyroidea, as in Graves' disease (an autoimmune disorder), causes a generalized metabolic acceleration, with irritability and weight loss. In the midst of the thyroid follicles are parafollicular cells (C cells), which secrete calcitonin. Calcitonin inhibits bone resorption and reduces the calcium concentration in the blood.

E Histology of the glandula parathyroidea
The chief cells of the gl. parathyroidea secrete parathormone which indirectly stimulates osteoclasts (via the osteoblasts) leading to increased bone resorption. As a result of bone resorption, the calcium concentration in the blood increases. Inadvertent removal of the gll. parathyroideae can lead to *hyoparathyroidism*. The body produces so little parathormone, the calcium concentration in the blood decreases which causes hypocalcemia, resulting in tetanic seizures involving skeletal muscle. Benign parathyroid tumors (adenoma) are associated with unregulated, excessive parathormone production resulting in increased calcium concentration in the blood (*hypercalcemia*) and excessive urinary calcium excretion (*hypercalciuria*). At the same time, phosphate metabolism is also affected given that parathormone stimulates renal phosphate excretion, resulting in a very low level of phosphate in the blood (*hypophosphatemia*) and very high levels of phosphate in the urine (*hypophosphaturia*). Clinical symptoms of hyperparathyroidism include muscle weakness, lethargy, small intestinal ulcers and pancreatitis.

5.42 Topography and Imaging of the Glandula Thyroidea

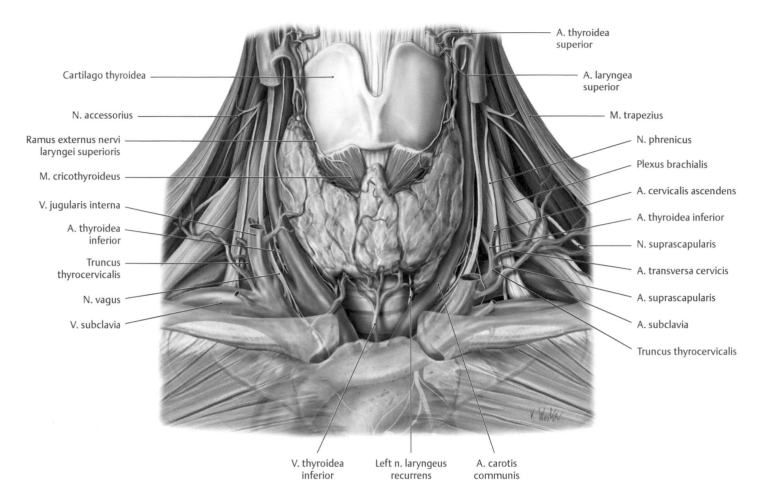

- A. thyroidea superior
- Cartilago thyroidea
- A. laryngea superior
- N. accessorius
- M. trapezius
- Ramus externus nervi laryngei superioris
- N. phrenicus
- Plexus brachialis
- M. cricothyroideus
- A. cervicalis ascendens
- V. jugularis interna
- A. thyroidea inferior
- A. thyroidea inferior
- N. suprascapularis
- Truncus thyrocervicalis
- A. transversa cervicis
- N. vagus
- A. suprascapularis
- V. subclavia
- A. subclavia
- Truncus thyrocervicalis
- V. thyroidea inferior
- Left n. laryngeus recurrens
- A. carotis communis

A Deep regio cervicalis anterior with the glandula thyroidea

Anterior view. The following neurovascular structures are clearly visible in their course through the apertura thoracis superior: the a. carotis communis, a. subclavia, v. subclavia, v. jugularis interna, v. thyroidea inferior, n. vagus, n. phrenicus, and n. laryngeus recurrens. It can be seen that a retrosternal goiter enlarging the inferior pole of the gl.

thyroidea can easily compress neurovascular structures at the apertura thoracis superior (see Fig. **E**, p. 7).

Note: Thyroid surgery represents the fifth most common surgical procedure in Germany, which is why it is important to be familiar with the topographical relationships between this gland and its surrounding structures.

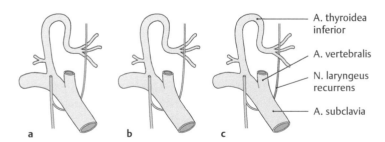

- A. thyroidea inferior
- A. vertebralis
- N. laryngeus recurrens
- A. subclavia

B Course of the right nervus laryngeus recurrens
   (after von Lanz and Wachsmuth)

Anterior view. The n. laryngeus recurrens is a special visceral efferent and sensory branch of the n. vagus, which among others innervates the m. cricoarytenoideus posterior. This is the only muscle to fully open the glottis (see p. 217). Unilateral damage to this nerve supply results in hoarseness, while bilateral damage leads to a closed glottis with severe dyspnea. The n. laryngeus recurrens may pass in front of (**a**), behind (**b**), or between (**c**) the branches of the a. thyroidea inferior. Its course should be noted during operative procedures on the gl. thyroidea.

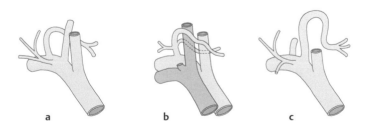

C Variations in the branching pattern of the right arteria thyroidea inferio (after Platzer)

The course of the a. thyroidea inferior is highly variable. It can run medially behind the a. vertebralis (**a**), divide immediately after arising from the truncus thyrocervicalis (sometimes, **b**) or it may arise as the first branch of the a. subclavia (**c**).

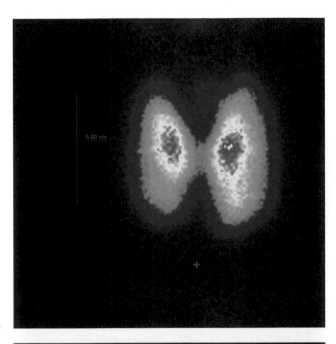

a

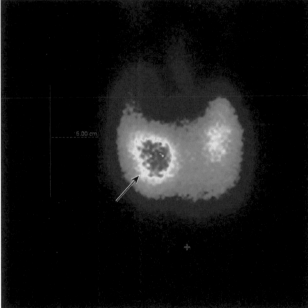

b

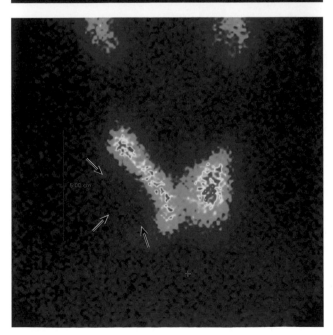

c

D Scintigrams of the thyroid gland

Frontal views. To perform gl. thyroidea scintigraphy, ^{99m}Tc pertechnetate (TcO$_4$) is injected intravenously. It is absorbed by the sodium-iodide symporter, which are characteristic to the gl. thyroidea, located in the principal cells. This uptake is visualized with the aid of a special gl. thyroidea camera (producing a gl. thyroidea scintigram). It forms the basis for evaluation of position, shape, size and storage capacity of the gl. thyroidea.

a ^{99m}TcO$_4$ uptake in the normally functioning gl. thyroidea.
b Warm nodule in the right lobe of the thyroid gland. The presence of a warm nodule means higher absorption of ^{99m}TcO$_4$. The technetium uptake is identifiable by the larger red-shaded area on the right lobe; the findings can indicate thyroid hyperfunction.
c Cold nodule in the right lobe of the gl. thyroidea. The presence of a cold nodule means that less radioactive material is taken up, identifiable by the lack of a red-shaded areas on the right. The findings can indicate a benign tumor or thyroid carcinoma.

(Images: Prof. Dr. J. Mester, Department of Nuclear Medicine, University Hospital Hamburg Eppendorf)

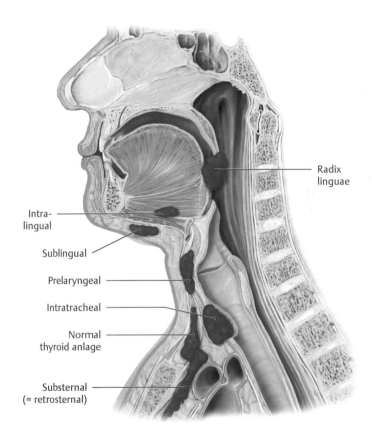

Radix
linguae

Intra-
lingual

Sublingual

Prelaryngeal

Intratracheal

Normal
thyroid anlage

Substernal
(= retrosternal)

E Glandula thyroidea ectopias

Median sagittal section, left lateral view. Gl. thyroidea ectopia describes the location of the gl. thyroidea other than the normal position. It is the result of an abnormal descent during its embryological development (see p. 11). These position anomalies can be visualized with the help of gl. thyroidea scintigraphy so that they can be surgically corrected if necessary.

6.1 Face: Nerves and Vessels

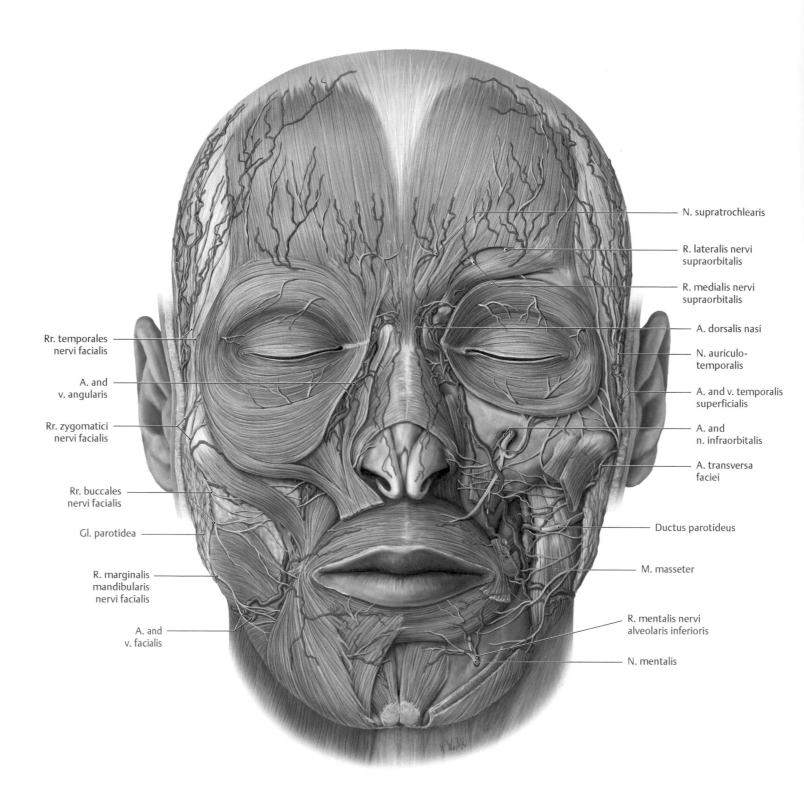

N. supratrochlearis

R. lateralis nervi supraorbitalis

R. medialis nervi supraorbitalis

A. dorsalis nasi

N. auriculo-temporalis

A. and v. temporalis superficialis

A. and n. infraorbitalis

A. transversa faciei

Ductus parotideus

M. masseter

R. mentalis nervi alveolaris inferioris

N. mentalis

Rr. temporales nervi facialis

A. and v. angularis

Rr. zygomatici nervi facialis

Rr. buccales nervi facialis

Gl. parotidea

R. marginalis mandibularis nervi facialis

A. and v. facialis

A Superficial nerves and vessels of the anterior facial region

The skin and fatty tissue have been removed to demonstrate the superficial muscular layer—the mm. faciei. This layer has been partially removed on the left side of the face to display underlying portions of the mm. masticatorii. The mm. faciei receive their motor innervation from the *n. facialis*, which emerges laterally from the gl. parotidea. The face receives its sensory innervation from the *n. trigeminus*, whose three terminal branches are shown here (see **E**). Branches from the third division of the n. trigeminus additionally supply motor innervation to the mm. masticatorii. The face receives most of its blood supply from the *a. carotis externa*. Only small areas around the medial and lateral canthi of the eyes and in the forehead are supplied by the *a. carotis interna* (see **B**).

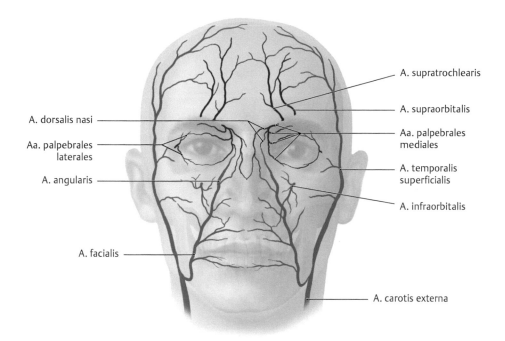

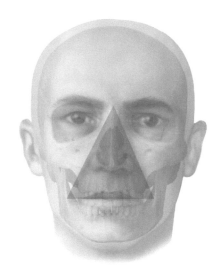

B Distribution of the arteria carotis externa (red) and arteria carotis interna (brown) in the face

Hemodynamically significant anastomoses may develop between these two arterial territories. Even a marked reduction of flow in the a. carotis interna by atherosclerosis may not lead to cerebral ischemia, as long as there is adequate compensatory flow through the a. temporalis superficialis. If this is the case, then ligation of the a. temporalis superficialis is contraindicated (the artery might otherwise be ligated, for example, in a biopsy to confirm the diagnosis of temporal arteritis; see p. 95).

C Triangular danger zone in the face

This zone is marked by the presence of venous connections from the face to the sinus durae matris. Because the veins in this region are valveless, there is a particularly high risk of bacterial dissemination into the cavitas cranii (a boil may lead to meningitis—see p. 101).

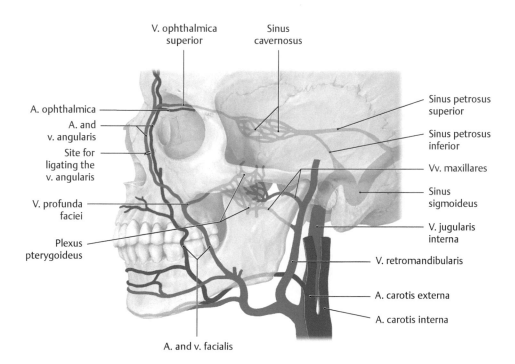

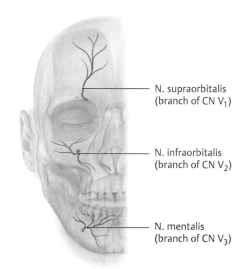

D Clinically important vascular relationships in the face

Note the connections between the exterior of the face and the sinus durae matris.

If a purulent inflammation develops in the "danger zone" (see **C**), the v̇. angularis can be ligated at a standard site to prevent the transmission of infectious organisms to the sinus cavernosus.

E Nerve exit point of the three trigeminal branches

The n. trigeminus (CN V) is the major somatic sensory nerve of the head. The diagram shows the sites of emergence of its three large sensory branches:

- branch of CN V$_1$: n. supraorbitalis (foramen supraorbitale)
- branch of CN V$_2$: n. infraorbitalis (foramen infraorbitale)
- branch of CN V$_3$: n. mentalis (foramen mentale); see also p. 123.

227

6.2 Neck, Ventral View: Superficial Layers

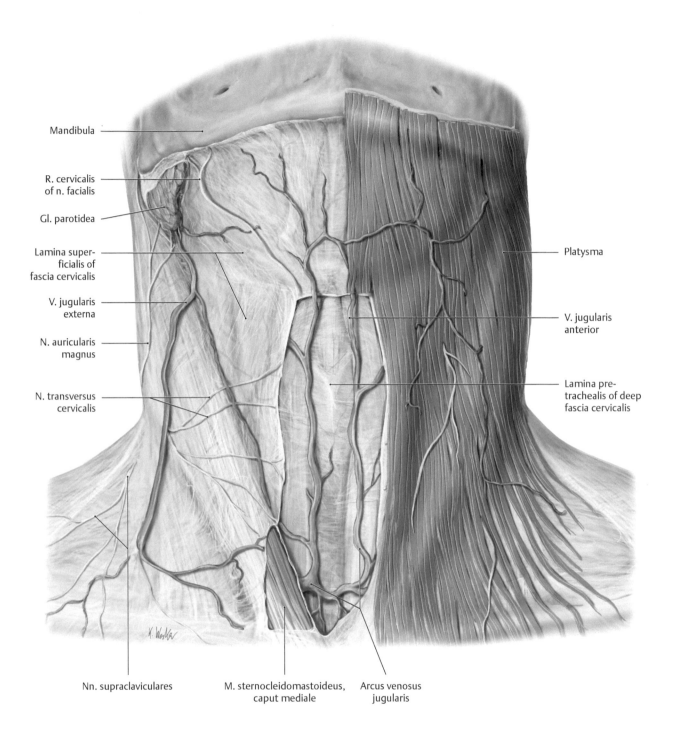

Mandibula

R. cervicalis of n. facialis

Gl. parotidea

Lamina super- ficialis of fascia cervicalis

V. jugularis externa

N. auricularis magnus

N. transversus cervicalis

Platysma

V. jugularis anterior

Lamina pre- trachealis of deep fascia cervicalis

Nn. supraclaviculares

M. sternocleidomastoideus, caput mediale

Arcus venosus jugularis

A The neck, superficial layer
Anterior view. The subcutaneous platysma has been removed on the right side, and the lamina superficialis of the fascia cervicalis (see p. 4 for cervical fascial structure) has been split in the midline and partially removed, exposing the caput mediale of the right m. sternocleidomastoideus. The trigonum cervicale anterius, which is bounded posteriorly by the m. sternocleidomastoideus and superiorly by the lower border of the mandibula, is particularly well delineated on the right side.

The v. jugularis anterior and arcus venosus jugularis can be identified. The inferior pole of the gl. parotidea projects inferior to the mandibula. When the gl. parotidea is inflamed (mumps), it causes conspicuous facial swelling and deformity in this region ("hamster cheeks" with prominent earlobes).
Note also the cutaneous nerves of the plexus cervicalis (n. auricularis magnus, n. transversus cervicalis, nn. supraclaviculares), which radiate from Erb's point (see p. 240).

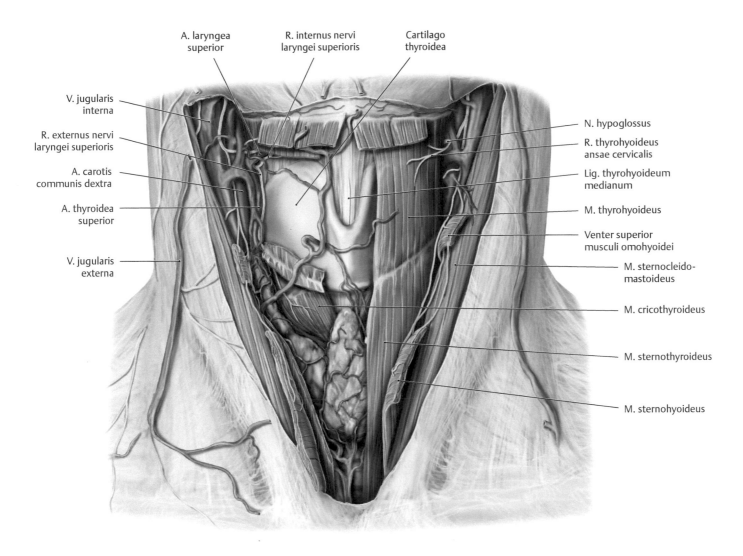

A. laryngea superior

R. internus nervi laryngei superioris

Cartilago thyroidea

V. jugularis interna

R. externus nervi laryngei superioris

A. carotis communis dextra

A. thyroidea superior

V. jugularis externa

N. hypoglossus

R. thyrohyoideus ansae cervicalis

Lig. thyrohyoideum medianum

M. thyrohyoideus

Venter superior musculi omohyoidei

M. sternocleido-mastoideus

M. cricothyroideus

M. sternothyroideus

M. sternohyoideus

B Neck, middle layer

Anterior view. The lamina pretrachealis (middle layer of fascia cervicalis) has been removed. The mm. infrahyoidei inserting on the lamina pretrachealis have been resected and the visceral fascia has been removed to expose the gl. thyroidea, which is posterior to the mm. infrahyoidei. The a. thyroidea superior, the first branch of the a. carotis externa, can be identified. The r. externus of the n. laryngeus superior, a branch of the n. vagus, courses with the a. thyroidea superior to the crim. cricothyroideus. The r. internus of the n. laryngeus superior passes through the membrana thyrohyoidea with the a. laryngea superior to supply the larynx.

6.3   Neck, Ventral View: Deep Layers

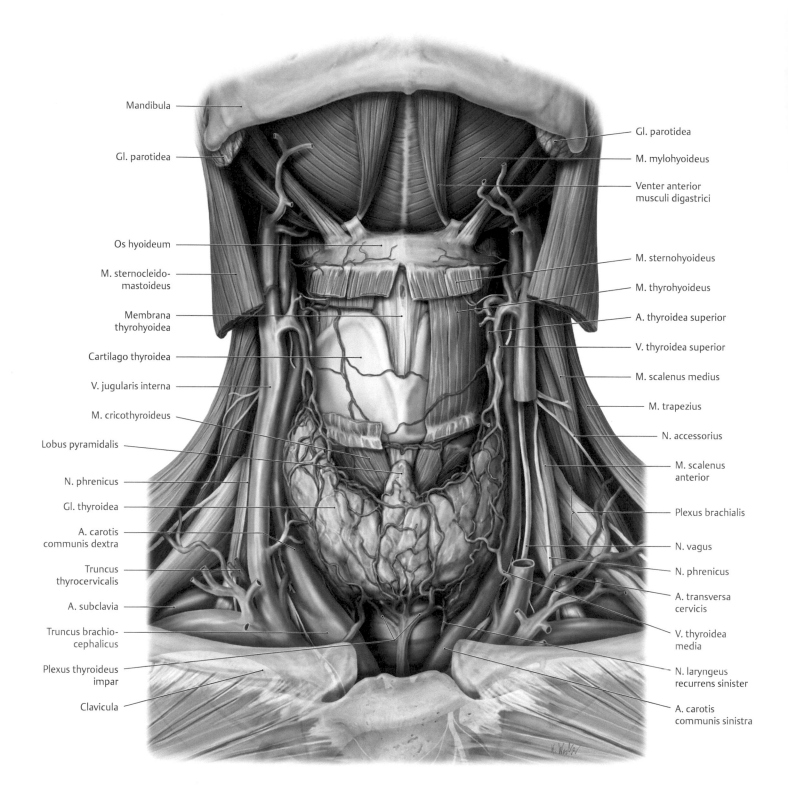

Mandibula

Gl. parotidea

Os hyoideum

M. sternocleido-
mastoideus

Membrana
thyrohyoidea

Cartilago thyroidea

V. jugularis interna

M. cricothyroideus

Lobus pyramidalis

N. phrenicus

Gl. thyroidea

A. carotis
communis dextra

Truncus
thyrocervicalis

A. subclavia

Truncus brachio-
cephalicus

Plexus thyroideus
impar

Clavicula

Gl. parotidea

M. mylohyoideus

Venter anterior
musculi digastrici

M. sternohyoideus

M. thyrohyoideus

A. thyroidea superior

V. thyroidea superior

M. scalenus medius

M. trapezius

N. accessorius

M. scalenus
anterior

Plexus brachialis

N. vagus

N. phrenicus

A. transversa
cervicis

V. thyroidea
media

N. laryngeus
recurrens sinister

A. carotis
communis sinistra

A Fascia cervicalis, ventral view

Identifiable are the viscera of the neck, larynx, and gl. thyroidea, located along and around the midline. Lateral to both, vertical pathways run to and from the head. The arterial blood supply to the gl. thyroidea is provided primarily by the cranially and posteriorly located a. thyroidea superior. Its venous drainage is carried out primarily by the caudally and anteriorly located plexus thyroideus impar. The discernible nerves include the n. vagus (CN X) and the n. phrenicus. The n. laryngeus recurrens comes from the apertura thoracis superior and runs lateral to the trachea behind the gl. thyroidea to the larynx, the muscles of which it innervates.

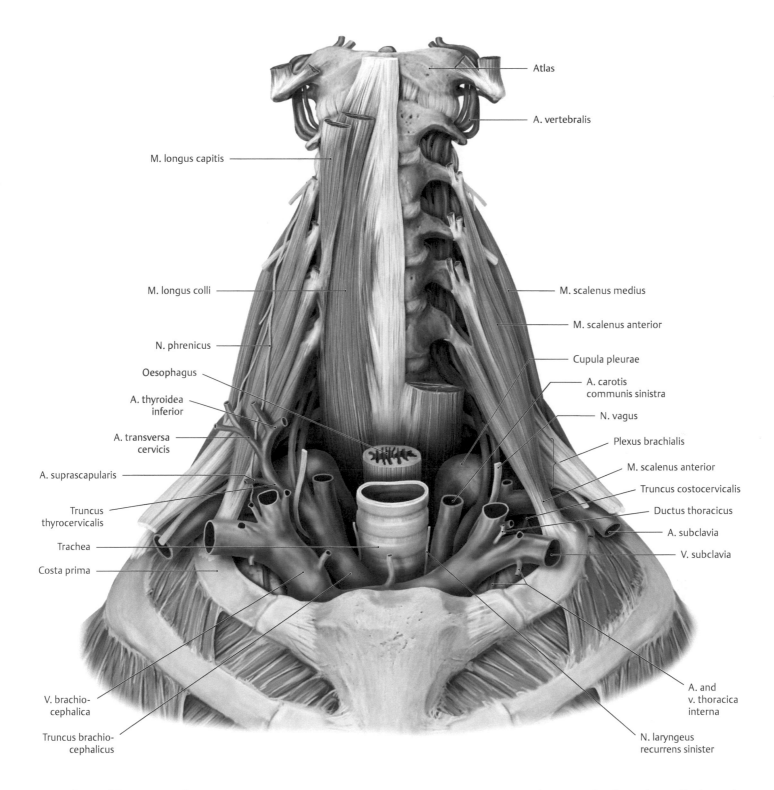

Atlas

A. vertebralis

M. longus capitis

M. longus colli

N. phrenicus

Oesophagus

A. thyroidea inferior

A. transversa cervicis

A. suprascapularis

Truncus thyrocervicalis

Trachea

Costa prima

M. scalenus medius

M. scalenus anterior

Cupula pleurae

A. carotis communis sinistra

N. vagus

Plexus brachialis

M. scalenus anterior

Truncus costocervicalis

Ductus thoracicus

A. subclavia

V. subclavia

A. and v. thoracica interna

V. brachio-cephalica

Truncus brachio-cephalicus

N. laryngeus recurrens sinister

B Deepest layer of fascia cervicalis

The viscera of the neck, larynx and gl. thyroidea, have been removed, also the trachea and oesophagus. The two large cervical vessels (a. carotis communis and v. jugularis interna) have been dissected on both sides. The deeper-lying a. vertebralis is now visible on the left side. On the right side, it is still covered by prevertebral muscles. The a. vertebralis runs through the foramen transversarium of the cervical vertebrae and travels across the arcus posterior atlantis (C1) to the inside of the skull (via the foramen magnum) where in particular it supplies the truncus encephali. The plexus cervicalis and n. phrenicus, is identifiable. It runs from the m. scalenus anterior in a caudal direction to the diaphragm, which it innervates. In this layer, two arterial trunks along with their branches are identifiable:

- on the right truncus thyrocervicalis with
  - A. thyroidea inferior

- A. transversa cervicis with its rr. profundus and superficialis, and
- A. suprascapularis

- on the left truncus costocervicalis with
  - A. cervicalis profunda
  - A. intercostalis suprema

In the scalene gap between the mm. scaleni anterior and medius runs the plexus brachialis and the a. subclavia, whereas the v. subclavia runs in front of the the m. scalenus anterior. The ductus thoracicus, which drains the lymph from ¾ of the body, empties into the left venous angle - the junction of left v. subclavia and left v. jugularis interna.

6.4　Head, Lateral View: Superficial Layer

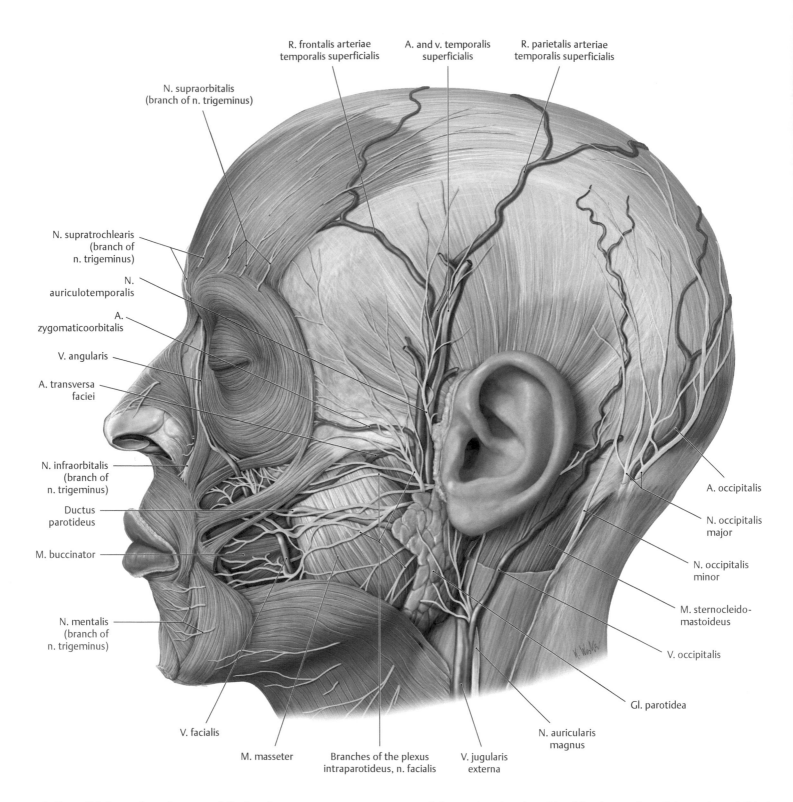

R. frontalis arteriae
temporalis superficialis

A. and v. temporalis
superficialis

R. parietalis arteriae
temporalis superficialis

N. supraorbitalis
(branch of n. trigeminus)

N. supratrochlearis
(branch of
n. trigeminus)

N.
auriculotemporalis

A.
zygomaticoorbitalis

V. angularis

A. transversa
faciei

N. infraorbitalis
(branch of
n. trigeminus)

Ductus
parotideus

M. buccinator

N. mentalis
(branch of
n. trigeminus)

A. occipitalis

N. occipitalis
major

N. occipitalis
minor

M. sternocleido-
mastoideus

V. occipitalis

Gl. parotidea

N. auricularis
magnus

V. facialis

M. masseter

Branches of the plexus
intraparotideus, n. facialis

V. jugularis
externa

A Superficial vessels and nerves of the head

Left lateral view. All the arteries visible in this diagram arise from the *a. carotis externa*, which is too deep to be visible in this superficial dissection. The lateral head region is drained by the *v. jugularis externa*. The v. facialis, however, drains into the deeper v. jugularis interna (not shown here). The *n. facialis* has divided in the gl. parotidea to form the plexus intraparotideus, whose branches leave the gl. parotidea at its anterior border and are distributed to the musculi faciei (facial muscles, see **C**). This lateral head region also receives sensory innervation from branches of the *n. trigeminus* (see **D**), while the portion of the occiput visible in the figure is supplied by the *nn. occipitales major* and *minor*. Unlike the n. trigeminus, the nn. occipitales originate from the nn. spinales of the plexus cervicalis (see **E**). The secretory duct of the gl. parotidea (the ductus parotideus) is easy to identify at dissection. It passes forward on the surface of the m. masseter, pierces the m. buccinator, and terminates in the oral cavity opposite the maxillary second molar (not shown).

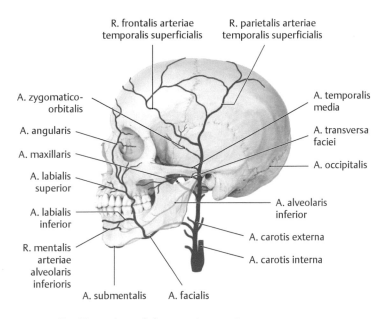

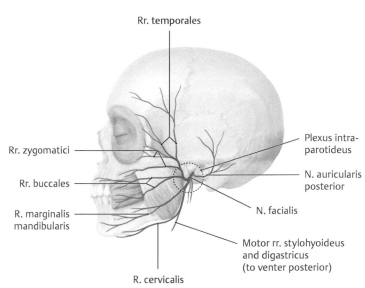

B Superficial branches of the arteria carotis externa

Left lateral view. This diagram shows the arteries in isolation to demonstrate their branches and their relationships to one another (cf. **A**; details see p. 94).

C Nervus facialis (CN VII)

Left lateral view. The mm. faciei receive all of their motor innervation from the seventh n. cranialis (see p. 125).

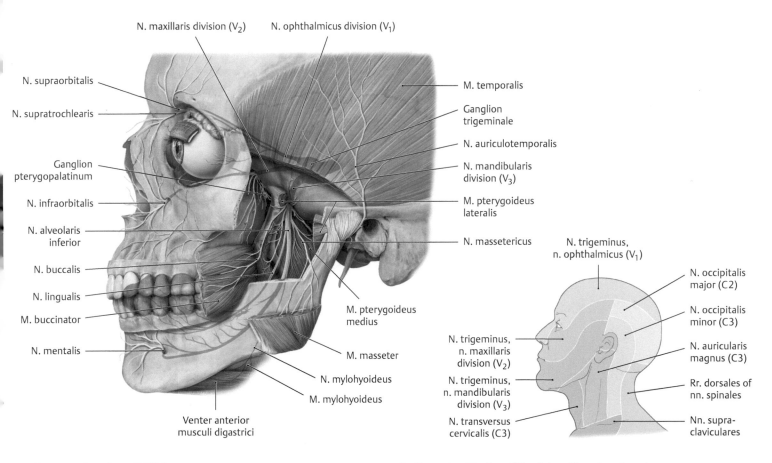

D Nervus trigeminus (CN V)

Left lateral view. In the region shown here, the head derives its somatic sensory supply from three large branches of the n. trigeminus (n. supraorbitalis, n. infraorbitalis, and n. mentalis). The diagram illustrates their course in the skull and their sites of emergence in the anterior facial region (see the anterior view on p. 226). The n. trigeminus is partly a mixed nerve because motor fibers travel with the n. mandibularis (= third division of the n. trigeminus) to supply the mm. masticatorii.

E Nerve territories of the lateral head and neck

Left lateral view.

Note: The lateral head and neck region receives its sensory supply from one n. cranialis (n. trigeminus and its branches), and from the rr. dorsales (n. occipitalis major) and rr. ventrales (n. occipitalis minor, n. auricularis magnus, n. transversus cervicalis) of nn. spinales.

The n. spinalis C1 has a radix anterior, containing motor fibers, but no radix posterior; it therefore provides no sensory innervation to the skin (i.e., it has no dermatome).

6.5   Head, Lateral View: Middle and Deep Layers

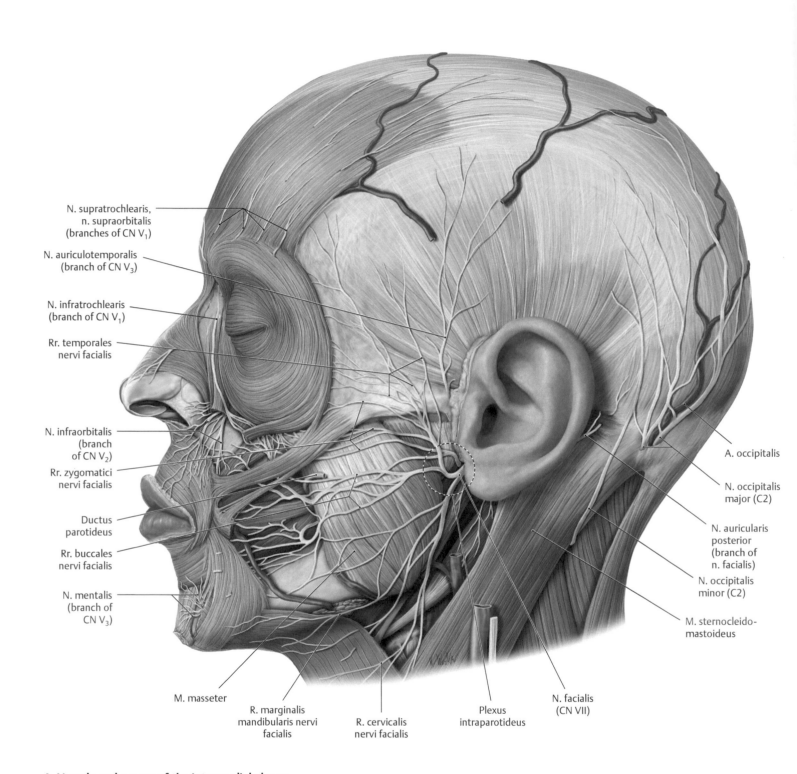

N. supratrochlearis,
n. supraorbitalis
(branches of CN V₁)

N. auriculotemporalis
(branch of CN V₃)

N. infratrochlearis
(branch of CN V₁)

Rr. temporales
nervi facialis

N. infraorbitalis
(branch
of CN V₂)

Rr. zygomatici
nervi facialis

Ductus
parotideus

Rr. buccales
nervi facialis

N. mentalis
(branch of
CN V₃)

A. occipitalis

N. occipitalis
major (C2)

N. auricularis
posterior
(branch of
n. facialis)

N. occipitalis
minor (C2)

M. sternocleido-
mastoideus

M. masseter

R. marginalis
mandibularis nervi
facialis

R. cervicalis
nervi facialis

Plexus
intraparotideus

N. facialis
(CN VII)

A   Vessels and nerves of the intermediale layer
Left lateral view. The gl. parotidea has been removed to demonstrate
the structure of the plexus intraparotideus of the n. facialis.
Note certain nerves have been described in previous units.
The veins have been removed for clarity.

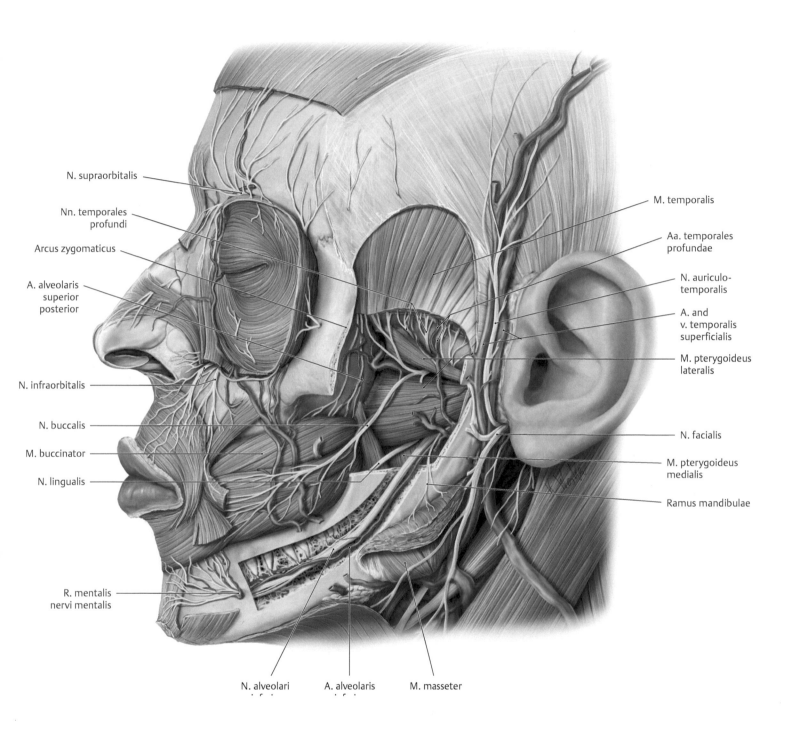

N. supraorbitalis

Nn. temporales profundi

Arcus zygomaticus

A. alveolaris superior posterior

N. infraorbitalis

N. buccalis

M. buccinator

N. lingualis

R. mentalis nervi mentalis

M. temporalis

Aa. temporales profundae

N. auriculo-temporalis

A. and v. temporalis superficialis

M. pterygoideus lateralis

N. facialis

M. pterygoideus medialis

Ramus mandibulae

N. alveolari... ...f...

A. alveolaris ...f...

M. masseter

B Vessels and nerves of the deep layer
Left lateral view. The m. masseter and arcus zygomaticus have been divided to gain access to the deep structures. Also, the ramus mandibulae has been opened to demonstrate the neurovascular structures that traverse it.

235

6.6 Infratemporal Fossa (Fossa Infratemporalis)

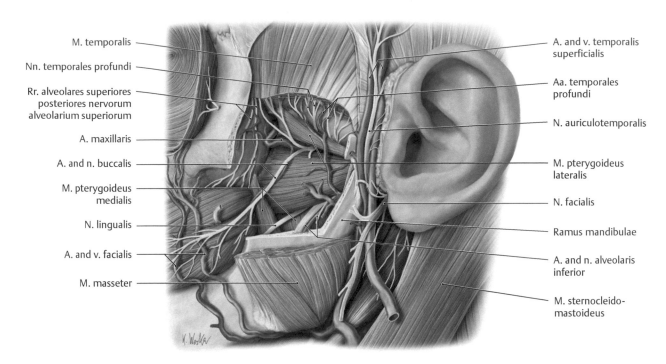

M. temporalis

Nn. temporales profundi

Rr. alveolares superiores posteriores nervorum alveolarium superiorum

A. maxillaris

A. and n. buccalis

M. pterygoideus medialis

N. lingualis

A. and v. facialis

M. masseter

A. and v. temporalis superficialis

Aa. temporales profundi

N. auriculotemporalis

M. pterygoideus lateralis

N. facialis

Ramus mandibulae

A. and n. alveolaris inferior

M. sternocleido-mastoideus

A Left fossa infratemporalis, superficial layer
Lateral view. A separate unit is devoted to the fossa infratemporalis because of the many structures that it contains. The arcus zygomaticus and the anterior half of the ramus mandibulae have been removed in this dissection to gain access to the fossa infratemporalis. The canalis mandibulae has been opened, and the a. and n. can be seen entering the canal (the accompanying vein has been removed). The a. maxillaris divides into its terminal branches deep within the fossa infratemporalis (see **B**).

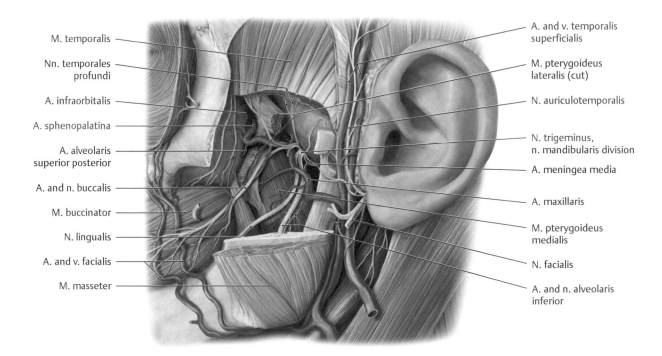

M. temporalis

Nn. temporales profundi

A. infraorbitalis

A. sphenopalatina

A. alveolaris superior posterior

A. and n. buccalis

M. buccinator

N. lingualis

A. and v. facialis

M. masseter

A. and v. temporalis superficialis

M. pterygoideus lateralis (cut)

N. auriculotemporalis

N. trigeminus, n. mandibularis division

A. meningea media

A. maxillaris

M. pterygoideus medialis

N. facialis

A. and n. alveolaris inferior

B Left fossa infratemporalis, deep layer
Lateral view. This differs from the previous dissection in that both heads of the m. pterygoideus lateralis have been partially removed, so that only their stumps are visible. The branches of the a. maxillaris and n. mandibularis division of the n. trigeminus (CN V) can be identified. By
careful dissection, it is possible to define the site where the n. auriculotemporalis (branch of the n. mandibularis division) splits around the a. meningea media before entering the fossa cranii media through the foramen spinosum (see p. 123).

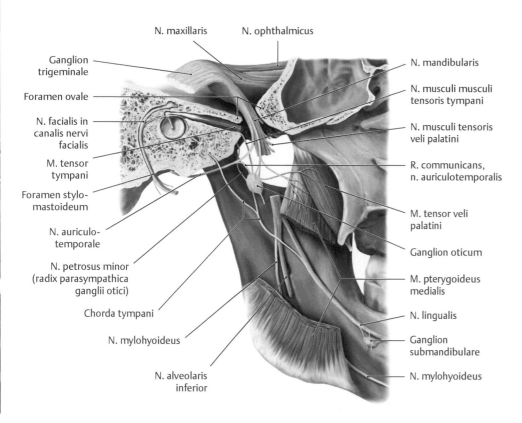

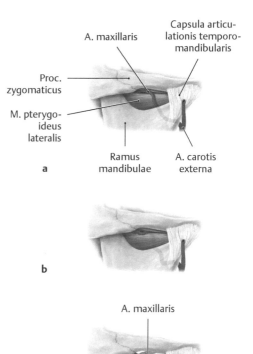

C Left ganglion oticum and its roots located deep in the fossa infratemporalis
Medial view. The small, flat ganglion oticum is located medial to the n. mandibularis just inferior to the foramen ovale. The parasympathetic fibers for the gl. parotidea are relayed in the ganglion.

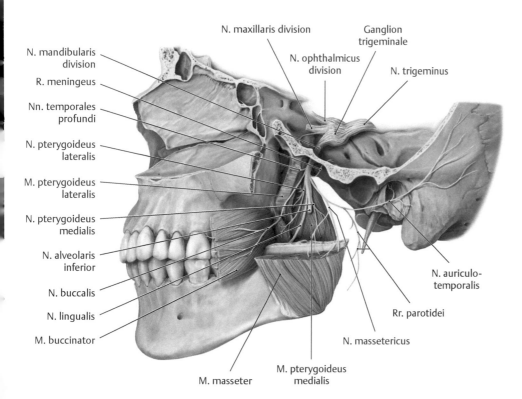

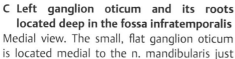

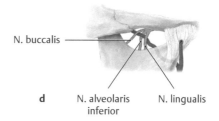

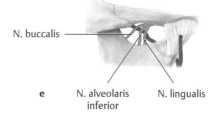

D Branches of the n. mandibularis division in the fossa infratemporalis
Left lateral view. The m. pterygoideus medialis can be identified deep within the fossa. The third division of the n. trigeminus passes through the foramen ovale from the fossa cranii media to enter the fossa infratemporalis. Traveling with it are motor fibers (motor root) that supply the mm. masticatorii (only a few of the fibers are illustrated here).

E Variants of the a. maxillaris sinistra
Lateral view. The course of the a. maxillaris exhibits numerous variations. The most common variants are listed below:

a Runs lateral to the m. pterygoideus lateralis (common).
b Runs medial to the m. pterygoideus lateralis.
c Runs medial to the n. buccalis but lateral to the n. lingualis and n. alveolaris inferior.
d Runs lateral to the n. alveolaris inferior and medial to the nn. buccalis and lingualis.
e Runs in medial direction from the trunk of the n. mandibularis.

6.7 Pterygopalatine Fossa (Fossa Pterygopalatina)

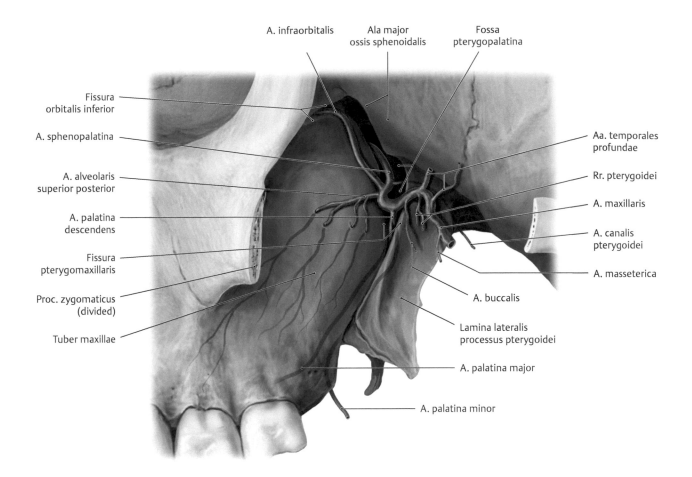

A Course of the arteries in the left fossa pterygopalatina

Lateral view. The fossa infratemporalis (see previous unit, p. 236) is continuous with the fossa pterygopalatina shown here, with no clear line of demarcation between them. The anatomical boundaries of the fossa pterygopalatina are listed in **B** (cf. p. 39). The fossa pterygopalatina is a crossroad for neurovascular structures traveling between the fossa cranii media, orbita, cavitas nasi, and cavitas oris (see the passageways in **E**). Because so many small arterial branches arise here, the arteries and veins have been shown separately for better clarity. The a. maxillaris divides into its terminal branches in the fossa pterygopalatina (see p. 100). The a. maxillaris can be ligated within the fossa for the control of severe nosebleed (epistaxis, see p. 185).

B Structures bordering the fossa pterygopalatina

Direction	Bordering structure
Anterior	Tuber maxillae
Posterior	Proc. pterygoideus (lamina lateralis)
Medial	Lamina perpendicularis of the os palatinum
Lateral	Communicates with the fossa infratemporalis via the fissura pterygomaxillaris
Superior	Ala major ossis sphenoidalis, junction with the fissura orbitalis inferior
Inferior	Opens into the spatium retropharyngeum

C Larger branches of the arteria maxillaris

The a. maxillaris consists of a mandibular part, pterygoid part, and pterygopalatine part. Because the vessels of the mandibular part lie outside the area of the dissection, they are not listed in the table below (see p. 100).

Branch	Distribution
Pterygoid part:	
• A. masseterica	• M. masseter
• Aa. temporales profundae	• M. temporalis
• Rr. pterygoidei	• Mm. pterygoidei
• A. buccalis	• Tunica mucosa buccalis
Pterygopalatine part:	
• A. alveolaris superior posterior	• Dentes molares sinus maxillaris, gingiva
• A. infraorbitalis	• Alveolae maxillares
• A. palatina descendens	
– A. palatina major	• Palatum durum
– A. palatina minor	• Palatum molle, tonsilla palatina, pharyngeal wall
• A. sphenopalatina	
– Aa. nasales posteriores laterales	• Lateral wall of cavitas nasi, choanae
– Rr. septales posteriores	• Septum nasi

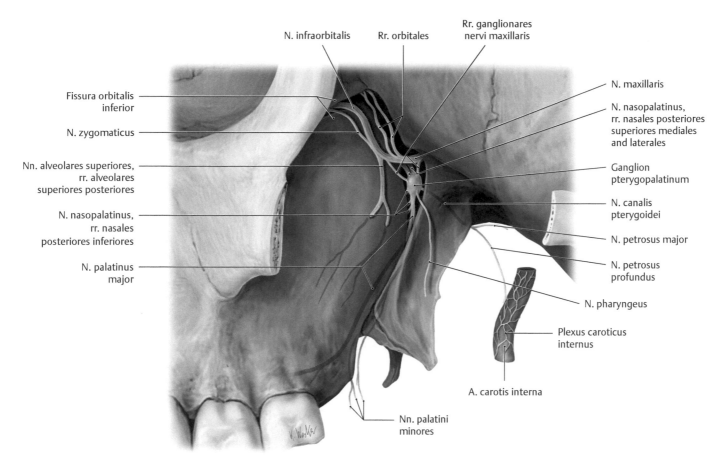

N. infraorbitalis

Rr. orbitales

Rr. ganglionares nervi maxillaris

Fissura orbitalis inferior

N. zygomaticus

Nn. alveolares superiores, rr. alveolares superiores posteriores

N. nasopalatinus, rr. nasales posteriores inferiores

N. palatinus major

N. maxillaris

N. nasopalatinus, rr. nasales posteriores superiores mediales and laterales

Ganglion pterygopalatinum

N. canalis pterygoidei

N. petrosus major

N. petrosus profundus

N. pharyngeus

Plexus caroticus internus

A. carotis interna

Nn. palatini minores

D Course of the nerves in the left fossa pterygopalatina

Lateral view. The n. maxillaris, the second division of CN V, passes from the fossa cranii media through the foramen rotundum into the fossa pterygopalatina. Closely related to the n. maxillaris is the parasympathetic ganglion pterygopalatinum, in which preganglionic fibers synapse with ganglion cells that, in turn, innervate the gll. lacrimales and the small gll. palatinae and gll. nasales. The ganglion pterygopalatinum receives its presynaptic fibers from the n. petrosus major. This nerve is the parasympathetic root of the n. intermedius branch of the n. facialis. The sympathetic fibers of the n. petrosus profundus (sympathetic root), like the sensory fibers of the n. maxillaris (sensory root), pass through the ganglion without synapsing.

E Passageways to the fossa pterygopalatina and transmitted neurovascular structures

Passageway	Comes from...	Transmitted structures
Foramen rotundum	Fossa cranii media	• N. maxillaris (CN V_2)
Canalis pterygoideus	Basis cranii (inferior aspect)	• A. canalis pterygoidei with accompanying veins • N. canalis pterygoidei (comes from the parasympathetic branch of the facial nerve—the n. petrosus major and sympathetic n. petrosus profundus in the canal)
Canalis palatinus major/ foramen palatinum majus	Palatum	• A. palatina major (from a. palatina descendens) • N. palatinus major
Canales palatini minores	Palatum	• Aa. palatinae minores (terminal branches of the a. palatina descendens) • Nn. palatini minores
Foramen sphenopalatinum	Cavitas nasi	• A. sphenopalatina (and accompanying veins) • Rr. nasales posteriores superiores mediales and laterales (from n. nasopalatinus, CN V_2)
Fissura orbitalis inferior	Orbita	• A. infraorbitalis (and accompanying veins) • V. ophthalmica inferior • N. infraorbitalis (plus accompanying veins) • N. zygomaticus (from CN V_2) • Rr. orbitales (from CN V_2)
Fissura pterygomaxillaris	Fossa infratemporalis	• A. maxillaris

6.8 Posterior Cervical Triangle (Trigonum Cervicale Posterius)

A Lateral view of the neck, subcutaneous layer

The trigonum cervicale posterius (regio cervicalis lateralis) is a topographically important region bounded by the clavicula, the anterior border of the m. trapezius, and the posterior border of the m. sternocleidomastoideus.

This and the following figures show progressively deeper dissections of the regio cervicalis lateralis. The adjacent regio sternocleidomastoidea and the regio cervicalis anterior are also exposed. The skin and subcutaneous fat have been removed to display the subcutaneous, purely sensory cutaneous nerves from the plexus cervicalis in the regio cervicalis lateralis. They perforate the lamina superficialis of the fascia cervicalis at the Erb's point to supply the anterior and lateral neck. Specifically these nerves are the nn. occipitalis minor, auricularis magnus, transversus cervicalis, and supraclaviculares (medial, intermediate, and lateral).

Note: The n. transversus cervicalis passes beneath the v. jugularis externa and forms an anastomosis with the r. cervicalis of the n. facialis. This mixed loop contains motor fibers from the n. facialis and sensory fibers for the neck from the n. transversus cervicalis.

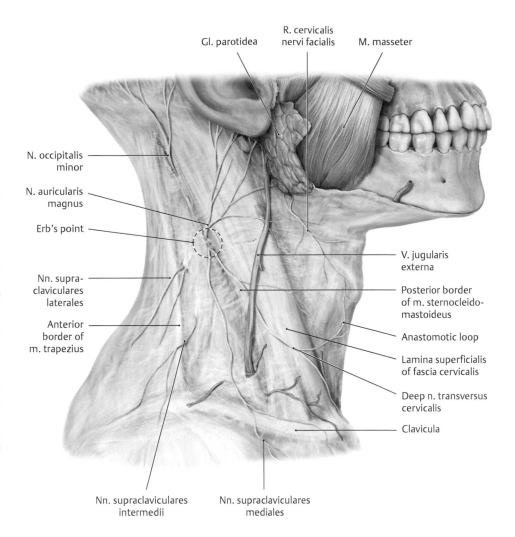

B Regio cervicalis lateralis (trigonum cervicale posterius), subfascial layer

Right lateral view. The lamina superficialis of the fascia cervicalis has been removed over the trigonum cervicale posterius to expose the lamina prevertebralis of the fascia cervicalis, which is fused to the lamina pretrachealis at the level of m. omohyoideus (see p. 5). The cutaneous nerves from the plexus cervicalis perforate the lamina superficialis of the fascia cervicalis at approximately the mid-posterior border of the m. sternocleidomastoideus (Erb's point) and are distributed in the subcutaneous plane.

Note the r. externus of the n. accessorius, which passes to the m. trapezius. A surgeon taking a lymph node biopsy may accidentally sever the r. externus. This injury restricts the mobility of the scapula, and the patient may be unable to elevate the upper limb beyond 90°.

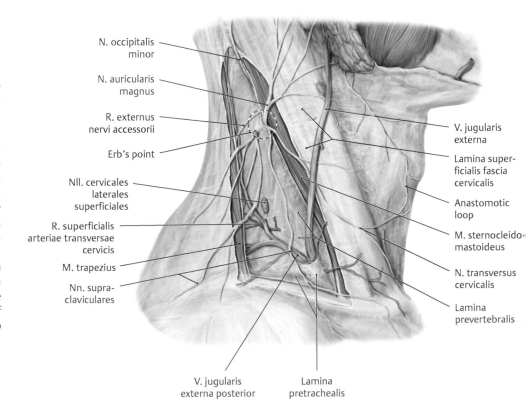

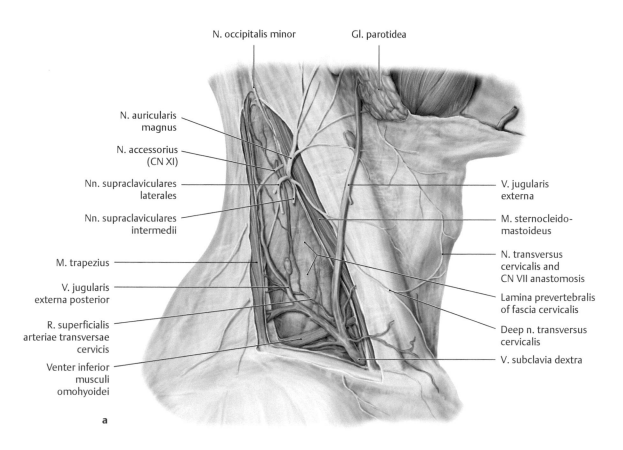

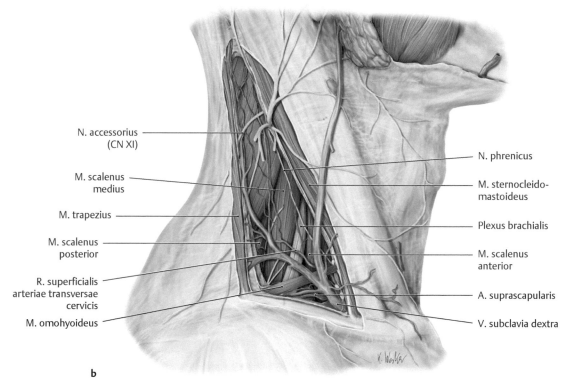

C Trigonum cervicale posterius

a Deeper layer, right lateral view. In this dissection, the lamina pretrachealis of the fascia cervicalis has additionally been removed to display the m. omohyoideus, which is enveloped by that fascia.

b Deepest layer with a view of the plexus brachialis. The lamina prevertebralis has been removed to expose the mm. scaleni.
Note the n. phrenicus, which runs obliquely over the m. scalenus anterior to the apertura thoracis superior.

6.9 Deep Lateral Cervical Region, Carotid Triangle (Trigonum Caroticum), and Thoracic Inlet (Apertura Thoracis Superior)

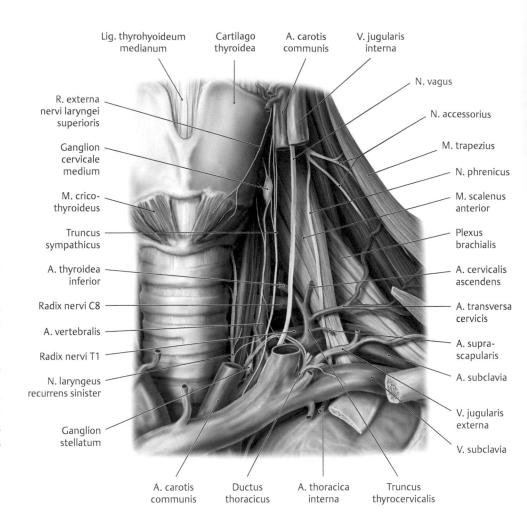

A Base of neck and apertura thoracis superior on the left side

Anterior view. The sternal end of the clavicula, the anterior end of the costa prima, the manubrium sterni, and the gl. thyroidea have been removed to expose the apertura thoracis superior. The a. subclavia and truncus thyrocervicalis can be identified.

Note the course of the following structures: The a. thoracica interna descends parallel to the sternum. It is of special clinical interest. In patients with coronary heart disease, the a. thoracica interna can be mobilized and anastomosed to the a. coronaria past the point of the stenosis. The truncus sympathicus, n. vagus, n. phrenicus, and portions of the plexus brachialis are visible, the latter passing through the interscalene space (see **C**).

Note also the termination of the ductus thoracicus at the jugulosubclavian venous junction and the left n. laryngeus recurrens. This branch of the n. vagus winds around the arcus aortae and ascends to the larynx.

Lig. thyrohyoideum medianum — Cartilago thyroidea — A. carotis communis — V. jugularis interna — N. vagus — N. accessorius — M. trapezius — N. phrenicus — M. scalenus anterior — Plexus brachialis — A. cervicalis ascendens — A. transversa cervicis — A. suprascapularis — A. subclavia — V. jugularis externa — V. subclavia

R. externa nervi laryngei superioris — Ganglion cervicale medium — M. cricothyroideus — Truncus sympathicus — A. thyroidea inferior — Radix nervi C8 — A. vertebralis — Radix nervi T1 — N. laryngeus recurrens sinister — Ganglion stellatum

A. carotis communis — Ductus thoracicus — A. thoracica interna — Truncus thyrocervicalis

B Trigonum caroticum

Right lateral view. The trigonum caroticum is a subregion of the trigonum cervicale anterius. It is bounded by the m. sternocleidomastoideus, the venter posterior of the m. digastricus, and the venter superior of the m. omohyoideus. The gl. submandibularis can be seen at the inferior border of the mandibula and the m. sternocleidomastoideus has been retracted posterolaterally. The following structures are located in the trigonum caroticum:

- Aa. carotides interna and externa (the aa. thyroidea superior and lingualis branch from the latter)
- N. hypoglossus (CN XII)
- N. vagus (CN X)
- N. accessorius (CN XI)
- Truncus sympathicus with associated ganglia.

Venter posterior musculi digastrici — A. carotis interna — A. carotis externa — A. facialis — A. lingualis — R. marginalis mandibulae of n. facialis — Gl. submandibularis — N. hypoglossus (CN XII) — Os hyoideum — R. internus nervi laryngei superioris — R. thyrohyoideus — A. thyroidea superior — M. thyrohyoideus — M. sternothyroideus — Gl. thyroidea — Ansa cervicalis

N. accessorius (CN XI) — Ganglion cervicale superius — V. jugularis interna — V. facialis communis — R. sternocleidomastoideus arteriae thyroideae superioris — N. vagus (CN X) — Radix superior of ansa cervicalis — Glomus caroticum — V. jugularis interna — M. sternocleidomastoideus

Venter superior musculi omohyoidei

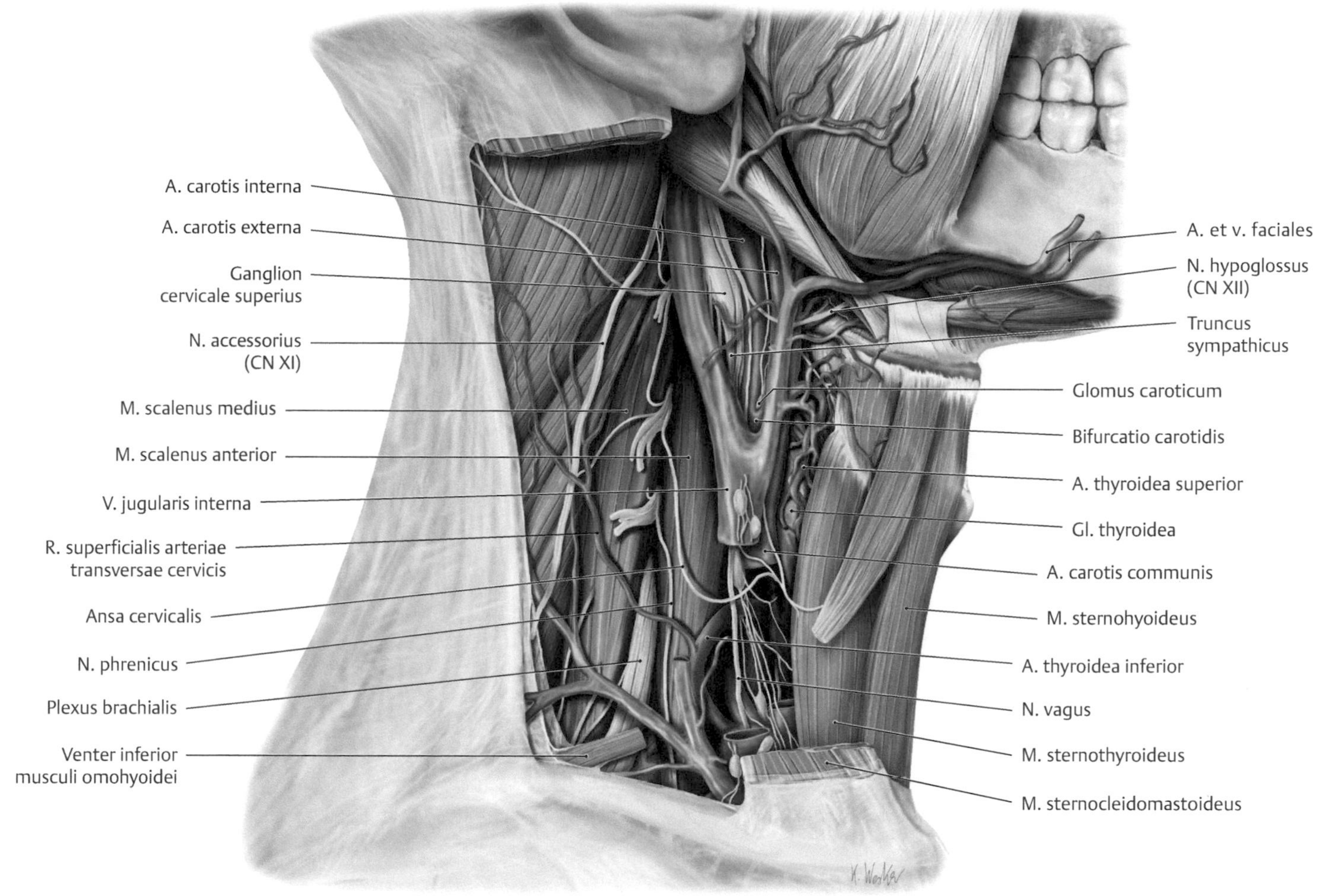
A. carotis interna
A. carotis externa
Ganglion cervicale superius
N. accessorius (CN XI)
M. scalenus medius
M. scalenus anterior
V. jugularis interna
R. superficialis arteriae transversae cervicis
Ansa cervicalis
N. phrenicus
Plexus brachialis
Venter inferior musculi omohyoidei
A. et v. faciales
N. hypoglossus (CN XII)
Truncus sympathicus
Glomus caroticum
Bifurcatio carotidis
A. thyroidea superior
Gl. thyroidea
A. carotis communis
M. sternohyoideus
A. thyroidea inferior
N. vagus
M. sternothyroideus
M. sternocleidomastoideus

C Deep regio cervicalis lateralis
Right lateral view. The regio sternocleidomastoidea and trigonum caroticum have been dissected along with adjacent portions of the trigona cervicalia posterius and anterius. The vagina carotica has been removed in this dissection along with the fasciae cervicales, m. sternocleidomastoideus, and m. omohyoideus to demonstrate all important neurovascular structures in the neck:

- A. carotis communis with its division into the aa. carotides interna and externa
- Aa. thyroideae superior and inferior
- V. jugularis interna
- Nll. cervicales laterales profundi along the v. jugularis interna
- Truncus sympathicus including its ganglia
- N. vagus
- N. hypoglossus
- N. accessorius
- Plexus brachialis
- N. phrenicus

The n. phrenicus originates from the C3–C5 segments and therefore is part of the plexus cervicalis. The muscular landmark for locating the n. phrenicus is the m. scalenus anterior, along which the nerve descends in the neck. The (posterior) interscalene space is located between the mm. scalenus anterior and medius and the costa prima and is traversed by the plexus brachialis and a. subclavia. The v. subclavia passes deeply through the interval formed by the m. scalenus anterior, the m. sternocleidomastoideus (resected), and the costa prima (the anterior interscalene space).

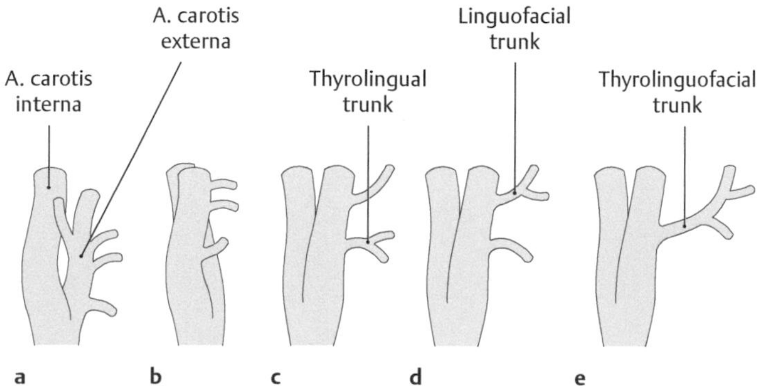
A. carotis externa
A. carotis interna
Thyrolingual trunk
Linguofacial trunk
Thyrolinguofacial trunk
a
b
c
d
e

D Variable position of the aa. carotides externa and interna and variants in the anterior branches of the a. carotis externa
(after Faller and Poisel-Golth)

a, b The a. carotis interna may arise from the a. carotis communis posterolateral (49%) or anteromedial (9%) to the a. carotis externa, or at other intermediate sites.

c–e The a. carotis externa may give origin to a thyrolingual trunk (4%), linguofacial trunk (23%), or thyrolinguofacial trunk (0.6%).

6.10 Posterior Cervical and Occipital Regions (Regiones Cervicalis Posterior and Occipitalis)

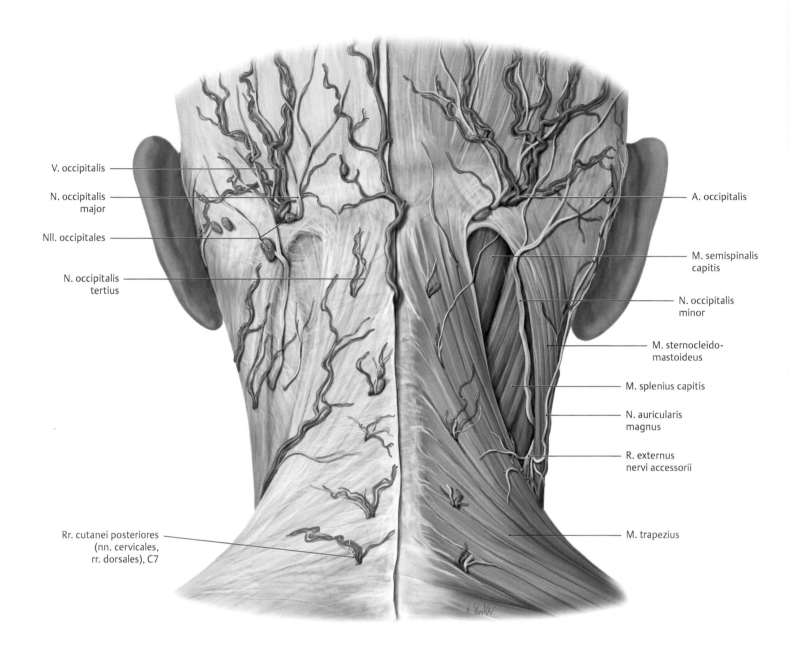

V. occipitalis

N. occipitalis major

Nll. occipitales

N. occipitalis tertius

Rr. cutanei posteriores (nn. cervicales, rr. dorsales), C7

A. occipitalis

M. semispinalis capitis

N. occipitalis minor

M. sternocleido-mastoideus

M. splenius capitis

N. auricularis magnus

R. externus nervi accessorii

M. trapezius

A Regio cervicalis posterior and regio occipitalis

Posterior view of the subcutaneous layer on the left side and the subfascial layer on the right side. Although the regio occipitalis is part of the head, it is discussed here because it borders on the regio cervicalis posterior. The principal arterial vessel in this region is the a. occipitalis, the second branch arising from the posterior side of the a. carotis externa. The medially situated n. occipitalis major is a dorsal ramus of the n. spinalis C2, while the laterally situated n. occipitalis minor is a *ventral* ramus of C2 that arises from the plexus cervicalis (see p. 139). The lymph nodes are located at the sites where the nerves and veins emerge through the fascia cervicalis.

Note the n. accessorius, which crosses the trigonum cervicale posterius at a relatively superficial level.

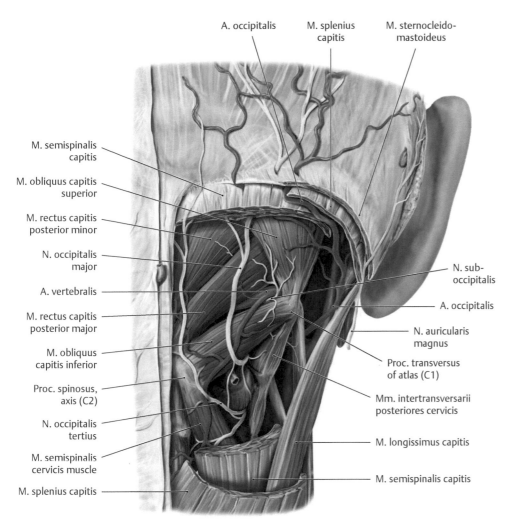

A. occipitalis   M. splenius capitis   M. sternocleido-mastoideus

M. semispinalis capitis

M. obliquus capitis superior

M. rectus capitis posterior minor

N. occipitalis major

A. vertebralis

M. rectus capitis posterior major

M. obliquus capitis inferior

Proc. spinosus, axis (C2)

N. occipitalis tertius

M. semispinalis cervicis muscle

M. splenius capitis

N. sub-occipitalis

A. occipitalis

N. auricularis magnus

Proc. transversus of atlas (C1)

Mm. intertransversarii posteriores cervicis

M. longissimus capitis

M. semispinalis capitis

B Right suboccipital triangle
Posterior view. The suboccipital triangle is bounded superiorly by the m. rectus capitis posterior major, laterally by the m. obliquus capitis superior, and inferiorly by the m. obliquus capitis inferior. This muscular triangle can be seen only after the mm. trapezius, splenius capitis, and semispinalis capitis have been removed. A short, free segment of the a. vertebralis runs through the deep part of the triangle after leaving the foramen transversarium and before exiting the triangle by perforating the membrana atlantooccipitalis (not visible here). That segment of the a. vertebralis gives off branches to the surrounding short nuchal muscles. Both aa. vertebrales unite intracranially to form the a. basilaris, which is a major contributor to cerebral blood flow.

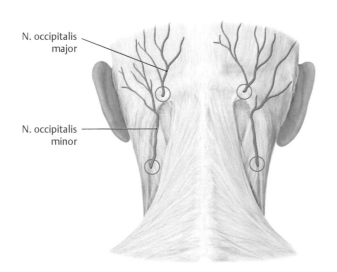

N. occipitalis major

N. occipitalis minor

N. ophthalmicus

C2

C3

C4

a

N. ophthalmicus

N. occipitalis major

N. occipitalis minor

Rr. posteriores

N. auricularis magnus

Nn. supra-claviculares

b

C Clinically important sites of emergence of the nn. occipitales
Posterior view. The sites where the nn. occipitales minor and major emerge from the fascia into the subcutaneous connective tissue are clinically important because they are tender to palpation in certain diseases (e.g., meningitis). The examiner tests the sensation of these nerves by pressing lightly on the circled points with the thumb. If these points (but not their surroundings) are painful, the finding is described, logically, as "tenderness over the occipital nerves."

D Cutaneous innervation of the neck
Posterior view. The pattern of segmental innervation is illustrated on the left, and the territorial assignments of specific cutaneous nerves on the right. The occiput and neck derive most of their segmental innervation from the second and third cervical segments. The n. ophthalmicus supplying the area above the C2 level is the first branch of the n. trigeminus (CN V).
Note that in the peripheral innervation pattern, the n. occipitalis major is a *dorsal* spinal nerve branch while the n. occipitalis minor is a *ventral* branch (see p. 22).

7.1 Coronal Sections: Anterior Orbital Margin and Retrobulbar Space

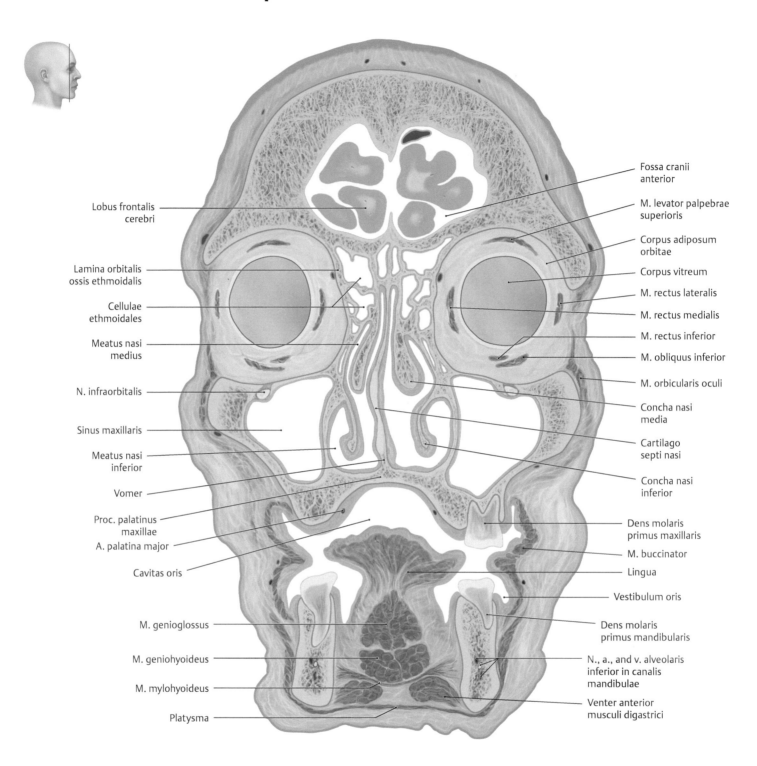

Lobus frontalis cerebri

Lamina orbitalis ossis ethmoidalis

Cellulae ethmoidales

Meatus nasi medius

N. infraorbitalis

Sinus maxillaris

Meatus nasi inferior

Vomer

Proc. palatinus maxillae

A. palatina major

Cavitas oris

M. genioglossus

M. geniohyoideus

M. mylohyoideus

Platysma

Fossa cranii anterior

M. levator palpebrae superioris

Corpus adiposum orbitae

Corpus vitreum

M. rectus lateralis

M. rectus medialis

M. rectus inferior

M. obliquus inferior

M. orbicularis oculi

Concha nasi media

Cartilago septi nasi

Concha nasi inferior

Dens molaris primus maxillaris

M. buccinator

Lingua

Vestibulum oris

Dens molaris primus mandibularis

N., a., and v. alveolaris inferior in canalis mandibulae

Venter anterior musculi digastrici

A Coronal section through the anterior orbital margin

Anterior view. This section of the skull can be roughly subdivided into four regions: the cavitas oris, the cavitas nasi and sinus, the orbita, and the fossa cranii anterior.

Inspecting the region in and around the **cavitas oris**, we observe the muscles of the oral floor, the apex linguae, the neurovascular structures in the canalis mandibulae, and the dens molaris primus. The palatum durum separates the cavitas oris from the **cavitas nasi**, which is divided into left and right halves by the septum nasi. The conchae nasi inferior and media can be identified along with the laterally situated sinus maxillaris. The structure bulging down into the roof of the sinus is the canalis infraorbitalis, which transmits the n. infraorbitalis (branch of the n. maxillaris division of the n. trigeminus, CN V$_2$). The plane of section is

so far anterior that it does not cut the lateral bony walls of the **orbitae** because of the lateral curvature of the skull. The section passes through the transparent corpus vitreum, and three of the six extraocular muscles can be identified in the corpus adiposum orbitae. Two additional muscles can be seen in the next deeper plane of section (see **B**). The space between the two orbitae is occupied by the cellulae ethmoidales.

Note: The bony lamina orbitalis (medial wall of the orbita) is very thin (lamina papyracea) and may be penetrated by infection, trauma, and neoplasms.

In the **fossa cranii anterior**, the section passes through both lobi frontales of the brain in the most anterior portions of the cerebral substantia grisea. Very little substantia alba is visible at this level.

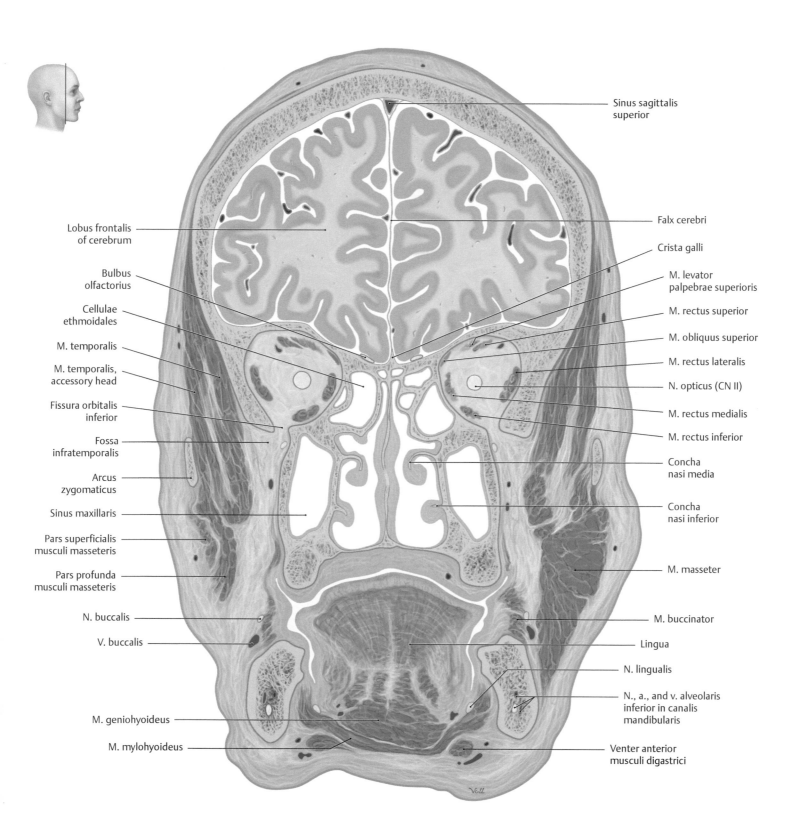

Sinus sagittalis superior

Lobus frontalis of cerebrum

Bulbus olfactorius

Cellulae ethmoidales

M. temporalis

M. temporalis, accessory head

Fissura orbitalis inferior

Fossa infratemporalis

Arcus zygomaticus

Sinus maxillaris

Pars superficialis musculi masseteris

Pars profunda musculi masseteris

N. buccalis

V. buccalis

M. geniohyoideus

M. mylohyoideus

Falx cerebri

Crista galli

M. levator palpebrae superioris

M. rectus superior

M. obliquus superior

M. rectus lateralis

N. opticus (CN II)

M. rectus medialis

M. rectus inferior

Concha nasi media

Concha nasi inferior

M. masseter

M. buccinator

Lingua

N. lingualis

N., a., and v. alveolaris inferior in canalis mandibularis

Venter anterior musculi digastrici

B Coronal section through the retrobulbar space
Anterior view. Here, the tongue is cut at a more posterior level than in **A** and therefore appears broader. In addition to the oral floor muscles, we see the mm. masticatorii on the sides of the skull. In the orbital region we can identify the retrobulbar space with its fatty tissue, the extraocular muscles, and the n. opticus. The orbita communicates laterally with the fossa infratemporalis through the fissura orbitalis anterior. This section cuts through both bulbi olfactorii in the fossa cranialis anterior, and the sinus sagittalis superior can be recognized in the midline.

247

7.2 Coronal Sections: Orbital Apex and Hypophysis

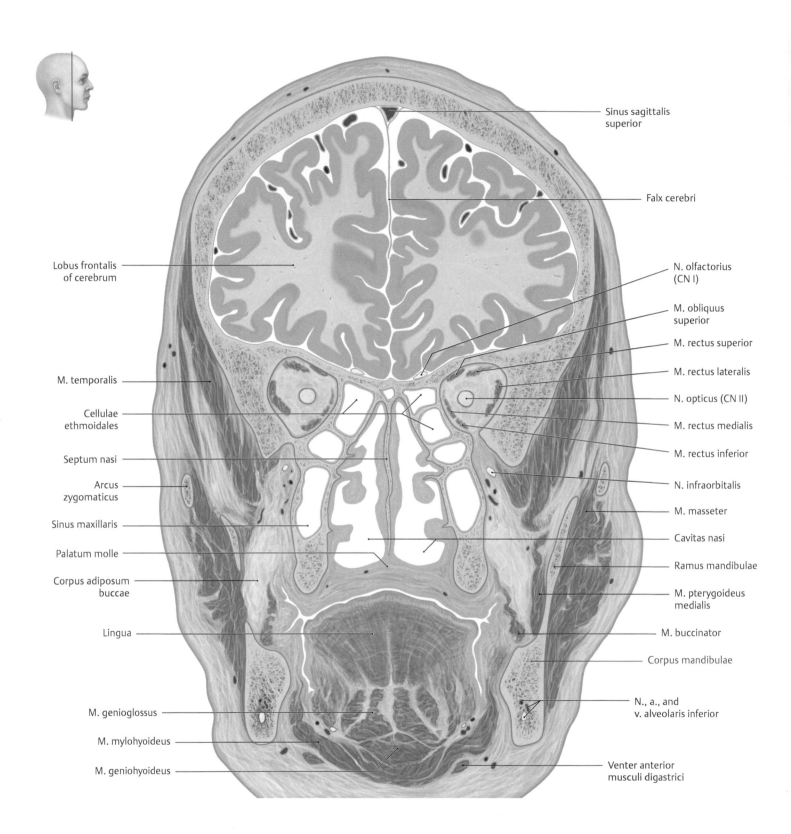

Sinus sagittalis superior

Falx cerebri

Lobus frontalis of cerebrum

N. olfactorius (CN I)

M. obliquus superior

M. rectus superior

M. temporalis

M. rectus lateralis

Cellulae ethmoidales

N. opticus (CN II)

Septum nasi

M. rectus medialis

M. rectus inferior

Arcus zygomaticus

N. infraorbitalis

Sinus maxillaris

M. masseter

Palatum molle

Cavitas nasi

Corpus adiposum buccae

Ramus mandibulae

M. pterygoideus medialis

Lingua

M. buccinator

Corpus mandibulae

N., a., and v. alveolaris inferior

M. genioglossus

M. mylohyoideus

Venter anterior musculi digastrici

M. geniohyoideus

A Coronal section through the orbital apex
Anterior view. The palatum molle replaces the palatum durum in this plane of section, and the septum nasi becomes osseous at this level. The corpus adiposum buccae is also visible in this plane. Because the corpus is composed of fat, it is attenuated in wasting diseases; this is why the cheeks are sunken in patients with end-stage cancer. This coronal section is slightly angled, producing an apparent discontinuity in the ramus mandibulae on the left side of the figure (compare with the continuous ramus on the right side).

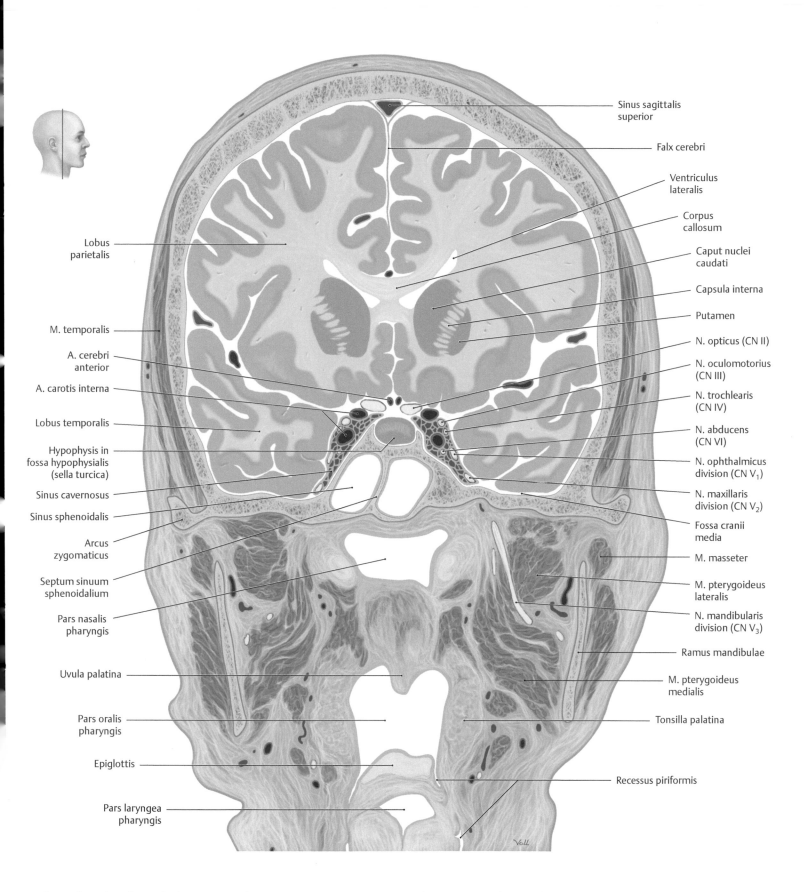

Sinus sagittalis superior

Falx cerebri

Ventriculus lateralis

Corpus callosum

Caput nuclei caudati

Capsula interna

Putamen

N. opticus (CN II)

N. oculomotorius (CN III)

N. trochlearis (CN IV)

N. abducens (CN VI)

N. ophthalmicus division (CN V₁)

N. maxillaris division (CN V₂)

Fossa cranii media

M. masseter

M. pterygoideus lateralis

N. mandibularis division (CN V₃)

Ramus mandibulae

M. pterygoideus medialis

Tonsilla palatina

Recessus piriformis

Lobus parietalis

M. temporalis

A. cerebri anterior

A. carotis interna

Lobus temporalis

Hypophysis in fossa hypophysialis (sella turcica)

Sinus cavernosus

Sinus sphenoidalis

Arcus zygomaticus

Septum sinuum sphenoidalium

Pars nasalis pharyngis

Uvula palatina

Pars oralis pharyngis

Epiglottis

Pars laryngea pharyngis

B Coronal section through the pituitary (hypophysis)

Anterior view. The pars nasalis pharyngis, pars oralis pharyngis, and pars laryngea pharyngis can now be identified. This section cuts the epiglottis, below which is the supraglottic space. The plane cuts the ramus mandibulae on both sides, and a relatively long segment of the n. mandibularis division (CN V₃) can be identified on the left side. The paired sinus sphenoidales are visible, separated by a median septum. Above the roof of the sinus sphenoidales is the hypophysis (pituitary), which lies in the fossa hypophysialis. In the cavitas cranii, the plane of section passes through the fossa cranii media. Due to the presence of the siphon caroticum (a 180° bend in the pars cavernosa of the a. carotis interna), the section cuts the a. carotis interna twice on each side. Nn. cranii can be seen passing through the sinus cavernosus on their way from the fossa cranii media to the orbita. The sinus sagittalis superior appears in cross-section at the attachment of the falx cerebri. At the level of the cerebrum, the plane of section passes through the lobi parietalis and temporalis. Intracerebral structures appearing in this section include the nucleus caudatus, the putamen, the capsula interna, and the cornu anterius (frontale) of each ventriculus lateralis.

249

7.3 Transverse Sections: Orbits (Orbitae) and Optic Nerve (Nervus Opticus)

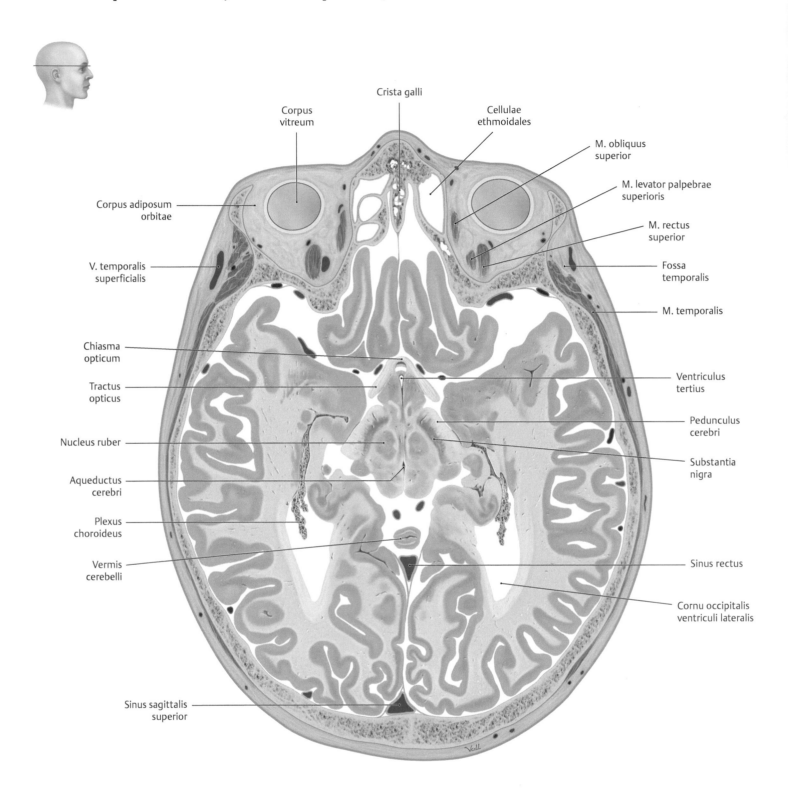

Crista galli

Corpus vitreum

Cellulae ethmoidales

M. obliquus superior

M. levator palpebrae superioris

M. rectus superior

Fossa temporalis

M. temporalis

Ventriculus tertius

Pedunculus cerebri

Substantia nigra

Sinus rectus

Cornu occipitalis ventriculi lateralis

Corpus adiposum orbitae

V. temporalis superficialis

Chiasma opticum

Tractus opticus

Nucleus ruber

Aqueductus cerebri

Plexus choroideus

Vermis cerebelli

Sinus sagittalis superior

A Transverse section through the upper level of the orbitae
Superior view. The highest section in this series displays the muscles in the upper level of the orbita (the orbital levels are described on p. 176 ff). The section cuts the bony crista galli in the fossa cranii anterior, flanked on each side by cellulae ethmoidales. The sections of the chiasma opticum and adjacent tractus opticus are parts of the diencephalon, which surrounds the ventriculus tertius at the center of the section. The nucleus ruber and substantia nigra are visible in the mesencephalon. The tractus pyramidalis descends in the pedunculi cerebri. The section passes through the cornua posteriora (occipitalia) of the ventriculi laterales and barely cuts the vermis cerebelli in the midline.

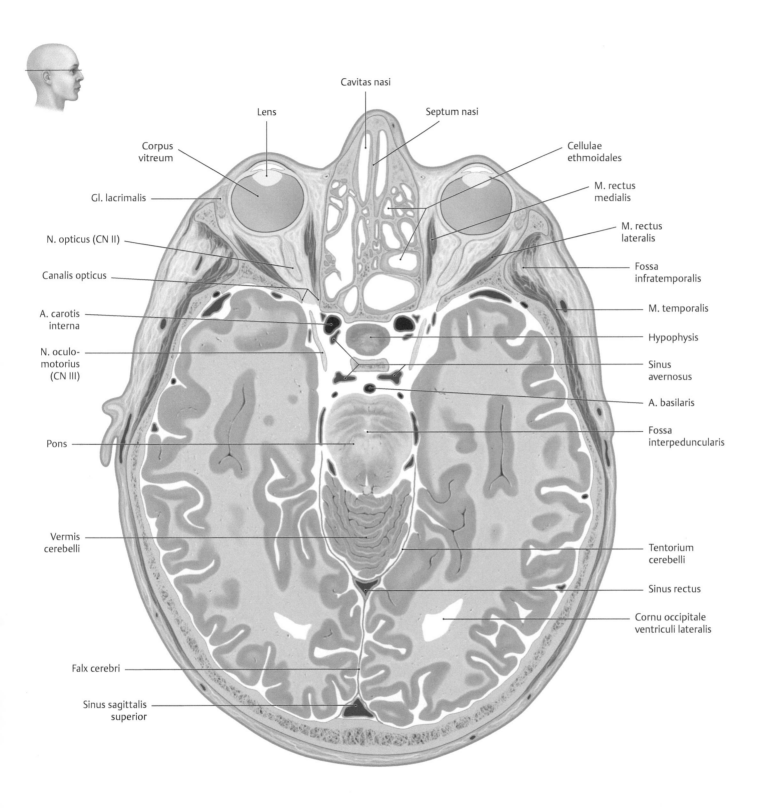

Cavitas nasi

Lens

Septum nasi

Corpus vitreum

Cellulae ethmoidales

Gl. lacrimalis

M. rectus medialis

N. opticus (CN II)

M. rectus lateralis

Canalis opticus

Fossa infratemporalis

A. carotis interna

M. temporalis

N. oculomotorius (CN III)

Hypophysis

Sinus avernosus

A. basilaris

Pons

Fossa interpeduncularis

Vermis cerebelli

Tentorium cerebelli

Sinus rectus

Cornu occipitale ventriculi lateralis

Falx cerebri

Sinus sagittalis superior

B Transverse section through the nervus opticus and hypophysis
Superior view. The n. opticus is seen just before its entry into the canalis opticus, indicating that the plane of section passes through the middle level of the orbita. Because the nerve completely fills the canal, growth disturbances of the bone at this level may cause pressure injury to the nerve. This plane cuts the lentes and the cellulae ethmoidales.

The a. carotis interna can be identified in the fossa cranii media, embedded in the sinus cavernosus. The section cuts the n. oculomotorius on either side, which courses in the lateral wall of the sinus cavernosus. The pons and vermis cerebelli are also seen. The falx cerebri and tentorium cerebelli appear as thin lines that come together at the sinus rectus.

251

7.4 Transverse Sections: Sphenoid Sinus (Sinus Sphenoidalis) and Middle Nasal Concha (Concha Nasalis Media)

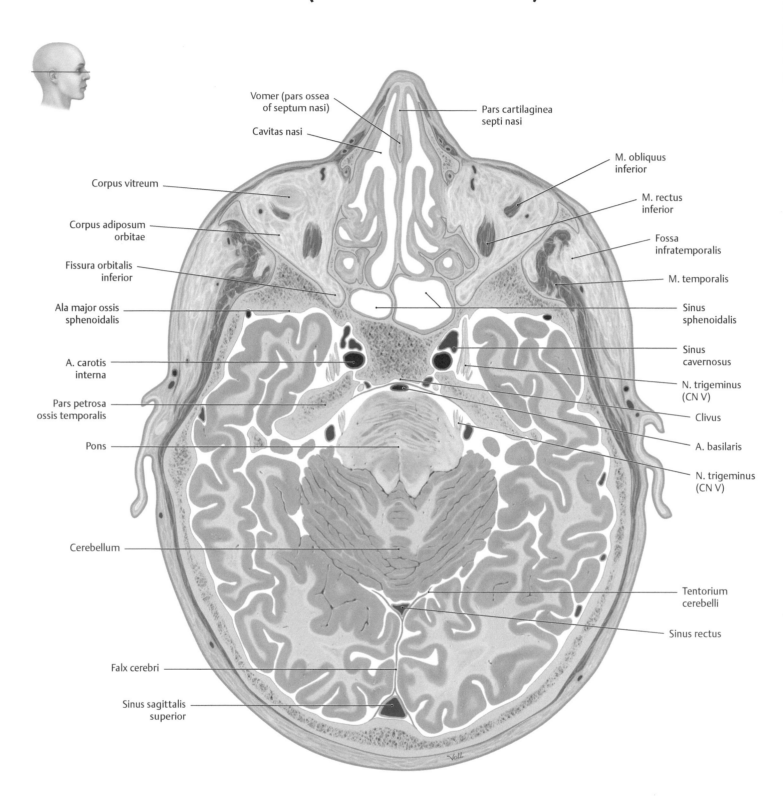

Vomer (pars ossea of septum nasi)

Pars cartilaginea septi nasi

Cavitas nasi

M. obliquus inferior

Corpus vitreum

M. rectus inferior

Corpus adiposum orbitae

Fossa infratemporalis

Fissura orbitalis inferior

M. temporalis

Ala major ossis sphenoidalis

Sinus sphenoidalis

A. carotis interna

Sinus cavernosus

Pars petrosa ossis temporalis

N. trigeminus (CN V)

Pons

Clivus

A. basilaris

N. trigeminus (CN V)

Cerebellum

Tentorium cerebelli

Sinus rectus

Falx cerebri

Sinus sagittalis superior

A Transverse section through the sinus sphenoidalis

Superior view. This section cuts the fossa infratemporalis on the lateral aspect of the skull and the m. temporalis that lies within it. The plane passes through the lower level of the orbita, and a small portion of the bulbus oculi is visible on the left side. The orbita is continuous posteriorly with the fissura orbitalis inferior. This section displays the anterior extension of the two alae majores of the os sphenoidalis and the posterior extension of the two "petrous bones" (partes petrosae of the ossa temporalia), which mark the boundary between the fossae cranii media and posterior (see p. 22 f). The clivus is part of the fossa cranii posterior and lies in contact with the a. basilaris. The pontine origin of the n. trigeminus and its intracranial course are clearly demonstrated.

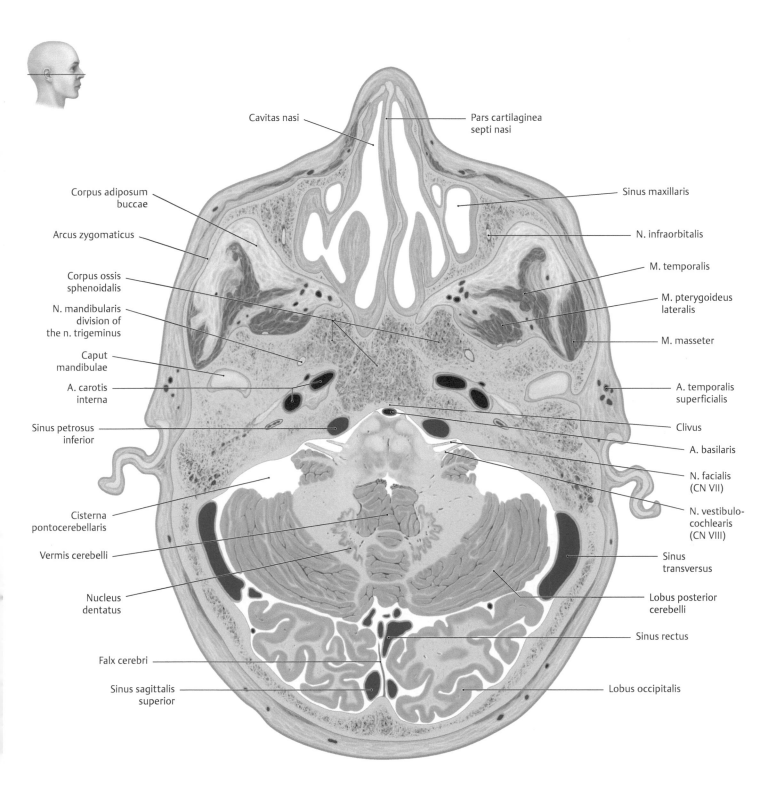

Cavitas nasi

Pars cartilaginea
septi nasi

Corpus adiposum
buccae

Sinus maxillaris

Arcus zygomaticus

N. infraorbitalis

Corpus ossis
sphenoidalis

M. temporalis

N. mandibularis
division of
the n. trigeminus

M. pterygoideus
lateralis

Caput
mandibulae

M. masseter

A. carotis
interna

A. temporalis
superficialis

Sinus petrosus
inferior

Clivus

A. basilaris

Cisterna
pontocerebellaris

N. facialis
(CN VII)

N. vestibulo-
cochlearis
(CN VIII)

Vermis cerebelli

Sinus
transversus

Nucleus
dentatus

Lobus posterior
cerebelli

Falx cerebri

Sinus rectus

Sinus sagittalis
superior

Lobus occipitalis

B Transverse section through the concha nasi media

Superior view. This section below the orbita passes through the n. infraorbitalis in the accordingly named canal. Medial to the n. infraorbitalis is the roof of the sinus maxillaris. The arcus zygomaticus is visible
in its entirety, and portions of the musculi masticatorii medial to the
arcus zygomaticus (mm. masseter, temporalis, and pterygoideus lateralis) can be seen. The plane of section passes through the upper part of
the caput mandibulae. The n. mandibularis division (CN V₃) appears in

cross-section in its bony canal, the foramen ovale. It is evident that the
corpus ossis sphenoidalis forms the bony center of the basis cranii. The
n. facialis and n. vestibulocochlearis emerge from the truncus encephali. The nucleus dentatus lies within the substantia alba of the cerebellum. The space around the anterior part of the cerebellum, the cisterna
pontocerebellaris, is filled with liquor cerebrospinalis in the living individual. The sinus transversus is prominent among the sinus durae matris
of the brain.

7.5 Transverse Sections: Nasopharynx (Pars Nasalis Pharyngis) and Median Atlantoaxial Joint (Articulatio Atlantoaxialis Mediana)

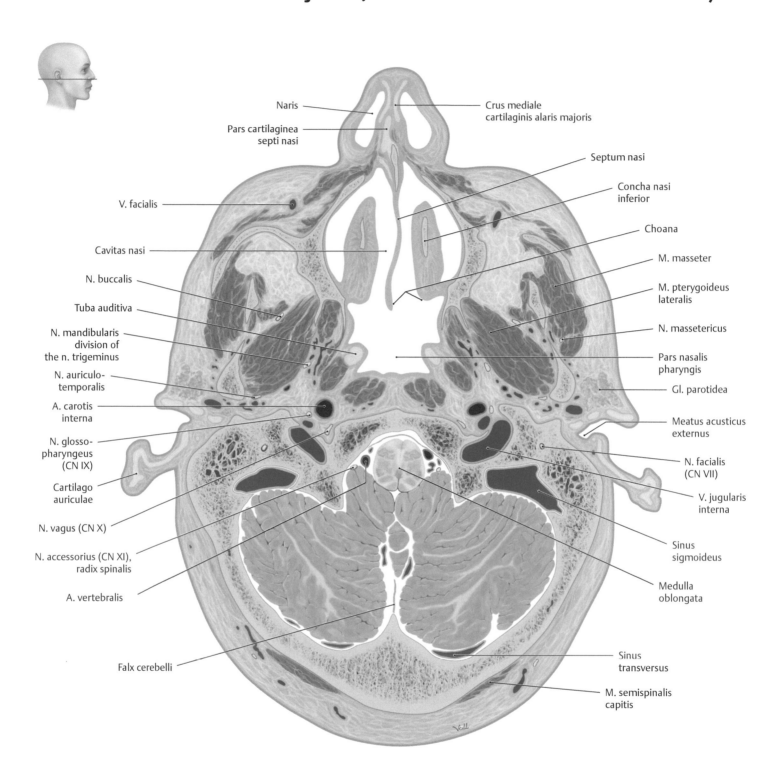

A Transverse section through the pars nasalis pharyngis
Superior view. This section passes through the external nose and portions of the cartilagines nasi. The cavitates nasi communicate with the pars nasalis pharyngis through the choanae. The partes cartilagines of the tubae auditivae project into the pars nasalis pharyngis. The arterial blood vessels that supply the brain can also be seen: the a. carotis interna and a. vertebralis.

Note the v. jugularis interna and n. vagus, which pass through the vagina carotica in company with the a. carotis interna.
A number of nn. craniales that emerge from the basis cranii are displayed in cross-section, such as the n. facialis coursing in the canalis nervi facialis. This section also cuts the auricula and portions of the meatus acusticus externus.

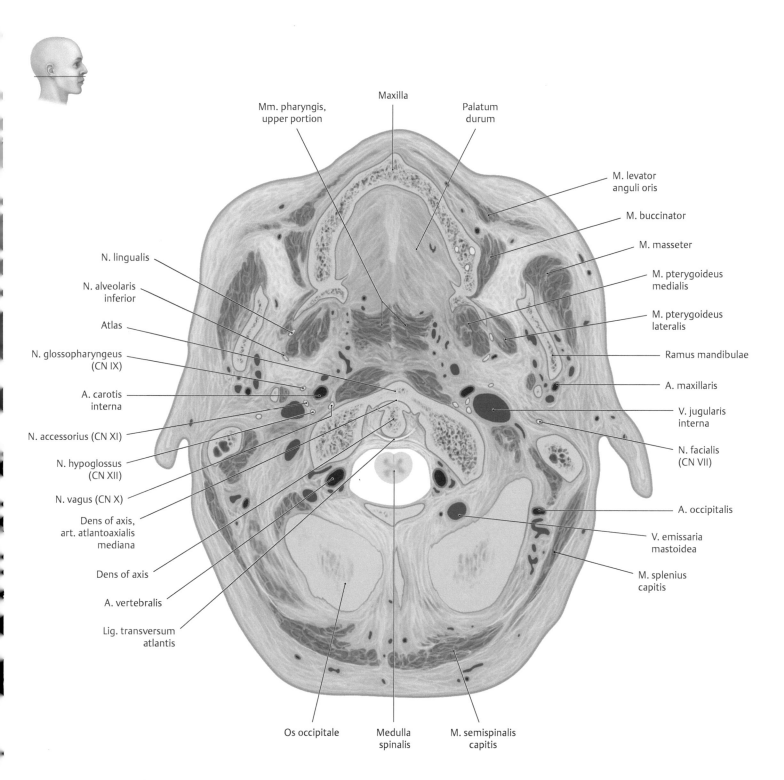

B Transverse section through the articulatio atlantoaxialis mediana

Superior view. The section at this level passes through the connectivetissue sheet that stretches over the bone of the palatum durum. Portions of the upper pharyngeal muscles are sectioned close to their origin. The neurovascular structures in the vagina carotica are also well displayed. The dens of the axis articulates in the art. atlantoaxialis mediana with the fovea dentis on the posterior surface of the arcus anterior atlantis. The lig. transversum of the atlas that helps to stabilize this joint can also be identified. The a. vertebralis and its accompanying veins are displayed in cross-section, as is the medulla spinalis. In the occipital region, the section passes through the upper portion of the posterior neck muscles.

7.6 Transverse Sections: C5–C6

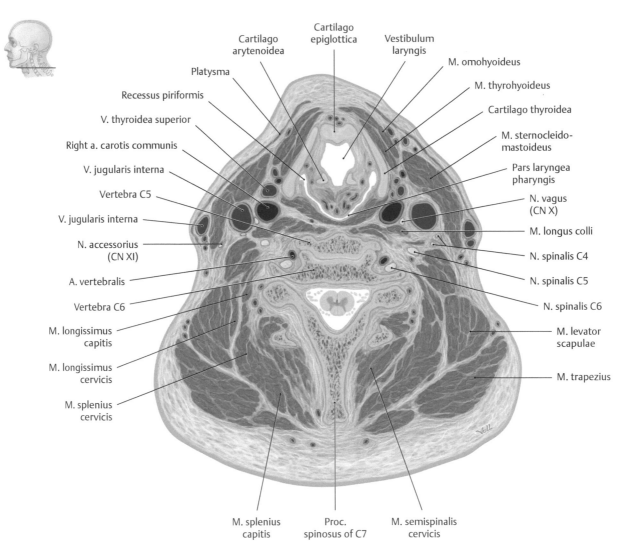

A Transverse cross-section at the level of the corpus vertebrae C5
Caudal view. The elongated proc. spinosus of the C7 vertebra (vertebra prominens) is also visible at this level owing to the lordotic curvature of the neck. The triangular shape of the cartilago arytenoidea is clearly demonstrated in the laryngeal cross-section. The vestibulum laryngis can also be identified. This view also shows the n. accessorius medial to the m. sternocleidomastoideus.

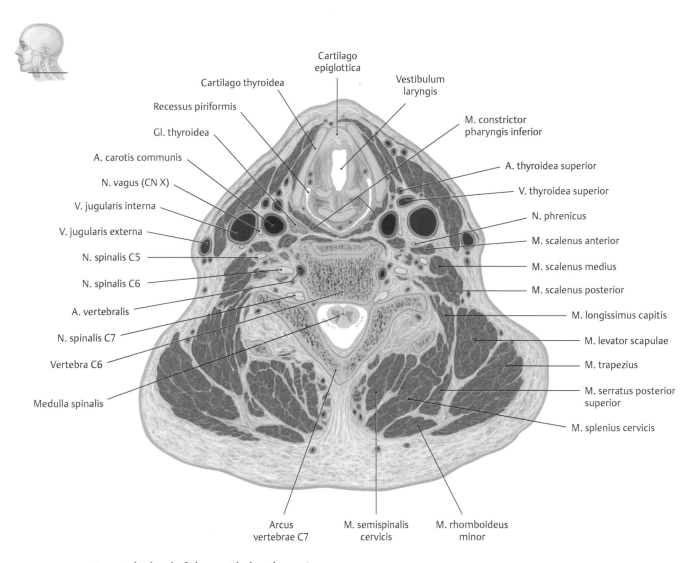

Cartilago epiglottica

Cartilago thyroidea

Recessus piriformis

Gl. thyroidea

A. carotis communis

N. vagus (CN X)

V. jugularis interna

V. jugularis externa

N. spinalis C5

N. spinalis C6

A. vertebralis

N. spinalis C7

Vertebra C6

Medulla spinalis

Vestibulum laryngis

M. constrictor pharyngis inferior

A. thyroidea superior

V. thyroidea superior

N. phrenicus

M. scalenus anterior

M. scalenus medius

M. scalenus posterior

M. longissimus capitis

M. levator scapulae

M. trapezius

M. serratus posterior superior

M. splenius cervicis

Arcus vertebrae C7

M. semispinalis cervicis

M. rhomboideus minor

B Transverse cross-section at the level of the vestibulum laryngis, demonstrating the epiglottis (corpus vertebrae C6)

Caudal view. The recessus piriformis can be identified at this level, and the a. vertebralis is visible in its course along the corpus vertebrae. The n. vagus lies in a posterior angle between the a. carotis communis and v. jugularis interna. This view shows the profile of the n. phrenicus on the m. scalenus anterior on the left side.

7.7 Transverse Sections: Anatomy of the Neck from the T 1/T 2 to C 6/C 7 Levels

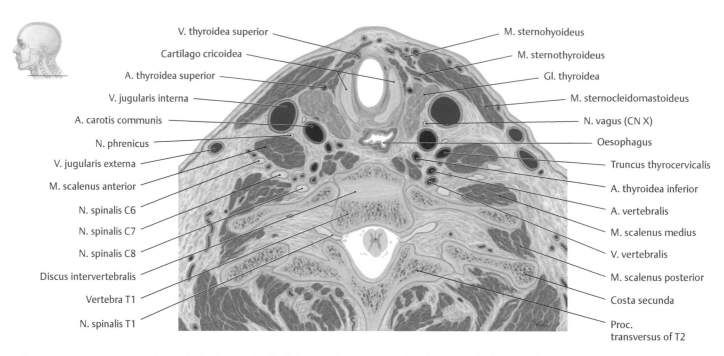

Labels (left, top to bottom): V. thyroidea superior · Cartilago cricoidea · A. thyroidea superior · V. jugularis interna · A. carotis communis · N. phrenicus · V. jugularis externa · M. scalenus anterior · N. spinalis C6 · N. spinalis C7 · N. spinalis C8 · Discus intervertebralis · Vertebra T1 · N. spinalis T1

Labels (right, top to bottom): M. sternohyoideus · M. sternothyroideus · Gl. thyroidea · M. sternocleidomastoideus · N. vagus (CN X) · Oesophagus · Truncus thyrocervicalis · A. thyroidea inferior · A. vertebralis · M. scalenus medius · V. vertebralis · M. scalenus posterior · Costa secunda · Proc. transversus of T2

A Transverse cross-section through the lower third of the cartilago thyroidea (junction of the T1/C7 vertebral bodies)
This cross-section clearly displays the mm. scalenus anterior and medius and the interval between them, which is traversed by the C6–C8 roots of the plexus brachialis. *Note* the neurovascular structures in the vagina carotica (a. carotis communis, v. jugularis interna, n. vagus).

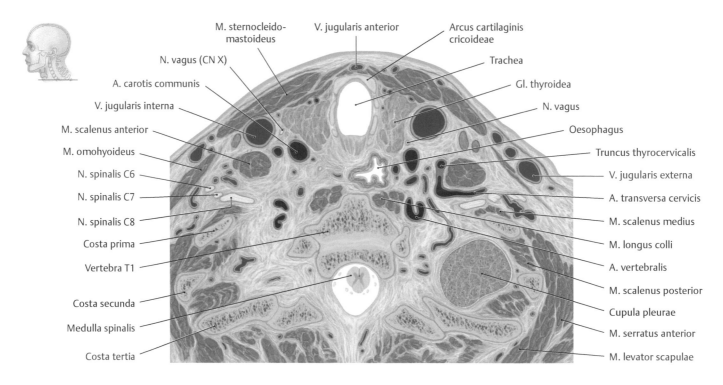

Labels (top): M. sternocleido-mastoideus · V. jugularis anterior · Arcus cartilaginis cricoideae

Labels (left, top to bottom): N. vagus (CN X) · A. carotis communis · V. jugularis interna · M. scalenus anterior · M. omohyoideus · N. spinalis C6 · N. spinalis C7 · N. spinalis C8 · Costa prima · Vertebra T1 · Costa secunda · Medulla spinalis · Costa tertia

Labels (right, top to bottom): Trachea · Gl. thyroidea · N. vagus · Oesophagus · Truncus thyrocervicalis · V. jugularis externa · A. transversa cervicis · M. scalenus medius · M. longus colli · A. vertebralis · M. scalenus posterior · Cupula pleurae · M. serratus anterior · M. levator scapulae

B Transverse cross-section of the neck at a level that just cuts the left cupula pleurae (level of the corpora vertebralia T1/T2)
Inferior view. Due to the curvature of the neck in this specimen, the section also cuts the discus intervertebralis between T1 and T2.
Note that the cross-section is viewed from below like a CT scan or MRI slice. The illustrations that follow are transverse cross-sections through the neck at progressively higher (more cranial) levels (Tiedemann series).

The section in **A** includes cross-sections of the C6–C8 nerve roots of the plexus brachialis and a small section of the left cupula pleurae. The proximity of the apex pulmonis to the plexus brachialis shows why the growth of an apical lung tumor may damage the plexus brachialis roots. *Note* also the gl. thyroidea and its proximity to the trachea and neurovascular bundle in the vagina carotica (a thin fibrous sheet which is not clearly discernible in these views).

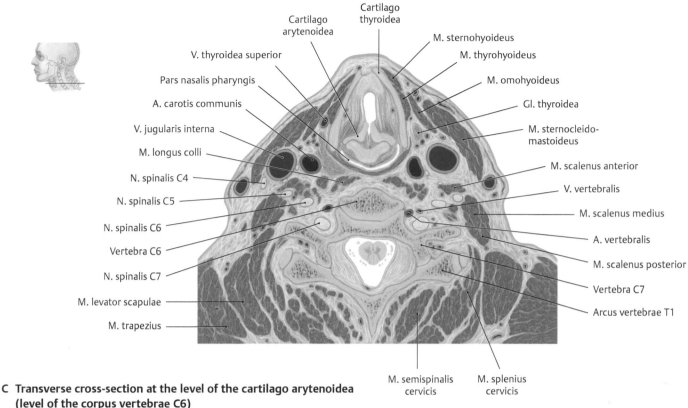

Cartilago thyroidea

Cartilago arytenoidea

V. thyroidea superior

Pars nasalis pharyngis

A. carotis communis

V. jugularis interna

M. longus colli

N. spinalis C4

N. spinalis C5

N. spinalis C6

Vertebra C6

N. spinalis C7

M. levator scapulae

M. trapezius

M. sternohyoideus

M. thyrohyoideus

M. omohyoideus

Gl. thyroidea

M. sternocleido-mastoideus

M. scalenus anterior

V. vertebralis

M. scalenus medius

A. vertebralis

M. scalenus posterior

Vertebra C7

Arcus vertebrae T1

M. semispinalis cervicis

M. splenius cervicis

C Transverse cross-section at the level of the cartilago arytenoidea (level of the corpus vertebrae C6)
Caudal view. This cross-section passes through the base of the cartilago arytenoidea in the larynx. The pars laryngea pharyngis appears as a narrow transverse cleft behind the larynx.

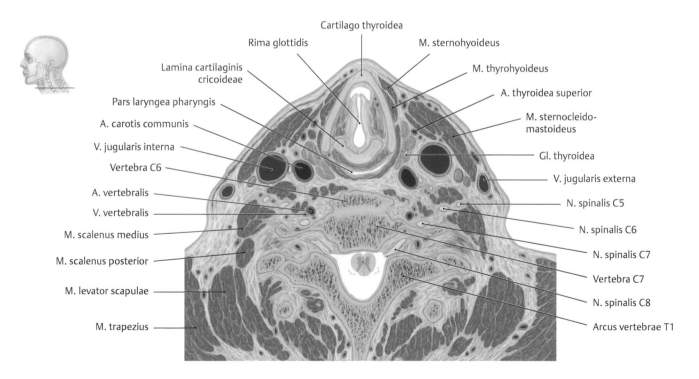

Cartilago thyroidea

Rima glottidis

Lamina cartilaginis cricoideae

Pars laryngea pharyngis

A. carotis communis

V. jugularis interna

Vertebra C6

A. vertebralis

V. vertebralis

M. scalenus medius

M. scalenus posterior

M. levator scapulae

M. trapezius

M. sternohyoideus

M. thyrohyoideus

A. thyroidea superior

M. sternocleido-mastoideus

Gl. thyroidea

V. jugularis externa

N. spinalis C5

N. spinalis C6

N. spinalis C7

Vertebra C7

N. spinalis C8

Arcus vertebrae T1

D Transverse cross-section at the level of the m. vocalis in the larynx (junction of the corpora vertebralia C6/C7)
Caudal view. This cross-section passes through the larynx at the level of the plicae vocales. The gl. thyroidea appears considerably smaller at this level than in views **A** and **B**.

7.8 Midsagittal Sections: Nasal Septum (Septum Nasi) and Medial Orbital Wall

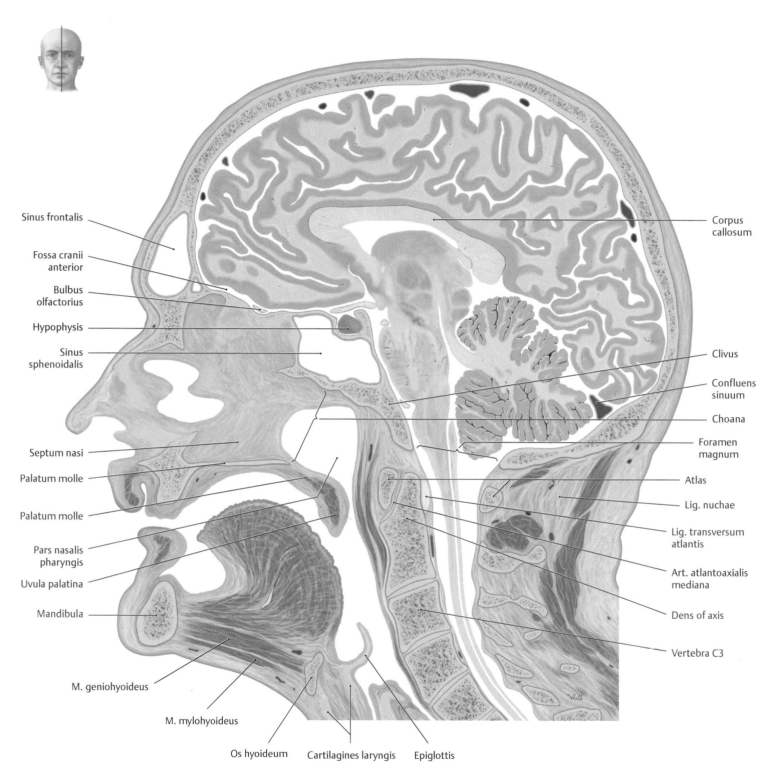

Sinus frontalis

Fossa cranii anterior

Bulbus olfactorius

Hypophysis

Sinus sphenoidalis

Septum nasi

Palatum molle

Palatum molle

Pars nasalis pharyngis

Uvula palatina

Mandibula

M. geniohyoideus

M. mylohyoideus

Os hyoideum   Cartilagines laryngis   Epiglottis

Corpus callosum

Clivus

Confluens sinuum

Choana

Foramen magnum

Atlas

Lig. nuchae

Lig. transversum atlantis

Art. atlantoaxialis mediana

Dens of axis

Vertebra C3

A Midsagittal section through the septum nasi

Left lateral view. The midline structures are particularly well displayed in this plane of section, and the anatomical structures at this level can be roughly assigned to the **facial skeleton** or neurocranium (cranial vault). The lowest level of the facial skeleton is formed by the oral floor muscles between the os hyoideum and mandibula and the overlying skin. This section also passes through the epiglottis and the larynx below it, which are considered part of the cervical viscera. The palata durum and molle with the uvula define the boundary between the cavitates oris and nasi. Posterior to the uvula palatina is the pars oralis pharyngis. The section includes the septum nasi, which divides the cavitas nasi into two cavities (sectioned above and in front of the septum) that communicate with the pars nasalis pharyngis through the choanae. Posterior to the sinus frontalis is the fossa cranii anterior, which is part of the **neurocranium**. This section passes through the medial surface of the brain (the falx cerebri has been removed). The cut edge of the corpus callosum, the bulbus olfactorius, and the hypophysis are also shown.

Note the art. atlantoaxialis mediana (whose stability must be evaluated after trauma to the cervical spine).

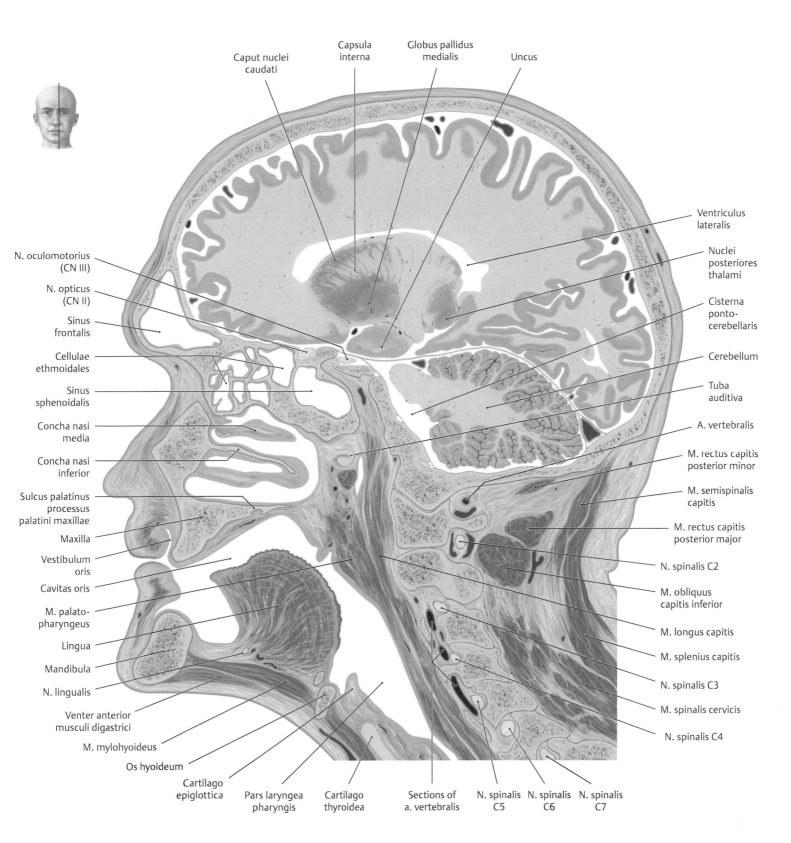

Caput nuclei caudati

Capsula interna

Globus pallidus medialis

Uncus

Ventriculus lateralis

N. oculomotorius (CN III)

N. opticus (CN II)

Sinus frontalis

Cellulae ethmoidales

Sinus sphenoidalis

Concha nasi media

Concha nasi inferior

Sulcus palatinus processus palatini maxillae

Maxilla

Vestibulum oris

Cavitas oris

M. palato-pharyngeus

Lingua

Mandibula

N. lingualis

Venter anterior musculi digastrici

M. mylohyoideus

Os hyoideum

Cartilago epiglottica

Pars laryngea pharyngis

Cartilago thyroidea

Sections of a. vertebralis

N. spinalis C5

N. spinalis C6

N. spinalis C7

Nuclei posteriores thalami

Cisterna ponto-cerebellaris

Cerebellum

Tuba auditiva

A. vertebralis

M. rectus capitis posterior minor

M. semispinalis capitis

M. rectus capitis posterior major

N. spinalis C2

M. obliquus capitis inferior

M. longus capitis

M. splenius capitis

N. spinalis C3

M. spinalis cervicis

N. spinalis C4

B Sagittal section through the medial orbital wall

Left lateral view. This section passes through the conchae nasi inferior and media within the cavitas nasi. Above the concha nasi media are the cellulae ethmoidalis. The only parts of the pars nasalis pharyngis visible in this section are a small luminal area and the lateral wall, which bears a section of the pars cartilaginea of the tuba auditiva. The sinus sphenoidalis is also displayed. In the region of the cervical spine, the section cuts the a. vertebralis at multiple levels. The lateral sites where the nn. spinales emerge from the foramina intervertebralia are clearly displayed.

7.9 Sagittal Sections: Inner Third and Center of the Orbit

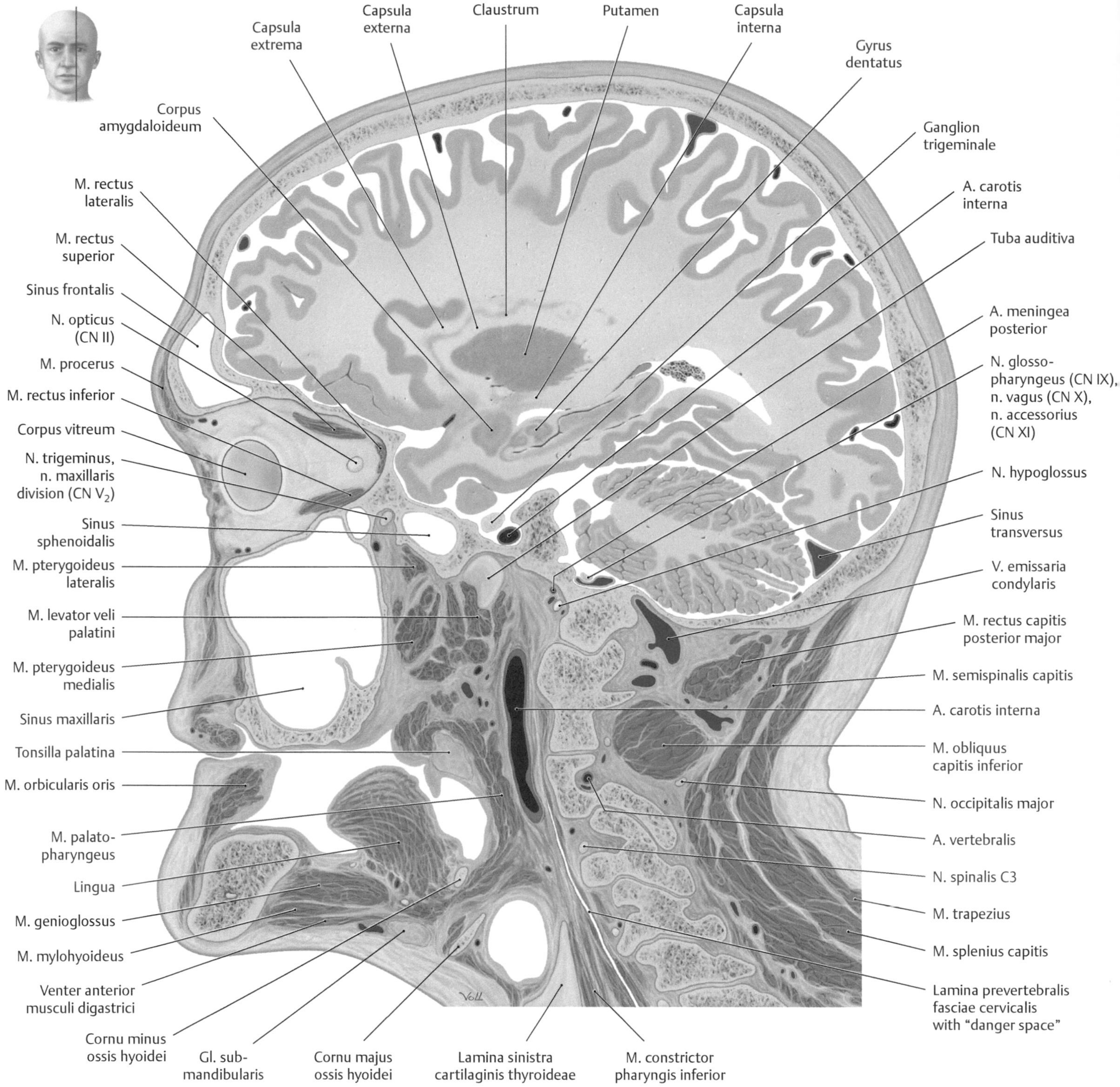

Capsula extrema
Capsula externa
Claustrum
Putamen
Capsula interna
Gyrus dentatus
Corpus amygdaloideum
Ganglion trigeminale
M. rectus lateralis
A. carotis interna
M. rectus superior
Tuba auditiva
Sinus frontalis
N. opticus (CN II)
A. meningea posterior
M. procerus
N. glosso-pharyngeus (CN IX), n. vagus (CN X), n. accessorius (CN XI)
M. rectus inferior
Corpus vitreum
N. trigeminus, n. maxillaris division (CN V2)
N. hypoglossus
Sinus sphenoidalis
Sinus transversus
M. pterygoideus lateralis
V. emissaria condylaris
M. levator veli palatini
M. rectus capitis posterior major
M. pterygoideus medialis
M. semispinalis capitis
Sinus maxillaris
A. carotis interna
Tonsilla palatina
M. obliquus capitis inferior
M. orbicularis oris
N. occipitalis major
M. palato-pharyngeus
A. vertebralis
Lingua
N. spinalis C3
M. genioglossus
M. trapezius
M. mylohyoideus
M. splenius capitis
Venter anterior musculi digastrici
Lamina prevertebralis fasciae cervicalis with “danger space”
Cornu minus ossis hyoidei
Gl. sub-mandibularis
Cornu majus ossis hyoidei
Lamina sinistra cartilaginis thyroideae
M. constrictor pharyngis inferior

A Sagittal section through the inner third of the orbita

Left lateral view. This section passes through the sinus maxillaris and frontalis while displaying one cellula ethmoidalis and the peripheral part of the sinus sphenoidalis. It passes through the medial portion of the a. carotis interna and gl. submandibularis. The mm. pharyngis and masticatorii are grouped about the pars cartilaginea of the tuba auditiva. The bulbus oculi and n. opticus are cut peripherally by the section, which displays relatively long segments of the mm. recti superior and inferior. Sectioned brain structures include the capsula externa and interna and the intervening putamen. The corpus amygdaloideum and hippocampus can be identified near the base of the brain. A section of the ganglion trigeminale appears below the cerebrum.

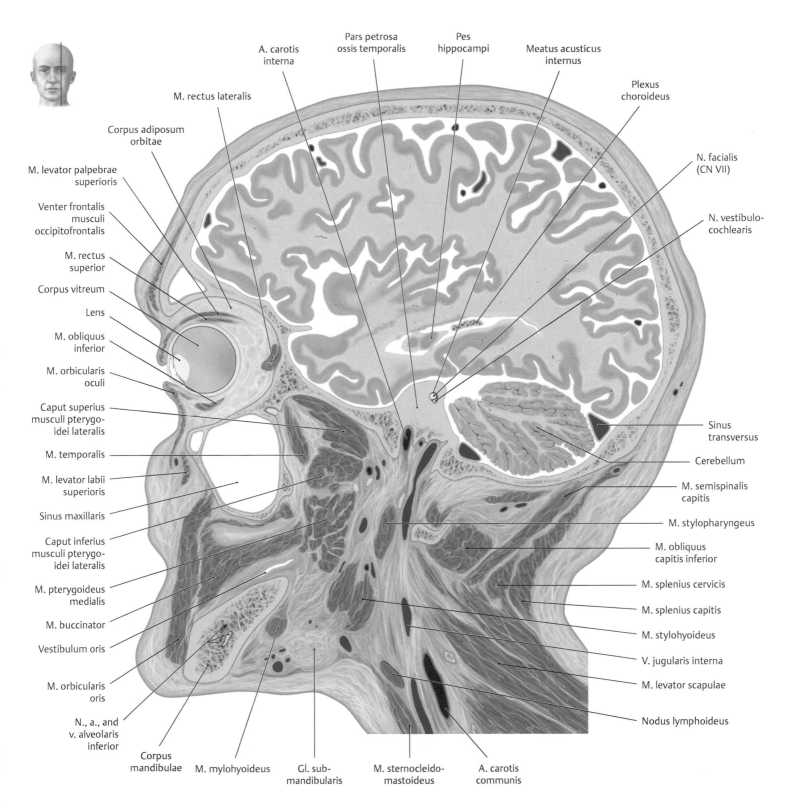

Pars petrosa
ossis temporalis

Pes
hippocampi

A. carotis
interna

Meatus acusticus
internus

Plexus
choroideus

M. rectus lateralis

Corpus adiposum
orbitae

N. facialis
(CN VII)

M. levator palpebrae
superioris

N. vestibulo-
cochlearis

Venter frontalis
musculi
occipitofrontalis

M. rectus
superior

Corpus vitreum

Lens

M. obliquus
inferior

M. orbicularis
oculi

Caput superius
musculi pterygo-
idei lateralis

Sinus
transversus

M. temporalis

Cerebellum

M. levator labii
superioris

M. semispinalis
capitis

Sinus maxillaris

M. stylopharyngeus

Caput inferius
musculi pterygo-
idei lateralis

M. obliquus
capitis inferior

M. pterygoideus
medialis

M. splenius cervicis

M. buccinator

M. splenius capitis

Vestibulum oris

M. stylohyoideus

V. jugularis interna

M. orbicularis
oris

M. levator scapulae

N., a., and
v. alveolaris
inferior

Nodus lymphoideus

Corpus
mandibulae

M. mylohyoideus

Gl. sub-
mandibularis

M. sternocleido-
mastoideus

A. carotis
communis

B Sagittal section through the approximate center of the orbita
Left lateral view. Due to the obliquity of this section, the dominant structure in the oral floor region is the mandibula while the vestibulum oris appears as a narrow slit. The mm. buccales and masticatorii are prominently displayed in this plane. Much of the orbita is occupied by the bulbus oculi, which appears in longitudinal section. Aside from a few sections of the extraocular muscles, the orbita in this plane is filled with fatty tissue. Both the a. carotis interna and the v. jugularis interna are demonstrated. Except for the pes hippocampi, the only visible cerebral structures are the substantia alba and cortex. The n. facialis and n. vestibulocochlearis can be identified in the meatus acusticus internus.

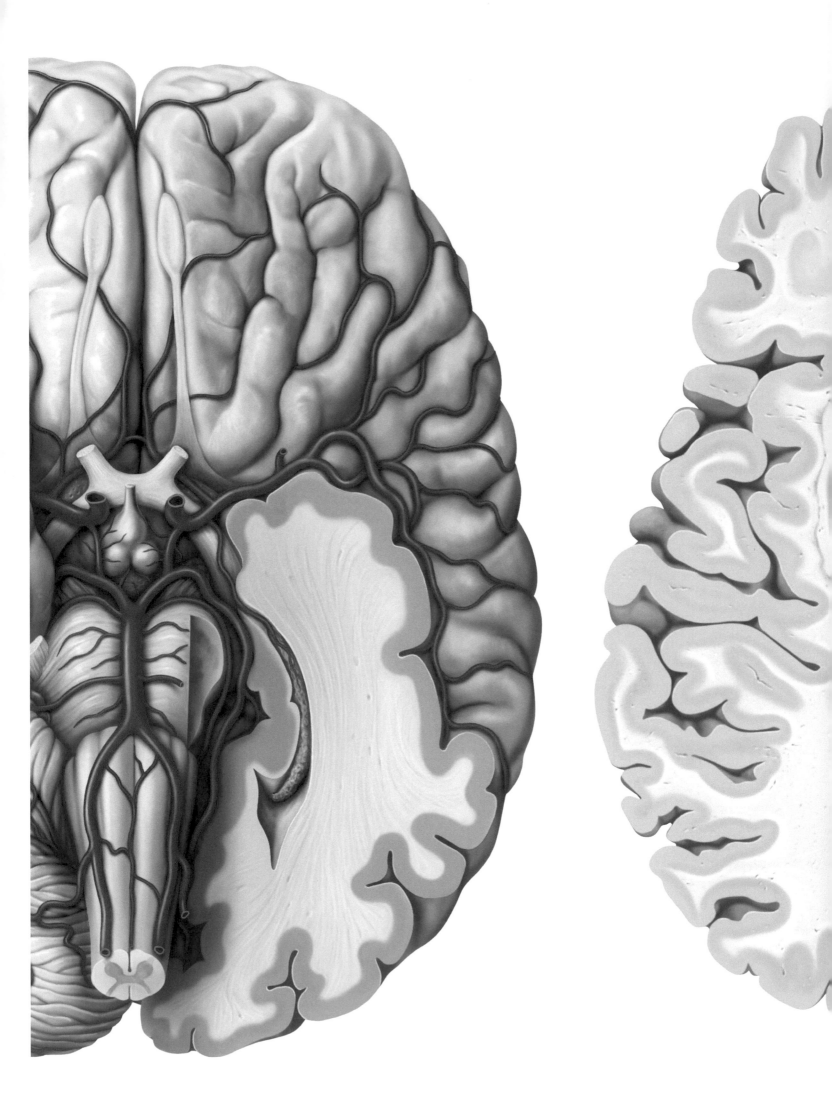

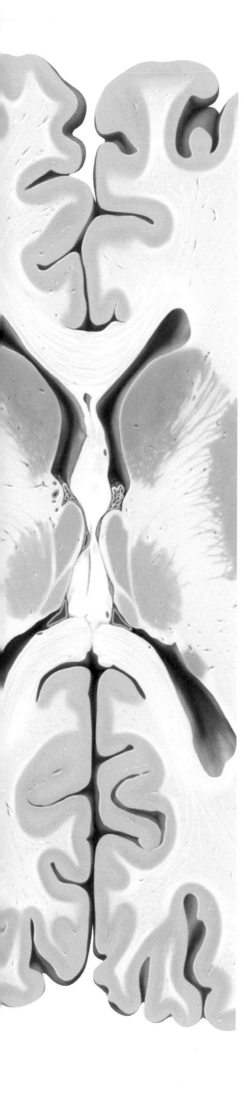

B Neuroanatomy

1.1 Organization and Basic Functions of the Nervous System

Introduction

The human nervous system is the most complex organ system to have developed in the evolution of life. Its function involves the perception of its surroundings and the detection of changes as they occur. It is responsible for responding to those changes with the help of other organ systems. At the same time, the nervous system is the only organ system with the ability to reflect upon itself and to consciously communicate with that of another human. It is this compexity and the aspect of self-awareness which makes the nervous system such an especially difficult subject of observation yet also explains our fascination with it.

Unlike the nervous system of animals, the human nervous system to a particularly large degree has the ability to learn, remember, conceptualize and show self-awareness as well as communicate with the nervous system of another individual through complex language. Disorders of the nervous system can significantly compromise the quality of life in affected patients. Thus, profound knowledge of the structure and the functions of the nervous system form the basis for prevention or treatment of diseases and are thus the foundation on which medical studies are based.

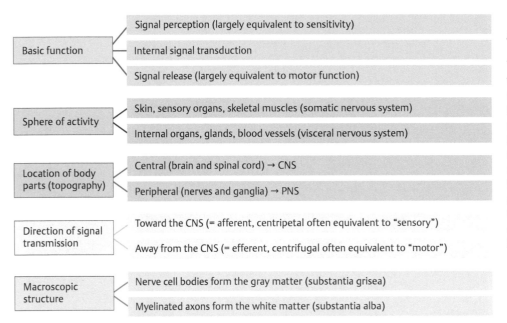

A Classification of the nervous system: Overview

The nervous system can be divided in various ways. It is this variety of criteria that makes an overall understanding of the nervous system seem initially difficult. In addition, every classification is artificial and always takes into account only specific aspects. Yet, knowledge of the structural classification makes for a much better understanding of the numerous interconnections of the nervous system without the need to memorize them all. The nervous system will be classified according to five different criteria. Each individual criterion will be explained diagramatically.

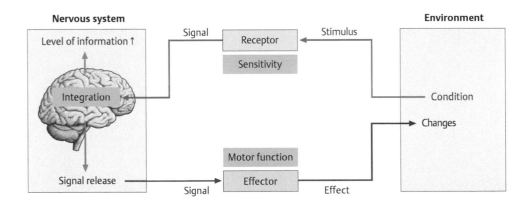

B Basic functions of the nervous system

The nervous system functions in processing information. It constantly communicates with the environment around us, both internal and external. The major functions of the nervous system are as follows:

- **Sensation** (sensory perception): The nervous system continously receives information from the surrounding environment, concerning physical and chemical stimuli. This information is
  - received by specialized receptors,
  - converted to a (mostly electrical) signal which is
  - transmitted through the nervous system.

- **Integration:** The nervous system
  - processes the information, which is coded as an electrical signal, within specialized, extremely complex structures in a very differentiated way, using electrical processing and
  - transmits it to effectors.

- **Motor function:** The effectors can now produce a response or an effect.

Note: The terms sensation, integration, and motor function are suitable to describe the basic functions of the CNS. That does not mean that every response initiated within the CNS can necessarily be attributed to motor function or that integration is always equivalent to signal transmission to an effector. Elevating the state of information within the nervous system (e.g., internal recognition memory, the formation of thoughts) is an integrative process, and the release of hormones is also an effect, which can be triggered by the CNS.

As a result of the diversity and complexity of particular stimuli in the environment, and receptors which are specialized in the reception of certain stimuli, comprise functional units—the sensory organs.

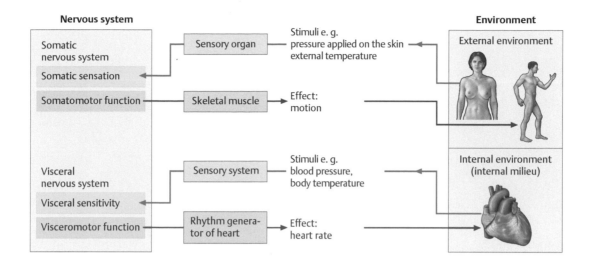

C Functional classification of the nervous system

Classifying the nervous system according to either the function (functional classification) or location (topographical classification, see **D**) of particular structures of the nervous system has proven successful, but take into consideration only certain aspects. The result is a certain degree of overlap in classifications. To a certain extent, the classification is somewhat artificial. Referring to the terms, sensation and motor function (as mentioned under **B**), requires a more precise definition of "environment":

- the "external environment" referring to the surrounding environment in which an organism lives
- the "internal environment," inside the body, with which the nervous system communicates, to maintain a state of homeostasis

Sensory perception (sensation), information about the external environment, is received through the skin or the sensory organs and the musculoskeletal system responds to those stimuli. The functional aspect of nervous system classification is represented through the somatic nervous system. The regulation of the internal environment occurs with the help of the viscera, with which the nervous system exchanges information. The part of the nervous system that communicates directly with the viscera is called the visceral nervous system. The combination of function (sensory, motor function) and location (somatic, visceral) can be subdivided:

- Interaction with the external environment is somatomotor function (see p. 286) or somatic sensation (see p. 284).
- Internal interaction is visceromotor function or visceral sensation.

Note: For visceral sensation, there are natural receptors, though they are usually not collected in their own group of sensory organs. The visceral nervous system is also commonly known as the autonomic nervous system (see p. 296).

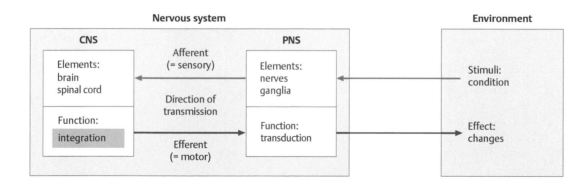

D Topographical classification and signal transmission

The nervous system can also be classified based on the location inside the body into

- the central nervous system (CNS) and
- the peripheral nervous system (PNS).

Note: Both the CNS and PNS contain portions of the somatic and visceral nervous system. The CNS consists of the brain and spinal cord, both of which are protected by being housed in bony enclosures (cranium and columna vertebralis respectively). The PNS consists of nerves and ganglia (see p. 269) located outside the CNS and enclosed in a connective tissue sheath. Except for a few restrictions, it can be said that the function of the PNS is to carry signals and act as a "mediator" between CNS and the external environment or between CNS and effector. The direction of signal transmission in the PNS is of particular importance: carrying sensory information to the CNS is referred to as afferent transmission; signal transmission away from the CNS carrying motor impulses is referred to as efferent transmission.

1.2 Cells, Signal Transmission, and Morphological Structure of the Nervous System

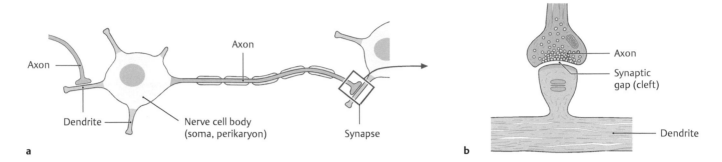

A Nerve cell and synapse

a Nerve cell: Both morphologically and functionally, the nerve cell (or neuron) is the basic structural element of the nervous system. Since nerve cells are found in both the CNS and PNS a distinction is drawn between central and peripheral neurons. Nerve cells generate electric signals, the action potential, and pass them on to other nerve or muscle cells. A number of types of nerve cells are classified based on their form and function. Their structure, however, is largely similar. Attached to the cell body, are at least two projections of different length:

- the dendrite (dendron = tree), is typically short and highly branched (arborized); a nerve cell can posess one or more dendrites;
- the axon (neurite), which is typically longer than the dendrites and does not taper in diamater or exhibit tree-like branching; a nerve cell only ever posesses a single axon. Axons can branch but these branches (collaterals) occur at roughly 90°.

In cases where there is a single dendrite it is typically located at the opposite end of the cell body from the axon, resulting in a structural polarization, which corresponds to the functional polarization of the neuron (see **A**, p. 292): In dendrites, the electric signal always flows toward the cell body while in the axon it flows away from it. This flow pattern remains constant even if a nerve cell posesses numerous dendrites, some of which are not located opposite the axon.

b Synapse: Functionally speaking, nerve cells never work alone but are grouped together and transmit electric signals that are passed from cell-to-cell via junctions called synapses. At synapses, the axon of one nerve cell comes into very close contact with other cells. The unusual feature of this conduction is that in most cases it is discontinuous: There is a gap (synaptic gap/cleft) between the axon and the receptor cell where the electric signal is converted into a chemical signal (or transmitter). Usually, this transmitter generates another electric signal in the downstream nerve cell. The order in which signals are transmitted are electric → chemical → electric.

Note: In terms of their functions, one differentiates between excitatory synpases, which enhance the transmission of signals, and inhibitory synapses, which slow down signal transmission. The nervous system is capable of producing excitatory and inhibitory signals (see **A**, p. 292).

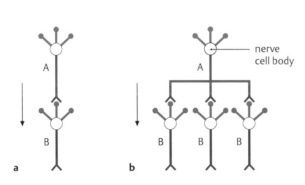

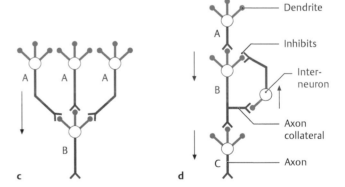

B Signal transmission within the nervous system: neural wiring

There are different ways in which neurons connect to each other to form neural networks:

a Neuron A sends its signal (projects to) neuron B: the transmission is 1:1.

b Neuron A sends its signal (via the axon's collateral branching) to multiple neurons B (here 3); the transmission is 1:3. There is a divergence as a result of the signal being passed to additional cells (the megaphone effect).

c Multiple neurons A (here 3) project to a neuron B, the transmission is 3:1. There is a convergence effect which can be used to filter information. For instance, neuron B will only pass on information if at least two A neurons send their signals simultaneously to neuron B (a threshold level or filtering effect).

d A nerve cell can be connected to other nerve cells via an interneuron. An example of this occurs in a phenomenon known as "recurrent" inhibition. A signal from neuron A stimulates neuron B, which passes it on to neuron C. However, through axon collaterals, neuron B can inhibit the A → B synapse. Neuron B is temporarily numb for additional signals sent by neuron A. A time filter has been integrated: Only after a certain amount of time has expired will neuron B pass on the signals it receives from neuron A. This prevents the nervous system from being overwhelmed by continuous stimulation.

Synapse and wiring, excitation and inhibition, are important functional terms used to describe the nervous system.

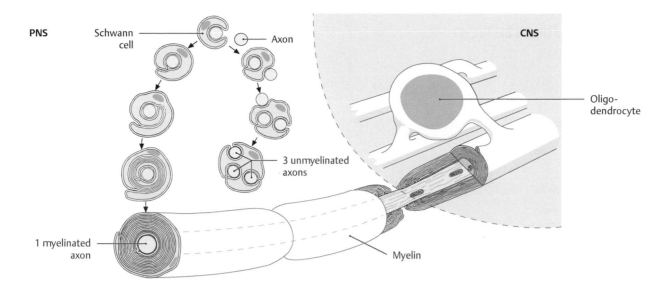

C Glial cells (neuroglia)

The other distinctive cell type of the nervous system is the glial cell (neuroglia), which can be found in both the CNS and PNS. Glial cells don't carry nerve impulses but they are a crucial factor in determining the speed with which impulses travel through the nervous system. They accomplish this by forming sheaths around the axons of nerve cells, giving the axons different names based on shape and size of the sheath:

- **Myelinated axons:** multiple lamellar layers of glial cell membrane surround a single axon forming a distinct myelin sheath.
- **Unmyelinated axon:** a glial cell surrounds/supports multiple axons without forming a myelin sheath.

Different glial cells are responsible for myelination in each division of the nervous system. In the CNS, myelination is accomplished by oligodendrocytes; in the PNS that function is carried out by Schwann cells. Myelinated axons constitute the vast majority, outnumbering the unmyelinated ones. Since the sheath formation influences conduction velocity (myelinated axons conduct faster), this sheath is of utmost importance to the neuron's function. Other types of glial cells also support neuron function. They play an important role in regulating the environment of the nervous system (e.g., blood-brain barrier) and in providing protection against harmful agents.

Note: The axon + its glial sheath (myelinated or unmyelinated) = a nerve fiber. This term is very important for the following microscopic observation of the nervous system.

D Structural classification of the nervous system: gray and white matter

Neuron cell bodies and axons are surrounded by neuroglial cells of differing types. Observed individually, they are visible only under a microscope. However, since they tend to group together, or form clusters, they are also macroscopically visible. Groups of nerve cell bodies appear gray and as such these areas are referred to as gray matter (substantia grisea). The clusters of myelinated fibers appear white and are referred to as white matter (substantia alba). Dendrites, which are usually very short, and the few unmyelinated fibers get lost in the mass of cell bodies and are not observable via macroscopic obervation. Depending on whether you are describing the CNS or PNS these grouops of neuron cell bodies and myelinated axons are described as follows (glossary, p. 502ff):

- In the **PNS**, Nerve fiber-rich regions/structures are referred to as a nerve. Regions containing neuron cell bodies are referred to as ganglia.
- In the **CNS**, white matter is divided into tracts while the gray matter is divided into the cortex and nuclei.

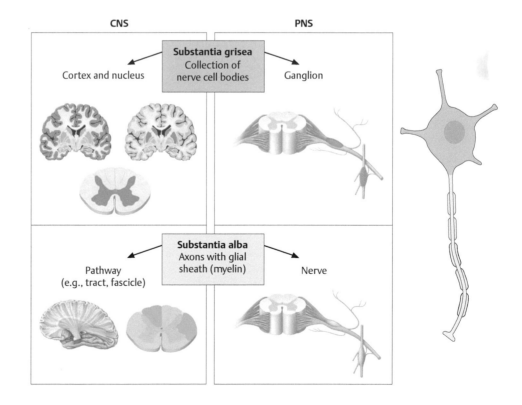

Note: Morphologically, the structure of gray and white matter in the CNS is analogous to their structure in the PNS. This is easy to forget given the precise descriptions and differentiation of the distinct parts (nerve, ganglia, tract etc.) making up the CNS and PNS.

1.3 Overview of the Entire Nervous System: Morphology and Spatial Orientation

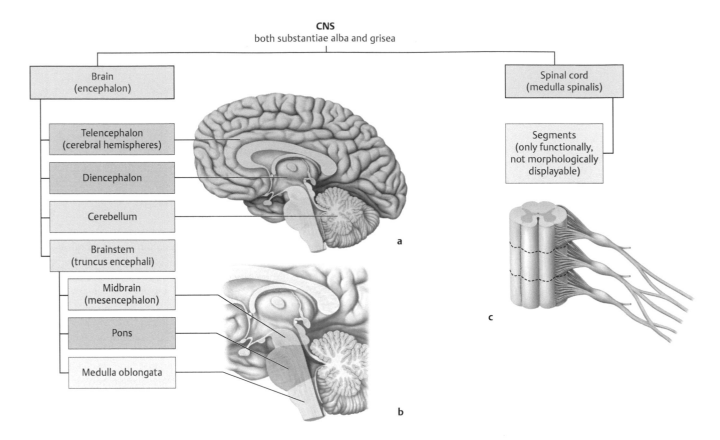

a

b

c

A Morphology of the central nervous system (CNS)

a and **b** Right side of the brain, medial view; **c** Ventral view of a section of the spinal cord. A general morphological overview of the entire nervous system is necessary to help with understanding the material that follows. The CNS is divided into the brain and the spinal cord with the **brain (encephalon)** subdivided into the following regions:

- Cerebral hemispheres (telencephalon or endbrain)
- Interbrain (diencephalon)
- Cerebellum
- Brainstem (truncus encephali) composed of the midbrain (mesencephalon), pons (bridge) and medulla oblongata

In contrast, the other part of the CNS, the **spinal cord (medulla spinalis)** appears morphologically rather as one homogenous structure. In terms of its functions, however, the spinal cord can also be divided into segments. The division of substantiae grisea and alba is clearly visible:

- substantia grisea: centrally located, butterfly-shaped structure
- substantia alba: substance that surrounds the "butterfly"

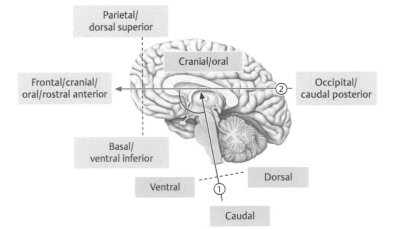

B Axes of the nervous system and directional terms

The same planes, axes and directional terms apply for both the entire body and the PNS. However, with the CNS, one differentiates between two axes:

- Axis No.1 = Meynert axis: It corresponds to the axes of the body and is used to designate locations in the spinal cord, brainstem (truncus encephali) and cerebellum.
- Axis No. 2 = Forel axis. It runs horizontally through the diencephalon and telencephalon and forms an a 80° angle to axis 1. As a result, the diencephalon and telencephalon lie "face down."

Note: In order to avoid topographical misunderstandings, the following directional terms for axis No. 2 (Forel axis) are used:

- basal instead of ventral
- parietal instead of dorsal
- frontal and oral/rostral respectively instead of cranial
- occipital instead of caudal

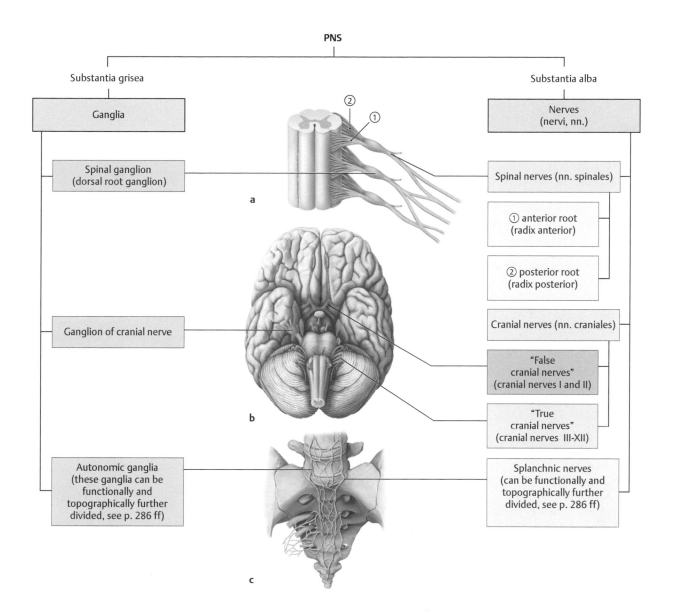

PNS

Substantia grisea

Ganglia

Spinal ganglion
(dorsal root ganglion)

Ganglion of cranial nerve

Autonomic ganglia
(these ganglia can be
functionally and
topographically further
divided, see p. 286 ff)

Substantia alba

Nerves
(nervi, nn.)

Spinal nerves (nn. spinales)

① anterior root
(radix anterior)

② posterior root
(radix posterior)

Cranial nerves (nn. craniales)

"False
cranial nerves"
(cranial nerves I and II)

"True
cranial nerves"
(cranial nerves III-XII)

Splanchnic nerves
(can be functionally and
topographically further
divided, see p. 286 ff)

a

b

c

C Morphology of the peripheral nervous system
a Ventral view of a segment of the medulla spinalis; **b** View of base of the brain; **c** View of sympathetic ganglia and nerves located anteriorly to the sacrum.

The nerves and ganglia forming the peripheral nervous system and are generally named for the part of the CNS with which they communicate:

- Nn. spinales (connect the periphery of the body with the spinal cord). Usually 31 or 32 pairs. Nn. spinales (except those related to vertebral levels T1 to T11 or T12) generally have their ventral rami form plexuses for reasons of functionality (see **A**, p. 398).
- Nn. craniales (connect the periphery of the body to the brain, see p. 112 ff). 12 pairs.

Nerve cells found within ganglia (in the PNS) can be classified based on their affiliation with a particular functional division of the nervous system:

- Sensory neurons can be found within either division of nervous system. In the PNS, sensory neurons are found within the sensory (dorsal root) ganglia on the radix posterior (dorsal root) of the nervus spinalis. In the CNS, sensory neurons are found within the sensory nuclei associated with the appropriate nervi craniales that contain sensory fibers.
- Ganglia of the autonomic nervous system contain postganglionic sympathetic and parasympathethic neurons that control the organs

of the body (see **C**, p. 297). Autonomic ganglia are associated with splanchnic nerves that take vasomotor fibers to the viscera. The autonomic nervous system also demonstrates characteristic plexus formation.

Note: The distinction discussed here applies except for a few special cases. These include the following:

- The optic nerve, which is not a true nerve but a part of the diencephalon. For historical reasons, it has been called a "nerve," which is systematically false.

- The olfactory system: The olfactory bulb and tract are components of the CNS (not the PNS) because they have a meningeal covering. The olfactory nerve (the aggregated filia olfactoria, which in turn are composed of fibers of the olfactory cells) does not belong to the CNS as the olfactory cells develop from the ectodermal olfactory placode. Its embryologic origin from the placode epithelium gives this structure a special status as well.

Because of these peculiarities, the nn. opticus et olfactorius are often referred to as "bogus" cranial nerves (shown here in red) and contrasted with the "true" cranial nerves (III-X and XII, shown here in yellow), which are clearly part of the PNS. Cranial nerve XI is currently considered a spinal nerve with an atypical trajectory. In the interest of clarity, further details are omitted at this point (see p. 116).

1.4 Embryological Development of the Nervous System

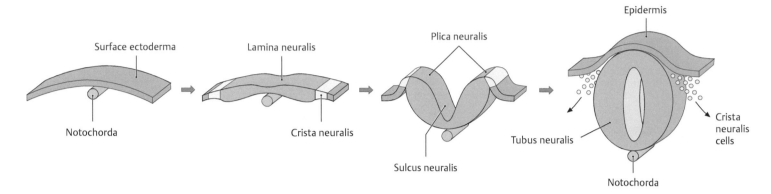

Surface ectoderma
Lamina neuralis
Plica neuralis
Epidermis
Notochorda
Crista neuralis
Sulcus neuralis
Tubus neuralis
Crista neuralis cells
Notochorda

A Development of the tubus neuralis, crista neuralis and their deriviatives

The entire nervous system develops from the ectoderma, which in the third week of gestation differentiates into the lamina neuralis and located laterally to it, the two cristae neurales. The lamina neuralis develops a central sulcus neuralis between two peripheral plicae neurales. The now heavily invaginated lamina neuralis detaches from the remaining ectoderma and closes over to form the tubus neuralis. The cells of both cristae neurales also exit the ectoderma and migrate to areas lateral to the tubus neuralis. The tubus neuralis gives rise to the following:

- In the central nervous system (CNS)
  - the encephalon
  - the medulla spinalis
  - neuroglial cells of the CNS
- In the peripheral nervous system (PNS)
  - the motor component of the nn. spinales (see **C**)

The **cellulae cristae neuralis** give rise only to parts of the PNS:

- the sensory component of the n. spinalis and the ganglion spinalis
- the entire visceral peripheral nervous system
- the suprarenal (adrenal) medulla
- glial cells of the PNS.

The cells of the crista neuralis give also rise to additional components such as melanoblasts (pigment cell precursors), which are not part of the nervous system.

Note: The tubus neuralis provides material for the CNS and PNS; the crista neuralis provides material only for the PNS. The suprarenal (adrenal) medulla (not the cortex) is phylogenetically considered to be a part of the peripheral nervous system.

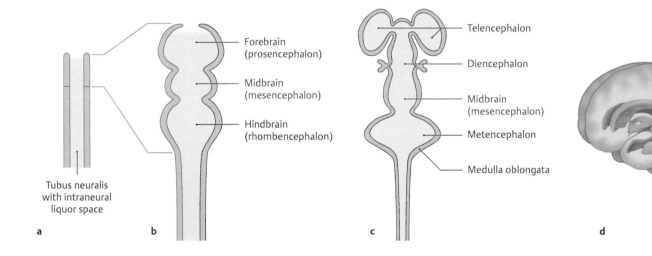

Forebrain (prosencephalon)
Midbrain (mesencephalon)
Hindbrain (rhombencephalon)
Tubus neuralis with intraneural liquor space

Telencephalon
Diencephalon
Midbrain (mesencephalon)
Metencephalon
Medulla oblongata

a   b   c   d

B Development of brain and spatia subarachnoidea from the tubus neuralis

Tubus neuralis and its deriviatives; dorsal view, In **a–c** the tubus neuralis is cut open; **d** Mature brain with spatia subarachnoidea in situ.

From the initially undifferentiated tubus neuralis, still open on both ends (**a**), develop three primary brain vesicles (**b**). From these the five secondary brain vesicles arise (**c**) from which differentiate the eventual brain regions. The lower part of the tubus neuralis which is not involved in the development of brain vesicles gives rise to the medulla spinalis.

In the regions of the medulla spinalis, the shape of the tubus neuralis is still visible (see **a**); in the regions of the brain, the shape of the tube is no longer discernible due to prominent vesicle formation.

Note: The cavity of the tubus neuralis also differentiates at the same time as the brain vesicles and the medulla spinalis. It develops into the intraneural liquor space composed of the four ventricles (I–IV) and the connecting aqueduct which eventually leads to the canalis centralis of the medulla spinalis, see p. 312.

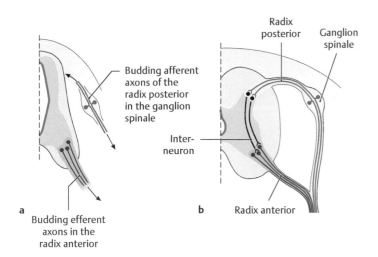

C Development of a nervus spinalis

Afferent (blue) and efferent (red) axons sprout separately from the cell bodies of neurons during the early developmental stage.

a The primary afferent (sensory) neurons develop in the spinal (sensory) ganglion, the α-motor neurons (cornu anterius motor cells) develop in the basal plate of the spinal cord.

b The interneurons (black), which form a functional connection between the two neuron types, develop at a later stage.

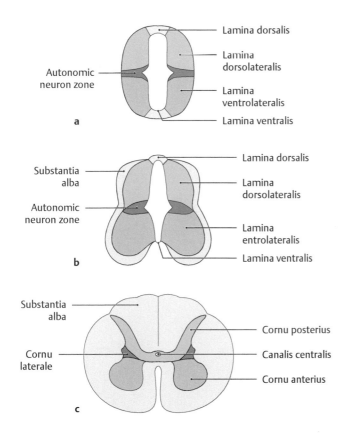

D Differentiation of the tubus neuralis in the medulla spinalis region during embryonic development

Cross-section, cranial view.

a Early tubus neuralis development; **b** Intermediate stage; **c** Adult medulla spinalis.

Neurons that originate in the lamina ventrolateralis of the spinal cord anlage are efferent (motor) neurons; neurons that originate in the lamina dorsolateralis, are afferent (sensory) neurons. In between—in the eventual thoracic, lumbar and sacral regions—lies an additional zone, from which the autonomic neurons originate. Laminae dorsalis and ventralis do not form neurons.

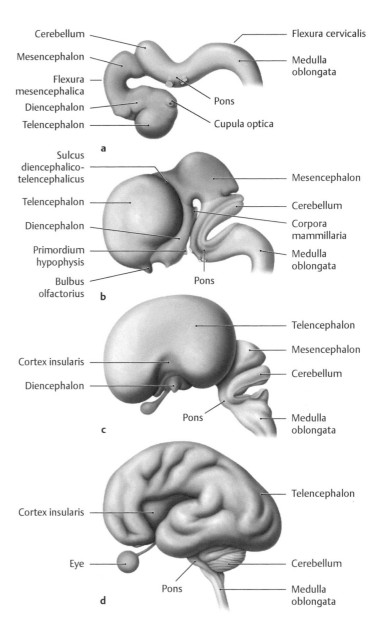

E Development of the encephalon from the tubus neuralis

a Embryo at a crown-rump-length of 10 cm, approx. second month of pregnancy. The eventual division of the encephalon (in its final form) is already visible:

- Red: endbrain or cerebrum (telencephalon)
- Dark yellow: interbrain (diencephalon)
- Dark blue: midbrain (mesencephalon)
- Light blue: cerebellum
- Gray: bridge (pons) and medulla oblongata

Note: Over the course of development, the telencephalon enlarges and covers all other regions of the brain.

b Fetus at a crown-rump-length of 27 mm, approx. third month of pregnancy. Telencephalon and diencephalon enlarge, the bulbus olfactorius develops in the telencephalon, the hypophysis (pituitary) anlage appears in the diencephalon.

c Fetus at a crown-rump-length of 53 mm, approx. fourth month of pregnancy. The telencephalon begins to overgrow the other brain sections. The insula, which later will be covered by the two hemispheria cerebri, is still located at the brain's surface (cf. **d**).

d Fetus at a crown-rump-length of 133 mm, approx. sixth month of pregnancy. Fissurae and gyri begin to form in the hemispherium cerebri.

1.5 Nervous System in situ

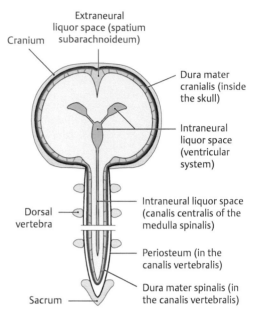

Extraneural liquor space (spatium subarachnoideum)

Cranium

Dura mater cranialis (inside the skull)

Intraneural liquor space (ventricular system)

Intraneural liquor space (canalis centralis of the medulla spinalis)

Dorsal vertebra

Periosteum (in the canalis vertebralis)

Dura mater spinalis (in the canalis vertebralis)

Sacrum

A Nervous system in situ

A simplified schematic diagram of the CNS and its surroundings, frontal cut. Like any other tissue or organ, the nervous system is built into the overall structure of the human body. This integration is achieved through specific types of connective tissue, which help to provide mechanical protection against strain on the nervous system:

- **CNS:** encephalon and medulla spinalis are located in cavities encased in bone, the cavitas cranii and the canalis vertebralis, respectively. The connective tissue responsible for their integration into the body are the meninges. These membranes completely cover the encephalon and medulla spinalis and can be divided into 3 different layers (see **B**). Meninges of the encephalon

and medulla spinalis define a space which is filled with a watery fluid (liquor cerebrospinalis). This extraneural liquor space (spatium subarachnoideum) can in topographic terms be contrasted with the intraneural liquor space (ventricular system within the CNS). Bony cavities, meninges, and the spatium subarachnoideum define the integration of the CNS into the body (for details see **B** and **C**).

- **PNS:** (not shown here, see **D**) has its nerves and ganglia surrounded by connective tissue, and as such is directly built into the body's cavities also lined with connective tissue. The outer layer of connective tissue (epineurium), communicates with the structures of the body also enveloped by connective tissue.

B The CNS and surrounding structures: The meninges

The calvarium has been removed. Superior view of the meninges; **a** and **b** Brain in situ; **c** View of the dural folds after brain has been removed; **d** Layers of meninges. The meninges of the brain and spinal cord—from outer to inner layer—are divided into

- **Dura mater (pachymeninx),** outermost layer surrounding the encephalon and medulla spinalis consists of tough, collagenous connective tissue. At the nerves' exit and entry points respectively, the dura mater merges with the epineurium covering these peripheral nerves. The dura mater participates in the formation of specialized sinus venosi, the intracranial sinus durae matris. In addition, one of its inward-directed folds (dural fold), the falx cerebri, connects to the tentorium cerebelli and separates the two cerebral hemispheres incompletely dividing the cranial cavity into compartments (see illustration **B**, p. 298). The dura mater does not form similar structures in the medulla spinalis where it forms only the outermost layer.

- **Leptomeninx,** which in addition to collagen fibers is composed of epithelioid cells (meningeal cells). No equivalent exists in the peripheral nerve. The leptomeninx itself divides into two layers:

  - Arachnoidea mater: It lies between the dura mater and the
  - pia mater: It is the innermost layer, intimately attached to the surface of the brain or spinal cord and is separated from the arachnoidea mater by the spatium subarachnoideum.

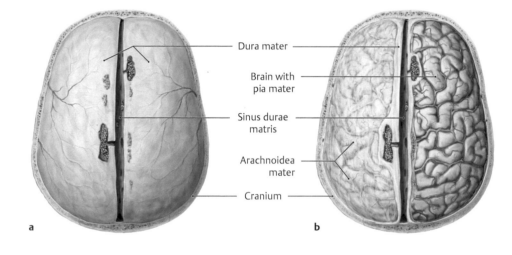

Dura mater

Brain with pia mater

Sinus durae matris

Arachnoidea mater

Cranium

a   b

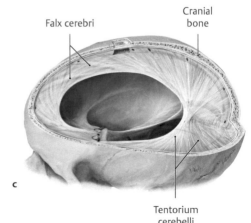

Falx cerebri

Cranial bone

c

Tentorium cerebelli

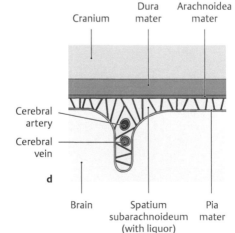

Cranium

Dura mater

Arachnoidea mater

Cerebral artery

Cerebral vein

d

Brain   Spatium subarachnoideum (with liquor)   Pia mater

Note: Generally, the sheaths covering the encephalon and medulla spinalis are analogous. However, the communication between the dura mater (outermost meningeal layer) and its environment in the cavitas cranii differs characteristically (and in clinically significant ways) when compared to the canalis vertebra-

lis. In the cavitas cranii, the endosteal (inner) layer of the dura mater also forms the inner periosteum of the cranial bone whereas in the canalis vertebralis, a real space—the spatium epidurale—separates the dura mater from the vertebral periosteum (for more details, see **D**, p. 311).

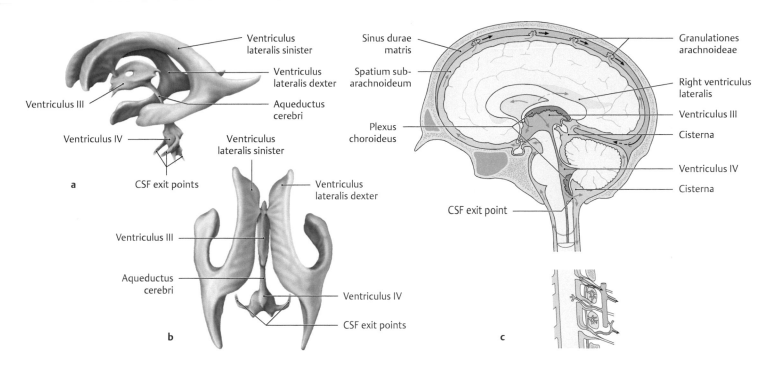

C The CNS and surrounding structures: Subarachnoid space

Ventricular System, left anterior view (**a**) and superior view (**b**); Schematic sagittal section through the encephalon with extraneural liquor space (**c**).

The spatium subarachnoideum, which surrounds both the encephalon and the medulla spinalis, lies between the arachnoidea mater and pia mater. Topographically, it represents the extraneural liquor space which is connected with the intraneural liquor space—the ventricular system composed of four ventriculi and aqueductus (in the encephalon) and the canalis centralis (in the medulla spinalis).

- In the four ventriculi of the **ventricular system,** cerebrospinal fluid (CSF; liquor cerebrospinalis) is continuously produced in functionally specialized blood vessels, the plexus choroideus. Due to the pressure gradient, liquor cerebrospinalis exits the ventriculus quartus, located in the truncus encephali, through specialized openings and flows into the spatium subarachnoideum. The red-colored areas in (**b**) mark the

junction/continuity of the ventricular system with the spatium subarachnoideum.
- In the spatium subarachnoideum, the liquor cerebrospinalis is constantly reabsorbed (lost) into the dural venous system through functionally specialized structures—the granulationes arachnoideae. Liquor cerebrospinalis is being constantly produced.

The cavity of the tubus neuralis and its folding forms the ventricular system and gives it its distinct shape (see **A**, p. 272). The spatium subarachnoideum is a result of the of the CNS being enveloped by the meningeal layers. Its distinct shape is derived from the form of the encephalon and medulla oblongata and how they are surrounded by the meninges. The convex surface of the brain does not conform everywhere to the internal concave surface of the cranium which leads to the creation of topographically characteristic "enlargements" of the spatia subarachnoidea, the cisternae. They do not serve a particular function but are the inevitable result of two shapes that are not wholly congruent.

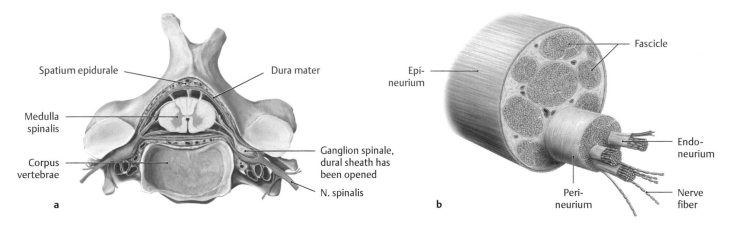

D The peripheral nerve and surrounding structures: The epineurium

a Cut through the canalis vertebralis with medulla spinalis; **b** Peripheral nerve, "pulled out like a telescope." The medulla spinalis (**a**) is surrounded by meninges in the same way as the brain (see **B**). It is clearly visible that

- the dura mater (red in **a**) merges with the epineurium of the peripheral nerve,
- the dura mater spinalis (unlike the dura mater cranialis) is not firmly attached to the bone or the inner periosteum. There is a distinct epidural space filled with fat and a venous plexus.

The peripheral nerve has a cable-like structure. Its outer surface is completely covered by connective tissue, the epineurium. The nerve is comprised of fascicles (nerve fiber bundles) which are covered by their own connective tissue sheath—the perineurium. In the fascicles, individual nerve fibers are covered by endoneurium. In nn. craniales and spinales, the epineurium is the continuation of dura mater. The connective tissue sheath that surrounds the peripheral ganglion corresponds to the epineurium.

1.6 Overview of the Brain: Telencephalon and Diencephalon

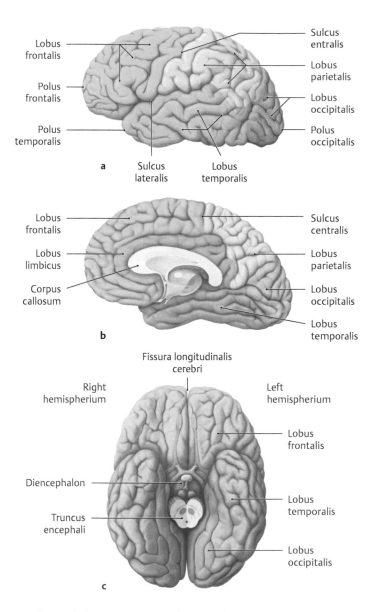

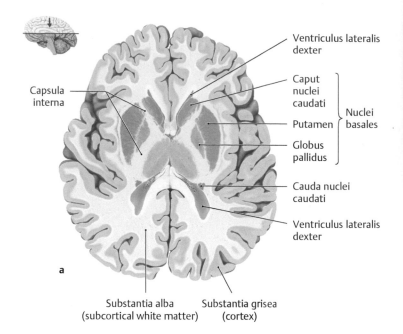

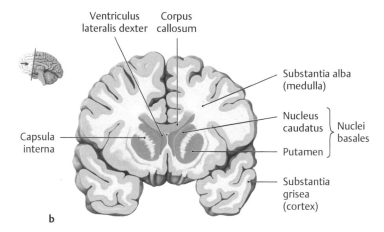

A Telencephalon: Overview and external structure

a Telencephalon, left lateral view; **b** Right hemispherium, left lateral view; **c** Telencephalon, basal view.

The telencephalon is the largest and most complex part of the CNS where the highest level of integration occurs in information processing. All complex motor functions, all perceptions as well as the emergence of consciousness, are tied to the functional integrity of the brain. With regard to morphology, the telencephalon is divided into two almost symmetric hemispheres which are incompletely separated by a longitudinal fissure. Each of the two hemiphere consists of six lobes: the lobi frontalis, temporalis, occipitalis, parietalis, limbicus, et insularis. Each of the first three lobes terminate in a pole. Characteristic deep furrows, or sulci, define most of the borders between lobes. The surface of each lobe is made up of folds or gyri, which in part are named for the lobe in which they are located. The insula (insular lobe) is located deep on the lateral surface of the hemisphere as it is covered by other lobes. It can only be viewed from the lateral aspect once the surrounding structures have been pushed aside (see p. 321). A medial view of the hemisphere includes gyri which are collectively referred to as the limbic lobe. Within the temporal lobe lies a part of the cortex called the hippocampus which is only visible after resection of surrounding parts of the brain (see **D**, p. 331).

B Telencephalon: Internal structure

a Horizontal cut, superior view; **b** Coronal cut, anterior view.

Like the entire CNS, the telencephalon consists of substantia grisea and alba:

- Substantia grisea forms the entire outer layer or cortex.
- Beneath the cortex lies the substantia alba or medulla.
- Embedded in the medulla are additional isolated islands of substantia grisea or nuclei. A nucleus is typically an aggregation of neurons in the CNS that have a similar function. An example would be the nuclei basales (nucleus caudatus, putamen, globus pallidus).

Portions of the ventricular system—the ventriculi laterales—are also visible in a horizontal cut. The substantia alba, the macroscopic appearance of which is largely homogeneous, can be functionally divided into tractus, which depending on their course can be further differentiated. The capsula interna is a white matter structure in which numerous tracts concerned with carrying sensory and motor infomation are closely grouped together. Phylogenetically, the cortex can be divided into paleocortex (the oldest part of the cortex cerebri), archicortex and neocortex (the most recent part of the cortex cerebri). The neocortex forms the largest part of the cortex. All parts of the cortex cerebri consist of multiple layers of neurons but there are microscopic differences between paleocortex, archicortex, and neocortex.

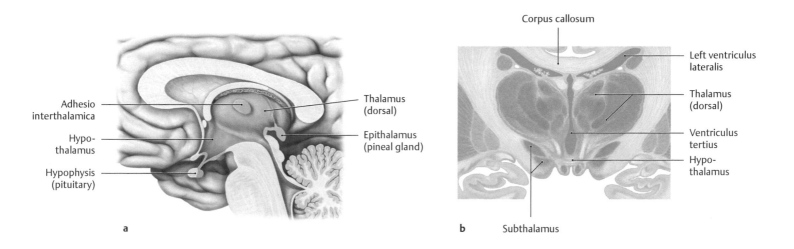

a — Mid-sagittal cut (left lateral view of right hemisphere)

Labels: Adhesio interthalamica; Hypo-thalamus; Hypophysis (pituitary); Thalamus (dorsal); Epithalamus (pineal gland)

b — Coronal cut, anterior view

Labels: Corpus callosum; Left ventriculus lateralis; Thalamus (dorsal); Ventriculus tertius; Hypo-thalamus; Subthalamus

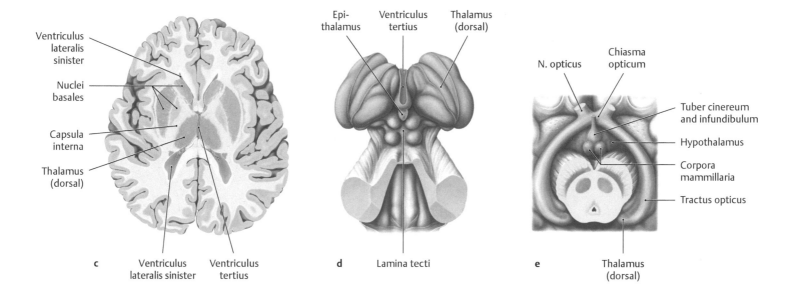

c — Horizontal cut, superior view

Labels: Ventriculus lateralis sinister; Nuclei basales; Capsula interna; Thalamus (dorsal); Ventriculus lateralis sinister; Ventriculus tertius

d — Superior and posterior view

Labels: Epi-thalamus; Ventriculus tertius; Thalamus (dorsal); Lamina tecti

e — View of the base of the diencephalon

Labels: N. opticus; Chiasma opticum; Tuber cinereum and infundibulum; Hypothalamus; Corpora mammillaria; Tractus opticus; Thalamus (dorsal)

C Diencephalon: Location and classification

a Mid-sagittal cut through the brain, left lateral view of the right hemisphere; **b** Coronal cut through the brain, anterior view; **c** Horizontal cut through the brain, superior view; **d** Superior and posterior view of the diencephalon; **e** View of the base of the diencephalon.

Topographically, the diencephalon consists of structures surrounding the ventriculus tertius found in the midline of the brain. During embryonic development, the diencephalon is covered by the fast growing hemispheria cerebri and sits above the truncus encephali. In an intact brain, only the very basal aspect of the diencephalon is visible. A mid-sagittal, coronal, or horizontal cut through the brain provides a good overview of the diencephalon using the ventriculus tertius as a reference point. Due to the location of the individual parts of the diencephalon related to the ventriculus tertius, none of the views allows for a complete overview where all the sections listed below are visible:

- In its upper section, the lateral wall of the ventriculus tertius is formed by a large paired structure, the **thalamus** (**a – d**). Both halves of the thalamus lie very closely together and occasionally touch in the region of the interthalamic adhesion (**a**). The thalamus relays sensory and motor signals to the cortex cerebri.
- The lower section of the lateral wall of the ventriculus tertius is formed by the **hypothalamus** (another region composed of nuclei) and the pituitary gland (hypophysis). The hypothalamus can be considered the primary autonomic control center for a number of body functions (blood pressure, water balance, temperature, food intake, hormone secretion).
- Lateral to the posterior part of hypothalamus, beneath the thalamus but not involved in forming the ventriculus, lies the **subthalamus** (**b**) a group of nuclei concerned with motor function.
- A small nuclear group—the epithalamus—is located superior and posterior to the thalamus (**d**). One of its components is the gl. pinealis. Both structures are involved in photoperiodic regulation.
- Looking at the intact diencephalon from below, at the base of the hypothalamus the hypophysis as well as a group of nuclei, the **corpora mammillaria** are visible. Also visible from below are the n. opticus, chiasma opticum and the tractus opticus—a portion of the visual pathway. All three structures are part of the diencephalon.
- The roof of the ventriculus tertius is formed by the body of the fornix, a pair of crura forming a pathway that extends on each side from the hippocampus (a part of the lobus temporalis of the cortex cerebri) to the hypothalamus.

Note: The capsula interna delineates the topographical border between the diencephalon and telencephalon.

1.7 Overview of the Brain: Brainstem (Truncus Encephali) and Cerebellum

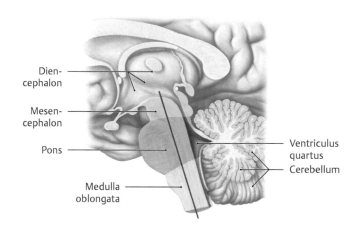

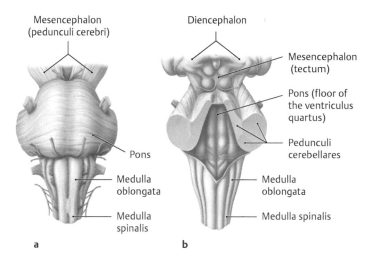

a   b

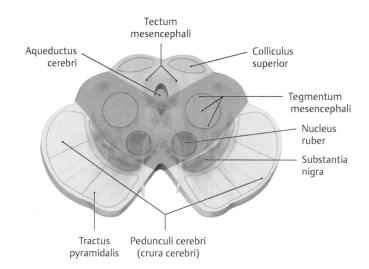

A Truncus encephali: Location and structure
Mid-sagittal cut through the brain, left lateral view.
In an intact brain, the truncus encephali is visible only from basal aspect since laterally and posteriorly it is surrounded by the cerebellum and the lobi temporales. It has an elongated shape which in situ has a cranial-caudal orientation that is ventrally slanted. The axis of the truncus encephali is described using the same terms of location and direction used for the longitudinal body axis. The truncus encephali consists of three brain sections, which from cranial to caudal are the mesencephalon, pons, and medulla oblongata. The cerebellum, which is not part of the truncus encephali, is located dorsal to the truncus encephali and attached to it by the pedunculi cerebellares. Inside the skull, the truncus encephali lies close to the clivus, a region of the os occipitale.

B Truncus encephali: External structure
The external structure of the brainstem is shaped by nuclei or pathways located within the structure. Visible from the outside in a **ventral view** (**a**) are

- the pedunculi cerebri (crura cerebri), composed of tracts descending to the pons, medulla oblongata and medulla spinalis,
- the pars basilaris pontis, containing a large tract that enters the cerebellum,
- the pyramis medullae oblongatae (formed by the tractus pyramidalis), and
- the oliva (a group of nuclei).

In **dorsal view** (**b**, visible only after the cerebellum has been removed):

- the lamina quadrigemina (tectum), with two paired nuclear groups for auditory and visual function, forming the roof plate (lamina tecti) of the mesencephalon,
- the medulla oblongata with two paired tubercula formed by the posterior funiculus nuclei,
- intersection of the three paired pedunculi cerebellares which border the truncus encephali and between which lies the diamond-shaped base of the ventriculus quartus (fossa rhomboidea). The fossa rhomboidea is formed partially by the pons and partially by the medulla oblongata.

Note: The truncus encephali is the point of entry and emergence for all true nn. craniales (for classification see p. 112 ff). Of the twelve pairs of nn. craniales, two nn. craniales (I: n. olfactorius and II: n. opticus) are not structurally nerves but tracts of the CNS (not shown here, because they don't emerge from the truncus encephali).

C Truncus encephali: Compartmental organization and internal structure
Cross-section of truncus encephali, superior view.
In anteroposterior direction, the truncus encephali can be divided into four segments. Although they can be found in all segments of the truncus encephali to a greater or lesser degree, they are most prominent in the mesencephalon. The terms for describing these segments in pons and medulla oblongata differ.

- The base, which at the mesencephalon appears as the pair of pedunculi cerebri (crura), is located ventrally. The base of the truncus encephali usually contains large motor tracts descending to the truncus encephali and the cerebellum, (e.g., the tractus pyramidalis). A continuous band of substantia grisea, the substantia nigra, is located directly above the pedunculi cerebri.
- Continuing dorsally, the base and substantia nigra is followed by the tegmentum mesencephali. Large groups of nuclei are found here that serve different functions (particularly prominent is the nucleus ruber). Multiple ascending (sensory) tracts to the telencephalon (over the thalamus in the diencephalon) and the cerebellum and a few descending tracts to the medulla spinalis also occupy the tegmentum.
- The tectum mesencephali sits dorsal to the tegmentum. Depending on its location in the mesencephalon it is either called lamina tecti or due to its distinct shape (see **Bb**) the lamina quadrigemina. This roof region contains two superior colliculi and two inferior colliculi, which play an important role in the visual and auditory pathways.
- Each section of the truncus encephali contains part of the ventricular system. In the mesencephalon this is the aqueductus cerebri.

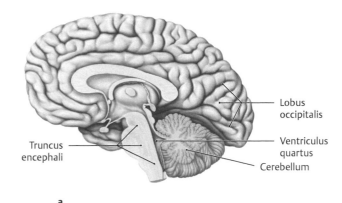

a

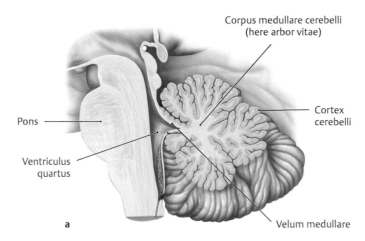

a

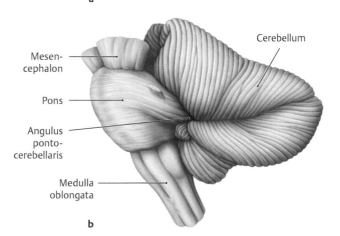

b

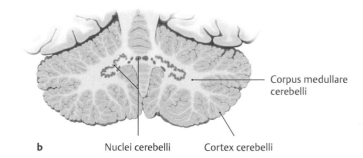

b

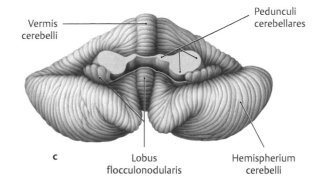

c

E Cerebellum: Internal structure

a Midsagittal cut through the cerebellum; left lateral view of the right hemispherium cerebelli; **b** Oblique section through the cerebellum; superior view.

Similar to the telencepahlon, the cerebellar vermis and hemispheri contain centrally located substantia alba (or medulla), surrounded by substantia grisea in the form of the cortex. The morphological appearance of medulla and cortex in a midsagittal section is called the abor vitae (tree of life). Embedded within the white matter are four paired deep nuclei cerebelli, composed of substantia grisea. The cerebellum is concerned with multiple functions including the unconscious control of balance and fine motor skills.

D Cerebellum: Positional relationship and external structure

a Midsagittal cut through truncus encephali and cerebellum, left lateral view of the right hemisphere; **b** Left lateral view of truncus encephali and cerebellum; **c** Cerebellum, anterior view after detachment from truncus encephali

The cerebellum is located dorsal to the truncus encephali and forms the roof of the ventriculus quartus (**a**). It lies beneath the lobus occipitalis of the telencephalon from which it is separated by a dural fold—the tentorium cerebelli (not shown here, see p. 274). Inside the skull, the cerebellum is situated in the fossa cranii posterior. Between the truncus encephali and cerebellum on both sides is a recess—the angulus pontocerebellaris (**b**) which is of clinical significance.

Like the telencephalon, the cerebellum consists of two hemispheria, which are separated by an unpaired vermis (**c**). The surface of hemispheria and vermis shows furrow-like depressions, the fissurae, which separate the very thin folia from one another. Fissurae and folia of the cerebellum correspond to the sulci and gyri of the telencephalon. Fissurae divide the cerebellum into lobi. The lobus flocculonodularis (**b**) one of the main subdivisions of the cerebellum, is located inferiorly and consists of the paired flocculi, their pedunculi, and the nodule of the vermis. All tracts to and from the cerebellum pass through the three paired pedunculi cerebellares.

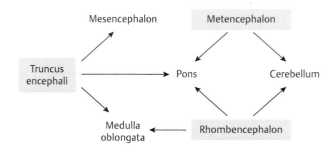

F Cerebellum and truncus encephali: Terminological peculiarities

Topographically, the cerebellum is not part of the truncus encephali, yet phylogenetically is derived from it. The pons and cerebellum are collectively known as the metencephalon. The combination of pons, cerebellum and medulla oblongata, the structures which surround the diamond-shaped ventriculus quartus, is called the hindbrain or rhombencephalon.

1.8 Overview of the Spinal Cord (Medulla Spinalis)

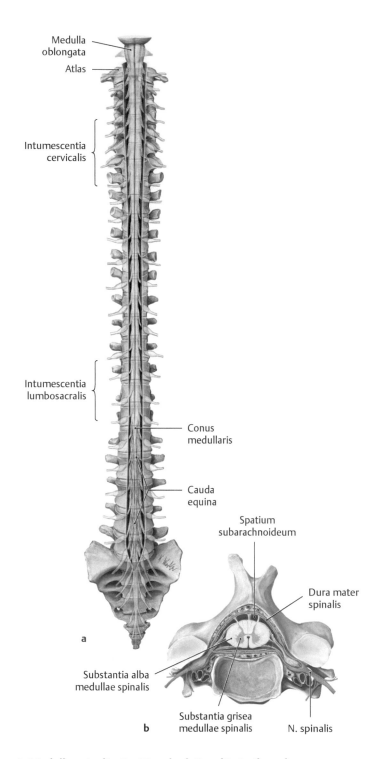

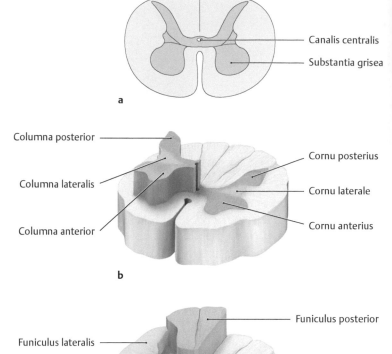

B Medulla spinalis: Internal structure

a Cross-section of the medulla spinalis, superior view; **b** Schematic, three-dimensional representation of the medulla spinalis with substantia grisea (**b**) and substantia alba (**c**) being highlighted; left anterior oblique and superior view. The medulla spinalis shows all characteristic structures of the CNS:

- **substantia grisea,** which in cross-section appears butterfly-shaped and typically is divided into a
  - cornu anterius,
  - cornu posterius (though only in the area surrounding the partes thoracica and sacral medullae spinalis), and
  - cornu laterale.

  All cornua substantiae griseae are paired, making the medulla spinalis symmetrical. The substantia grisea contains neurons. The three-dimensional representation (**b**) shows that the term "cornu" is used to describe the three-dimensional nature of the columnae anterior, posterior, and lateralis of substantia grisea. At the central core of substantia grisea lies part of the ventricular system, the canalis centralis of the medulla spinalis. The substantia grisea of the medulla spinalis is surrounded by

- **substantia alba,** which is composed of tracts (funiculi) clearly visible in the three-dimensional representation (**c**) which are analogous to the columnae griseae and are called the funiculi anterior, posterior, and lateralis. Occasionally, funiculi anterior and lateralis are collectively called the anterolateral funiculus.

A Medulla spinalis: Positional relationship in the columna vertebralis

a Ventral (anterior) view of the opened medulla spinalis; **b** Cross-section of a vertebra and the medulla spinalis.

The spinal cord (medulla spinalis) lies within the canalis vertebralis, which is formed by the foramina vertebralia of all the vertebrae stacked on top of one another and the ligaments of the columna vertebralis traversing the vertebrae. The medulla spinalis which is the most caudal part of the CNS, extends caudally from the first vertebra cervicalis, called the atlas, to the second vertebra lumbalis. From there, only certain parts of the medulla spinalis, the roots, extend further caudally. They are equivalent to the nn. spinales (see **D**) and are part of the PNS. Within the canalis vertebralis the medulla spinalis, as part of the CNS, is also surrounded by meninges and the spatium subarachnoideum (see p. 311).

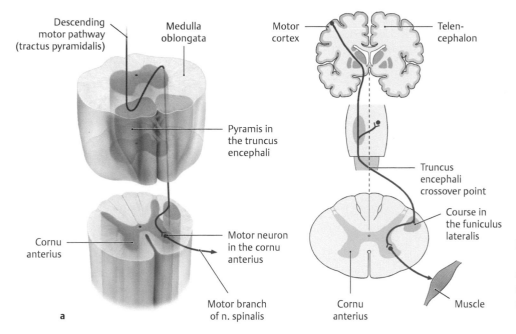

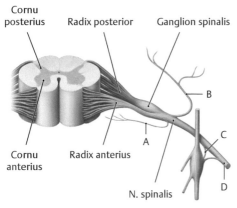

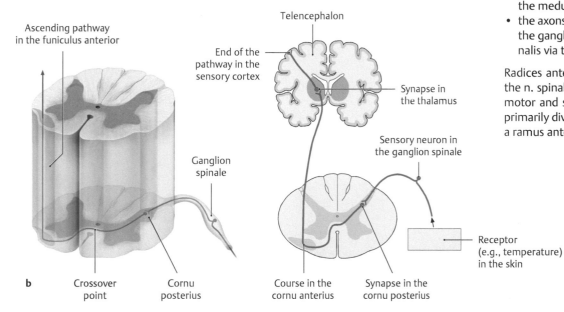

a

b Crossover point   Cornu posterius   Course in the cornu anterius   Synapse in the cornu posterius

D Relationship between CNS and PNS at the medulla spinalis

Cross section of medulla spinalis, anterior oblique and superior view. All parts of the PNS are in green.

- The axons of motor neurons, located in the cornu anterius, exit the anterior portion of the medulla spinalis via the radix anterior.
- the axons of the sensory neurons, located in the ganglion spinalis, enter the medulla spinalis via the radix posterior.

Radices anterior and posterior merge to form the n. spinalis which is mixed, containing both motor and sensory modalities. The n. spinalis primarily divides into a ramus posterior (**B**) and a ramus anterior (**D**).

C Tractus of the medulla spinalis

The tractus of the medulla spinalis run within the funiculi substantiae albae (see **Bc**). Depending on their course, they are either descending (**a**) or ascending (**b**). Descending tractus mainly affect motor function and usually originate in the higher centers of the CNS, such as the motor cortex of the cortex cerebri. Ascending tractus typically serve sensory functions and transmit the information of a sensory receptor to higher centers in the CNS.

a One example of a motor tract is the tractus corticospinalis lateralis, or motor tract of the funiculus lateralis, and as shown here is responsible for voluntary motor function. It originates in the (motor) cortex cerebri and runs within the funiculi anterior and lateralis of the medulla spinalis and extends to the cornu anterius where it terminates and projects to a motor neuron of the medulla spinalis. From this motor neuron originates the radix motorius of a nerve, which extends to the skeletal muscle;

b displays a sensory pathway, which runs within the anterolateral system of the medulla spinalis. It comes from the skin and extends to the (somatosensory) cortex cerebri passing through intermediate regions (mainly the thalamus in the diencephalon). The first neuron of this tract lies in the ganglion spinale and is therefore a neuron of the peripheral nervous system.

The course of both pathways helps illustrate the particular role of the medulla spinalis as a "conductor for information" between the CNS and PNS:

- The first sensory neuron with the body (in the ganglion spinale), the axons of which enters the CNS
- The alpha (lower) motor neuron in the cornu anterius of the CNS, the axon of which extends in the PNS

However, the medulla spinalis as part of the CNS can exercise its own integrative function, playing an important role in reflexes. For this purpose, the medulla spinalis contains intersegmental fibers (lateral proper fasciculi, not shown here) located in the white matter, which are responsible for relaying information within the medulla spinalis without exiting it. These are intersegmental fibers which arise from cells in the gray matter, and, after a longer or shorter course, reenter the gray matter and ramify in it. In terms of their function, the tracts running through the medulla spinalis are called extrinsic apparatus and the intersegmental fibers intrinsic apparatus. Knowledge of location, course and function of tracts of the medulla spinalis is essential for understanding clinical symptoms in case of injuries to, or diseases of, the medulla spinalis.

1.9 Blood Supply of the Brain and Spinal Cord

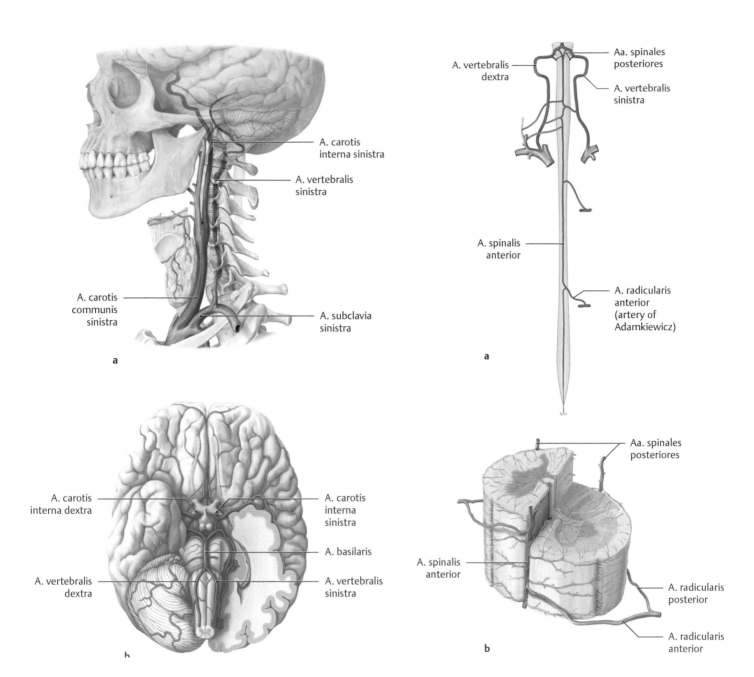

A Arterial supply to the encephalon

a Transparent skull viewed from the left; **b** Basal view of encephalon.
The encephalon has a very high demand for oxygen. While it represents only 2 % of the body's weight it receives 15 % of the cardiac output. The necessary blood supply is ensured by two paired arteries (**a**): The larger a. carotis interna and the smaller caliber a. vertebralis, which reach the cavitas cranii by passing through the canalis caroticus and the foramen magnum respectively. At the base of the brain—within the spatium subarachnoideum—the branches of these four arteries merge to form a vascular ring, the circulus arteriosus cerebri (of Willis) (**b**): The circulus arterius cerebri gives off branches that supply the encephalon (e.g., aa. cerebri or aa. cerebelli are all off the aa. vertebrales and a. basilaris, not off the circulus). Note that the circulus arteriosus cerebri is essentially fed by 3 main vessels—the two aa. carotides internae (sinister and dexter) and the a. basilaris formed by the fusion of the two aa. vertebrales (sinister and dexter). The blood supply from these three sources is connected by aa. communicantes posteriores and anteriores that result in the formation of the circulus arteriosus cerebri. In case of impaired circulation, the merging of these arteries in a vascular ring, to a certain extent allows for compensation of decreased blood flow in one vessel with increased blood flow through another vessel.

B Arterial supply to the medulla spinalis

a Schematic representation of blood supply to the medulla spinalis; **b** Cross-section of medulla spinalis, left lateral and superior view.
The great length of the medulla spinalis, which lies within the narrow canalis vertebralis, poses significant logistical problems with regard to blood supply. The medulla spinalis is supplied by various branches of the a. vertebralis on both sides (**a**). The a. spinalis anterior and aa. spinales posteriores extend from cranial to caudal. However, the ventricular filling pressure through the a. vertebralis is not sufficient to supply the entire medulla spinalis caudally. Segmentally derived smaller arteries, the aa. radiculares anterior and posterior, derived from the aa. intercostales, reach the medulla spinalis and constantly supply the aa. spinales. From cranial to caudal direction (due to the decreasing filling pressure in this direction by the a. vertebralis), these small segmental arteries become increasingly important. The goal is to guarantee a sufficient supply to the aa. spinales which extend the length of the medulla spinalis and send their branches into the medulla spinalis (**b**).

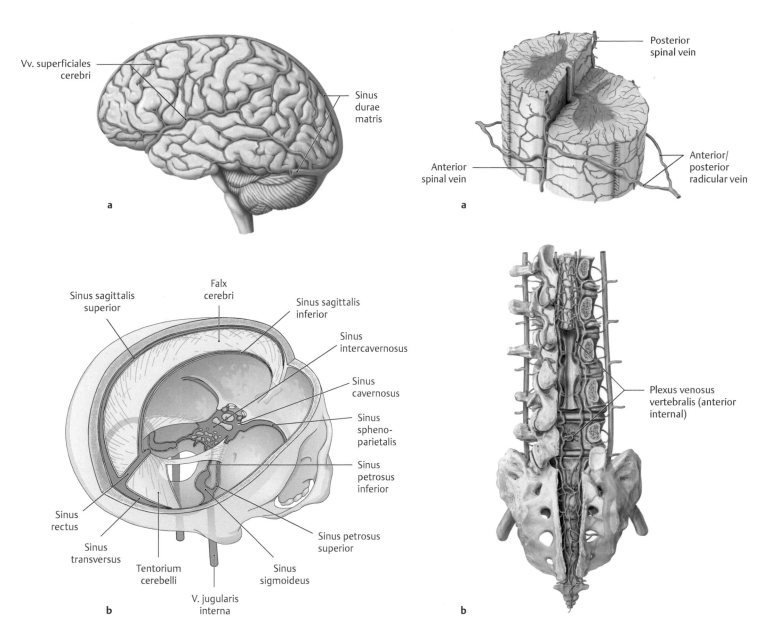

C Venous drainage of the encephalon

a Schematic representation of vv. superficiales cerebri, lateral view; **b** View of the sinus durae matris system, right, posterosuperior view of the skull after the calvarium has been removed.

Vv. superficiales cerebri collect and direct the blood to a series of venous sinuses generally, but not always, formed in the attached edges of dural folds in the cavitas cranii. These sinus durae matris are formed by separation of the two layers of dura generally unseparable except in these regions. Unlike true veins, there is no muscle tissue found in the walls of these venous sinuses, the dura is lined internally by only a layer of endothelium. Vv. profundae cerebri (not visible here) collect the blood from deeper brain regions and take it to the sinus durae matris system. The sinus durae matris system delivers the collected blood mainly to the v. jugularis interna that forms at the foramen jugulare of the cavitas cranii. In a similar fashion to the the true veins of the head, the sinus durae matris do not have valves. Blood can flow in either direction exclusively controlled by the existing pressure gradient.

Note: Sinus durae matris are found only in the encephalon and not in the medulla spinalis, even though dura mater also exists in the medulla spinalis. The connection between the sinus durae matris system and true veins outside the skull allow bacteria to enter the skull from outside even without injury to the bone or the meninges (see p. 385).

D Venous drainage of the medulla spinalis

a Cross-section of the medulla spinalis, left, anterior and superior view; **b** Anterior view of the canalis vertebralis which has been opened and the medulla spinalis.

The venous blood of the medulla spinalis is collected by the vv. spinales anteriores and posteriores and delivered to large plexus venosi located in the the spatium epidurale of the canalis vertebralis or directly to the vv. intercostales. Unlike the encephalon in the skull, there is no sinus durae matris system surrounding the medulla spinalis within the canalis vertebralis.

Note: The complex venous system of the plexus venosi vertebrales contains many more veins than what would be required for routine blood drainage supporting medulla spinalis metabolism. This plexus system serves an additional function acting as a pressure equalizer in the canalis vertebralis. By moving large amounts of blood between plexus venosi vertebrales internales and externales (both of which have no valves), fluctuations in blood pressure in the canalis vertebralis can be accommodated (see **B** and **C,** p. 417).

1.10 Somatic Sensation

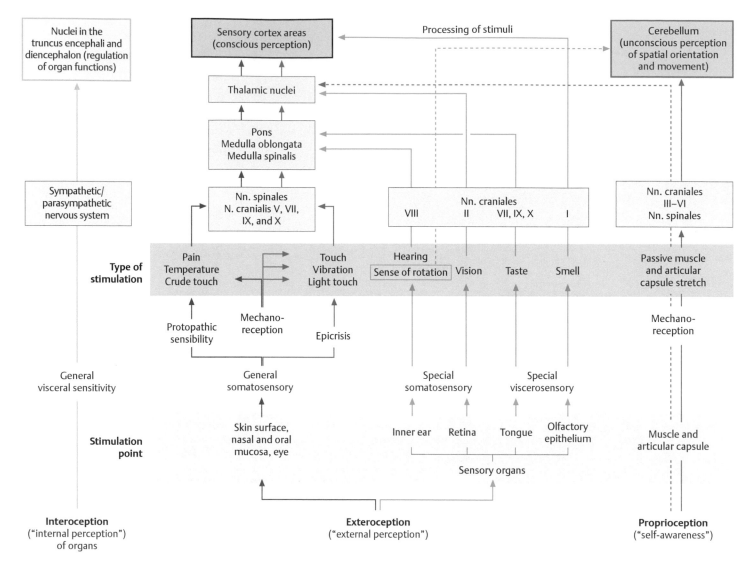

A Somatic sensation: Classification and overview

There are two kinds of sensation: somatic and visceral. The common visceral sensation—the processing of stimuli from viscera inside the body (interoception)—is explained on p. 297 along with visceral motor function and is only mentioned here for the sake of completeness. Somatic sensation can be distinguished based on location and type of stimulus. This distinction is important because the location and type determines the pathway via which the somatic signals are transmitted.

- Sensory signals originating on the skin, the tunica mucosa nasi or oris, or the ocular surface (not vision) are referred to as external perception (exteroception, superficial/cutaneous sensation).
- If the stimulus location is a stretch receptor (strain measurement) within a muscle, a tendon or an articular capsule, it is referred to as proprioception—deep sensation of the musculoskeletal system important for controlling the body position sense.

Classification based on type of stimulus: Only the external perception, meaning exteroception, is further divided into

- epicritic sensation (sense of touch, vibration, light touch, light pressure (or subtle mechanoreception) is contrasted with
- protopathic sensation (pain, temperature, crude mechanical stimuli) or crude mechanoreception.

Although proprioception is a form of mechanoreception, it is not further differentiated.

Both exteroception and proprioception are conveyed via nn. spinales (information from torso, neck, limbs) or in the case of the head, the n. trigeminus.

Perception through the sensory organs is ultimately a form of exteroception (red) and therefore a form of somatic sensation. It is transmitted exclusively via nn. craniales. However, for phylogenic reasons, not all sensory organs and their perception are referred to as somatic sensation. Regarding the sensory organs, chemical stimuli (taste, smell) and electromagnetic waves (optics) in addition to mechanic stimuli (acoustics) play a role.

The different ways of processing stimuli in the CNS—conscious or subconscious—is a factor in distinguishing various types of sensation. For a sensory stimulus to reach consciousness (conscious sensation), it has to reach the sensory cortex of the telencephalon. Usually, the stimuli are conveyed via the thalamus. Sensory stimuli, which are not transmitted to the cortex cerebri, but only reach other, secondary regions of the CNS are not perceived consciously (unconscious sensation). In addition to location and type of stimulus, the final destination of the signal transmission can be distinguished in sensory stimuli. Analogous to somatomotor function, specific terms for specific sensory perceptions are used to describe somatic sensation.

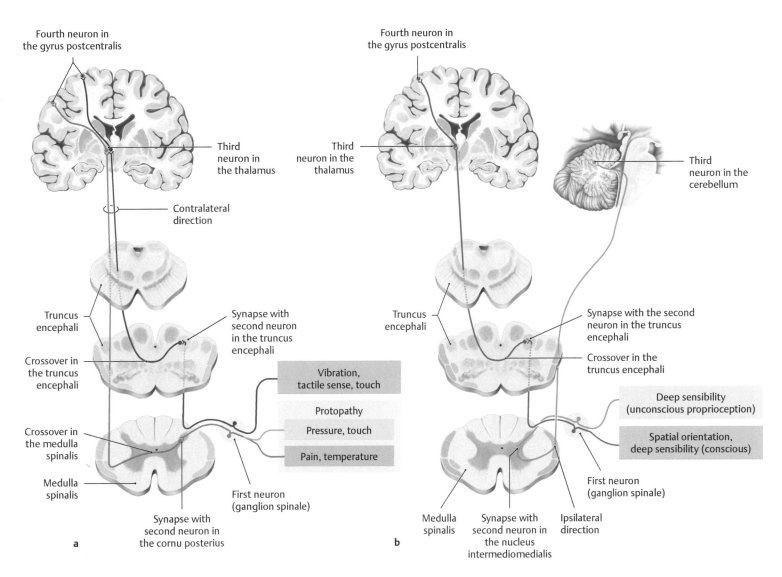

Fourth neuron in the gyrus postcentralis

Third neuron in the thalamus

Contralateral direction

Truncus encephali

Crossover in the truncus encephali

Crossover in the medulla spinalis

Medulla spinalis

Synapse with second neuron in the truncus encephali

Vibration, tactile sense, touch

Protopathy

Pressure, touch

Pain, temperature

First neuron (ganglion spinale)

Synapse with second neuron in the cornu posterius

a

Fourth neuron in the gyrus postcentralis

Third neuron in the thalamus

Truncus encephali

Synapse with the second neuron in the truncus encephali

Crossover in the truncus encephali

Third neuron in the cerebellum

Deep sensibility (unconscious proprioception)

Spatial orientation, deep sensibility (conscious)

First neuron (ganglion spinale)

Medulla spinalis

Synapse with second neuron in the nucleus intermediomedialis

Ipsilateral direction

b

B Somatic sensation: Interconnections and the anatomical structures involved

The CNS, PNS and a receptor are involved in somatic sensation.

a Transmission of a sensory stimulus from the skin to the telencephalon (epicritic and protopathic, conscious perception)
b Transmission of a signal from skeletal muscle (stretch in muscle), which is perceived via specialized stretch receptors (proprioception) to the cerebellum (unconscious) and to the telencephalon (conscious)

A n. cranialis or spinalis transmits the signal from the respective sensory receptor. The impulse is conveyed to the CNS, via afferent transmission. Like the motor neurons, the somatic neurons are numbered and defined using a signal chronology:

• Four neurons carry information to the telencephalon (conscious).
• Three neurons carry information to the cerebellum (unconscious).

In each instance, the first neuron in the PNS lies in a ganglion spinale or a ganglion nervi cranialis (not shown here), the second neuron is located in the CNS (medulla spinalis or the nuclei trunci encephali). From this point, the number of neurons differ. The reason for an additional neuron carrying information to the telencephalon is that all impulses conducted by neurons to the telencephalon first pass through a particular group of nuclei located in the diencephalon—the thalamus. This is the central relay station for conscious sensation, and also plays an important role in filtering information ("what has the highest priority?"). The third neuron is found In the thalamus (the "filter neuron"). The fourth neuron is the sensory endpoint. It is located in the gyrus postcentralis

of the telencepahlon. For signals that are relayed to the cerebellum, by only three neurons, the third neuron lies in the cerebellar cortex.
Note: Signals to the cerebellum don't pass through the thalamus and are therefore relayed by only three neurons.
Pain, temperature, and crude mechanoreception (pressure) of the skin and tunicae mucosae are transmitted in the medulla spinalis via the sensory tractus spinothalamicus. Subtle mechanoreception (vibration, light touch) is transmitted in the medulla spinalis via the funiculus posterior (fasciculus gracilis and cuneatus).
Note:

• All tracts that carry exteroceptive impulses cross over to the opposite side in the CNS. It is always the axon of the second neuron that crosses over. Thus, a stimulus in the left arm will pass through the thalamus and be relayed to, and received by, the right cortex cerebri.
• In the medulla spinalis, proprioceptive impulses are mainly transmitted via the tractus spinocerebellaris. First and second neurons lie in the ganglion spinale or in the medulla spinalis; the axon of the second neuron reaches a third neuron in the cerebellar cortex. This information processing is not conscious.

Within the head, all parts of somatic sensation pass via the n. trigeminus (CN V) and the tractus spinalis nervi trigemini.
Note: To a lesser extent, proprioceptive impulses can also be relayed to the cortex cerebri to perceive positional sense via the funiculus posterior: Epicrisis (as part of exteroception) and proprioception run parallel in the same tract, but terminate at different nuclei. For more details see p. 402 ff.

1.11 Somatomotor Function

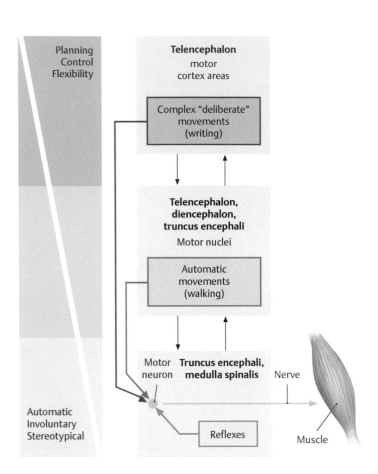

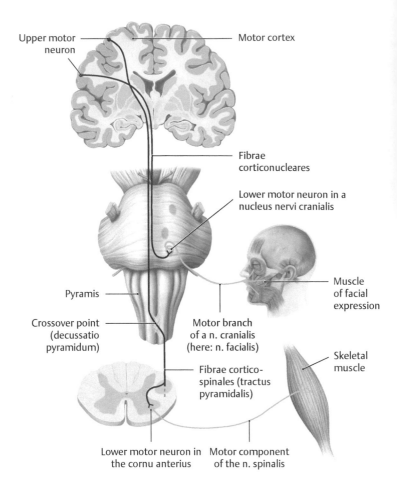

A Somatomotor function: An overview

The classification of somatomotor function is less complex than that of somatic sensation. Somatomotor function is the activation of skeletal muscle fibers. This process is mainly associated with the musculoskeletal system. However, muscles used for facial expression, mastication, or movement of the eyeball, are also skeletal muscle, but are in a stricter sense not part of the musculoskeletal system even if they move something such as the mandibula. Occasionally specific terms (see p. 112) are used to describe those specific somatomotor movements. Only the somatomotor function is described here; for visceromotor function, also refered to as organ motility see p. 296.

Somatomotor function can be characterized based on whether the movement happens entirely automatically or is deliberately controlled, both of which are linked to a high degree of flexibility in movement pattern.

Typically, movements are combinations of automatic movements and deliberate, controlled actions. All necessary interconnections in the CNS for such somatomotor functions share a common final segment/pathway: They terminate at a motor neuron which lies in the medulla spinalis (for nn. spinales) and in truncus encephali motor nuclei (for nn. craniales). This motor neuron sends signals to the muscle. Physiologically a distinction is drawn between α- and γ-motor neurons. To put it simply, the α-motor neuron causes muscle contractions that generate movement whereas the γ-motor neuron, independent of concrete movement, regulates normal muscle tone. The differing complexity of movements corresponds with the unequal participation of different complex parts of the nervous system concerned with interconnections. Simple reflexes occur only at the medulla spinalis level, the more complex voluntary motor functions involve particpation of the cortex cerebri and cerebellum.

B Somatomotor function: Neuronal wiring

The CNS and the PNS are involved in somatomotor function. Shown here is the deliberate activation of a muscle—the effector—by the telencephalon.

A neuron in the CNS sends a signal via its axon to another neuron in a different part of the CNS. This second neuron receives the signal and transmits it via its own axon through the PNS to the effector organ. Due to the direction of signal transmission (away from the CNS), it is considered to be an efferent transmission (see p. 266) and the participating neurons can be named in hierarchical order: upper and lower motor neurons. In the substantia alba of the CNS, the axons of many first neurons form a tract (e.g., cerebral or spinal cord tract). The axons of many second neurons, since they exit the CNS, form a nerve in the PNS (see **C** p. 295). The axon of the lower motor neuron terminates at the muscle in a specific structure at the motor endplate, where the signal transfer from nerve to muscle takes place.

The upper motor neuron lies in a motor area of the telencephalon in the motor cortex. A lower motor neuron found in the substantia grisea of the medulla spinalis has its axon reaching the muscle of the musculoskeletal system via a n. spinalis. If the lower motor neuron lies in a specific nucleus trunci encephali, its axon reaches the muscles of the head and neck, used for facial expression, mastication or movement of the eyeball and tongue, via a n. cranialis. Therefore, nn. craniales—but for a single exception—do not control the musculoskeletal system.

Note: The somatomotor system has only centrally located neurons. Only the axon of the lower motor neuron extends in the PNS.

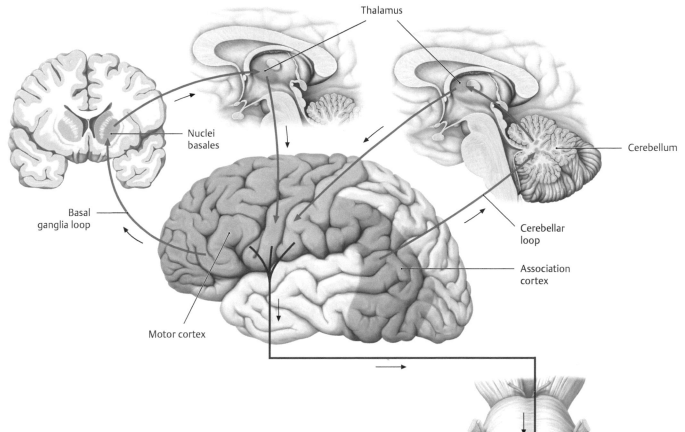

Thalamus

Nuclei basales

Basal ganglia loop

Motor cortex

Cerebellum

Cerebellar loop

Association cortex

C Somatomotor function: The anatomical structures involved

The general planning and initiation of movement takes place in different areas of the cortex cerebri, e.g., in the motor cortex and the association cortex. To eventually carry out the movement however, the participation of additional neuronal centers, such as the cerebellum (for balance control) and nuclei in other different brain regions is required. The latter are referred to as subcortical motor centers, since topographically, they are all located beneath the motor cortex. They include

- the nuclei basales in the telencephalon,
- motor areas of the thalamus in the diencephalon,
- the red nucleus (nucleus ruber), the substantia nigra (not shown here), and the oliva in the truncus encephali.

The subcortical motor centers are responsible for muscular coordination and fine motor control. Feedback loops link the cortex cerebri with the cerebellum and the nuclei basales. The tract of the motor cortex to the medulla spinalis, shown in fig. **B**, passes in the truncus encephali through a structure which, due to its shape, is called the pyramid (pyramis), the tract is referred to as the tractus pyramidalis. Tracts of the subcortical centers of the brainstem do not travel through the pyramid and are therefore called extrapyramidal tracts. Both types of tracts reach the medulla spinalis by descending and eventually terminating in the cornu anterius of the medulla spinalis at the neuron, the axon of which extends to the muscle. The tractus pyramidalis (fibrae corticospinales) is the tract which in the end generates movement. Extrapyramidal tracts of the subcortical centers in the brainstem play a role in planning and fine-tuning the movement.

Note: The fibrae corticonucleares, which like the fibrae corticospinales come from the motor cortex, terminate at motor nuclei of the truncus encephali, which functionally correspond to the cornua anteriora of the

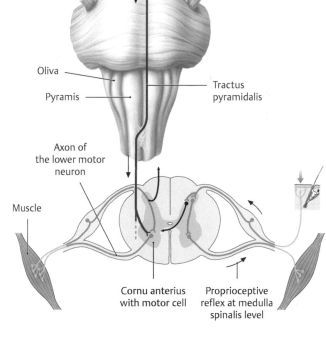

Oliva

Pyramis

Tractus pyramidalis

Axon of the lower motor neuron

Muscle

Cornu anterius with motor cell

Proprioceptive reflex at medulla spinalis level

medulla spinalis. They convey the same type of motor function as the fibrae corticospinales. However, they do not travel through the pyramid but terminate above it (the pyramid is located in the lowest part of the truncus encephali). Due to their analogous motor function, the fibrae corticonucleares are usually referred to as part of the tractus pyramidalis. The axons of the upper motor neuron typically cross. Motor impulses of the right hemispherium travel to the left side of the medulla spinalis and reach via the left n. spinalis, an effector organ located on the left side of the medulla spinalis. Very simple motor processes such as reflexes can be carried out directly at the medulla spinalis level (spinal cord reflexes) or the truncus encephali (brainstem reflexes) without including higher centers of the CNS.

1.12 Sensory Organs

Overview

Sensory organs are specialized for detecting stimuli. Specific receptors are grouped together forming the organ—a morphologically definable unit—and are not scattered across the skin. Typically, sensory organs are able to perceive very complex stimulus patterns, referred to as higher senses, contrasted to the more simple sensory functions performed by the skin. Detection of the stimulus, however, exhibits no difference between the sensory organs and sensory functions of the skin. However, detecting particularly complex stimuli, an ability that only sensory organs have, in most cases requires complex central nervous system processing. The level of sensory integration (see p. 256) for such stimuli is usually very high. The five classic senses include olfaction (smell), vision, gustation (taste), auditory sense (hearing), and vestibular sense (balance and sense of acceleration).

Note: The order in which the senses have been outlined above, which also matches the following descriptions, is based on the sequence of participating neuronal structures—in this case the nn. craniales involved. Smell and taste, which are often mentioned together, are separated here as they are processed by completely different parts of the nervous system.

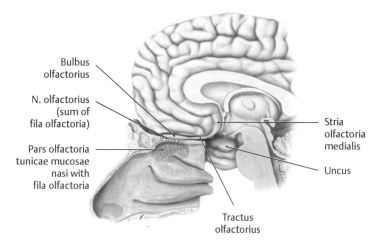

A Olfactory sense

Olfactory stimuli are detected by specific receptors in olfactory cells in the tunica mucosa nasi. The axons of these olfactory cells combine to form fila olfactoria. The receptor cells transmit their information directly to the CNS without involvement of a ganglion. The two other readily visible components of the olfactory system, the *bulbus olfactorius* and *tractus olfactorius*, are extensions of the brain and thus integral components of the CNS (not the PNS). From the olfactory n., the olfactory information is carried via different relay stations (olfactory bulb, olfactory tract) to very old cortex portions (the paleocortex, mainly located in the temporal lobe close to the uncus) in both cerebral hemispheres where it is consciously processed. In perception of odors the olfactory sense is triggered by a chemical stimulus, the odorant—that attaches to a receptor in the nasal mucosa.

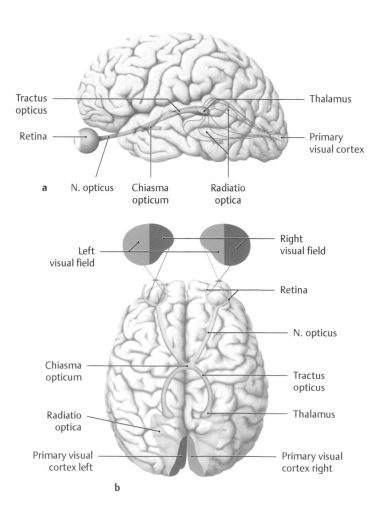

B Visual sense

Light stimuli (in the form of photons) are also exclusively received by the CNS: the light sensitive retina of the eye is an evaginated part of the diencephalon and again, the n. opticus (CN II) is considered not to be a true nerve but structurally a tract. There is also no ganglion. From the retina (first to third neuron) where a neuronal processing of the light stimulus has already taken place, the axons (of the third neuron) extend via the n. opticus and the tractus opticus to the thalamus (fourth neuron) in the cerebellum and from there as radiatio optica to the so-called primary visual cortex (fifth neuron) at the polus occipitalis (**a**). The visual information crosses over to the opposite side at the chiasma opticum. Visual impressions from the left visual field reach, and are interpreted in, the right hemisphere, and vice versa (**b**).

Note: The retina has a concave surface resembling the structure of a concave mirror. This means the images formed on the retina are upside down—up and down is reversed. Through a neuronal process up and down are placed in the correct position again. In terms of perception, the visual sense is triggered by a physical stimulus, electromagnetic waves, in a certain frequency range. The perception of warmth on the skin is a physical stimulus, also triggered by electromagnetic waves. Light in the infrared region (which receptors in the eye can't detect) stimulates temperature receptors. Some animals (e.g., some types of snakes) possess infrared receptors and are able to see the warmth radiating off their prey.

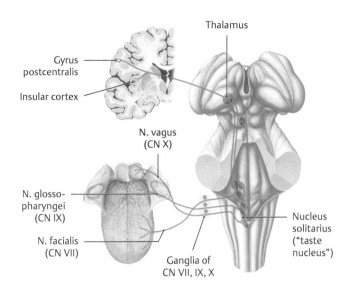

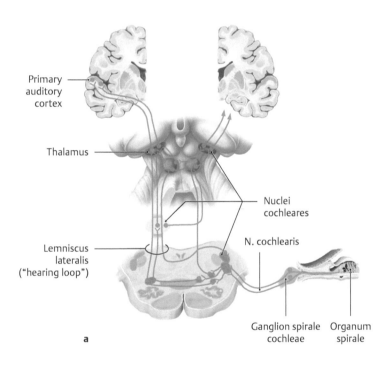

a

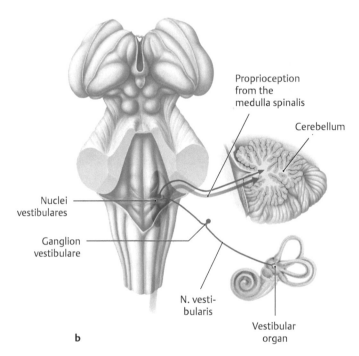

b

C Gustatory sense (of taste)

Taste perception takes place in the gemmae gustatoriae of the tongue. Three nn. craniales are responsible for the sense of taste: CN VII (n. facialis) covers the anterior two thirds of the dorsum linguae; CN IX (n. glossopharyngeus) covers the posterior one third of the tongue, and CN X (n. vagus) covers the epiglottic region. From this distribution, it is evident that the n. facialis (CN VII) plays the largest role in taste perception. All three nerves are true nn. craniales and as such, the first neuron lies in a sensory ganglion, and the second neuron is located in a nucleus trunci encephali shared by the three nerves, the nucleus solitarius. The third neuron of the gustatory tract uses the thalamus to reach the cortex cerebri of both hemispheria where the fourth neuron is located. The interesting point to note is that they terminate on both sides of two cortical regions—the gyrus postcentralis and the lobus insularis. In terms of perception, the gustatory sense is triggered by a chemical stimulus, a chemical compound or flavor, that attaches to a receptor in a gemma gustatoria on the surface of the tongue. Among the five senses, the gustatory sense is the simplest.

D Auditory and vestibular senses

In each case, information comes from an organ in the inner ear and is transmitted via the n. vestibulocochlearis which why they are discussed together here.

a Auditory sense: the auditory sense is a specific form of mechanoreception: air pressure fluctuations are perceived and analyzed. Loud music in the bass range can even be felt as vibration in visceral organs. The auditory sense is usually not considered part of mechanoreception. The perception of acoustic stimuli, which are transmitted to the inner ear through the middle ear in the form of pressure fluctuation, is achieved through sensory cells in the inner ear—auditory cells in the organum spirale (organ of Corti)—and is carried to the CNS via the n. cochlearis. The n. cochlearis is a peripheral nerve, the first neuron lies in the ganglion spirale cochleae. The axon of this first neuron enters the CNS at the truncus encephali. Via neuronal pathways in the nuclei cochleares in the truncus encephali (primarily pons and mesencephalon), the information reaches the primary auditory cortex in the lobi temporales of both hemispheria after passing through the thalamus. This is where conscious auditory perception takes place. The entire auditory pathway in the truncus encephali is referred to as the lemniscus lateralis which crosses multiple times in certain areas. The fact that auditory information from the ear reaches both hemispheria is a precondition for directional hearing.

b Vestibular sense: The term "vestibular sense" is not precise, as balance is not a sensory perception triggered by one single stimulus, but the inner representation of a state of motion or rest of the body. It is based on the processing of different sensory impressions. The most vital region for maintenance of balance is the cerebellum. From the auris interna, the vestibular organ provides information about angular acceleration (circular motion) or transverse acceleration (e.g., through gravitational force) via the n. vestibularis. The first neuron is located in the ganglion vestibulare the axon of which passes to the nuclei vestibulares to the cerebellum. Through proprioception, the cerebellum receives information about the position of head and limbs and their alignment to the trunk from receptors in skeletal muscle. Based on body posture and its spatial orientation, the cerebellum calculates the desired movement to control balance. Together the n. cochlearis (hearing) and n. vestibularis (acceleration) form the n. vestibulocochlearis. Auditory and vestibular sense in the vestibular apparatus are referred to as specific somatic sensation.

289

1.13   Principles of the Neurological Examination

In order to conduct a neurological examination and interpret its findings, the examiner has to be knowledgeable about basic neuroanatomy. This learning unit describes selected aspects of the neuroanatomical examination and explains why a neuroanatomical background is essential and indispensable for detecting and analyzing symptoms. The neurological examination as described below is a part of the general examination of a patient.

A Testing sensation

Sensation is the perception of different stimuli on the skin, mucosae, muscles, joints and internal organs. When assessing sensation, different qualities of sensory are being tested. Different receptors are responsible for different stimuli, which are transmitted to the brain via different pathways. The receptors and their pathways will be discussed in greater detail later on. For now, knowledge about the different sensory qualities and how to test them is sufficient. During all tests described here, the patient should keep the eyes closed in order to prevent a correction of the results by being able to see them. In addition, all tests should be conducted on both sides to detect damage affecting only one side of the body.

Note: All tests described here require the cooperation of the patient. They can only be conducted on a patient who is alert.

a **Touch sensation** is assessed using a paintbrush, a cotton ball, or the fingertips. The examiner strokes the skin and the patient has to say whether they can feel the touch. A reduced sensation is referred to as hypesthesia; a total loss of sensation is referred to as anesthesia.

b **Sensation of pain** is assessed using the pointed tip of an injection needle. A reduced sensation is referred to as hypalgesia, a loss of sensation is referred to as analgesia.

c **Temperature sensation** is assessed using a warm or cold metallic object or a test tube filled with either cold or warm water. It is important that the water is not so hot that it generates temperature and in addition, pain sensation. Impaired temperature sensation is referred to as thermohypesthesia; a total loss of sensation is referred to as thermoanesthesia. Pain and temperature sensitivity are referred to as *protopathic sensitivity* (see p. 284).

d The **vibratory sensation** is assessed using a tuning fork (64 or 128 Hz). A vibrating tuning fork is placed near the patient's ankle or held above the tibia. The patient is asked if they feel a vibration in their bones. A reduced sensation is referred to as pallhypesthesia; a total loss of sensation is referred to as pallesthesia.

Another sensory quality not described here is the **sense of position** (proprioception). It provides information about the spatial position of the limbs. The examiner moves one limb and asks the patient about the its position (e.g., bent or extended). The decisive stimulus is the elongation (tension) of muscles and articular capsules. The stimulus does not come from the body's surface but from deep within (deep sensation).

The sensory qualities listed here are found all over the body. In classical neuroanatomy, they are referred to as "sensitivity." The senses perceived by specific sensory organs (the five "classical" senses: olfactory, visual, gustatory, auditory and vestibular, see p. 288) were initially referred to as "sensation." However, since perception and transmission of impulses are in principle the same for sensitivity and sensation, they are both referred to now as sensation.

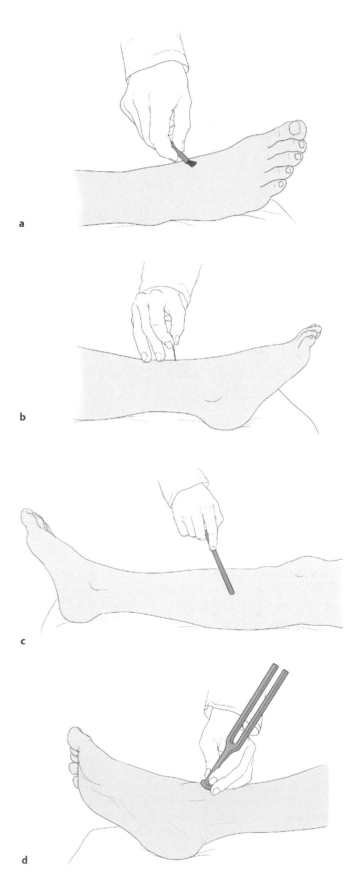

a

b

c

d

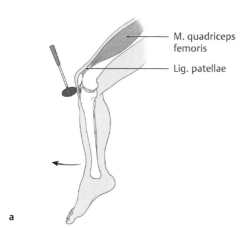

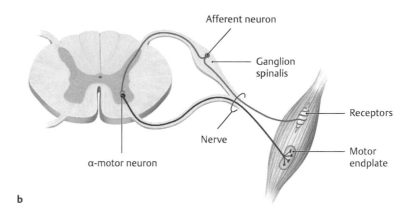

M. quadriceps femoris

Lig. patellae

Afferent neuron

Ganglion spinalis

Receptors

Nerve

α-motor neuron

Motor endplate

a

b

B Testing motor function

The efferent systems, which generate movements of the skeletal muscles, are referred to as "motor systems" or "motor function." They are assessed by examining the reflexes. One example listed here is the patellar tendon reflex (**a**). When tapping the lig. patellae with a reflex hammer, the m. quadriceps femoris shortens to such an extent that it causes the knee to extend. If that happens, the reflex arc is intact (**b**). By tapping the tendon, the muscle is pulled and elongates. This muscle elongation is perceived by muscle receptors and relayed to the medulla spinalis. The cell body of the stimulated afferent neuron lies in the ganglion spinale. Its axon releases a transmitter at the α-motor neuron in the medulla spinalis. This transmitter stimulates the α-motor neuron, which itself releases transmitters at the motor endplate. This transmitter stimulates the muscle which will then contract and the knee extends. The leg kicks forward.

Note: For the α-motor neuron to be stimulated, sensory input pathways must be intact. With regard to reflexes, sensation and motor function are closely related, which is why in physiology the term *sensorimotor function* is often used. Intact sensation is a precondition for intact motor function, and has been described in a previous chapter in this book.

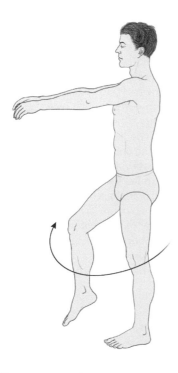

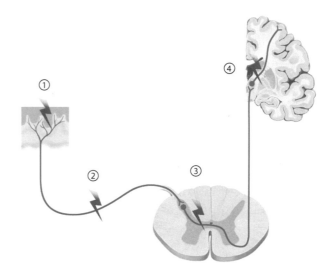

① ④ ② ③

C Coordination assessment

In addition to tests for assessing sensation and reflexes, the neurological exam also includes the assessment of more complex pathways of information processing. One example is Unterberger's stepping test. With eyes closed and arms extended forward, the patient is asked to walk on the spot. Performing this task requires the coordination of several sensory systems. It is especially challenging to provide information about the position of the head for which the inner ear is responsible (see p. 289). A malfunctioning of the vestibular parts of the inner ear (the canales semicirculares) leads to increased spinning of the affected side. In the example shown here, a turn to the right (illustrated by the arrow) is caused by right inner ear malfunction.

D Problems in neurological-topical diagnostics

The figure illustrates a pain pathway extending from the body surface to the sensory cortex. If the pathway is disrupted, the pain information does not reach the sensory cortex. Location of the disruption can be in either the receptive field (1), in the peripheral nerve (2), in the medulla spinalis (3), or the encephalon itself (4). Disruption in any of these locations prevents the sensory cortex from perceiving the pain. This explains why the brain always localizes disruption in the receptive field (1) even though the disruption can be located in the medulla spinalis (3). The physician is confronted with the problem of "tricking" the brain and to identify the location of the disruption, since the therapy differs depending on where the pathway has been damaged. The process of identifying the damaged location is referred to as neurological-topical diagnostics. This is why intimate knowledge of important pathways is essential when examining a patient.

2.1 Neurons

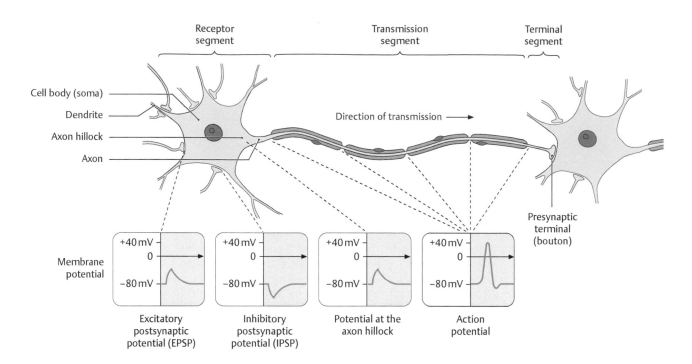

A **The nerve cell (neuron)**

The basic structure of a nerve cell (neuron) has already been explained on p. 268, fig. **A**. The terms "signal input," "signal output," and "signal exchange" as mentioned in the previous chapter can also be used to describe the "functional classification" of neurons. The three segments are as follows:

- The receptor segment; corresponds to the cell body and the dendrites.
- The transmission segment; carries the information to the target cell. Physiologically and morphologically, this segment is called the axon. Where a rapid transfer of information is required, the axon has a myelin sheath (for structure see **C**, p. 295). Fast reaction speed is usually needed in the CNS.
- The terminal segment is responsible for relaying the information to the target cell. It is identical to the structures that form a synapse.

The axons of other neurons, which also form synapses with the target neuron, (cf. **D**) terminate at the receptor segment of the target cell. It is in these synapses that the release of either excitatory or inhibitory neurotransmitters occurs. These transmitters released at the end of the axon bind to receptors at the cell membrane of the target cell, creating either a local increase in membrane potential (excitatory postsynaptic potential

EPSP) or a decrease (inhibitory postsynaptic potential IPSP).

A neuron constantly receives inhibitory and excitatory signals. The integration of these local potentials takes place at the axon hillock. A preponderance of excitatory over inhibitory signals leads to action potential generation at the axon hillock. The action potential arrives at the axon terminal (bouton) and triggers the release of transmitters at this axonal site. Receptors at the target cell recognize the released transmitters and the local membrane potential is either decreased (IPSP) or increased (EPSP) depending on the transmitter and its receptor. This last portion represents the terminal segment, the synapse.

Note: The transfer of information between nerve cells is made possible through neurotransmitters. The presynaptic neuron releases the transmitter, which is detected by a receptor on a postsynaptic membrane. As a result, the local membrane potential of a nerve cell increases (EPSP) or decreases (IPSP). These local potential changes occur only in dendrites and the neuron cell body.

In the axon, during the transfer of information, potential changes occur according to the all-or-none principle. In a myelinated axon, the potential change can be measured only at specific myelin-free sections (the nodes of Ranvier, see **B**, p. 294).

B **Electron microscopy of the neuron**

The organelles of neurons can be resolved with an electron microscope. Neurons are rich in rough endoplasmic reticulum (protein synthesis, active metabolism). This endoplasmic reticulum (called *Nissl substance* under a light microscope) is easily demonstrated by light microscopy when it is stained with cationic dyes (which bind to the anionic mRNA and nRNA of the ribosomes). The distribution pattern of the Nissl substance is used in neuropathology to evaluate the functional integrity of neurons. The neurotubules and neurofilaments that are visible by electron microscopy are referred to collectively in *light microscopy* as neurofibrils, as they are too fine to be resolved as separate structures under the light microscope. Neurofibrils can be demonstrated in light microscopy by impregnating the nerve tissue with silver salts. This is important in neuropathology, for example, because the clumping of neurofibrils is an important histological feature of Alzheimer's disease.

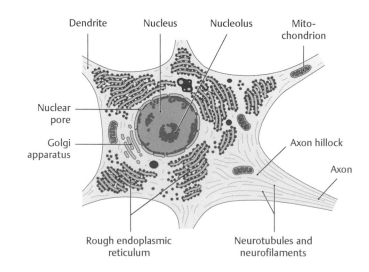

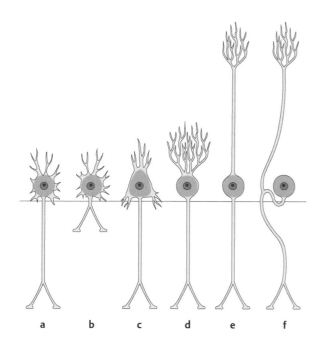

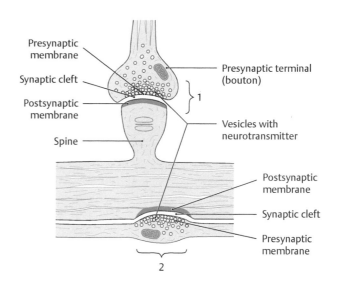

C Basic forms of the neuron and its functionally adapted variants

The horizontal line marks the region of the axon hillock, which represents the initial segment of the axon. (The structure of a peripheral nerve, which consists only of axons and sheath tissue, is shown on p. 275, see **D**)

a Multipolar neuron (multiple dendrites) with a long axon (= long transmission path). Examples are projection neurons such as alpha motor neurons in the medulla spinalis.
b Multipolar neuron with a short axon (= short transmission path). Examples are interneurons like those in the gray matter of the brain and medulla spinalis.
c Pyramidal cell: Dendrites are present only at the apex and base of the triangular cell body, and the axon is long. Examples are efferent neurons of the cerebral motor cortex (see pp. 327 and 457).
d Purkinje cell: An elaborately branched dendritic tree arises from one circumscribed site on the cell body. The Purkinje cell of the cerebellum has many synaptic contacts with other neurons (see p. 369).
e Bipolar neuron: The dendrite arborizes in the periphery. The bipolar cells of the retina are an example (see. **Ab**, S. 476).
f Pseudounipolar neuron: The dendrite and axon are not separated by the cell body. An example is the primary afferent (sensory) neuron in the spinal (dorsal root) ganglion (see p. 444 and **C**, p. 273).
Note: In pseudounipolar cells, the single dendrite also has a myelin sheath for fast signal transduction, and unlike the usually short dendrite of multipolar neurons, the dendrite of a unipolar neuron is generally long (e.g., from a receptor at the sole of the foot to the neuron in the spinal ganglion is about 1 meter in length). In these cells the axon and dendrite cannot be distinguished from each other based on their structure but their stimulus conduction can be used. The dendrite moves stimuli to the nerve cell body; the axon takes it away from the nerve cell body.

D Electron microscopic appearance of the two most common types of synapse in the CNS

Synapses—in terms of their structure correlate to the terminal segment (see **A**)—display a structure visible under the electron microscope. They consist of a presynaptic membrane, a synaptic gap and a postsynaptic membrane. In case of a synapse with a dendritic spine (1), the terminal bouton of the axon contacts a specialized protrusion (or spine) found on a dendrite of the target cell. The side-by-side synapse of an axon with the flat surface of a target neuron is called a parallel contact or *bouton en passage* (2). The vesicles in the presynaptic expansions contain the neurotransmitters that are released into the synaptic cleft by exocytosis when the axon fires. From there the neurotransmitters diffuse to the postsynaptic membrane, where their receptors are located. A variety of drugs and toxins act upon synaptic transmission (antidepressants, muscle relaxants, nerve gases, botulinum toxin).

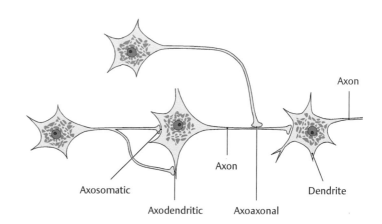

E Synaptic patterns in a small group of neurons

Axons may terminate at various sites on the target neuron and form synapses there. The synaptic patterns are described as axodendritic, axosomatic, or axoaxonal. Axodendritic synapses are the most common (see also **A**). The cortex cerebri consists of many small groups of neurons that are collected into functional units called columns (see p. 317).

2.2 Neuroglia and Myelination

A Cells of the neuroglia in the CNS

Neuroglial cells surround the neurons, providing them with structural and functional support (see **D**). Various staining methods are used in light microscopy to define specific portions of the neuroglial cells:

a Cell nuclei demonstrated with a basic stain
b Cell body demonstrated by silver impregnation

Recent studies have found that in the CNS neurons and neuroglia exist at a ratio ranging from 1:1 up to 1.6. Neuroglial cells provide critical support functions for neurons. For example, astrocytes absorb excess neurotransmitters from the extracellular milieu, helping to maintain a constant internal environment. While neurons are, almost without exception, permanently post-mitotic, some neuroglial cells continue to divide throughout life. For this reason, most primary brain tumors originate from neuroglial cells and are named for their morphological similarity to normal neuroglial cells: astrocytoma, oligodendroglioma, and glioblastoma. Developmentally, most neuroglial cells arise from the same progenitor cells as neurons. This may not apply to microglial cells, which develop from precursor cells in the blood from the monocyte lineage.

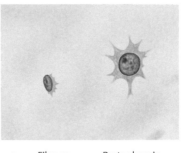
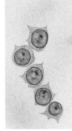
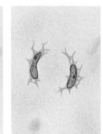

a   Fibrous astrocyte   Protoplasmic astrocyte   Oligo-dendrocytes   Microglia

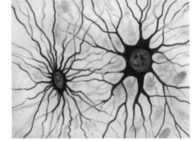
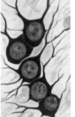
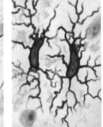

b

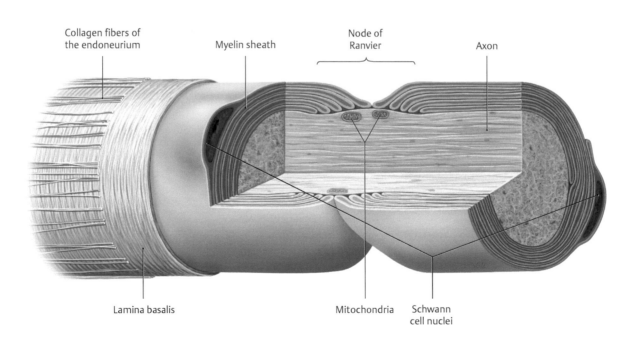

Collagen fibers of the endoneurium · Myelin sheath · Node of Ranvier · Axon

Lamina basalis · Mitochondria · Schwann cell nuclei

B Myelinated axon in the PNS

Most axons in the peripheral nervous system are insulated by a myelin sheath, although unmyelinated axons are also found in the PNS (see **C**).

The myelin sheath enables impulses to travel faster along the axon as they "jump" from one node of Ranvier to the next (saltatory nerve conduction), rather than travel continuously as in an unmyelinated axon.

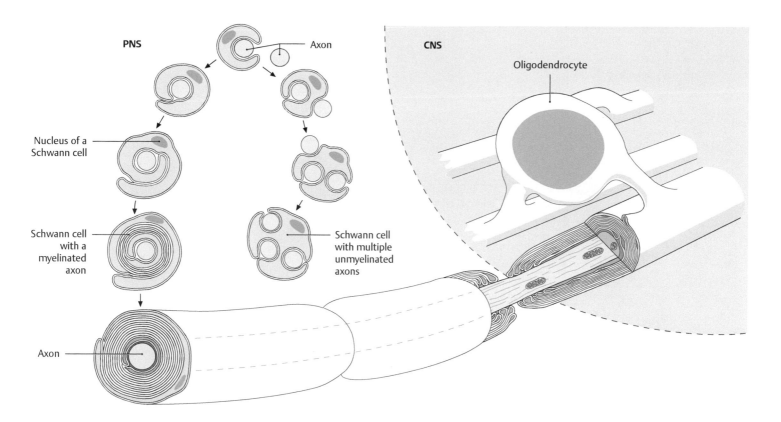

C Myelination differences in the PNS and CNS

The purpose of myelination is to insulate the axons electrically. This significantly boosts the nerve conduction velocity as a result of saltatory conduction (i.e., potentials jumping from one node of Ranvier to the next). While almost all axons in the CNS are myelinated, this is not the case in the PNS. The axons of the PNS are myelinated in regions where fast reaction speeds are needed (e.g., skeletal muscle contraction) and unmyelinated in regions that do not require rapid information transfer (e.g., the transmission of muscle spindle and tendon tension sensation). The very lipid-rich membranes of myelinating cells are wrapped around the axons to insulate them. There are differences between the myelinating cells of the central and peripheral nervous systems. Schwann cells (left) myelinate the axons in the PNS, whereas oligodendrocytes (right) form the myelin sheaths in the CNS.

Note: In the CNS, one oligodendrocyte always wraps around multiple axons; however, Schwann cells ensheathe either one myelinated axon or multiple unmyelinated axons.

This difference in myelination has important clinical implications. In multiple sclerosis, the oligodendrocytes are damaged but the Schwann cells are not. As a result, the peripheral myelin sheaths remain intact in MS while the central myelin sheaths degenerate.

D Summary: Cells of the central nervous system (CNS) and peripheral nervous system (PNS) and their functional importance

Cell type	Function
Neurons (CNS and PNS)	1. Impulse formation 2. Impulse conduction 3. Information processing
Glial cells	
Astrocytes (CNS only) (also called *macroglia*)	1. Maintain a constant internal milieu in the CNS 2. Help to form the blood–brain barrier 3. Phagocytosis of nonfunctioning synapses 4. Scar formation in the CNS (e.g., after cerebral infarction or in multiple sclerosis) 5. Absorb excess neurotransmitters and K^+
Microglial cells (CNS only)	Cells specialized for phagocytosis and antigen processing (brain macrophages, part of the mononuclear phagocyte system); secrete cytokines and growth factors
Oligodendrocytes (CNS only)	Form the myelin sheaths in the CNS
Ependymal cells (CNS only)	Line ventricular system cavities in the CNS
Cells of the plexus choroideus (CNS only)	Secrete cerebrospinal fluid
Schwann cells (PNS only)	Form the myelin sheaths in the PNS
Satellite cells (PNS only) (also called *mantle cells*)	Modified Schwann cells; surround the cell body of neurons in PNS ganglia

3.1 Sympathetic and Parasympathetic Nervous Systems, Organization

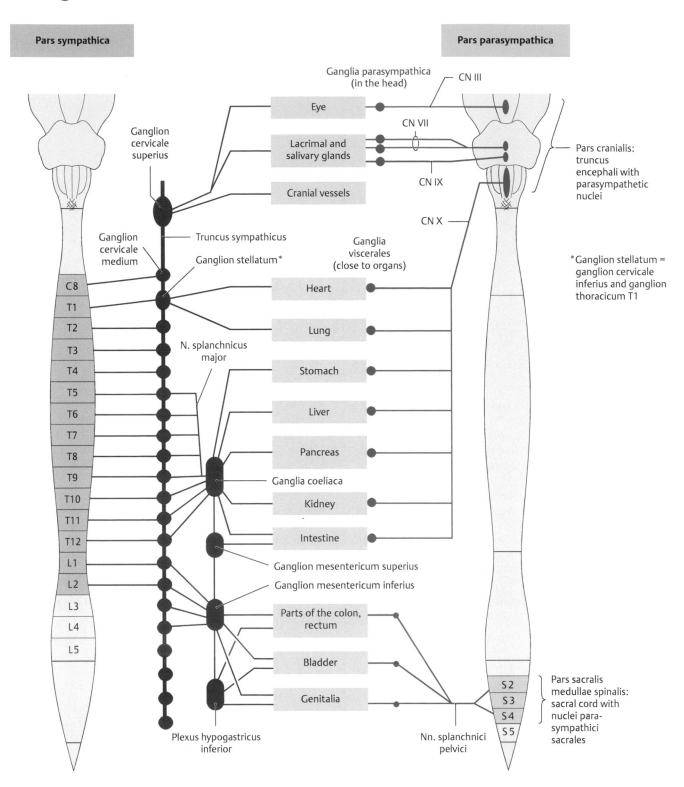

Pars sympathica

Pars parasympathica

Ganglia parasympathica (in the head) — CN III

Ganglion cervicale superius

Eye

CN VII

Lacrimal and salivary glands

Pars cranialis: truncus encephali with parasympathetic nuclei

Cranial vessels

CN IX

Ganglion cervicale medium — Truncus sympathicus

CN X

Ganglion stellatum*

Ganglia viscerales (close to organs)

*Ganglion stellatum = ganglion cervicale inferius and ganglion thoracicum T1

C8
T1   Heart
T2
T3   Lung
T4
T5   Stomach

N. splanchnicus major

T6   Liver
T7
T8   Pancreas
T9   Ganglia coeliaca
T10   Kidney
T11
T12   Intestine
L1
L2   Ganglion mesentericum superius
L3   Ganglion mesentericum inferius
L4   Parts of the colon, rectum
L5

Bladder

Pars sacralis medullae spinalis: sacral cord with nuclei para-sympathici sacrales

S2
S3
S4
S5

Genitalia

Plexus hypogastricus inferior

Nn. splanchnici pelvici

A Structure of the autonomic nervous system

The somatic nervous system, which innervates skeletal muscles, is contrasted with the autonomic nervous system. This is further subdivided into the partes sympathica (red) and parasympathica (blue) nervous systems (for their function see **C**). The neurons of the pars sympathica are located in the cornua lateralia of thoracic and lumbar medulla spinalis. The neurons of the pars parasympathica are located in parts of the truncus encephali and in the sacral medulla spinalis. Axons of the sympathetic neurons form the nn. splanchnici (visceral nerves). In the pars sympathica, first order neurons synapse with second order neurons in ganglia sympathica (paravertebral ganglia), prevertebral ganglia or in ganglia near or within the target organ and in the pars parasympathica in the head ganglia or ganglia within the target organ. Langley (1905) restricted the terms sympathetic and parasympathetic systems to the efferent neurons and their axons (visceral efferent fibers; only those are shown here). Meanwhile, it has been proven that the partes sympathica and parasympathica contain also afferent fibers (visceral afferents, pain and stretch receptors; not shown here, see p. 302). The enteric nervous system is now regarded as an independent part of the autonomic nervous system (see p. 304).

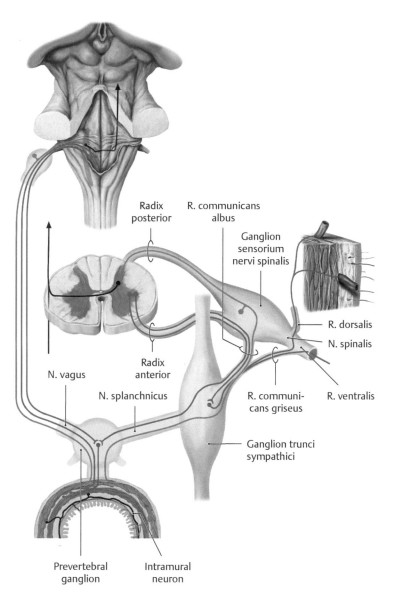

Radix posterior

R. communicans albus

Ganglion sensorium nervi spinalis

R. dorsalis

N. spinalis

N. vagus

Radix anterior

N. splanchnicus

R. communicans griseus

R. ventralis

Ganglion trunci sympathici

Prevertebral ganglion

Intramural neuron

B Synaptic organization of the autonomic nervous system

The partes sympathica and parasympathica portions of the nervous systems innervate many of the same targets, but use different transmitters, often with antagonistic effects (see **C**). These antagonistic systems also have differing patterns of organization, including unique paths to their targets and connections to the CNS. The cell bodies of the presynaptic motor neurons of the **pars sympathica** are located in the cornu laterale of medulla spinalis segments T1 to L2. Their axons leave the medulla spinalis through thoracolumbar radices anteriores, briefly travel in nn. spinales, and enter the paravertebral truncus sympathicus via rr. communicantes albi (white = myelinated). These axons terminate in synapses with postsynaptic neurons at three different levels:

1. Ganglia trunci sympathici along the paravertebral chain: The postsynaptic neurons send their axons back into the nn. spinales via rr. communicantes grisei (gray = unmyelinated). These axons travel in the nn. spinales to innervate local blood vessels, sweat glands, etc.
2. Prevertebral ganglia sympathica: These ganglion cells send their axons along arterial plexuses to the bowel, kidneys, etc., providing innervation to both the organs and their vasculature (see p. 304).
3. Adrenal medulla (not shown): Adrenal medullary (endocrine) cells are developmentally related to sympathetic ganglion cells, and receive direct innervation from presynaptic sympathetic axons.

In contrast, the presynaptic neurons of the **pars parasympathica** are located in the CNS in the truncus encephali (nn. craniales III, VII, IX, and X) and sacral medulla spinalis (S2–S4). The presynaptic axons leave the CNS via the nn. craniales noted above (the n. vagus [CN X] is the example shown here), and nn. splanchnici pelvici. These presynaptic axons synapse with postsynaptic neurons in discrete cranial ganglia (ciliare, pterygopalatinum, submandibulare, and oticum), which in turn send their axons in other nn. craniales to the target organ. Some presynaptic axons, particularly the n. vagus, synapse on postsynaptic neurons found in small ganglia within the wall of the effector organ. Afferent fibers (shown in green), originating from pseudounipolar neurons in ganglia sensoria nervorum spinalium (dorsal root) and ganglia sensoria nervorum cranialium, travel with autonomic motor axons. These sensory fibers carry information from visceral nociceptors (pain) and stretch receptors into the CNS. Efferent fibers are shown in purple, the ascending pain pathway in gray. For detailed description of the autonomic innervation of the viscera, see *Volume II, Internal Organs*.

C Synopsis of the partes sympathica and parasympathica of the autonomic nervous systems

This table summarizes the effects of the partes sympathica and parasympathica on specific organs.

1. The *pars sympathica* is the excitatory part of the autonomic nervous system (fight or flight).
2. The *pars parasympathica* coordinates rest and digestive processes (rest and digest).
3. Although the two systems have separate nuclei, they establish close anatomical and functional connections in the periphery.
4. The transmitter at the target organ is *acetylcholine* in the pars parasympathica and *norepinephrine* in the pars sympathica (except for the adrenal medulla).
5. Stimulation of the pars sympathica or parasympathica produces the following effects in specific organs (see table):

Organ	Pars sympathica	Pars parasympathica
Eye	Pupillary dilation	Pupillary constriction and increased curvature of the lens
Gll. salivariae	Decreased salivation (scant, viscous)	Increased salivation (copious, watery)
Heart	Increased heart rate	Decreased heart rate
Lungs	Decreased bronchial secretions and bronchodilation	Increased bronchial secretions and bronchoconstriction
Gastrointestinal tract	Decrease in secretions and motility	Increase in secretions and motility
Pancreas	Decreased exocrine secretions	Increased exocrine secretions
Male sex organs	Ejaculation	Erection
Skin	Vasoconstriction, sweating, piloerection	No effect

3.2 Autonomic Nervous System, Actions and Regulation

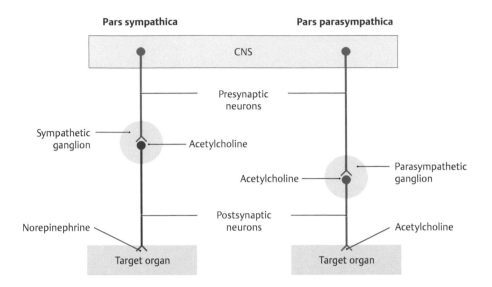

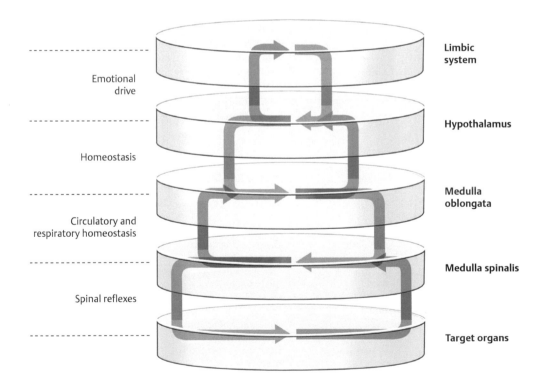

A Circuit diagram of the autonomic nervous system
The central first (presynaptic) neuron uses acetylcholine as a transmitter in both the pars sympathica and pars parasympathica (cholinergic neuron, shown in blue). Acetylcholine is also used as a neurotransmitter by the second (postsynaptic) neuron in the pars parasympathica. In the pars sympathica, norepinephrine is used by the noradrenergic neuron (shown in red).

Note: the target cell membrane contains different types of receptors (= transmitter sensors) for acetylcholine and norepinephrine. Each transmitter can produce entirely different effects, depending on the type of receptor.

B Control of the peripheral autonomic nervous system
   (after Klinke and Silbernagl)
The peripheral actions of the autonomic nervous system are subject to control at various levels, the highest being the limbic system, whose efferent fibers act on the peripheral target organs (e.g., heart, lung,

bowel; also affects sympathetic tone and cutaneous blood flow) through centers in the hypothalamus, medulla oblongata, and medulla spinalis. The higher the control center, the more subtle and complex its effect on the target organ. The limbic system receives signals from its target organs via afferent feedback mechanisms.

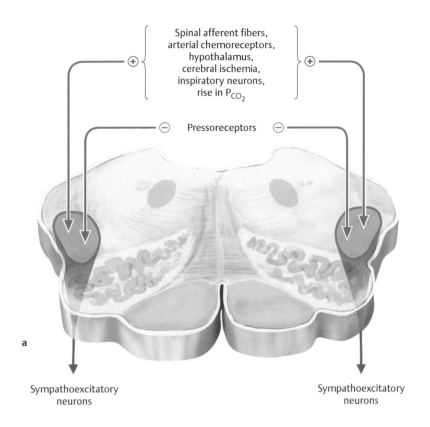

Spinal afferent fibers,
arterial chemoreceptors,
hypothalamus,
cerebral ischemia,
inspiratory neurons,
rise in P_{CO_2}

⊖ Pressoreceptors ⊖

a

Sympathoexcitatory
neurons

Sympathoexcitatory
neurons

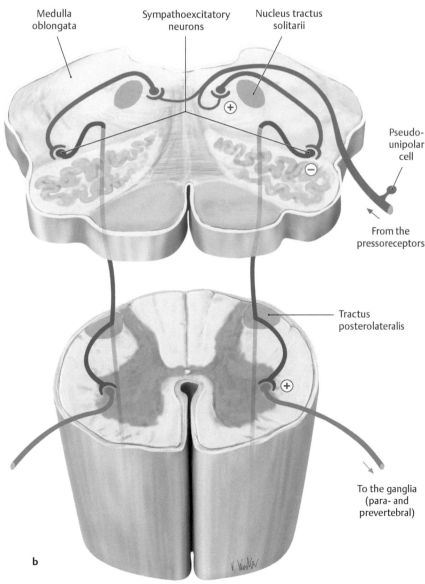

Medulla
oblongata

Sympathoexcitatory
neurons

Nucleus tractus
solitarii

Pseudo-
unipolar
cell

From the
pressoreceptors

Tractus
posterolateralis

To the ganglia
(para- and
prevertebral)

b

C Excitatory and inhibitory effects on sympathoexcitatory neurons in the medulla oblongata

a Cross-section through the truncus encephali (brainstem) at the level of the medulla oblongata. To generate a baseline level of sympathetic outflow, the presynaptic visceral efferent sympathetic neurons in the medulla spinalis (nuclei intermediolateralis and intermediomedialis) must be stimulated by sympathoexcitatory neurons in the anterolateral part of the medulla oblongata. Numerous factors can inhibit or enhance the activity of these neurons which play a critical role in the regulation of blood pressure. If the blood pressure is too high, for example, afferent impulses from the pressoreceptors will inhibit sympathetic outflow.

b Afferent impulses from the factors listed in **a** are relayed in the nucleus medialis solitarius of the nucleus tractus solitarii to secondary neurons, whose axons project back to the sympathoexcitatory neurons. When these neurons are inhibited, the peripheral resistance vessels relax and the blood pressure falls. The axons from these sympathoexcitatory neurons pass ipsilaterally through the tractus posterolateralis to presynaptic sympathetic neurons in the cornu laterale of the medulla spinalis. Sensory neurons are shown in orange, motor neurons in green.

3.3 Parasympathetic Nervous System, Overview and Connections

A Overview: parasympathetic nervous system (cranial part)

There are four parasympathetic nuclei in the truncus encephali. The visceral efferent fibers of these nuclei travel along particular nn. craniales, listed below.

- Nucleus visceralis nervi oculomotorii (Edinger–Westphal nucleus): n. oculomotorius (CN III)
- Nucleus salivatorius superior: n. facialis (CN VII)
- Nucleus salivatorius inferior: n. glossopharyngeus (CN IX)
- Nucleus posterior nervi vagi: n. vagus (CN X)

The presynaptic parasympathetic fibers often travel with multiple nn. craniales to reach their target organs (for details see p. 528 and **E**, S. 130). The n. vagus supplies all of the thoracic and abdominal organs as far as a point near the flexura coli sinistra. *Note:* The sympathetic fibers to the head travel along the arteries to their target organs.

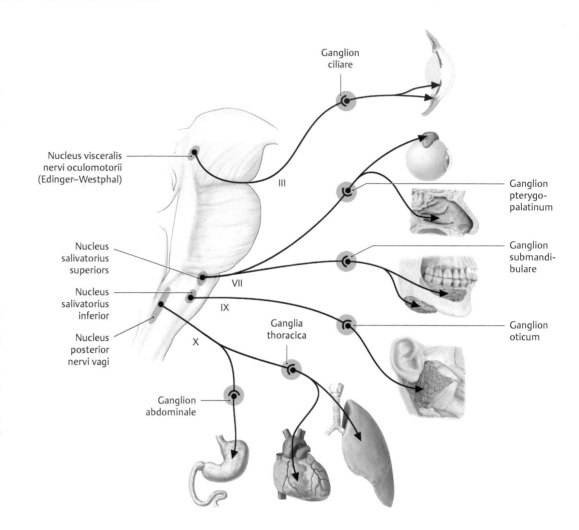

B Parasympathetic ganglia in the head

Nucleus	Path of presynaptic fibers	Ganglion	Postsynaptic fibers	Target organs
• Nucleus visceralis nervi oculomotorii (Edinger-Westphal)	• N. oculomotorius	• Ganglion ciliare	• Nn. ciliares breves	• M. ciliaris (accommodation) • M. sphincter pupillae (miosis)
• Nucleus salivatorius superior	• N. intermedius (n. facialis root) divides into:		• N. maxillaris → n. zygomaticus → anastomosis → n. lacrimalis	• Gl. lacrimalis

	1. N. petrosus major → n. canalis pterygoidei	• Ganglion pterygopalatinum	• Orbital branches
			• Rr. nasales posteriores superiores laterales
			• N. nasopalatinus
			• Nn. palatini
				• Glands on
				  – cellulae ethmoidales posteriores
				  – conchae nasi
				  – anterior palatum
				  – palata durum and molle

	2. Chorda tympani → n. lingualis	• Ganglion submandibulare	• Glandular branches	• Gl. submandibularis • Gl. sublingualis
• Nucleus salivatorius inferior	• N. glossopharyngeus → n. tympanicus → n. petrosus minor	• Ganglion oticum	• N. auriculotemporalis (CN V$_3$)	• Gl. parotidea
• Nucleus posterior nervi vagi	• N. vagus	• Ganglia near organs	• Fine fibers in organs, not individually named	• Thoracic and abdominal viscera

→ = is continuous with

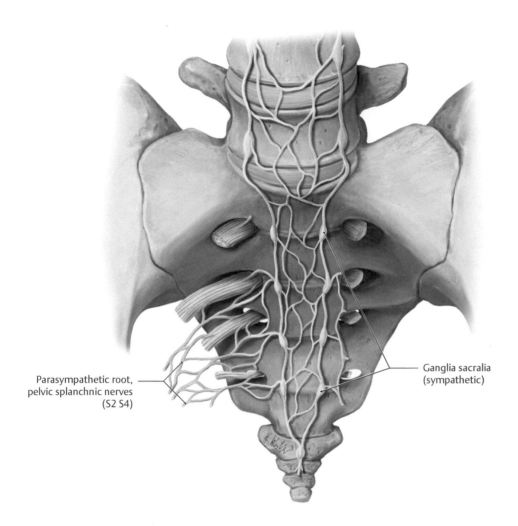

Parasympathetic root, pelvic splanchnic nerves (S2 S4)

Ganglia sacralia (sympathetic)

C Overview: parasympathetic nervous system (lumbrosacral part)
The portions of the bowel past the flexura coli sinistra and the pelvic viscera are supplied by the sacral part of the pars parasympathica of the autonomic nervous system. Efferent fibers emerge from the foramina sacralia anteriora in the radices anteriores (ventrales) of segments S2–S4. The fibers are collected into bundles to form the nn. splanchnici pelvici. They blend with the sympathetic fibers and synapse in the ganglia in or near the organs.

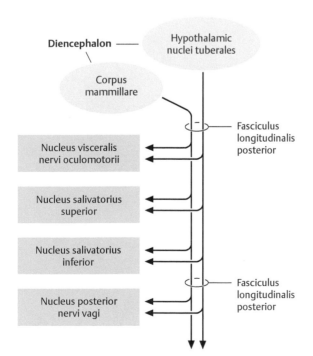

Diencephalon

Hypothalamic nuclei tuberales

Corpus mammillare

Nucleus visceralis nervi oculomotorii

Nucleus salivatorius superior

Nucleus salivatorius inferior

Nucleus posterior nervi vagi

Fasciculus longitudinalis posterior

Fasciculus longitudinalis posterior

D Connections of the fasciculus longitudinalis posterior
Increased salivation during eating results from stimulation of the gll. salivariae by the parasympathetic nervous system. To produce the coordinated stimulation of various glands, the cranial parasympathetic nuclei require excitatory impulses from higher centers (nuclei tuberales, corpora mammillaria). The parasympathetic nuclei are then stimulated to increase the flow of saliva. The fasciculus longitudinalis posterior establishes the necessary connections with the higher centers. Besides the fibers that coordinate the parasympathetic nuclei, the fasciculus contains other fiber systems that are not shown in the diagram.

301

3.4 Autonomic Nervous System: Pain Conduction

A Pain afferents conducted from the viscera by the partes sympathica and parasympathica of the autonomous nervous system (after Jänig)

a Sympathetic pain fibers, **b** parasympathetic pain fibers

It was originally thought that the partes sympathica and parasympathica conveyed only efferent fibers to the viscera. More recent research has shown, however, that both systems also carry afferent nociceptive (pain) fibers (shown in green), many running parallel to visceral efferent fibers (shown in purple). It is likely that many of these fibers (which make up only 5 % of all the afferent pain fibers in the body) are inactive during normal processes and may become active in response to organ lesions, for example.

a The pain-conducting (nociceptive) axons from the viscera course in the nn. splanchnici to the ganglia trunci sympathici and reach the n. spinalis by way of the rr. communicantes albi. The cell bodies of these neurons are located in the ganglion spinale. From the n. spinalis, the neurons pass through the radices posteriores to the cornu posterius of the medulla spinalis. There they are relayed to establish a connection with the ascending pain pathway. Alternatively, a reflex arc may be established through interneurons (see **B**). *Note:* Unlike the efferent system, the afferent nociceptive fibers of the partes sympathica and parasympathica are not relayed in the peripheral ganglia.

b The cell bodies of the pain-conducting pseudounipolar neurons in the cranial pars sympathica are located in the ganglion inferius or superius of the n. vagus (CN X). Those of the sacral pars parasympathica are located in the sacral ganglia spinalia of S2–S4. Their fibers run parallel to the efferent vagal fibers and establish a central connection with the pain-processing systems.

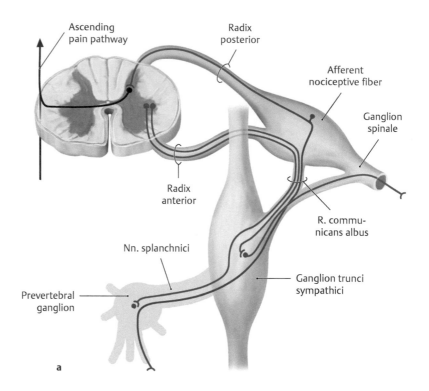

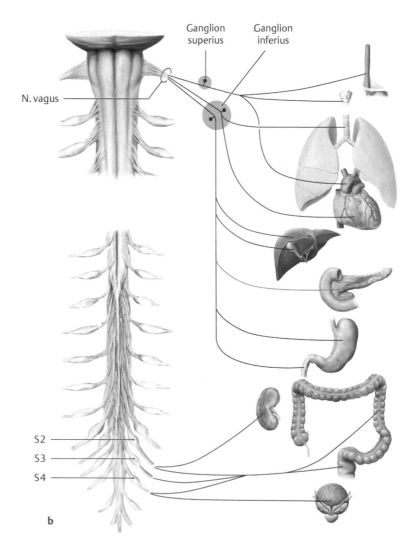

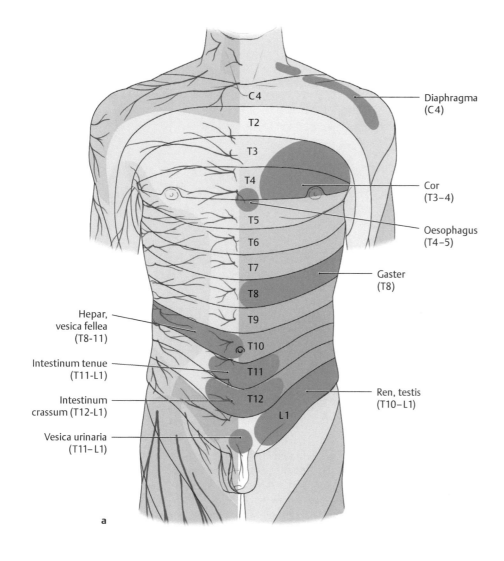

a

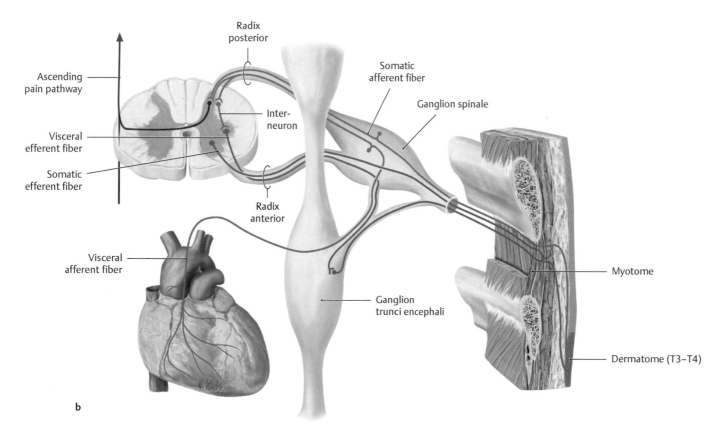

b

B Referred pain

It is believed that nociceptive afferent fibers from dermatomes (somatic pain) and internal organs (visceral pain) terminate on the same relay neurons in the cornu posterius of the medulla spinalis. The convergence of somatic and visceral afferent fibers (see **b**) confuses the relationship between the perceived and actual sites of pain, a phenomenon known as referred pain. The pain is typically perceived at the somatic site given that somatic pain is well-localized while visceral pain is not. Pain impulses from a particular internal organ are consistently projected to the same well-defined skin area (**a**); the pattern of pain projection is very helpful in determining the affected organ. In this figure, main areas of the dermatomes are marked. Due to the diffuse nature of pain, it can extend to the adjacent dermatomes (see numbers).

3.5 Enteric Nervous System (Plexus Entericus)

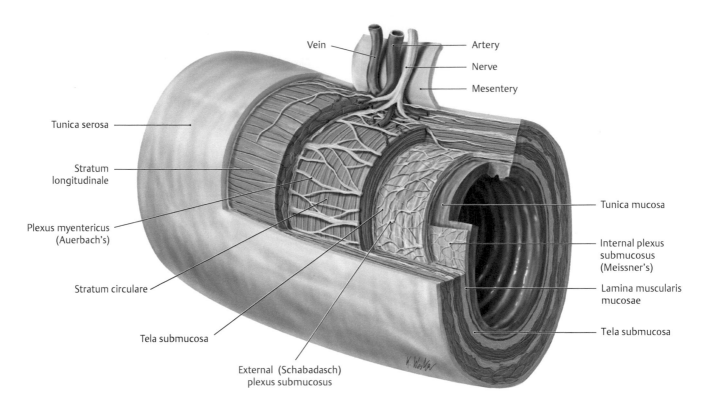

Vein
Artery
Nerve
Mesentery
Tunica serosa
Stratum longitudinale
Plexus myentericus (Auerbach's)
Stratum circulare
Tela submucosa
External (Schabadasch) plexus submucosus
Tunica mucosa
Internal plexus submucosus (Meissner's)
Lamina muscularis mucosae
Tela submucosa

A Enteric nervous system (plexus entericus) in the intestinum tenue

The plexus entericus is the intrinsic nervous system of the bowel, consisting of small groups of neurons that form interconnected, microscopically visible ganglia in the wall of the digestive tube. Its two main divisions are the *plexus myentericus* (Auerbach) (located between the strata longitudinale and circulare of muscle fibers) and the *plexus submucosus* (located in the submucosa), which is subdivided into external (Schabadasch) and *internal* (Meissner) *plexus submucosi.* (Details on the fine lamination of the enteric nervous system can be found in textbooks of histology.) These networks of neurons are the foundation for autonomic reflex pathways. In principle they can function without external innervation, but their activity is intensely modulated by the partes sympathica and parasympathica. Activities influenced by the plexus entericus include enteric motility, secretion into the digestive tube, and local intestinal blood flow.

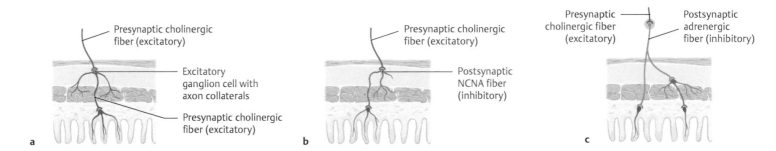

Presynaptic cholinergic fiber (excitatory)
Excitatory ganglion cell with axon collaterals
Presynaptic cholinergic fiber (excitatory)

a

Presynaptic cholinergic fiber (excitatory)
Postsynaptic NCNA fiber (inhibitory)

b

Presynaptic cholinergic fiber (excitatory)
Postsynaptic adrenergic fiber (inhibitory)

c

B Modulation of intestinal innervation by the autonomic nervous system

Although the pars parasympathica ("rest and digest") generally promotes the activities of the digestive tube (secretion, motility), it may also produce inhibitory effects.

a Excitatory presynaptic cholinergic parasympathetic fibers terminate on excitatory cholinergic neurons that promote intestinal motility (mixing of the bowel contents to facilitate absorption).

b An inhibitory parasympathetic fiber synapses with an inhibitory ganglion cell that uses noncholinergic, nonadrenergic (NCNA) transmitters. These NCNA transmitters are usually neuropeptides that inhibit intestinal motility.

c Sympathetic fibers are not abundant in the muscular layers of the bowel wall. Postsynaptic adrenergic fibers inhibit the motor and secretory neurons in the plexuses.

The clinical importance of autonomic bowel innervation is illustrated below:

- During shock, the vessels in the bowel are constricted and the intestinal tunica mucosa is accordingly deprived of oxygen. This results in disruption of the epithelial barrier, which may then be penetrated by microorganisms from the bowel lumen. This is an important mechanism contributing to multisystem failure in shock.
- There may be a cessation of intestinal motility (atonic bowel) after intestinal operations involving surgical manipulation of the digestive tube.
- Medications (especially opiates) may suppress the motility of the enteric nervous system, causing constipation.

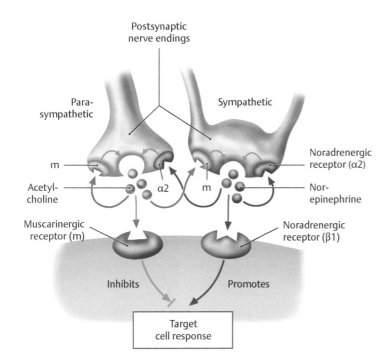

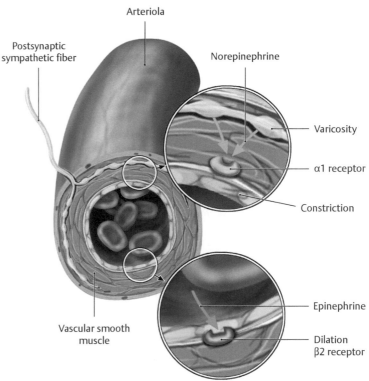

C Functional interactions of the partes sympathica and parasympathica of the autonomic nervous systems at the target organ

The transmitters of the partes sympathica and parasympathica of the autonomic nervous systems (norepinephrine and acetylcholine, respectively) act upon both the target organ and the (para)sympathetic nerve endings at the synapse. Noradrenergic receptors on the target tissue (β1, shown in blue) and nerve endings themselves (α2, shown in pink) modulate target cell responses on two levels: norepinephrine binding to the β1 receptor directly promotes a cellular response in heart tissue, while similar binding to the α2 receptors on the postsynaptic nerve endings allows for regulation of subsequent neurotransmitter release, through positive and negative feedback loops. The muscarinergic receptors (m, shown in green) mediate a similar process upon binding of acetylcholine. The neurotransmitters of the autonomic nervous system can therefore self- and cross-regulate in a multifaceted control mechanism.

D Sympathetic effects on arteries

An important function of the sympathetic nervous system is to regulate the caliber of the arterioles (blood pressure regulation). When sympathetic fibers release norepinephrine into the media of the arterioles, the α1 receptor mediates contraction of the vascular smooth muscle, and the blood pressure rises. Meanwhile, epinephrine from the blood acts on the β2 receptors in the sarcolemma of the same vascular smooth muscle cells, inducing vasodilation and a corresponding drop in blood pressure.

Note: Parasympathetic fibers do not terminate on blood vessels.

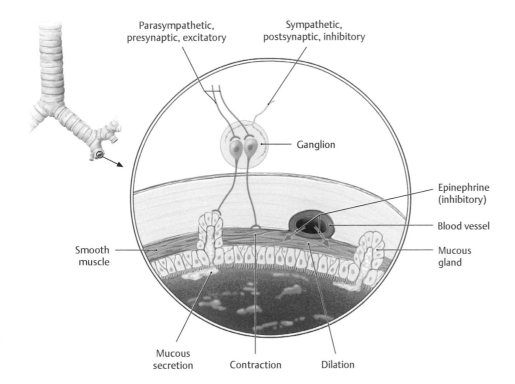

E Autonomic innervation of the trachea and bronchi

Parasympathetic stimulation of the local ganglia promotes secretion by the gll. bronchiales and narrowing of the bronchial passages. For this reason, the preparations for bronchoscopy include the administration of a drug (atropine) which blocks parasympathetic innervation, ensuring that mucous secretions will not obscure the bronchial mucosa. A similar reduction in bronchial secretions can be achieved through *sympathetic* stimulation. Epinephrine from the bloodstream acts on adrenergic β2 receptors to induce bronchodilation. This effect is used to treat severe asthma attacks.

4.1 Brain and Meninges in situ

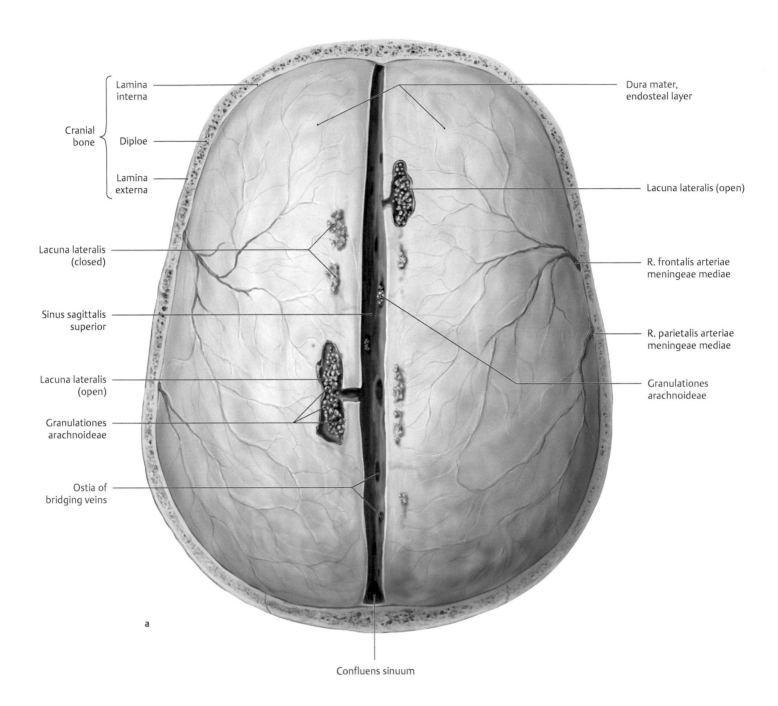

Lamina interna

Cranial bone — Diploe

Lamina externa

Lacuna lateralis (closed)

Sinus sagittalis superior

Lacuna lateralis (open)

Granulationes arachnoideae

Ostia of bridging veins

Dura mater, endosteal layer

Lacuna lateralis (open)

R. frontalis arteriae meningeae mediae

R. parietalis arteriae meningeae mediae

Granulationes arachnoideae

a

Confluens sinuum

A Brain and meninges in situ
Superior view of the cavitas cranii with the calvarium removed. **a** The calvarium has been removed, and the sinus sagittalis superior and its lacunae laterales have been opened; **b** After removal of dura mater (left hemisphere) and dura mater and arachnoidea mater (right hemisphere).

a The first structure encountered when the calvarium has been removed is the outer layer of the meninges, the endosteal (periosteal) layer of the dura mater. It contains a very dense network of collagen fibers that lend mechanical strength and make it impossible to tear without scissors or a scalpel. Hair-like collagen fibers can be seen torn out of the calvarium—

Sharpey's fibers of the outermost endosteal layer of dura. On its surface, branches of the epidurally located aa. meningeae are visible. They run in grooves—sulci arteriosi (see fig. **A**, p. 18)—on the internal surface of the calvarial bones. They are located directly between dura and bone, which is significant with regard to the localization and spreading of epidural hematomas (see **Aa**, p. 390) which are caused by ruptured or injured aa. meningeae. The dura mater of the cavitas cranii is formed of two inseparable layers—the outer endosteal (periosteal) layer (seen here) and the inner meningeal layer (not visible here, see **C**, p. 311). In certain regions the layers separate to form a dural venous sinus (sinus durae matris)—the sinus sagittalis superior, one of the largest venous sinuses, is seen here opened along its entire length.

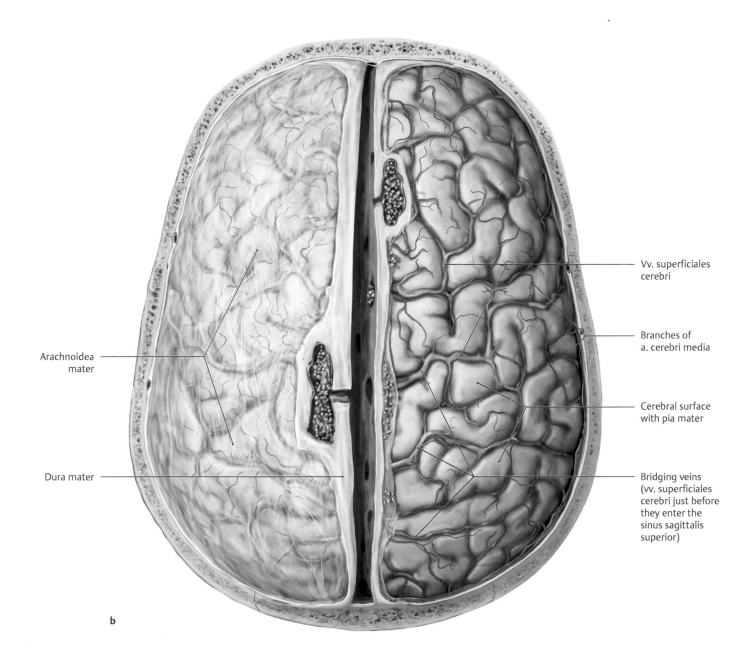

Arachnoidea mater

Dura mater

Vv. superficiales cerebri

Branches of a. cerebri media

Cerebral surface with pia mater

Bridging veins (vv. superficiales cerebri just before they enter the sinus sagittalis superior)

b

In figure **b** the arachnoidea mater is now visible after removal of the dura mater from the left hemispherium cerebri. On the right side, the arachnoidea mater has also been removed so that the brain enclosed by pia mater (the innermost layer) is visible. Unlike the arachnoidea mater, the pia mater extends into the sulci. The spatium subarachnoideum, which is filled with liquor cerebrospinalis (CSF), lies between the arachnoidea and the pia mater (see fig. **C**, p. 311). The space remains covered on the left side but opened on the right. In addition to the aa. cerebri, the vv. superficiales cerebri pass through the spatium subarachnoideum. The veins open into the sinus sagittalis superior via bridging veins. Some open into pools or lacunae laterales that then drain into the sinus sagittalis superior. Protuding into the sinus and the lacunae

are granulationes arachnoideae. These structures are important for the reabsorption of CSF (for further details see **A**, p. 314).

Note: Unlike the CNS which develops from the tubus neuralis, the meninges originate from embryonic connective tissue (mesenchyma) which surrounds the tubus neuralis. Therefore, the meninges are not brain tissue derivatives. In the CNS the pia mater is separated from the surface of the brain by a layer of glial cells (astrocytes) which are derived from the tubus neuralis in the form of a superficial glial membrane. This membrane is only visible under the microscope. The pia mater appears intimately applied to the surface of the brain and cannot be separated from it.

4.2 Meninges and Dural Septa

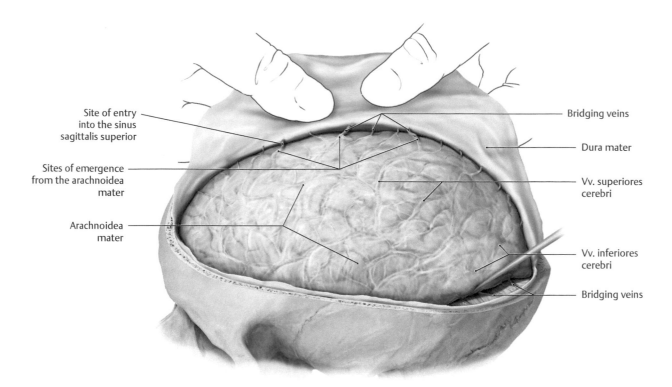

A Brain in situ with the dura mater partially dissected from the arachnoidea mater

Viewed from upper left. The dura mater has been opened and reflected upward, leaving the underlying arachnoidea mater and pia mater on the brain. Because the arachnoidea mater is so thin, we can see the underlying spatium subarachnoideum and the vessels that lie within it (see **C**). The spatium subarachnoideum no longer contains liquor cerebrospinalis at this stage of the dissection and is therefore collapsed. Before the vv. superficiales cerebri terminate in the sinus, they leave the spatium subarachnoideum for a short distance and course between the neurothelium of the arachnoidea mater and the meningeal layer of the dura mater to the sinus sagittalis superior. These segments of the cerebral veins are called *bridging veins* (see **C**). Some of the bridging veins, especially the vv. inferiores cerebri, open into the sinus transversus. Injury to the bridging veins leads to subdural hemorrhage (see pp. 311 and notes, p. 390).

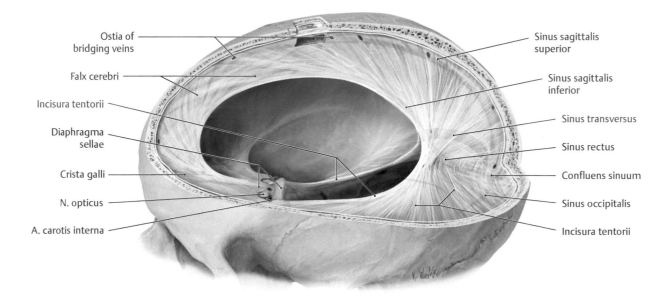

B Dural (folds) septa

Left anterior oblique view. The brain has been removed to demonstrate the dural folds or septa. The falx cerebri appears as a fibrous sheet that arises from the crista galli of the os ethmoidale and separates the two hemispheria cerebri. At its site of attachment to the calvaria, the falx cerebri separates to form the sinus sagittalis superior. Additional septa are the tentorium cerebelli and falx cerebelli (not shown here). The tentorium cerebelli fans out into the groove between the cerebrum and cerebellum and houses the sinus transversus in its attached margin. The falx cerebelli separates the two hemispheres of the cerebellum and has the sinus occipitalis in its attached margin. Because the dural septa are rigid structures, portions of the brain may herniate beneath their free edges (see **D**). The mesencephalon passes through an opening in the tentorium cerebelli called the incisura tentorii.

Sinus sagittalis superior

Dura mater, periosteal layer

V. emissaria

Galea aponeurotica

Scalp

Lamina externa

Diploe

Lamina interna

Lacuna lateralis with granulationes arachnoideae (arachnoid villi)

Scalp veins

Foveola granularis

Vv. diploicae

See b

Trabeculae arachnoideae

Dura mater, meningeal layer

Sinus endothelium

Falx cerebri

Bridging vein

Vv. superiores cerebri

Tight junctions

Spatium subarachnoideum with liquor cerebrospinalis

Dura mater

Neurothelium

Arachnoidea mater

Trabecula arachnoidea

V. superior cerebri

Superficial cerebral artery

Pia mater

Cortex cerebri

Glial limiting membrane with astrocytic end-feet

Basement membrane

C Relationship of the meninges to the calvarium

a Coronal section through the vertex of the skull, anterior view. The dura mater and internal periosteum of the skull form an inseparable structural unit. They are composed of a tough meshwork of collagen fibers. The part of the dura facing the bone takes on the task of the periosteum (periosteal/endosteal layer). The meningeal layer of dura, facing the brain, forms septa that extend between cerebral areas—dural folds. A dural fold is said to be composed of two layers of meningeal dura. In the vertex region pictured here, the septum shown is the falx cerebri (other septa are shown in **B**). Located within the dura, between its endosteal and meningeal layers, are the principal venous channels of the brain, the sinus durae matris (e.g., the sinus sagittalis superior). Their walls are composed of dura and endothelium. Granulationes arachnoideae, which protrude into the sinus durae matris, provide drainage of liquor cerebrospinalis from the spatium subarachnoideum into the blood stream (details see p. 314 ff). With age, the granulationes arachnoideae grow across the sinus and produce pits in the lamina interna of the skull (foveolae granulares, see p. 18). A schematic close-up (**b**) shows the relationship of the pia mater and arachnoidea mater, which contains the slit-like spatium subarachnoideum. This space is subdivided by trabeculae arachnoideae that extend from the outer layer (arachnoidea mater) to the inner layer (pia mater). At its boundary with the dura, the arachnoidea mater is covered by flat cells which, unlike other meningeal cells, are joined together by "tight junctions" (neurothelium) to create a diffusion barrier between the blood and liquor cerebrospinalis (see p. 317).

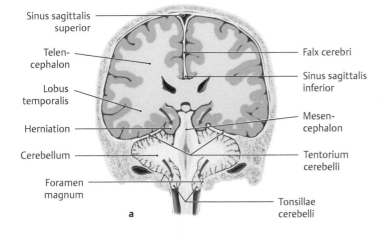

Sinus sagittalis superior

Telencephalon

Lobus temporalis

Herniation

Cerebellum

Foramen magnum

Falx cerebri

Sinus sagittalis inferior

Mesencephalon

Tentorium cerebelli

Tonsillae cerebelli

a

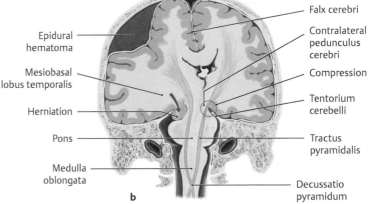

Epidural hematoma

Mesiobasal lobus temporalis

Herniation

Pons

Medulla oblongata

Falx cerebri

Contralateral pedunculus cerebri

Compression

Tentorium cerebelli

Tractus pyramidalis

Decussatio pyramidum

b

D Potential sites of brain herniation beneath the free edges of the menines

Coronal section, anterior view. The tentorium cerebelli divides the cavitas cranii into a supratentorial and an infratentorial space. The telencephalon is supratentorial, and the cerebellum is infratentorial (**a**). Because the dura is composed of tough, collagenous connective tissue, it creates a rigid intracranial framework. As a result, a mass lesion within the cranium may displace the cerebral tissue and cause portions of the cerebrum to become entrapped (herniate) beneath the rigid dural septa (duplication of the meningeal layer of the dura).

a Axial herniation. This type of herniation is usually caused by generalized brain edema. It is a symmetrical herniation in which the middle and lower portions of both lobi temporales of the cerebrum herniate down through the incisura tentorii, exerting pressure on the upper portion of the mesencephalon (bilateral uncal herniation). If the pressure persists, it will force the tonsillae cerebelli through the foramen magnum and also compress the lower part of the truncus encephali (tonsillar herniation). Because respiratory and circulatory centers are located in the truncus encephali, this type of herniation is life-threatening. Concomitant vascular compression may cause truncus encephali infarction.

b Lateral herniation. This type is caused by a unilateral mass effect (e.g., from a brain tumor or intracranial hematoma), as illustrated here on the right side. Compression of the ipsilateral pedunculus cerebri usually produces contralateral hemiparesis. Sometimes, the herniating mesiobasal portions of the lobus temporalis press the opposite pedunculus cerebri against the sharp edge of the tentorium. This damages the tractus pyramidalis above the level of its decussation, causing hemiparesis to develop on the side opposite the injury (compression).

4.3 Meninges of the Brain and Spinal Cord

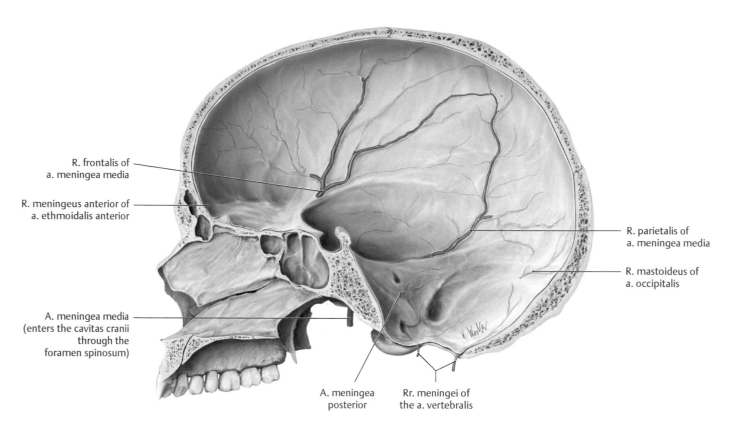

R. frontalis of
a. meningea media

R. meningeus anterior of
a. ethmoidalis anterior

A. meningea media
(enters the cavitas cranii
through the
foramen spinosum)

R. parietalis of
a. meningea media

R. mastoideus of
a. occipitalis

A. meningea
posterior

Rr. meningei of
the a. vertebralis

A Blood supply of the dura mater
Midsagittal section, left lateral view with branches of the a. meningea media exposed at several sites. Most of the dura mater in the cavitas cranii receives its blood supply from the a. meningea media, a branch of the a. maxillaris within the fossa infratemporalis. The other vessels shown here are of minor clinical importance. The essential function of the a. meningea media is to supply the calvarium. Head injuries may cause the a. meningea media to rupture, leading to life-threatening complications (epidural hematoma; see **C**, and pp. 309 and 390).

B Innervation of the dura mater in the cavitas cranii
(after von Lanz and Wachsmuth) Superior view with the tentorium cerebelli removed on the right side. The intracranial meninges are supplied by rr. meningei from all three divisions of the n. trigeminus and also by branches of the n. vagus and the first two nn. cervicales. Irritation of these sensory fibers due to meningitis is manifested clinically by headache and reflex nuchal stiffness (the neck is hyperextended in an attempt to relieve tension on the inflamed meninges). The brain itself is insensitive to pain.

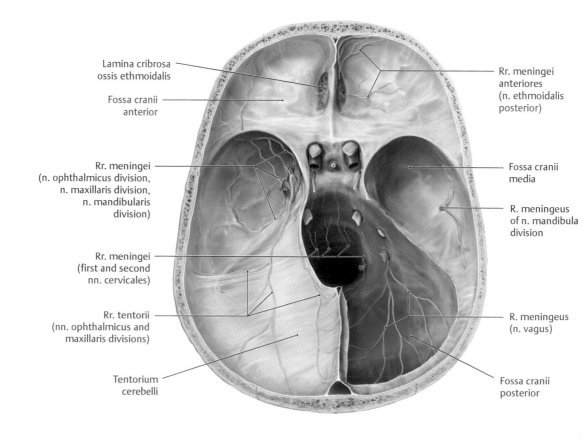

Lamina cribrosa
ossis ethmoidalis

Fossa cranii
anterior

Rr. meningei
(n. ophthalmicus division,
n. maxillaris division,
n. mandibularis
division)

Rr. meningei
(first and second
nn. cervicales)

Rr. tentorii
(nn. ophthalmicus and
maxillaris divisions)

Tentorium
cerebelli

Rr. meningei
anteriores
(n. ethmoidalis
posterior)

Fossa cranii
media

R. meningeus
of n. mandibula
division

R. meningeus
(n. vagus)

Fossa cranii
posterior

C Meninges and their spaces

Transverse section through the calvaria (schematic). The meninges have two spaces that do not exist under normal conditions, as well as one physiological space:

- **Spatium epidurale:** This space is not normally present in the brain (contrast with **E**, which shows the physiological spatium epidurale in the canalis vertebralis). It develops in response to bleeding from the a. meningea media or one of its branches (arterial bleeding). The extravasated blood separates the dura mater from the bone, dissecting a spatium epidurale between the lamina interna of the calvaria and the dura (epidural hematoma, see p. 390).
- **Spatium subdurale:** Bleeding from the bridging veins artificially opens the spatium subdurale between the meningeal layer of the dura mater and upper layer of the arachnoidea mater (subdural hematoma, see p. 390). The cells of the uppermost layer of the arachnoidea mater (neurothelium)

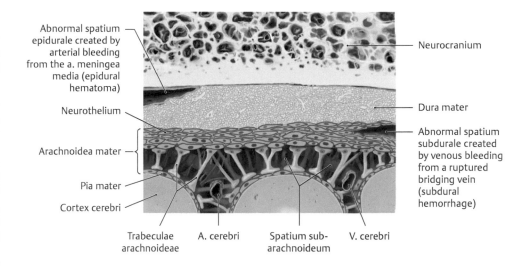

are interconnected by a dense network of tight junctions, creating a tissue barrier (blood-cerebrospinal fluid barrier).

- **Spatium subarachnoideum:** This physiologically normal space lies just beneath the arachnoidea mater. It is filled with liquor

cerebrospinalis and is traversed by blood vessels. Bleeding into this space (subarachnoid hemorrhage) is usually arterial bleeding from an aneurysm (abnormal circumscribed dilation) of the basal cerebral arteries (see p. 390).

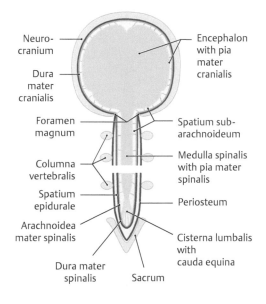

D Meninges in the cavitas cranii and canalis vertebralis

The two layers of the dura mater (meningeal and endosteal) form one inseparable structural unit in the cavitas cranii. The dura mater of the canalis vertebralis is separated from the periosteum beginning at the foramen magnum. Due to the mobility of the columna vertebralis, the periosteum of the vertebrae must be free to move relative to the dural sac. This is accomplished by the presence of the spatium epidurale, which exists physiologically only within the canalis vertebralis. It contains fat and venous plexuses (see **E**). This space has major clinical importance because it is the compartment into which epidural anesthetics are injected.

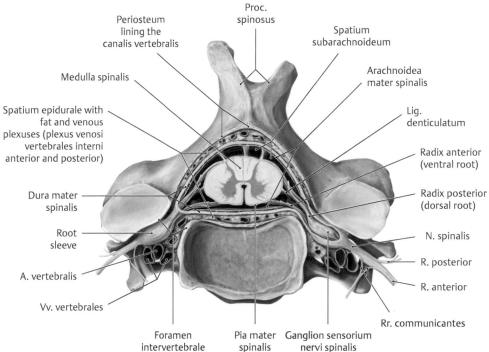

E Medulla spinalis in cross-section

Cross-section of a cervical vertebra, cranial view. The dura mater and periosteum in the canalis vertebralis separate from each other to define the spatium epidurale. This space is occupied by fatty tissue and venous plexuses functioning to cushion the medulla spinalis when it moves within the canalis vertebralis as a result of movements of the columna vertebralis. The radices posteriores and anteriores of the nn. spinales course within the dural sac of the medulla spinalis and collectively form the cauda equina in the lower part of the sac

(not shown here). The radices posteriores and anteriores unite within a dural sleeve at the foramina intervertebralia to form the nn. spinales. After the two roots have fused lateral to the ganglion sensorium nervi spinalis, the n. spinalis emerges from the dural sac. The pia mater invests the surfaces of the encephalon and medulla spinalis in the same fashion. The ligg. denticulata are sheets of pial connective tissue that pass from the medulla spinalis to the dura mater and are oriented in the coronal plane.

5.1 Ventricular System, Overview

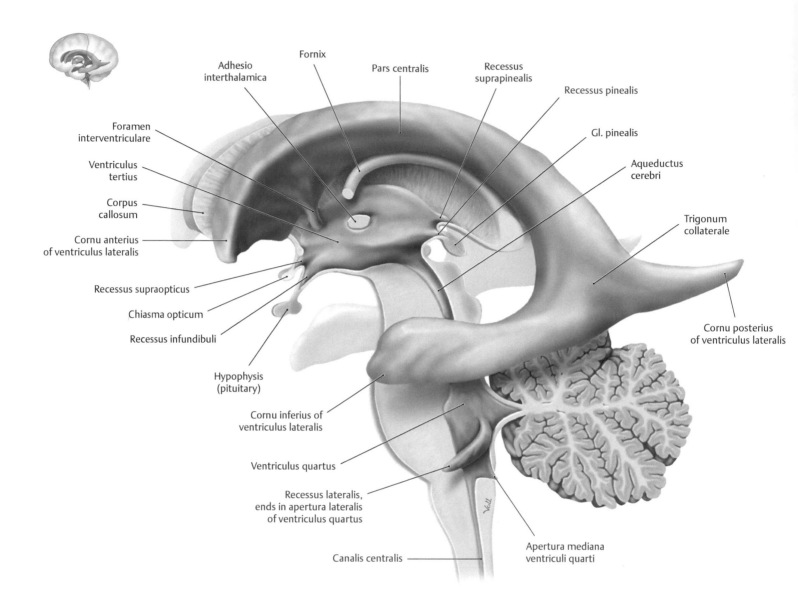

Fornix

Adhesio interthalamica

Pars centralis

Recessus suprapinealis

Recessus pinealis

Foramen interventriculare

Gl. pinealis

Ventriculus tertius

Aqueductus cerebri

Corpus callosum

Cornu anterius of ventriculus lateralis

Trigonum collaterale

Recessus supraopticus

Chiasma opticum

Recessus infundibuli

Cornu posterius of ventriculus lateralis

Hypophysis (pituitary)

Cornu inferius of ventriculus lateralis

Ventriculus quartus

Recessus lateralis, ends in apertura lateralis of ventriculus quartus

Canalis centralis

Apertura mediana ventriculi quarti

A Overview of the ventricular system and neighboring structures
Left lateral view. The ventricular system in the encephalon and the canalis centralis in the medulla spinalis develops from the cavity of the tubus neuralis. Topographically, they form what is referred to as the intraneural liquor space. The complex form of the ventriculi results from the development of brain vesicles. Ventriculi and canalis centralis are lined with a specialized type of epithelium, the ependyma (see fig. **D**, p. 317), which prevents direct contact between the liquor cerebrospinalis and the surrounding brain tissue. The four ventriculi are as follows:

- The *two* ventriculi laterales, each of which communicates through a foramen interventriculare with the
- ventriculus tertius, which in turn communicates through the aqueductus cerebri with the
- ventriculus quartus. This ventriculus communicates with the spatium subarachnoideum via aperturae mediana and laterales (cf. **B**).

The largest ventriculi are the ventriculi laterales, each of which consists of cornua anterius, inferius, and posterius and a pars centralis. Certain portions of the ventricular system can be assigned to specific parts of the brain: the cornu anterius (frontale) to the lobus frontalis of the

cerebrum, the cornu inferius (temporale) to the lobus temporalis, the cornu posterius (occipitale) to the lobus occipitalis, the ventriculus tertius to the diencephalon, the aqueduct to the midbrain (mesencephalon), and the ventriculus quartus to the hindbrain (rhombencephalon). The anatomical relationships of the ventricular system can also be appreciated in coronal and transverse sections (see pp. 420 ff and 432 ff).

Liquor cerebrospinalis is formed mainly by the plexus choroideus, a network of vessels that is present to some degree in each of the four ventriculi (see p. 315). Another site of liquor cerebrospinalis production is the ependyma. Certain diseases (e.g., atrophy of brain tissue in Alzheimer disease and internal hydrocephalus) are characterized by abnormal enlargement of the ventricular system and are diagnosed from the size of the ventriculi in sectional images of the brain.

This unit deals with the ventricular system and neighboring structures. The next unit will trace the path of the liquor cerebrospinalis from its production to its reabsorption. The last unit on the liquor cerebrospinalis spaces will deal with the specialized functions of the ependyma, the circumventricular organs, and the physiological tissue barriers in the brain.

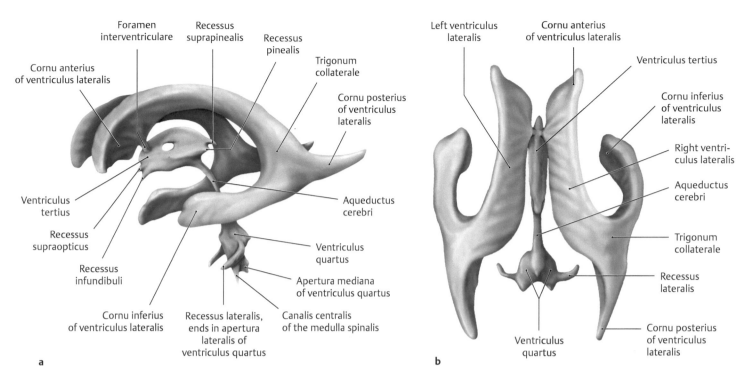

B Cast of the ventricular system
Left lateral view (**a**) and superior view (**b**). Cast specimens are used to demonstrate the connections between the ventricular cavities. Each ventriculus lateralis communicates with the ventriculus tertius through a foramen interventriculare. The ventriculus tertius communicates through the aqueductus cerebri with the ventriculus quartus in the rhombencephalon. The ventricular system has a fluid capacity of approximately 30 ml, while the spatium subarachnoideum has a capacity of approximately 120 ml.

Note the three apertures (paired aperturae laterales [foramina of Luschka] and an unpaired apertura mediana [foramen of Magendie]), through which liquor cerebrospinalis flows from the deeper ventricular system into the more superficial spatium subarachnoideum.

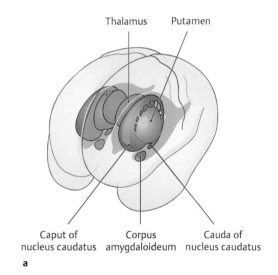

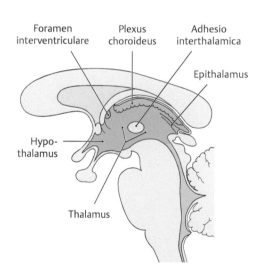

C Important structures neighboring the ventriculi laterales
a View of the brain from upper left.
b View of the cornu inferius of the left ventriculus lateralis in the opened lobus temporalis.

a The following brain structures border on the ventriculi laterales:
- The nucleus caudatus (anterolateral wall of the cornu anterius)
- The thalamus (posterolateral wall of the cornu anterius)

- The putamen, which is lateral to the ventriculus lateralis and does not border it directly

b The hippocampus (see p. 323) is visible in the anterior part of the floor of the cornu inferius. Its anterior portions with the digitationes hippocampi protrude into the ventricular cavity.

D Lateral wall of the ventriculus tertius
Midsagittal section, left lateral view. The lateral wall of the ventriculus tertius is formed by structures of the diencephalon (epithalamus, thalamus, hypothalamus). Protrusions of the thalami on both sides may touch each other (adhesio interthalamica) but are not functionally or anatomically connected and thus do not constitute a commissural tract.

313

5.2 Cerebrospinal Fluid (Liquor Cerebrospinalis), Circulation and Cisternae

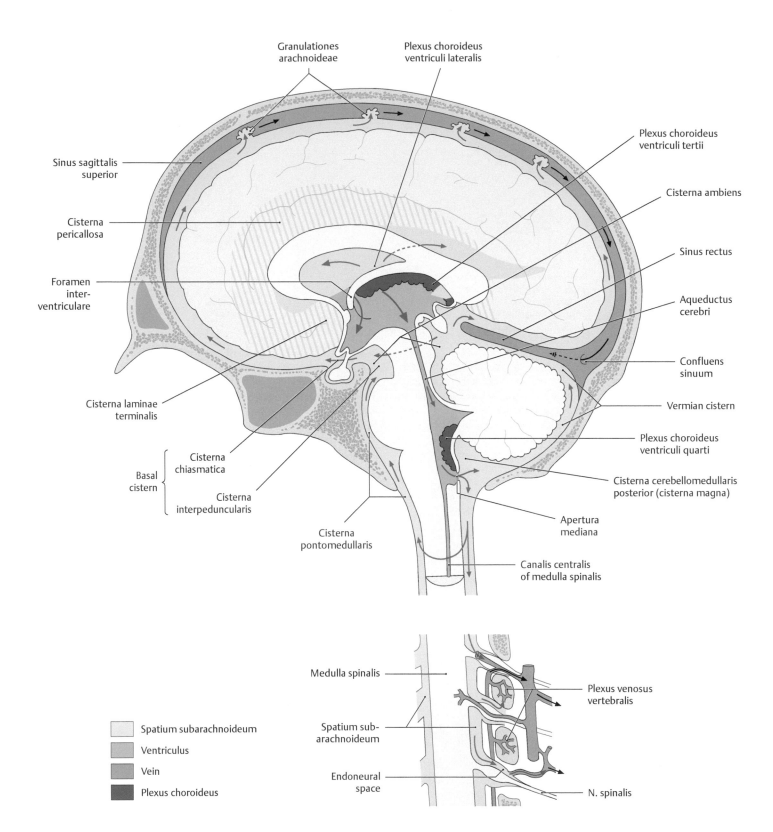

Granulationes arachnoideae

Plexus choroideus ventriculi lateralis

Plexus choroideus ventriculi tertii

Sinus sagittalis superior

Cisterna ambiens

Cisterna pericallosa

Sinus rectus

Foramen inter-ventriculare

Aqueductus cerebri

Confluens sinuum

Cisterna laminae terminalis

Vermian cistern

Basal cistern
- Cisterna chiasmatica
- Cisterna interpeduncularis

Plexus choroideus ventriculi quarti

Cisterna cerebellomedullaris posterior (cisterna magna)

Cisterna pontomedullaris

Apertura mediana

Canalis centralis of medulla spinalis

Medulla spinalis

Plexus venosus vertebralis

Spatium sub-arachnoideum

Spatium subarachnoideum

Endoneural space

N. spinalis

- Spatium subarachnoideum
- Ventriculus
- Vein
- Plexus choroideus

A Cerebrospinal fluid circulation and the cisternae

Liquor cerebrospinalis (cerebrospinal fluid, CSF) is produced in the plexus choroideus, which is present to some extent in each of the four cerebral ventriculi. It flows through the apertura mediana and paired aperturae laterales (not shown; see p. 302 for location) into the spatium subarachnoideum, which contains expansions called cisternae. The liquor cerebrospinalis drains from the spatium subarachnoideum through the granulationes arachnoideae in the cavitas cranii or along the n. spinalis root sleeves into the plexus venosi or lymphatic pathways of the spatium epidurale in the medulla spinalis. Recent studies have initiated a discussion about additional drainage of the CSF in the cavitas cranii through capillaries and vv. superficiales cerebri (not shown here). The cerebral ventriculi and spatium subarachnoideum have a combined capacity of approximately 150 ml of CSF (20% in the ventriculi and 80% in the spatium subarachnoideum). This volume is completely replaced two to four times daily, so that approximately 500 ml of CSF are produced each day. Obstruction of CSF drainage will therefore cause a rise in intracranial pressure (see **E**, p. 317).

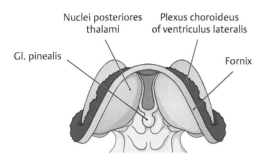

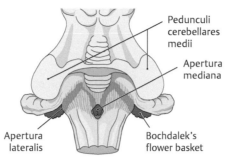

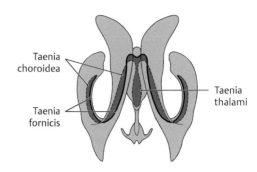

B Plexus choroideus in the ventriculi laterales

Rear view of the thalamus. Surrounding brain tissue has been removed down to the floor of the ventriculi laterales, where the plexus choroideus originates. The plexus is adherent to the ventricular wall at only one site (see **D**) and can thus float freely in the ventricular system.

C Plexus choroideus in the ventriculus quartus

Posterior view of the partially opened fossa rhomboidea (with the cerebellum removed). Portions of the plexus choroideus are attached to the roof of the ventriculus quartus and run along the apertura lateralis. Free ends of the plexus choroideus may extend through the aperturae laterales into the spatium subarachnoideum on both sides ("Bochdalek's flower basket").

D Taeniae of the plexus choroideus

Superior view of the ventricular system. The plexus choroideus is formed by the ingrowth of vascular loops into the ependyma, which firmly attach it to the wall of the associated ventriculus (see **F**). When the plexus tissue is removed with a forceps, its lines of attachment, called taeniae, can be seen.

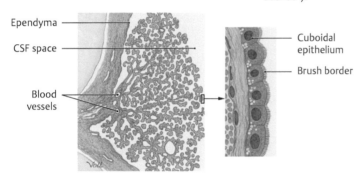

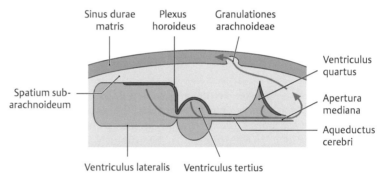

E Histological section of the plexus choroideus, with a detail showing the structure of the plexus epithelium (after Kahle)

The plexus choroideus is a protrusion of the ventricular wall. It is often likened to a cauliflower because of its extensive surface folds. The epithelium of the plexus choroideus consists of a single layer of cuboidal cells and has a brush border on its apical surface (to increase the surface area).

F Schematic diagram of liquor cerebrospinalis circulation

As noted earlier, the plexus choroideus is present to some extent in each of the four cerebral ventriculi. It produces CSF, which flows through the two aperturae laterales (not shown) and apertura mediana into the spatium subarachnoideum. At this point, the largest amout of CSF enters the systemic circulation (lymphatic vessels, venous blood) by escaping at the dural sleeve of each nervus spinalis exiting the foramen intervertebrale.

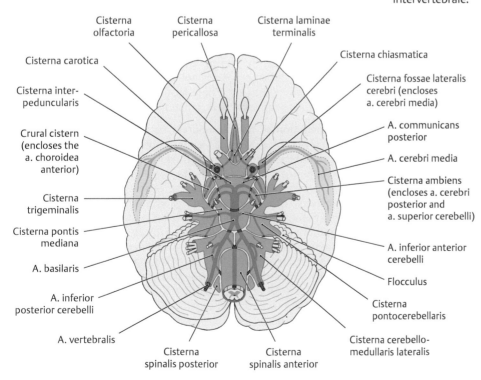

G Subarachnoid cisternae

(after Rauber and Kopsch)
Basal view. The cisternae are CSF-filled expansions of the spatium subarachnoideum. They contain the proximal portions of some nn. craniales and basal cerebral arteries (veins are not shown). When arterial bleeding occurs (as from a ruptured aneurysm), blood will leak into the spatium subarachnoideum and enter the CSF. A ruptured intracranial aneurysm is a frequent cause of blood in the CSF (methods of sampling the CSF are described on p. 317).

5.3 Circumventricular Organs and Tissue Barriers in the Brain

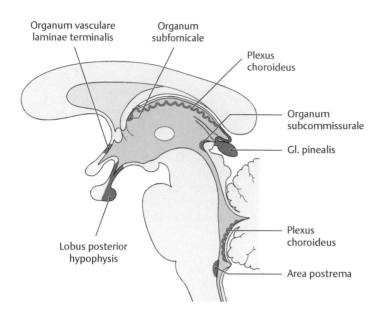

Organum vasculare laminae terminalis

Organum subfornicale

Plexus choroideus

Organum subcommissurale

Gl. pinealis

Plexus choroideus

Lobus posterior hypophysis

Area postrema

A Location of the circumventricular organs
Midsagittal section, left lateral view. The circumventricular organs include the following:

- Lobus posterior hypophysis with the neurohemal region (see p. 350)
- Plexus choroideus (see p. 315)
- Gl. pinealis (see **D** on p. 353)
- Organum vasculosum laminae terminalis, organum subfornicale, organum subcommissurale, and area postrema (see **B**)

The circumventricular or ependymal organs all have several features in common. They are composed of modified ependyma, they usually border on the ventricular and subarachnoid CSF spaces, and they are located in the median plane (except the plexus choroideus, though it does develop from an unpaired primordium in the median plane). The blood-brain barrier is usually absent in these organs (see **C** and **D**; except the organum subcommissurale).

B Summary of the smaller circumventricular organs
In addition to the four regions listed below, the circumventricular organs include the lobus posterior hypophysis, plexus choroideus, and gl. pinealis. The functional descriptions are based largely on experimental studies in animals.

Organ	Location	Function
Organum vasculosum laminae terminalis (VOLT)	Vascular loops in the rostral wall of the ventriculus tertius (lamina terminalis); rudimentary in humans	Secretes the regulatory hormones somatostatin, luliberin, and motilin; contains cells sensitive to angiotensin II; is a neuroendocrine mediator
Organum subfornicale (SFO)	Fenestrated capillaries between the foramina interventricularia and below the fornices	Secretes somatostatin and luliberin from nerve endings; contains cells sensitive to angiotensin II; plays a central role in the regulation of fluid balance ("organ of thirst")
Organum subcommissurale (SCO)	Borders on the gl. pinealis; overlies the commissura posterior at the junction of the ventriculus tertius and aqueductus cerebri	Secretes glycoproteins into the aqueductus that condense to form the Reissner fiber, which may extend into the canalis centralis of the medulla spinalis; blood-brain barrier is intact; function is not completely understood
Area postrema (AP)	Paired organs in the floor of the caudal end of the fossa rhomboidea, richly vascularized	Trigger zone for the emetic reflex (absence of the blood-brain barrier); atrophies in humans after middle age

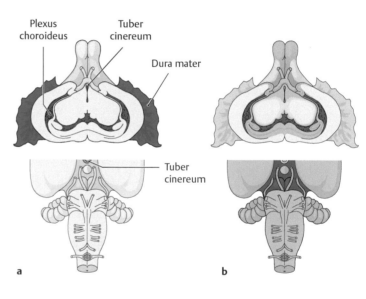

Plexus choroideus

Tuber cinereum

Dura mater

Tuber cinereum

a   b

C Demonstration of tissue barriers in the brain (after Kahle)
a Blood-brain barrier, **b** blood-CSF barrier. The upper drawings show an inferior view of a transverse section through a rabbit brain, and the lower drawings show the truncus encephali from the basal aspect. The function of these barriers is to protect the brain from harmful substances in the bloodstream. These include macromolecular as well as small molecular pharmaceutical compounds.

a Demonstration of the blood-brain barrier: The *intravenous injection* of trypan blue dye (first Goldmann test) stains almost all organs blue except the encephalon and medulla spinalis. Even the dura and choroid plexus show heavy blue staining. Faint blue staining is noted in the tuber cinereum (neurohemal region of the lobus posterior hypophysis), area postrema, and ganglia sensoria nervorum spinalium (absence of the blood-brain barrier in these regions). The same pattern of color distribution occurs naturally in *jaundice*, where bile pigment stains all organs but the encephalon and medulla spinalis, analogous to trypan blue in the first Goldmann test.
b Demonstration of the blood-CSF barrier: When the dye is injected *into the* CSF (second Goldmann test), the encephalon and medulla spinalis (CNS) show diffuse superficial staining while the rest of the body remains unstained. This shows that a barrier exists between the CSF and blood, but not between the CSF and the CNS.

D Blood-brain barrier and blood-CSF barrier

a Normal brain tissue with an intact blood-brain barrier; **b** Blood-CSF barrier in the plexus choroideus.

a The blood-brain barrier in normal brain tissue consists mainly of the tight junctions between capillary endothelial cells. It prevents the paracellular diffusion of hydrophilic substances from CNS capillaries into surrounding tissues and in the opposite direction as well. Essential hydrophilic substances that are needed by CNS must be channeled through the barrier with the aid of specific transport mechanisms (e.g., glucose through the insulin-independent transporter GLUT 1).

b The blood-brain barrier is absent at fenestrated capillary endothelial cells in the plexus choroideus and other circumventricular organs (see **A**), which allow substances to pass freely from the bloodstream into the brain tissue and vice versa. Tight junctions in the overlying ependyma (plexus choroideus epithelium) create a two-way barrier between the brain tissue and ventricular CSF in these regions. The diffusion barrier shifts from the vascular endothelium to the cells of the ependyma and plexus choroideus.

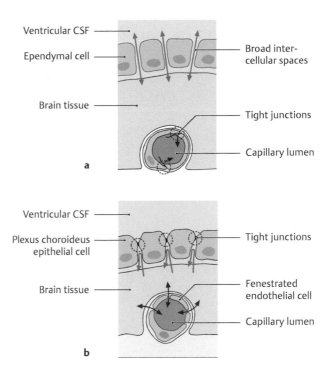

E Obtaining liquor cerebrospinalis samples

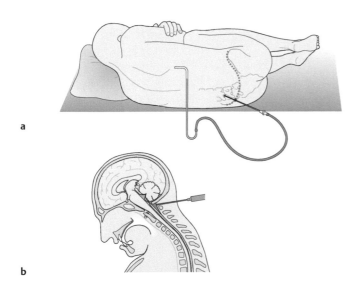

a **Lumbar puncture:** This is the *method of choice* for sampling the CSF. A needle is inserted precisely in the midline between the procc. spinosi of L3 and L4 and is advanced into the dural sac (cisterna lumbalis). At this time a fluid sample can be drawn and the CSF pressure can be measured for diagnostic purposes by connecting a manometer to the needle. Lumbar puncture is contraindicated if the intracranial pressure is markedly increased because it may cause a precipitous cranial to spinal pressure gradient, causing the truncus encephali and/or tonsillae cerebelli to herniate through the foramen magnum. This would exert pressure on vitally important centers in the medulla oblongata, with a potentially fatal outcome. Thus, the physician should always check for signs of increased intracranial pressure (e.g., papilledema, see p. 171) before performing a lumbar puncture.

b **Suboccipital puncture:** This technique should be used only in *exceptional cases* where a lumbar puncture is contraindicated (e.g., by a medulla spinalis tumor), because it may, in rare cases, produce a fatal complication. The mortality risk results from the need to pass a needle through the cisterna cerebellomedullaris posterior (cisterna magna), which may endanger vital centers in the medulla oblongata.

F Comparison of liquor cerebrospinalis and blood serum

Infection of the encephalon and its coverings (meningitis), subarachnoid hemorrhage, and tumor metastases can all be diagnosed by CSF examination. As the table indicates, CSF is more than a simple ultrafiltrate of blood serum. Its primary function is to impart buoyancy of the brain (the brain has an effective weight of only about 50 g despite a mass of 1300 g). Decreased CSF production therefore increases pressure on the spine and also renders the brain more susceptible to injury (less cushioning).

	CSF	Serum
Pressure	50–180 mm H$_2$O	
Volume	100–160 mL	
Osmolarity	292–297 mOsm/L	285–295 mOsm/L
Electrolytes		
Sodium	137–145 mM	136–145 mM
Potassium	2.7–3.9 mM	3.5–5.0 mM
Calcium	1–1.5 mM	2.2–2.6 mM
Chloride	116–122 mM	98–106 mM
pH	7.31–7.34	7.38–7.44
Glucose	2.2–3.9 mM	4.2–6.4 mM
CSF/serum glucose ratio	> 0.5–0.6	
Lactate	1–2 mM	0.6–1.7 mM
Total protein	0.2–0.5 g/L	55–80 g/L
Albumin	56–75 %	50–60 %
IgG	0.01–0.014 g/L	8–15 g/L
Leukocytes	< 4 cells/µL	
Lymphocytes	60–70 %	

5.4 In situ Projection of the Ventricular and Dural Venous Sinus Systems in the Cranial Cavity

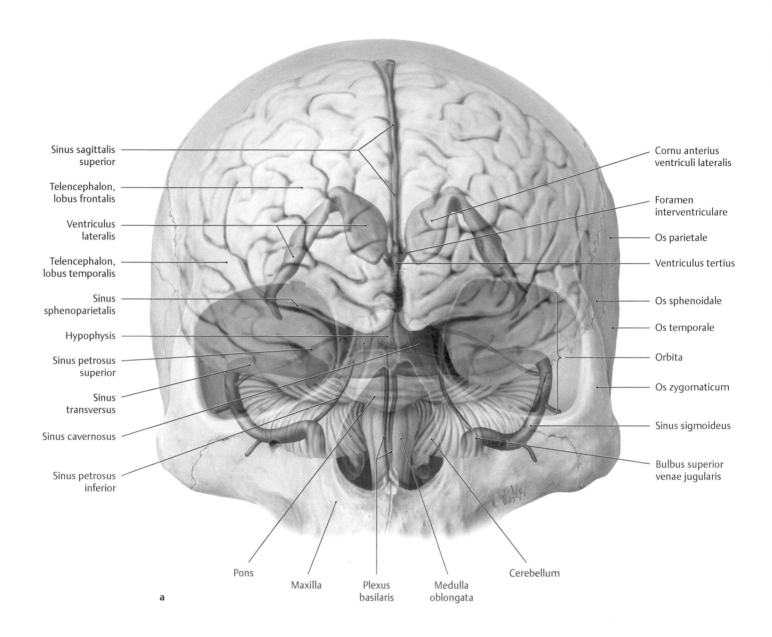

Sinus sagittalis superior

Telencephalon, lobus frontalis

Ventriculus lateralis

Telencephalon, lobus temporalis

Sinus sphenoparietalis

Hypophysis

Sinus petrosus superior

Sinus transversus

Sinus cavernosus

Sinus petrosus inferior

Cornu anterius ventriculi lateralis

Foramen interventriculare

Os parietale

Ventriculus tertius

Os sphenoidale

Os temporale

Orbita

Os zygomaticum

Sinus sigmoideus

Bulbus superior venae jugularis

Pons   Maxilla   Plexus basilaris   Medulla oblongata   Cerebellum

a

A Projection of important brain structures onto the skull

a Anterior view; **b** Left lateral view.

The largest structures of the cerebrum (telencephalon) are the lobi frontalis and temporalis. The falx cerebri separates the two hemispheria cerebri in the midline (not visible here). In the truncus encephali, we can identify the pons and medulla oblongata on both sides of the midline below the telencephalon. The sinus sagittalis superior and the paired sinus sigmoidei can also be seen. The cornua anteriora of the two ventriculi laterales are projected onto the forehead.

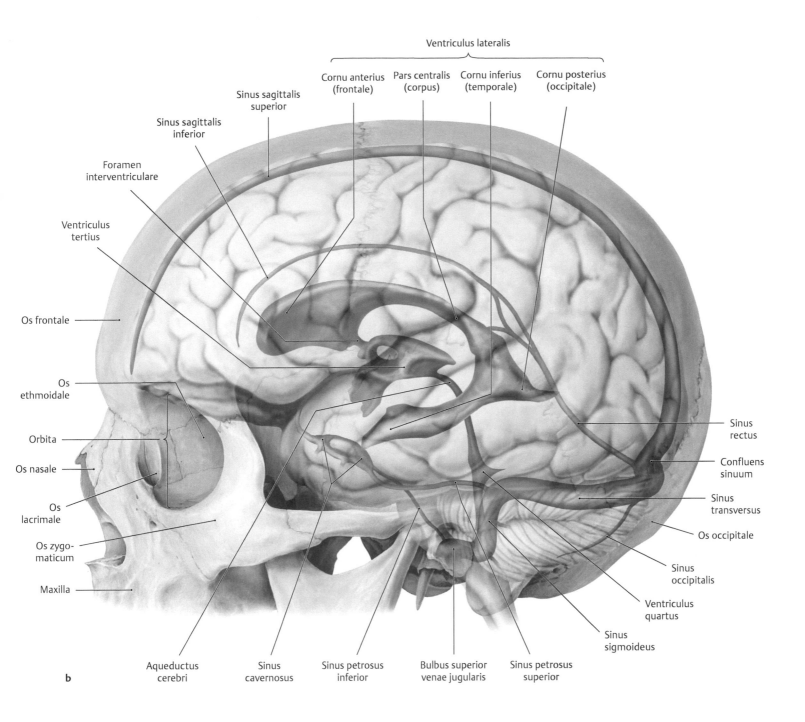

Ventriculus lateralis

Cornu anterius (frontale)
Pars centralis (corpus)
Cornu inferius (temporale)
Cornu posterius (occipitale)

Sinus sagittalis superior

Sinus sagittalis inferior

Foramen interventriculare

Ventriculus tertius

Os frontale

Os ethmoidale

Orbita

Os nasale

Os lacrimale

Os zygomaticum

Maxilla

Sinus rectus

Confluens sinuum

Sinus transversus

Os occipitale

Sinus occipitalis

Ventriculus quartus

Sinus sigmoideus

b

Aqueductus cerebri

Sinus cavernosus

Sinus petrosus inferior

Bulbus superior venae jugularis

Sinus petrosus superior

Viewed from left (**b**), the additional relationship between individual brain lobes and the fossae cranii becomes visible. The lobus frontalis lies in the fossa cranii anterior, the lobus temporalis in the fossa cranii media, and the cerebellum in the fossa cranii posterior. The following sinus durae matris can be identified: the sinus sagittales superior and inferior, sinus rectus, sinus transversus, sinus sigmoideus, sinus cavernosus, sinus petrosi superior and inferior, and sinus occipitalis.

6.1 Telencephalon, Development and External Structure

A Division of the hemispheria cerebri into lobes

a Lateral view of the left hemispherium; **b** Medial view of the right hemispherium; **c** Basal view of the intact telencephalon; n. opticus cut off on both sides, truncus encephali removed showing the cut surface of the mesencephalon.

Although morphologically both hemispheria are roughly symmetrical, textbooks more commonly depict the left hemispherium because of the functional asymmetry of the encephalon: some functions—for instance speech production and speech comprehension—are localized in only one hemispherium and more often in the left than in the right. The left hemispherium is considered to be dominant since in most people it contains the person's language centers. The sulci and gyri which are visible on the hemispheria increase the cortical surface area to roughly 2200 cm². Some anatomic landmarks are well suited to serve as reference points:

- Gyri precentrales and postcentrales are separated by the sulcus centralis.
- Above the gyrus temporalis superior lies the sulcus lateralis which terminates blindly at the gyrus supramarginalis (see p. 322).
- Close to the posterior end of each cerebral hemisphere—visible on the medial surface—lies the sulcus parietooccipitalis.
- The medial surface of the hemispherium shows the corpus callosum and the gyrus cinguli that is located above it.

With the help of these structures, the telencephalon can be divided into 6 lobi. This distinction is based in part on phylogenetic grounds but is also arbitrary in a topographical sense

- Topographically: the sulcus centralis separates the *lobi frontalis and parietalis* (**a**); the sulcus lateralis defines the superior border of the *lobus temporalis* (**a**); the *lobus insularis* (Insula, **Ba**) is located deep within the sulcus lateralis; the sulcus parietooccipitalis separates the lobi occipitalis and parietalis (**b**).
- Phylogenetically: the *lobus limbicus*—mainly visible on the medial surface through the gyrus cinguli (**b**)—is older than the previously mentioned lobes.

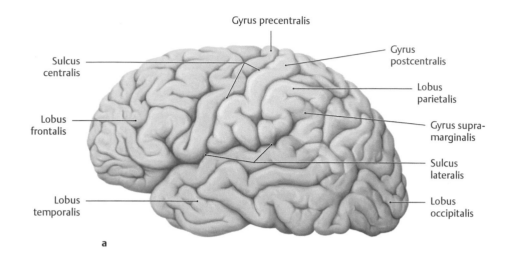

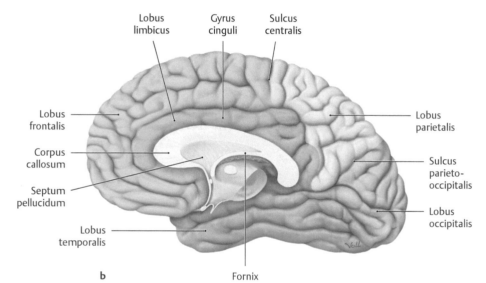

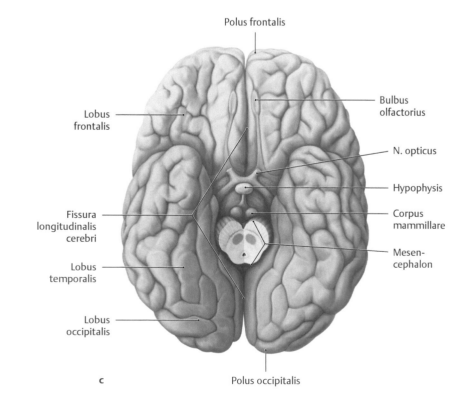

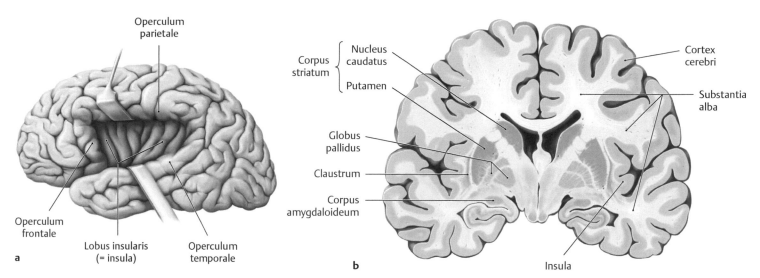

B Substantia grisea and alba in the telencephalon

a Left hemispherium cerebri, lateral view, sulcus lateralis spread open;
b Coronal section of the brain.

a The insula located in the depth of the hemispherium cerebri becomes visible only after the sulcus lateralis has been spread open. In an intact brain it is covered by neighboring lobi. These parts are referred to as little lids (opercula).

b The coronal section shows the distribution of substantia grisea and alba. Based on the division of the pallium, the cortex is divided into neo-, archi-, and paleocortex. The modern neocortex (also called isocortex) is composed of six layers. The archi- and paleocortex (collectively called allocortex) consist of fewer layers. For further detail see p. 326 and 330. Embedded subcortically in the substantia alba are the neuron groups or nuclei. Due to their location at the base of the telencephalon, the nucleus caudatus (having a tail), putamen (or shell, owing to the striation collectively called corpus striatum [or striped body]) and globus pallidus (pale globe) are also referred to as nuclei basales and are often misnamed basal ganglia. Additional nuclei, which anatomically are part of the nuclei basales, are the corpus amygdaloideum (amygdala, an almond-shaped structure) in the lobus temporalis and the claustrum (front wall) a subcortical structure found deep to the lobus insularis. Thus the insula, the previoususly mentioned nuclei, and the exposed ventriculi laterales dominate the cross-section.

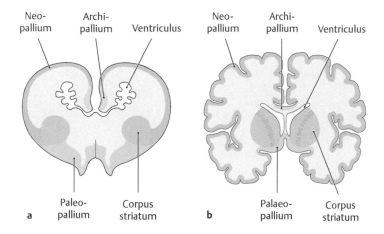

C Development of cortex cerebri and nuclei basales

a Embryonic brain; b Adult brain; frontal sections.

Phylogenetically, the entire telencephalon can be roughly divided into 3 parts of varying age. For this purpose, substantia alba and the overlying substantia grisea (cortex) are collectively referred to as mantle or pallium. In chronological order, a distinction is drawn between *paleopallium, archipallium,* and *neopallium* (for further detail see D). The newer the part of the pallium, the larger its share of the telencephalon. During embryonic development, a large part of the neopallium is invaginated to form the insula (see a). Additionally, neurons from the neopallium migrate into the deeper regions where they form a portion of the nuclei basales (the striatum, see p. 336). Insula and nuclei basales are thus anatomical reference structures on a frontal section.

D Phylogenetic origins of major components of the telencephalon

Phylogenetic term	Structure in the embryonic brain	Structure(s) in the adult brain	Cortical structure
Paleopallium (oldest part)	Floor of the hemispheria	• Rhinencephalon (bulbus olfactorius plus surrounding region)	Allocortex (see p. 330)
Archipallium (old part)	Medial portion of hemispheric wall	• Cornu ammonis (largest part, not shown here) • Indusium griseum • Fornix (see p. 332f)	Allocortex
Neopallium (newest part)	Most of the brain surface plus the deeper corpus striatum	• Neocortex (cortex), largest part of the cortex cerebri • Insula • Corpus striatum	Isocortex (see p. 326)

6.2 Gyri and Sulci of the Telencephalon: Convex Surface of the Cerebral Hemispheres and Base of the Brain

Introduction

Morphologically, the surface of the telencephalon is defined by numerous ridges or *gyri* which are separated from one another by furrows or *sulci*. This form follows a basic pattern in humans which can vary significantly from one individual to another. Some brains even show differences between the left and right hemispherium. This explains why the surface morphology of the brain is not the same in every textbook. A textbook can only present an average anatomical image of the brain. The following illustrations show the gyri and sulci that are officially recognized by the *Terminologia Anatomica*.

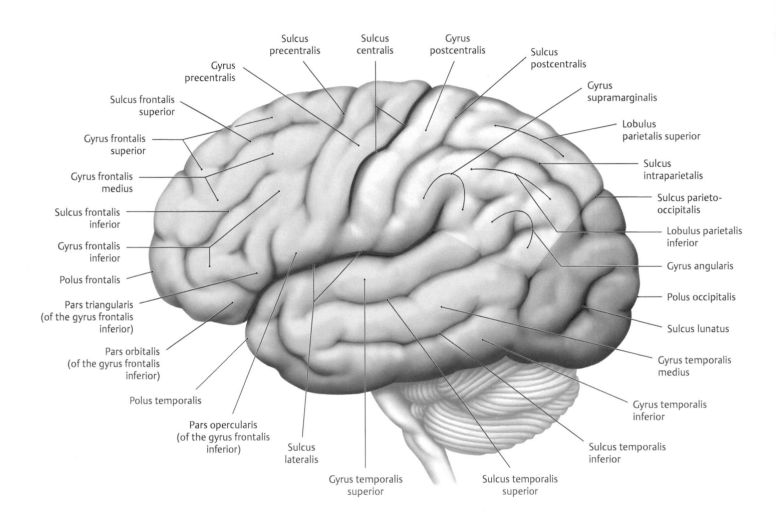

A Gyri and sulci of the convex surface

Left hemisphere, lateral view. The important reference point of the brain is the sulcus centralis, which is clearly visible here. It should not be confused with the neighboring sulci pre- and postcentralis. Often three morphological characteristics are ascribed to the sulcus centralis:

- it is the longest sulcus of the brain,
- it extends across the superior margin of the brain,
- it is joined by the sulcus lateralis, which is also clearly visible here.

In actuality, the sulcus centralis rarely exhibits all these three characteristics. In this case, it helps to use the "two finger rule" to locate the sulcus centralis on the surface of the brain. With the index and middle finger of one hand held close together, they are placed above the hemispherium so that the fingers are above the convolutions which most closely correspond to the longitudinal direction of the fingers and as such run more or less parallel. The index finger is located on the gyrus postcentralis and the middle finger lies on the gyrus precentralis. The gap between the fingers corresponds to the sulcus centralis.

Note: Many gyri are named for their location in a specific lobe (e.g., the gyrus frontalis superior is located on the superior portion of the lobus frontalis).

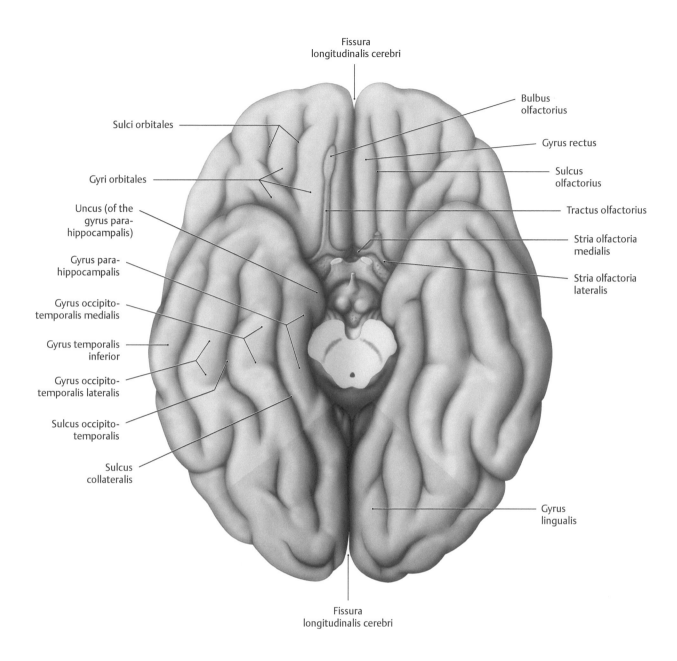

Fissura
longitudinalis cerebri

Sulci orbitales

Gyri orbitales

Uncus (of the
gyrus para-
hippocampalis)

Gyrus para-
hippocampalis

Gyrus occipito-
temporalis medialis

Gyrus temporalis
inferior

Gyrus occipito-
temporalis lateralis

Sulcus occipito-
temporalis

Sulcus
collateralis

Bulbus
olfactorius

Gyrus rectus

Sulcus
olfactorius

Tractus olfactorius

Stria olfactoria
medialis

Stria olfactoria
lateralis

Gyrus
lingualis

Fissura
longitudinalis cerebri

B Gyri and sulci at the base of the brain
Basal view of the telencephalon (from below).
The gyri at the base of the lobus temporalis are sometimes topographically barely distinguishable. This is the case with both the gyri occipitotemporales. For this reason the anatomical illustrations in textbooks may differ. In contrast, the gyri recti are located in the lobus frontalis and the gyri orbitales are situated in the cranium directly above the roof of the orbita. The comparison with **Aa** shows the "edge position" of the gyrus temporalis inferior: it is visible in both the lateral view (as the lower border of the lobus temporalis) and the basal view (as lateral border of the lobus temporalis). What is apparent at the base of the encephalon, is a paleocortical part of the telencephalon, which

morphologically resembles a nerve rather than a part of the cortex since it does not have any gyri: the bulbus and tractus olfactorii. Histologically, this part of the paleocortex does not exhibit a cortical structure.
Note: In the lobus occipitalis very close to the fissura longitudinalis cerebri lies the gyrus lingualis. Its shape, which resembles the tongue, is only visible when viewed from medial aspect (see **A**, p. 324). Although morphologically, it seems to be the posterior extension of the gyrus parahippocampalis (which is the most medial of the gyri) functionally these gyri have nothing to do with each other: The gyrus parahippocampalis is part of the limbic system, while the gyrus lingualis is part of visual cortex. The separation between the two gyri is visible in fig. **A**, p. 324.

6.3 Gyri and Sulci of the Telencephalon: Medial Surface and Insula

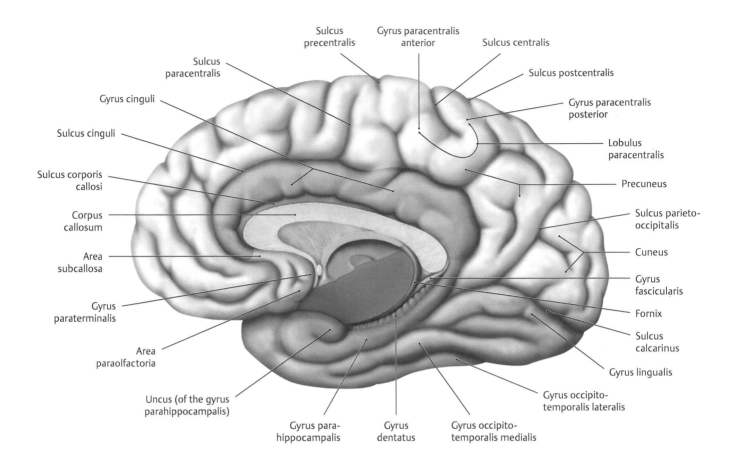

A Gyri and sulci of the medial surface
Right hemispherium, medial view; truncus encephali and basal parts of the diencephalon have been removed.
This midsagittal section provides a view of the medial surface of the encephalon. The corpus callosum serves as an anatomical reference point. Clearly visible are the following structures:

- Located directly above the corpus callosum and surrounding it like a clamp (= cingulum: clamp, yoke) is the gyrus cinguli, which is part of the limbic system.
- Located ventral to the corpus callosum are structures which are often referred to as the "hippocampal formation." The sections of the hippocampal formation are not easily visible from the outside. They are the hippocampus proprius (and the gyrus dentatus with its tooth-like surface). To provide an unobstucted view of the gyrus dentatus, in this specimen the neighboring gyri would have to be either removed or pushed out of the way. The gyrus dentatus lies above and somewhat medial to the hippocampus proprius, which is why the latter is still not visible here. The gyrus dentatus and in particular the hippocampus proprius are almost rolled up in the lobus temporalis of the brain; both structures are part of the limbic system and process information related to learning, memory, and emotions (for a description

of the hippocampus proprius see pp. 330–333). The fornix, which is also clearly visible, is a tract of the limbic system which extends from the hippocampus to the diencephalon.

The midsagittal section also shows additional morphological characteristics, which are less clearly visible when looking at the convex or basal cerebral surfaces:

- The gyrus cinguli has a tongue-like shape. Its superior border is marked by the sulcus calcarinus which separates it from the cuneus (= wedge). At the superior border of the gyrus lingualis and the lower margin of the cuneus—thus demarcating the sulcus calcarinus—lies the primary visual cortex (see p. 329).
- The separation between the gyri lingualis and parahippocampalis is visible.
- The gyrus parahippocampalis continues posteriorly and superiorly with the gyrus cinguli. Both gyri are connected through a long association tract—the cingulum—which is located in the substantia alba of the gyri and therefore not visible here.
- The anterior end of the gyrus parahippocampalis is uncinated or bent like a hook.

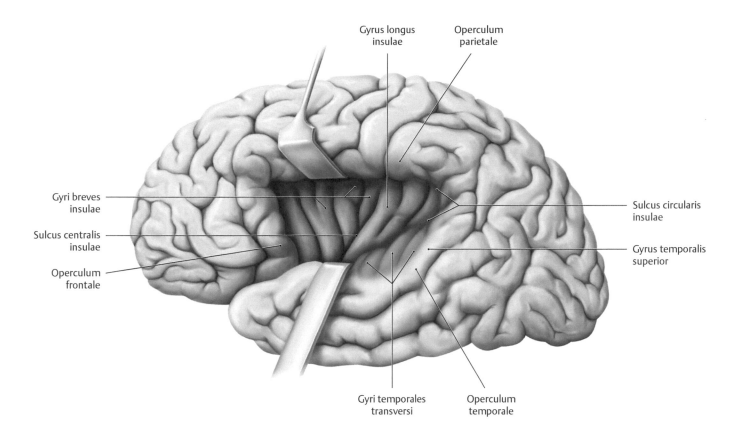

Gyrus longus insulae

Operculum parietale

Gyri breves insulae

Sulcus centralis insulae

Operculum frontale

Sulcus circularis insulae

Gyrus temporalis superior

Gyri temporales transversi

Operculum temporale

B Gyri and sulci of the insula

Left hemisphere, lateral view; sulcus lateralis spread open by retractors. As a result, the following structures become visible:

- the insula (not visible in an intact brain) along with the gyri insulae as well as
- the gyri temporales transversi (transverse gyri of Heschl—the primary auditory cortex) on the surface of the gyrus temporalis superior at its posterior end.

Gyri temporales transversi and gyri insulae do not touch but are separated by the sulcus circularis insulae. The insula is not isolated as its cortex connects it to the cortices of the neighboring lobi. The portions of those lobi which cover the insula in an intact brain from above and below like "little lids" (opercula) have been pulled aside with retractors:

- The operculum parietale (part of the lobus parietalis, which covers the superior part of the insula)
- The operculum temporale (part of the lobus temporalis which covers the inferior part of the insula)
- A small part of the lobus frontalis, which covers the anterior part of the insula, the operculum frontale, has been left in its place. It is significant in that in the operculum frontale—found in most people on the left side—is where the motor speech center of *Broca* is located.

C Gyri and sulci: variants

The previous illustrations depicting gyri and sulci (cf. p. 322 f) show a quasi-standardized basic arrangement pattern. However, there are significant individual variants regarding both the form of the gyri and the shape of the sulci located between them. In particular, the sulci can show enormous differences in depth but neighboring gyri are always connected at the bottom of the sulci. At points where sulci are typically much less dense, the range of variation can make them difficult to identify. Thus, gyri which are seemingly separated by such a sulcus are no longer recognizable as two separate units. The connection between these gyri is visible at the surface. In such a brain, it can be impossible to identify individual gyri due to a lack of demarcations between them. This is most often the case at the base of the encephalon where a demarcation between the gyri occipitotemporales does not exist. Assigning names to individual gyri here might not be possible.

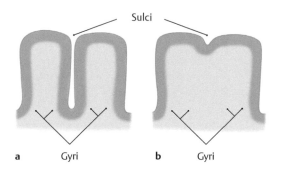

Sulci

a Gyri   b Gyri

The diagram shows a cross-section of two neighboring gyri with the sulcus located between them: In **a**, the sulcus is very deep and both gyri are clearly separated; in **b**, the sulcus is so shallow that it might not even be recognizable when viewed from the surface; in such a case, the morphological distinction of the two gyri would be impossible.

6.4 Cortex Cerebri, Histological Structure and Functional Organization

A Histological structure of the cortex cerebri

A six-layered (laminar) structure is found throughout most of the neocortex. The silver impregnation (**a**) or Nissl staining of the cell bodies (**b**) allows for histological division of the neocortex according to the dominant structure of each layer:

I   Lamina molecularis: (outermost layer); relatively few neurons
II   Lamina granularis externa: mostly stellate and scattered small pyramidal neurons
III   Lamina pyramidalis externa: small pyramidal neurons
IV   Lamina granularis interna: stellate and small pyramidal neurons
V   Lamina pyramidalis interna: large pyramidal neurons
VI   Lamina multiformis: (innermost layer); neurons of varied shape and size

Cortical areas that are concerned primarily with information processing (e.g., primary somatosensory cortex) are rich in granule cells; the lamina granulares of these regions (*granular cortex*, see **Ba**) are also exceptionally thick. Areas in which information is transmitted out of the cortex (e.g., the primary motor cortex) are distinguished by prominent layers of pyramidal cells and known as the *agranular cortex* (see **Bb**). Analysis of the distribution of nerve cells in the cortex cerebri allows for identification of functionally distinct areas (*cytoarchitectonics*, see **A,** p. 328).

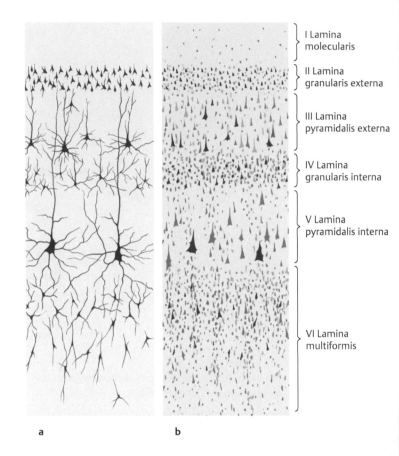

I Lamina molecularis
II Lamina granularis externa
III Lamina pyramidalis externa
IV Lamina granularis interna
V Lamina pyramidalis interna
VI Lamina multiformis

a   b

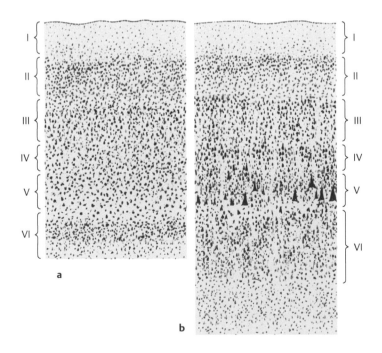

B Examples of granular and agranular cortex

a Granular cortex (koniocortex from the Greek konis = sand): The primary somatosensory cortex, in which the afferents from the thalamus terminate (at layer IV), is located in the gyrus postcentralis. It is thinner overall than the primary somatomotor cortex (see **b**). A striking feature in the primary somatosensory cortex is that the laminae granulares externa and interna (II and IV) where the large sensory tracts terminate are markedly widened. By contrast, the laminae pyramidales (III and V) are thinned.

b Agranular cortex: The efferent fibers that project to the nuclei motorii of the nervi craniales and columnae motorii of the medulla spinalis originate in the primary somatomotor cortex, located in the gyrus precentralis. Its laminae pyramidales (III and V) are greatly enlarged. Exceptionally large pyramidal neurons (Betz cells after the author who first described them) are found in the some areas of layer V. Their long axons extend as far as the sacral medulla spinalis.

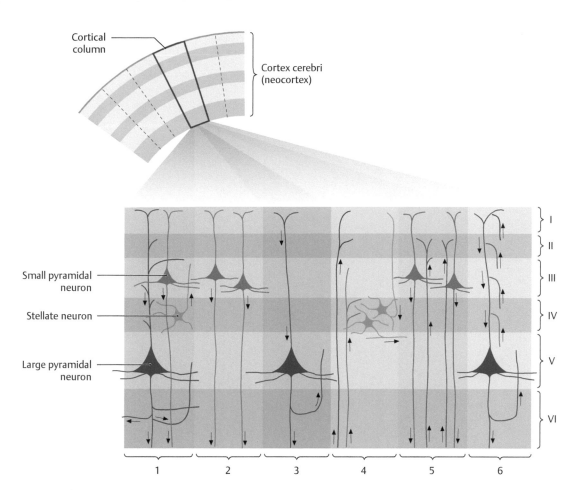

Cortical column

Cortex cerebri (neocortex)

Small pyramidal neuron

Stellate neuron

Large pyramidal neuron

I
II
III
IV
V
VI

1   2   3   4   5   6

C Columnar organization of the cortex (after Klinke and Silbernagl)
While morphological considerations divide the cortex cerebri into horizontal laminae (see **A**), functional considerations lead to its division into distinct units or modules (see **C**). Encompassing all six laminae, these modules consist of vertically-arranged *cortical columns* of neurons that are interconnected to serve a common function, despite showing no distinct histological boundaries. In total, there are several million of such modules in the cortex cerebri, with a variable width between 50 and 500 μm each. One cortical column has been magnified here to display its constituent neurons and connections in separate panels. Panels **a–c** show the principal types of cells participating in a cortical column: several thousand *stellate neurons* of various subtypes and one hundred or so large and small pyramidal neurons (panel **a**). Panel **b** isolates the small pyramidal cells whose axons tend to terminate within the cortex

itself. In contrast, the deeper, large pyramidal neurons (panel **c**) have axons that generally project to subcortical structures. Large pyramidal cells are responsible for tracts of corticobulbar and corticospinal motor axons, which project to the truncus encephali and medulla spinalis, respectively. They may also send recurrent collateral fibers which end in the local cortex. Panels **d–f** contain axons projecting *into* the cortex cerebri. Panel **d** isolates thalamocortical projections that enter from the thalamus and synapse mostly on the stellate neurons of layer IV. Incoming association fibers of the nearby cortex and commissural fibers of the contralateral hemisphere frequently terminate on the dendrites of the small pyramidal neurons (panel **e**). Panel **f** shows the large pyramidal neurons whose apical dendrites reach from layer V to layer I. These large pyramidal neurons integrate inputs from various other local neurons and incoming fibers.

D Types of neuron in the cortex cerebri (simplified)

Neuron	Definition	Properties
Stellate neuron (layers II and IV)	Cell with short axon for local information processing; various types: basket, candelabra, double-bouquet cells	Inhibitory interneuron in most cortical areas; primary information-processing neuron (in layer II), especially in primary sensory areas
Small pyramidal neuron (layer III)	Cell with long axon that often ends within the cortex, either as • Association fiber: axon ends in same hemispherium but different cortical area, or as • Commissural fiber: axon ends in opposite hemispherium but cortical area of similar function	Projection neuron whose axons end within the cortex
Large pyramidal neuron (layer V)	Cell with very long axon that projects outside the cortex, sometimes reaching distant structures	Excitatory projection neuron whose axons end outside the cortex
Granule cell (layers II and IV)	Generic term for small neuron, most often with stellate morphology	Depends on the cell type (see entries for stellate and small pyramidal neurons)

6.5 Neocortex, Cortical Areas

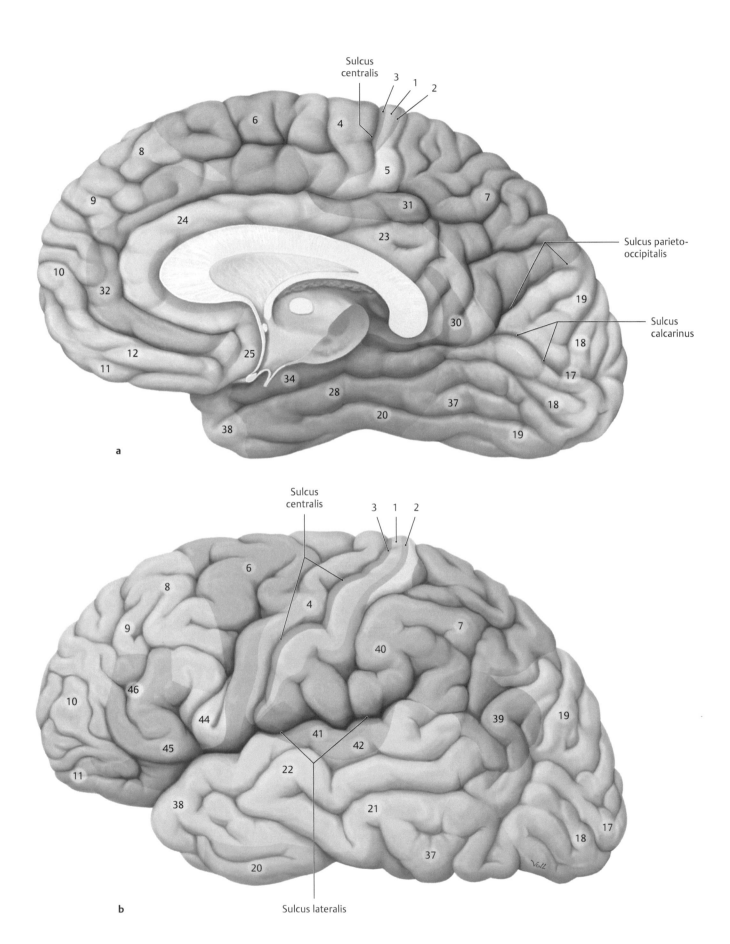

a

Sulcus centralis

Sulcus parieto-occipitalis

Sulcus calcarinus

b

Sulcus centralis

Sulcus lateralis

A Brodmann areas in the neocortex

a Midsagittal section of the right hemispherium cerebri, viewed from the left side; **b** Lateral view of the left hemispherium cerebri.

As noted earlier, the surface of the brain consists macroscopically of lobi, gyri, and sulci. Microscopically, however, subtle differences can be found in the distribution of the cortical neurons, and some of these differences do not conform to the gross surface anatomy of the brain. Portions of the cortex cerebri that have the same basic microscopic features are called *cortical areas* or *cortical fields*. This organization into cortical areas is based on the distribution of neurons in the different layers of the cortex (*cytoarchitectonics*, see **A**, p. 326). In the brain map shown at left, these areas are indicated by different colors. Although the size of the cortical areas may vary between individuals, the brain map pictured here is still used today as a standard reference chart. It was developed

in the early 20th century by the anatomist Korbinian Brodmann (1868–1918), who spent years painstakingly examining the cellular architecture of the cortex in a single brain. It has long been thought that the map created by Brodmann accurately reflects the functional organization of the cortex, and indeed, modern imaging techniques have shown that many of the cytologically defined areas are associated with specific functions. There is no need, of course, to memorize the location of all the cortical areas, but the following areas are of special interest:

- Areas 1, 2, and 3: primary somatosensory cortex
- Area 4: primary motor cortex
- Area 17: primary visual cortex (striate area, the extent of which is best appreciated in the midsagittal section)
- Areas 41 and 42: auditory cortex

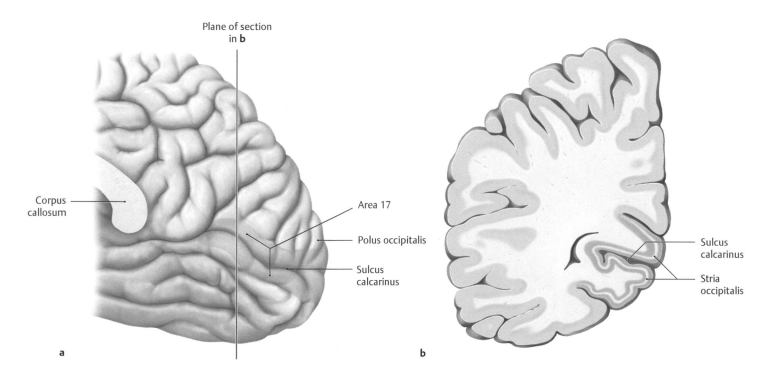

Plane of section in **b**

Corpus callosum

Area 17

Polus occipitalis

Sulcus calcarinus

Sulcus calcarinus

Stria occipitalis

a

b

B Visual cortex (striate area)

a Medial aspect of the right hemisphere viewed from the left side; **b** Coronal section (plane of section shown in **a**), anterior view.

The primary visual cortex (striate area, shaded yellow) is the only cortical area that can be clearly recognized by its macroscopic appearance. It extends along both sides of the sulcus calcarinus at the polus occipitalis. In an unstained coronal section (**b**), the *stria occipitalis* (stria of Gennari)

can be identified as a prominent white stripe within the gray cortical area. This stripe contains cortical association fibers that synapse with the neurons of the lamina granularis interna (IV, see p. 201). The laminae pyramidales (efferent fibers) are attenuated in the visual cortex, while the laminae granulares where the afferent fibers from the corpus geniculatum laterale terminate are markedly enlarged.

6.6 Allocortex, Overview

A Overview of the allocortex

View of the base of the encephalon (**a**) and the medial surface of the right hemispherium (**b**). Structures belonging to the allocortex are indicated by colored shading.

The allocortex consists of the phylogenetically old part of the cortex cerebri. It is very small in relation to the cortex as a whole. Unlike the isocortex, which has a six-layered structure, the allocortex (*allo* = "other") usually consists of *three* layers that encompass the paleo- and archicortexes. Additionally, there exist *four*-layered transitional areas between the allocortex and isocortex: the *peri*paleocortex (not indicated separately in the drawing) and the *peri*archicortex (indicated by pink shading). An important part of the allocortex is the *rhinencephalon* ("olfactory brain"). Olfactory impulses that are perceived by the bulbus olfactorius are the only sensory afferent impulses that do not reach the cortex cerebri by way of the nuclei dorsales thalami. Another important part of the allocortex is the hippocampus and its associated nuclei (see p. 332). As in the isocortex, the gyral patterns of the allocortex do not always conform to its histological organization.

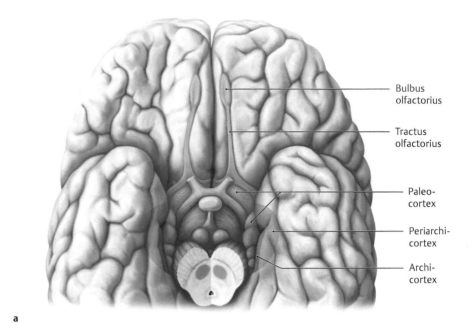

Bulbus olfactorius

Tractus olfactorius

Paleo-cortex

Periarchi-cortex

Archi-cortex

a

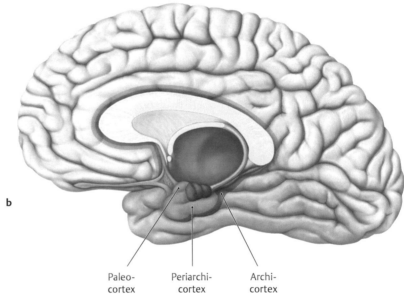

b

Paleo-cortex Periarchi-cortex Archi-cortex

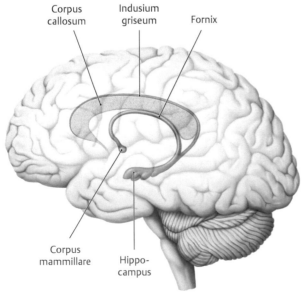

Corpus callosum   Indusium griseum   Fornix

Corpus mammillare   Hippo-campus

B Organization of the archipallium: deeper parts

Lateral view of the left hemispherium. The archicortex described in A is the *only* part of the archipallium that is located on the brain surface. The deeper parts of the archipallium, which lie within the white matter, are the hippocampus ("sea horse"), indusium griseum ("gray covering"), and fornix ("arch"). All three structures are part of the *limbic system* (see p. 492), and together form a border ("limbus") around the corpus callosum as a result of their arrangement during development.

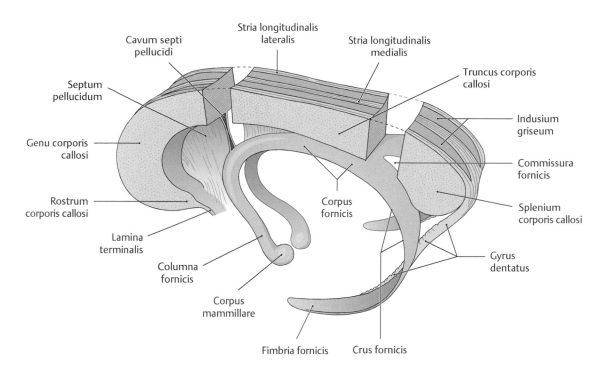

C Topography of the fornix, corpus callosum, and septum pellucidum (after Feneis)

Occipital view from upper left. The fornix is a tract of the archicortex that is closely apposed but functionally unrelated to the corpus callosum. The corpus callosum is the largest neocortical commissural tract between the hemispheria, serving to interconnect cortical areas of similar function in the two hemispheria (see **D**, p. 335). The septum pellucidum is a thin plate that stretches between the corpus callosum and fornix, forming the medial boundary of the ventriculi laterales. Between the two septa is a cavity of variable size, the *cavum septi pellucidi*. The cholinergic nuclei in the septa, which are involved in the organization of memory, are connected to the hippocampus by the fornix (see p. 332).

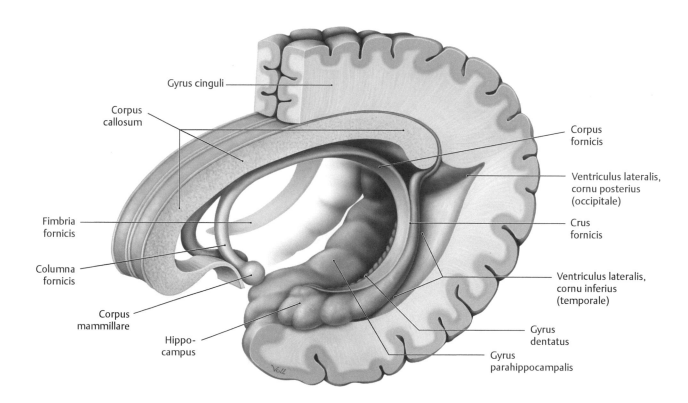

D Topography of the hippocampus, fornix, and corpus callosum

Viewed from the upper left and anterior aspect. This drawing shows the hippocampus on the floor of the cornu inferior of the ventriculus lateralis. The left and right *crura fornices* unite to form the *commissura fornicis* (see **C**) and the *corpus fornicis*, which divides anteriorly into left and right bundles, the *columnae fornices*. The fornix is a white matter tract connecting the hippocampus to the corpora mammillaria in the diencephalon. Contained within the fornix are hippocampal neurons whose axons project to the septum, corpora mammillaria, contralateral hippocampus, and other structures. In it run efferent pathways between hippocampus and hypothalamus. This important pathway is part of the *limbic system*.

331

6.7 Allocortex: Hippocampus and Amygdala

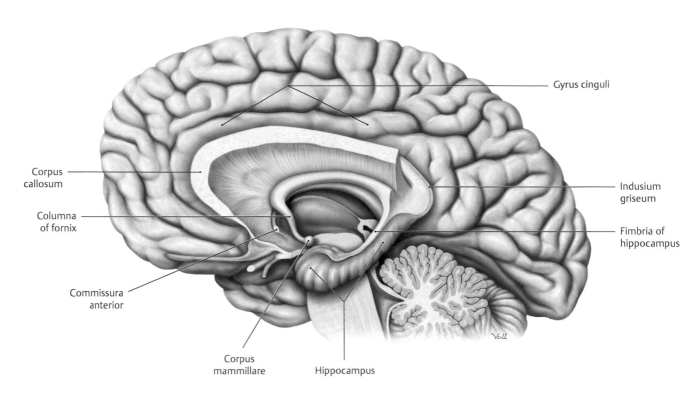

Gyrus cinguli

Corpus callosum

Indusium griseum

Columna of fornix

Fimbria of hippocampus

Commissura anterior

Corpus mammillare

Hippocampus

A Left hippocampal formation

Lateral view of hippocampus and fornix. Most of the left hemispherium has been dissected and removed, leaving only the corpus callosum, fornix, and hippocampus. The intact right hemispherium is visible in the background.

The hippocampal formation is an important component of the *limbic system* (see p. 492). It consists of three parts:

- Subiculum (see **Cb**)
- Hippocampus proprius (cornu ammonis)
- Gyrus dentatus (fascia dentata)

The fiber tract of the fornix connects the hippocampus to the corpus mammillare. The hippocampus integrates information from various brain areas and influences endocrine, visceral, and emotional processes via its efferent output. It is particulary associated with the establishment of short-term memory. Lesions of the hippocampus can therefore cause specific defects in memory formation (see **B**, p. 498).

Besides the hippocampus, which is the largest part of the archicortex, we can recognize another component of the archicortex, the indusium griseum.

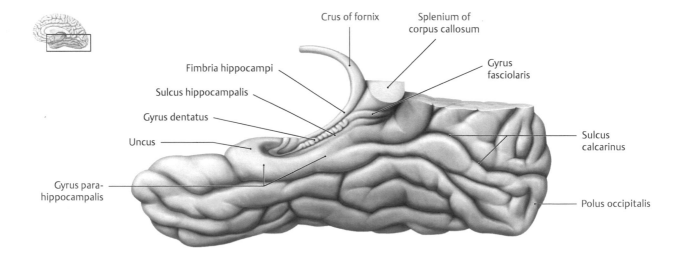

Crus of fornix

Splenium of corpus callosum

Fimbria hippocampi

Gyrus fasciolaris

Sulcus hippocampalis

Gyrus dentatus

Uncus

Sulcus calcarinus

Gyrus para-hippocampalis

Polus occipitalis

B Right hippocampal formation and the caudal part of the fornix

Medial view. Compare this medial view of the right hippocampal formation with the lateral view in **A** above. A useful landmark is the sulcus calcarinus, which leads to the polus occipitalis. The cortical areas that border the hippocampus (e.g., the gyrus parahippocampalis) are particulary visible in this view.

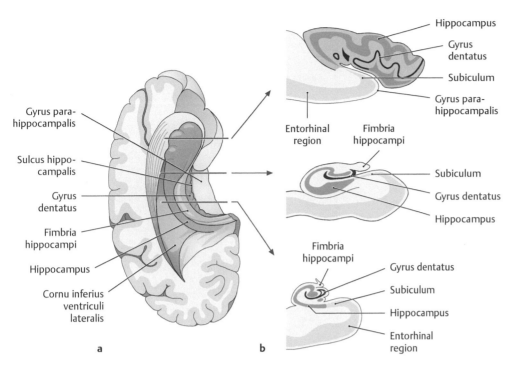

C Left lobus temporalis with the cornu inferior of the ventriculus lateralis exposed

a Transverse section, posterior view of the hippocampus on the floor of the cornu inferius (temporale). The following structures can be identified from lateral to medial: hippocampus, fimbria, gyrus dentatus, sulcus hippocampalis, and gyrus parahippocampalis.

b Coronal sections of the left hippocampus. The hippocampus appears here as a curled band (cornu ammonis = the hippocampus proprius), which shows considerable structural diversity in its different portions. The junction between the entorhinal cortex (entorhinal region) in the gyrus parahippocampalis and cornu ammonis is formed by a transitional area, the subiculum. The entorhinal region is the "gateway" to the hippocampus, through which the hippocampus receives most of its afferent fibers.

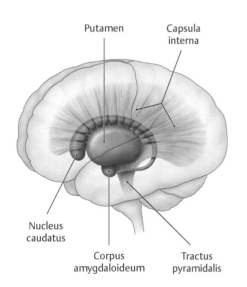

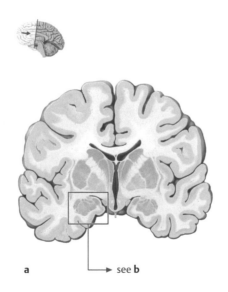

D Relationship of the corpus amygdaloideum to internal brain structures

Lateral view of the left hemispherium. The amygdala (corpus amygdaloideum) is located below the putamen and anterior to the cauda of the nucleus caudatus. The fibers of the nucleus caudatus run posterior and medial to the corpus amygdaloideum.

E Corpus amygdaloideum

a Coronal section at the level of the foramen interventriculare. The corpus amygdaloideum extends medially to the inferior surface of the cortex of the lobus temporalis. For this reason, it is considered to be part of the cortex as well as a nuclear complex that has migrated into the substantia alba. Stimulation of the corpus amygdaloideum in humans leads to changes in mood, ranging from rage and fear to rest and relaxation depending on the emotional state of the patient immediately prior to stimulation. Since the corpus amygdaloideum functions as an "emotional amplifier," lesions affect the patient's evaluation of events' emotional significance. The surrounding cortex periamygdaloideus and the corticomedial half of the corpus amygda-

loideum are part of the primary olfactory cortex. Hence these portions of the corpus amygdaloideum are considered part of the paleocortex, while the deeper portion is characterized as "nuclear."

b Detail from a showing the two main groups of nuclei in the corpus amygdaloideum:

- Phylogenetically old corticomedial group:
  - Nucleus amygdalae corticalis
  - Nucleus amygdalae centralis
- Phylogenetically new basolateral group:
  - Nuclei amygdalae basales
  - Nucleus amygdalae lateralis

The nuclei amygdalae basales can be subdivided into a parvocellular nucleus amygdalae basalis medialis and a macrocellular nucleus amygdalae basalis lateralis.

333

6.8 The White Matter (Substantia Alba)

A Substantia alba in the telencephalon

a Midsagittal view of the right hemispherium viewed from the left; **b** Parasagittal view of left hemisphere viewed from the left, a *fiber dissection specimen*.

In the intact central nervous system, the substantia alba appears structurally homogeneous. With the help of special preparation techniques that utilize the different water content of various structures of the CNS, it can be shown that the substantia alba is composed of tracts (tractus, see **D**, p. 269), of myelinated axons. Axons are responsible for signal transduction. Tracts are therefore "data highways" for the rapid signal transmission in the CNS. Although all of the substantia alba in the CNS consists of tracts, they can be most easily shown in the substantia alba of the telencephalon. The tracts are distinguished based on the direction of information flow and the localization of the tract connecting parts of the CNS:

* projection tracts
* commissural tracts (see **D**)
* association tracts (see **C**)

If tracts are destroyed (e.g., in the case of multiple sclerosis) the functions assigned to one tract are no longer executed. Due to the functional variety of tracts, the disruption can lead to a range of symptoms including paralysis, impaired somatosensation, visual disturbances, and/or memory loss. Since tracts always connect two structures in the CNS, it is very important when studying those tracts, to learn the involved structures, signal sender and signal receiver. For more detail see **B**.

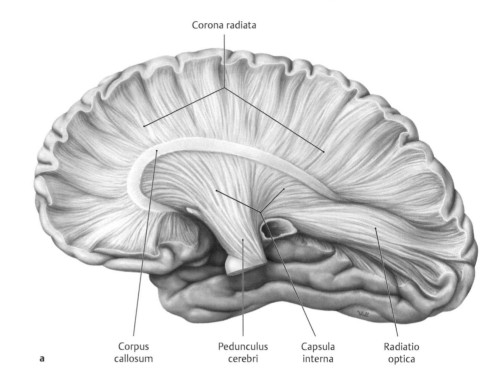

Corona radiata

a Corpus callosum | Pedunculus cerebri | Capsula interna | Radiatio optica

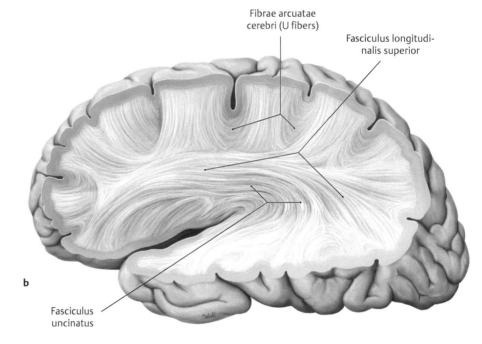

Fibrae arcuatae cerebri (U fibers)

Fasciculus longitudinalis superior

b Fasciculus uncinatus

B Pathways of the CNS

Classification of pathways. Two pathways are ususally macroscopically visible in a brain even if it has not been specifically prepared: fornix (vault) and corpus callosum.

Projection fibers	Connect the cortex cerebri to subcortical centers, either ascending or descending (Fornix = special projection tract of the limbic system)
• **Ascending fibers**	Connect subcortical centers to the cortex cerebri
• **Descending fibers**	Connect the cortex cerebri to deeper/lower centers
Fibrae associationis	Connect different cortical areas within one hemispherium (see **C**)
Fibrae commissurales	Connect similar cortical areas in both hemispheria (see **D**) (= interhemispheric association fibers); Corpus callosum = largest commissural tract in the brain

Fasciculus orbitofrontalis

Fasciculus occipito-frontalis superior

Fasciculus longitudinalis superior

Fasciculi occipitales verticales

Fasciculus uncinatus

Fasciculus occipitofrontalis inferior

Fasciculus longitudinalis inferior

a

Cingulum

Fasciculus occipitofrontalis superior

Fasciculus longitudinalis superior

Fasciculus occipito-frontalis inferior

b

Fibrae arcuatae cerebri

Fibrae associationis telencephali

c

C Fibrae associationis
a Lateral view of the left hemispherium. **b** Anterior view of coronal section of the right hemispherium. **c** Anterior view of fibrae associationis breves. Fibrae associationis longae interconnect different brain areas that are located in different lobi, whereas fibrae associationis breves interconnect cortical areas within the same lobus. Adjacent cortical areas are interconnected by short, U-shaped fibrae arcuatae cerebri, which run just below the cortex.

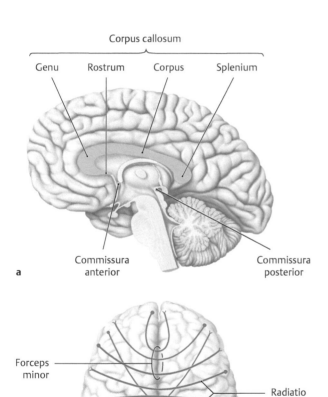

Corpus callosum

Genu Rostrum Corpus Splenium

Commissura anterior

Commissura posterior

a

Forceps minor

Radiatio corpus callosi

Forceps major

b

D Fibrae commissurales
a Medial view of the right hemispherium. **b** Superior view of the transparent brain.
Fibrae commissurales interconnect the two hemispheria of the brain. The most important connecting structure between the hemispheria is the corpus callosum. If the corpus callosum is intentionally divided, as in a neurosurgical procedure, the two halves of the brain can no longer communicate with each other ("split-brain" patient, see p. 496). There are other, smaller commissural tracts besides the corpus callosum (commissura anterior, commissura fornicis).

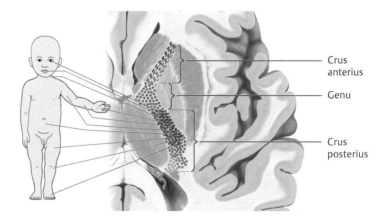

Crus anterius

Genu

Crus posterius

E Projection tracts
Horizontal section through the right hemispherium, superior view of the capsula interna. Both ascending and descending projection fibers pass through the capsula interna. If blood flow to the capsula interna is interrupted, as by a stroke, these ascending and descending tracts undergo irreversible damage. The figure of the child shows how the sites where the tractus pyramidalis fibers pass through the capsula interna can be assigned to peripheral areas of the human body. Thus, we see that smaller lesions of the capsula interna may cause a loss of upper motor neuron control (= spastic paralysis) of certain areas of the body. This accounts for the great clinical importance of this structure. The capsula interna is bounded medially by the thalamus and the caput of the nucleus caudatus, and laterally by the globus pallidus and putamen. The capsula interna consists of a crus anterius, a genu, and a crus posterius, which are traversed by specific tracts:

Crus anterius	• Tractus frontopontinus (red dashes)
	• Radiatio thalami anterior (blue dashes)
Genu capsulae internae	• Radiatio thalami centralis (blue dots)
Crus posterius	• Fibrae corticonucleares (red dots)
	• Fibrae corticospinales (red dots)
	• Radiatio thalamica posterior (blue dots)
	• Fibrae temporopontinae (orange dots)
	• Fibrae occipitopontinae (green dots)

6.9 Basal Nuclei (Nuclei Basales)

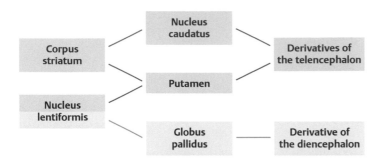

A Definition and classification of nuclei basales
The term "nuclei basales" includes three paired large nuclear regions, which are topographically located at the base of the telencephalon at its border with the diencephalon. The "official" term is telencephalic basal nuclei to explicitly distinguish them from the thalamic basal nuclei located in the diencephalon. *Anatomically,* the nuclei basales include the nucleus caudatus (tail), the putamen (dish), and the globus pallidus (pale globe). Based purely on morphological grounds, two nuclei

basales are grouped together under one name: Putamen and nucleus caudatus are collectively called corpus striatum (striated body) and putamen and globus pallidus are referred to as nucleus lentiformis (lentil-shaped nucleus). Developmentally significant is the fact that the nucleus caudatus and putamen are derived from the cortex cerebri (see **D**, p. 323), whereas the phylogenetically older globus pallidus is derived from the diencephalon (from a region referred to as "subthalamic"), see **D**, p. 329. It is not uncommon, especially in the clinical literature, to find the term "basal ganglia" used. From a strictly anatomic point of view, this is incorrect because "ganglia" are only found in the PNS. Here in the CNS, true nuclei exist.
Note: The nuclei basales are involved in motor control. They share these functions with other central areas (e.g., the substantia nigra and the nucleus ruber in the truncus encephali). Thus physiologically, these two truncus encephali nuclei are occasionally considered—exclusively due to their shared functions—as part of the group of nuclei basales. This is functionally justified. In the following chapters, the term "nuclei basales" exlusively refers to the nuclear complex as that anatomically defined above.

B Location and projection of nuclei basales
Telencephalon. **a** Left lateral view of the brain: nuclei basales located anteriorly; **b** Left anterior oblique view.
The location of the nuclei basales leads to complex topographical relationships, which can be best understood with the help of a conceptual combination of three-dimensional representations and parts (see **C**). The nucleus caudatus with its sections caput, corpus, and cauda virtually "nestles" into the concave wall of the ventriculus lateralis and follows it along its entire length down to the lobus temporalis (**a**). Located on the concave side of the nucleus caudatus is the putamen. The comparatively small globus pallidus lies hidden medially to the putamen and is not visible here. The oblique view (**b**) additionally shows the thalamus which is part of the diencephalon. In the lateral view (**a**) the thalamus is also hidden by the putamen. The thalamus is not a nucleus basalis, yet it is located adjacent to the nuclei basales, since they lie at the base of the telencephalon at the border with the diencephalon. The thalamus is mentioned here because it is a significant anatomical landmark for the demarcation of the capsula interna.
Note: In both horizontal and coronal sections, with a suitable sectional plane, the nucleus caudate can be cut twice (green arrows in **a**) due to its curved nature.

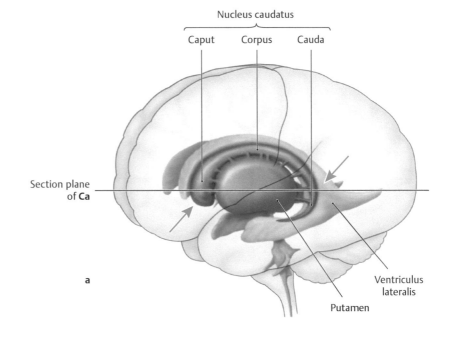

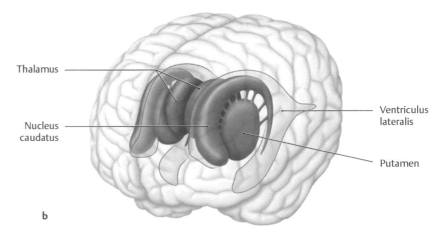

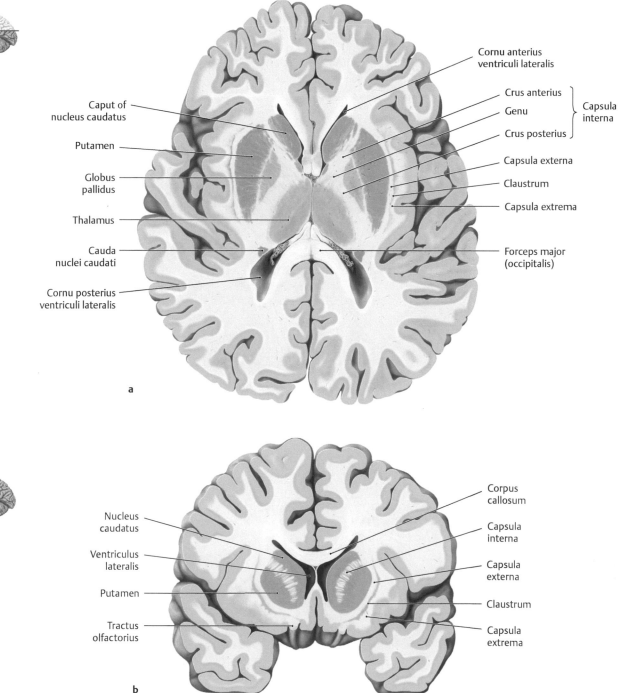

Labels on figure **a**:
- Caput of nucleus caudatus
- Putamen
- Globus pallidus
- Thalamus
- Cauda nuclei caudati
- Cornu posterius ventriculi lateralis
- Cornu anterius ventriculi lateralis
- Crus anterius ⎫
- Genu ⎬ Capsula interna
- Crus posterius ⎭
- Capsula externa
- Claustrum
- Capsula extrema
- Forceps major (occipitalis)

Labels on figure **b**:
- Nucleus caudatus
- Ventriculus lateralis
- Putamen
- Tractus olfactorius
- Corpus callosum
- Capsula interna
- Capsula externa
- Claustrum
- Capsula extrema

C Nuclei basales on the brain section: neighborhood relationships
a Horizontal section through the brain at the telencephalon-diencephalon border, superior view; **b** Coronal section through the telencephalon, anterior view.

If the encephalon is cut horizontally at the border between telencephalon and diencephalon, all nuclei basales are visible. The nucleus caudatus is cut twice (caput and cauda and topographically closely associated with the cornua anterius and posterius of the ventriculus lateralis). The small globus pallidus is located medially to the putamen (thus not visible in the lateral view, see **B**). The thalamus lies on both sides of the very narrow ventriculus tertius. The capsula interna, a boomerang-shaped area of substantia alba, which contains ascending and descending projection tracts, is surrounded by nuclei basales and the thalamus (see **A**, p. 334). The crus anterius of the capsula interna, runs between the caput of the nucleus caudatus and nucleus lentiformis; the genu, and the crus posterius are located between the thalamus and the nucleus lentiformis, thus at the border between telencephalon and diencephalon.

Note: Lateral to the putamen, directly medial to the insular cortex, lies a nucleus that is referred to as claustrum (front wall). It is surrounded by substantia alba of the capsulae externa and extrema. The claustrum is not a nucleus basalis (though it once was referred to as one); its function is largely unknown; it is believed to be involved in regulating sexual behavior.

The coronal section that was chosen here, cuts though the caput of the nucleus caudatus, which protrudes into the cornu anterius of the ventriculus lateralis. In this section, no parts of the diencephalon are visible. Ventriculus tertius, thalamus, and globus pallidus are not present in this section. The acrus anterius of the capsula interna passes between the nuclei basales, which are located close to one another, and due to the alternating arrangement of substantia grisea and alba gives the substantia grisea of the nuclei a striated appearance (corpus striatum). The coronal section (**b**) illustrates the close topographical relationship between the nucleus caudatus and the corpus callosum, which in this image is located supero-medial to the nucleus caudatus and forms the roof of the ventriculus lateralis.

7.1 Diencephalon, Overview and Development

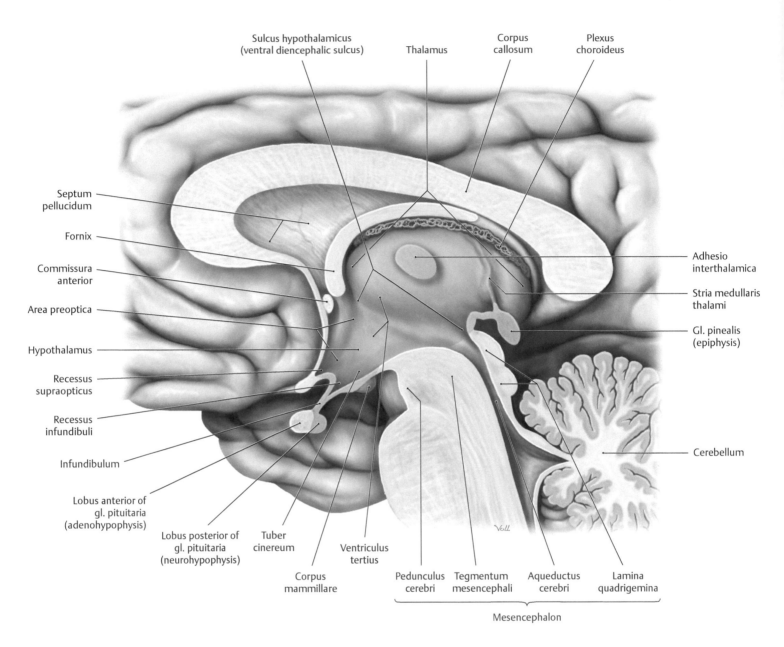

Sulcus hypothalamicus (ventral diencephalic sulcus)
Thalamus
Corpus callosum
Plexus choroideus
Septum pellucidum
Fornix
Commissura anterior
Area preoptica
Hypothalamus
Recessus supraopticus
Recessus infundibuli
Infundibulum
Lobus anterior of gl. pituitaria (adenohypophysis)
Lobus posterior of gl. pituitaria (neurohypophysis)
Tuber cinereum
Corpus mammillare
Ventriculus tertius
Adhesio interthalamica
Stria medullaris thalami
Gl. pinealis (epiphysis)
Cerebellum
Pedunculus cerebri
Tegmentum mesencephali
Aqueductus cerebri
Lamina quadrigemina
Mesencephalon

A The diencephalon in situ

Midsagittal section; left lateral view of right hemispherium. The diencephalon is located beneath the two hemispheria cerebri and above the truncus encephali. The anterior, superior, and lateral parts of the diencephalon directly adjoin the telencephalon. Posteriorly a small section in the area around the pineal gland (see also fig. **B**, p. 352) lies exposed. The base of the diencephalon is composed of two parts. The posterior part of the base is located at the poorly defined border with the mesencephalon, the anterior part—defined by the hypothalamus—has been exposed. The ventriculus tertius located in the median plane divides the diencephalon into symmetrical halves which contain either paired structures (in the lateral wall of the ventriculus tertius, e.g., the thalamus, which are not cut in midsagittal sections), or unpaired structures (located in the midline; therefore they always appear cut on a midsagittal section). As a result of the position of the individual parts of the diencephalon, the ventriculus tertius has several extensions, or recesses. The corpus callosum and the septum pellucidum (the partition between the ventriculi laterales) are clearly visible and therefore helpful anatomical reference points. Located beneath the corpus callosum, the thalamus occupies the largest area of the lateral wall of the ventriculus tertius. Due to its projection into the ventricular lumen, the ventriculus tertius is separated from the smooth wall of the hypothalamus by a furrow: the sulcus hypothalamicus. The fornix (arch) is an arch-shaped structure that passes above the thalamus and surrounds it. It extends between the hippocampus (which is part of the telencephalon) and the corpora mammillaria. As a projection tract, it is, topographically and functionally, part of both the telencephalon and the diencephalon. Topographically, the fornix is occasionally referred to as the roof of the ventriculus tertius. Functionally, the diencephalon is extremely multifaceted: it acts as a relay station for most sensorial modalities, represents a station for the control of motor functions, regulates the circadian rhythm and endocrine activity and is the supreme authority for important autonomic functions of the body.

Note: One part of the diencephalon, which is particularly important for motor functions, the subthalamus, due to its far lateral location, can never be seen on the midsagittal section but only on coronal (see **B**, p. 343; **E**, p. 353; and p. 420 ff and p. 433 f) or horizontal sections.

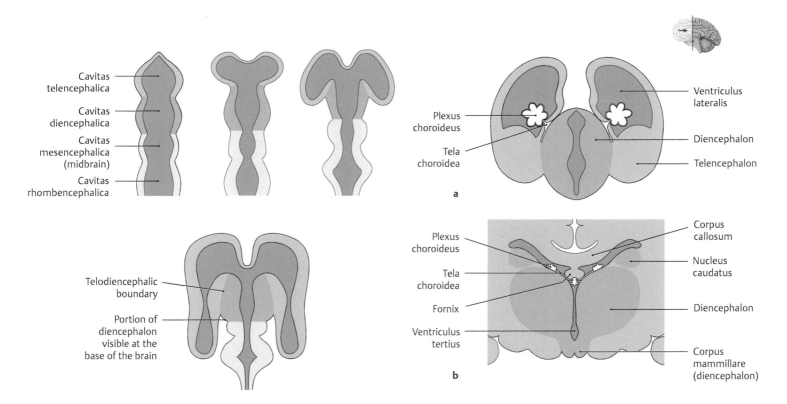

B Development of the diencephalon from the cranial tubus neuralis

Anterior view. To understand the location and extent of the diencephalon in the adult brain, it is necessary to know how it develops from the tubus neuralis. The diencephalon and telencephalon both develop from the prosencephalon, or forebrain (see p. 273). As development proceeds, the two hemispheria of the cavitas telencephalica (red) expand, overgrowing the cavitas diencephalica (blue). This process shifts the boundary between the telencephalon and diencephalon until only a small area of the diencephalon can be seen at the base of the developed brain (see **A**).

C Posterior telodiencephalic boundary

Coronal sections.

a **Embryonic brain.** The development of the telencephalon (red) has progressed considerably in relation to **B**. The ventriculi laterales containing the plexus choroideus have already completely overgrown the diencephalon (blue) from behind. The medial wall of the ventriculi laterales is very thin and has not yet fused to the diencephalon. Between the telencephalon and diencephalon is a vascularized sheet of connective tissue, the tela choroidea.

b **Adult brain.** By the adult stage, the tela choroidea and the medial wall of the ventriculus lateralis have become fused to the diencephalon. Removing the plexus choroideus and the thin tela choroidea affords a direct view of the posteromedial boundary of the diencephalon (see **B**, p. 340).

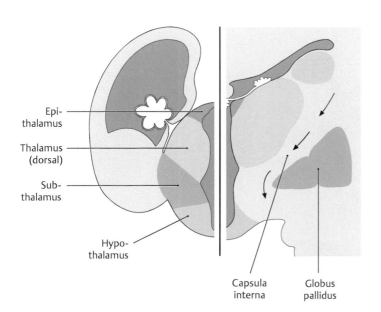

D Organization of the diencephalon during embryonic development

Coronal section of an embryonic brain (left) and an adult brain (right) demonstrating the parts of the diencephalon.

Because the diencephalon of the adult brain lies between the telencephalon and mesencephalon, the ascending and descending axons must penetrate this part of the brain during development, forming the capsula interna. As development proceeds, the axon bundles that form the capsula interna pass through the subthalamus (black arrows), displacing the greater portion of it laterally. This laterally displaced part of the subthalamus is called the *globus pallidus*. Although the globus pallidus is displaced anatomically into the telencephalon and is considered part of the telencephalon in a topographical sense, it still retains close functional ties with the subthalamus because both are part of the extrapyramidal motor system. The *medial* part of the subthalamus remains in the diencephalon as the true *subthalamus* (not visible in this plane of section). As a result, the capsula interna of the telencephalon forms the lateral boundary of the diencephalon. The different parts of the diencephalon grow to reach different definitive sizes. The thalamus grows disproportionately and eventually occupies four-fifths of the mature diencephalon.

339

7.2 Diencephalon, External Structure

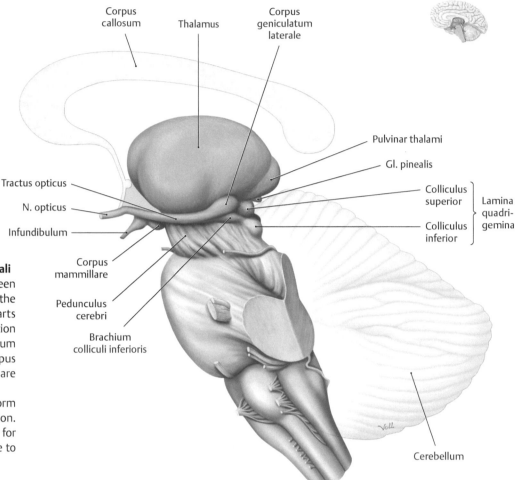

Corpus callosum

Thalamus

Corpus geniculatum laterale

Pulvinar thalami

Gl. pinealis

Tractus opticus

N. opticus

Infundibulum

Colliculus superior

Colliculus inferior

Lamina quadri-gemina

Corpus mammillare

Pedunculus cerebri

Brachium colliculi inferioris

Cerebellum

A The diencephalon and truncus encephali

Left lateral view. The telencephalon has been removed from around the thalamus, and the cerebellum has also been removed. The parts of the diencephalon visible in this dissection are the thalamus, the corpus geniculatum laterale, and the tractus opticus. The corpus geniculatum laterale and tractus opticus are components of the visual pathway.

Note: The retina and associated n. opticus form an anterior extension of the diencephalon. Departing from the convention of yellow for nerves, we have colored the n. opticus blue to emphasize this relationship.

B Arrangement of the diencephalon around the ventriculus tertius

Posterior superior view of an oblique transverse section through the telencephalon with the corpus callosum, fornix, and plexus choroideus removed. Removal of the plexus choroideus leaves behind its line of attachment, the *taenia choroidea*. The thin wall of the ventriculus tertius has been removed with the plexus choroideus to expose the thalamic surface medial to the boundary line of the taenia choroidea. The thin ventricular wall has been left on the thalamus lateral to the taenia choroidea. This thin layer of telencephalon, called the *lamina affixa*, is colored brown in the drawing and covers the thalamus (part of the diencephalon), shown in blue. Because the v. thalamostriata marks this boundary between the diencephalon and telencephalon, it is featured prominently in the drawing. Lateral to the vein is the nucleus caudatus, which is part of the telencephalon (compare with **D**, p. 339).

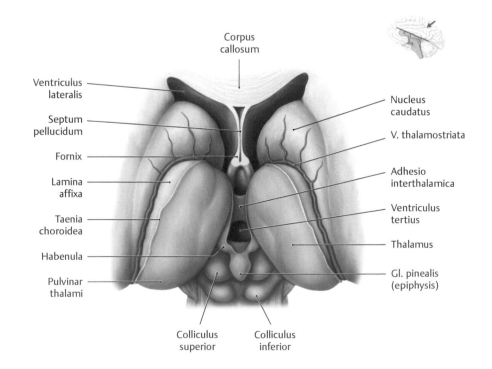

Corpus callosum

Ventriculus lateralis

Septum pellucidum

Fornix

Lamina affixa

Taenia choroidea

Habenula

Pulvinar thalami

Nucleus caudatus

V. thalamostriata

Adhesio interthalamica

Ventriculus tertius

Thalamus

Gl. pinealis (epiphysis)

Colliculus superior

Colliculus inferior

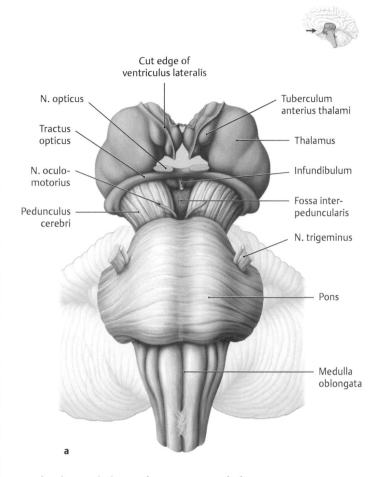

Cut edge of ventriculus lateralis

N. opticus

Tractus opticus

N. oculo-motorius

Pedunculus cerebri

Tuberculum anterius thalami

Thalamus

Infundibulum

Fossa inter-peduncularis

N. trigeminus

Pons

Medulla oblongata

a

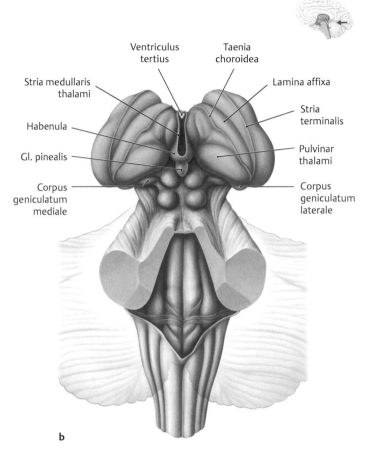

Ventriculus tertius

Taenia choroidea

Stria medullaris thalami

Lamina affixa

Habenula

Stria terminalis

Gl. pinealis

Pulvinar thalami

Corpus geniculatum mediale

Corpus geniculatum laterale

b

C The diencephalon and truncus encephali

a Anterior view, **b** posterior view with the cerebellum and telencephalon removed.

a The tractus opticus marks the lateral boundary of the diencephalon. It winds around the pedunculi cerebri (crura cerebri), which are part of the adjacent midbrain (mesencephalon).

b The epithalamus, which is formed by the gl. pinealis and the two habenulae ("reins"), is well displayed in this posterior view. The corpus geniculatum laterale is an important relay station in the visual

pathway, just as the corpus geniculatum medialis is an important relay station in the auditory pathway. The corpora geniculata are also collectively referred to as metathalamus and represent an extension of the nuclear regions of the thalamus proper. There are close functional connections with regard to the auditory pathway, particularly between the corpus geniculatum medialis and the colliculus inferior of the mesencephalon. The pulvinar ("pillow"), which encompasses the nuclei posteriores thalami, is seen particularly well in this section. It too is assigned complex functions, including relations with the visual and auditory connectivity.

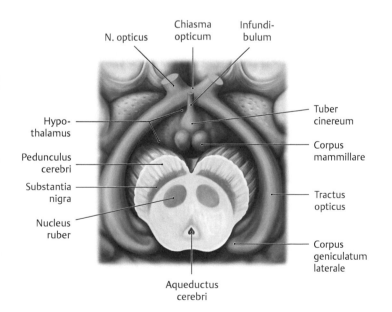

Chiasma opticum

Infundi-bulum

N. opticus

Hypo-thalamus

Pedunculus cerebri

Substantia nigra

Nucleus ruber

Tuber cinereum

Corpus mammillare

Tractus opticus

Corpus geniculatum laterale

Aqueductus cerebri

D Location of the diencephalon in the adult brain

Basal view of the brain (the truncus encephali has been sectioned at the level of the mesencephalon). The structures that can be identified in this view represent the parts of the diencephalon situated on the basal surface of the brain. This view also demonstrates how the tractus opticus, which is part of the diencephalon, winds around the pedunculi cerebri of the mesencephalon (see **Ca**). Due to the expansion of the telencephalon, only a few structures of the diencephalon can be seen on the undersurface of the brain:

• N. opticus
• Chiasma opticum
• Tractus opticus
• Tuber cinereum with the infundibulum
• Corpora mammillaria
• Corpus geniculatum mediale (see **Cb**)
• Corpus geniculatum laterale
• Lobus posterior of the hypophysis (neurohypophysis, see p. 350)

This view also demonstrates how the tractus opticus, which is part of the diencephalon, winds around the pedunculi cerebri of the mesencephalon (see **Ca**).

341

7.3 Diencephalon, Internal Structure

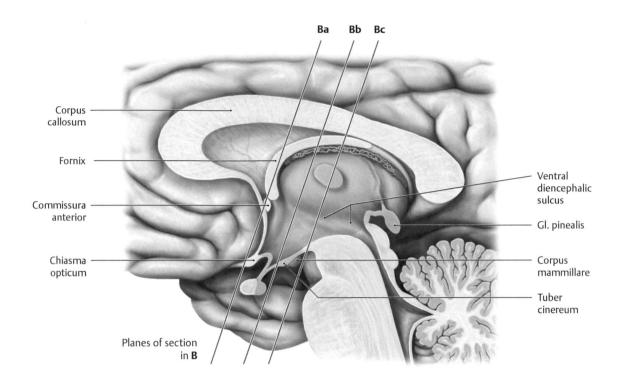

Ba   Bb   Bc

Corpus callosum

Fornix

Commissura anterior

Chiasma opticum

Planes of section in **B**

Ventral diencephalic sulcus

Gl. pinealis

Corpus mammillare

Tuber cinereum

A The four parts of the diencephalon

Boundary line	Part	Structure	Function
Dorsal diencephalic sulcus	**Epithalamus**	• Gl. pinealis • Habenulae	• Regulation of circadian rhythms; linking of olfactory system to truncus encephali
	Thalamus	• Thalamus	• Relay of sensory information; assistance in regulation of motor function
Middle diencephalic sulcus	**Subthalamus**	• Nucleus thalamicus • Zona incerta • Globus pallidus (see **E**, p. 353)	• Relay of sensory information (somatomotor zone of diencephalon)
Ventral diencephalic sulcus (= sulcus hypothalamicus)*	**Hypothalamus**	• Chiasma opticum, tractus opticus • Tuber cinereum, neurohypophysis • Corpora mammillaria	• Coordination of autonomic nervous system with endocrine system; participation in visual pathway

* This is the only sulcus shown in **A**

B Coronal sections through the diencephalon at three different levels

a Level of the optic chiasm: Portions of the diencephalon and telencephalon appear in this section, which clearly shows the position of the diencephalon on both sides of the ventriculus tertius. An outpouching of the ventriculus tertius, the recessus supraopticus, is located above the chiasma opticum. Its connection to the ventriculus tertius lies outside this plane of section.

b Level of the tuber cinereum, just behind the foramen interventriculare: The boundary between the diencephalon and telencephalon is clearly defined only in the region about the ventriculi; the underlying nuclear areas blend together with no apparent boundary. Along the ventriculi laterales, the boundary between the diencephalon and telencephalon is marked by the lamina affixa, a narrow strip of telencephalon that overlies the thalamus. It can be seen that layers of substantia grisea permeate the capsula interna in its dorsal portion.

c Level of the corpora mammillaria: This section displays the thalamic nuclei. More than 120 separate nuclei may be counted, depending on the system of nomenclature used. Most of these nuclei cannot be grossly identified in anatomical specimens. Their classification is reviewed on p. 344 (after Kahle and Frotscher, quoted from Villinger and Ludwig).

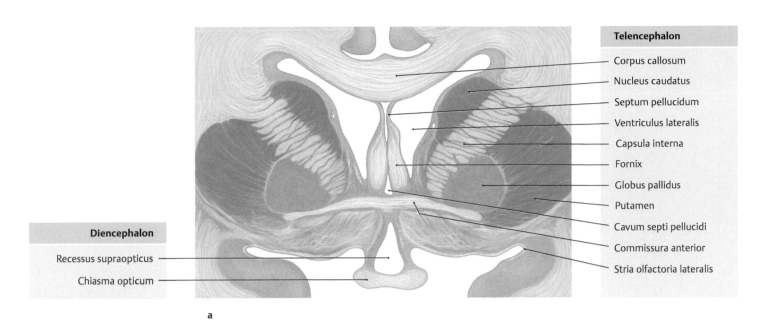

Telencephalon

- Corpus callosum
- Nucleus caudatus
- Septum pellucidum
- Ventriculus lateralis
- Capsula interna
- Fornix
- Globus pallidus
- Putamen
- Cavum septi pellucidi
- Commissura anterior
- Stria olfactoria lateralis

Diencephalon

- Recessus supraopticus
- Chiasma opticum

a

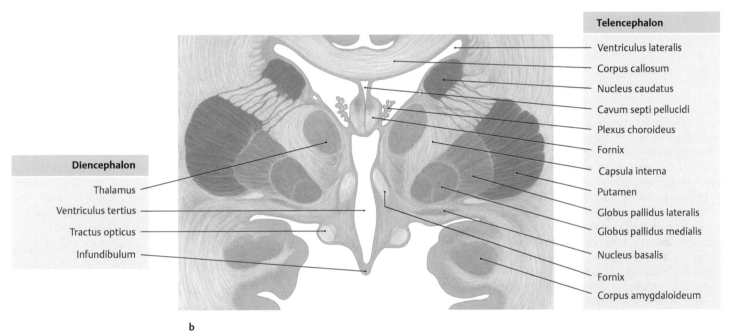

Telencephalon

- Ventriculus lateralis
- Corpus callosum
- Nucleus caudatus
- Cavum septi pellucidi
- Plexus choroideus
- Fornix
- Capsula interna
- Putamen
- Globus pallidus lateralis
- Globus pallidus medialis
- Nucleus basalis
- Fornix
- Corpus amygdaloideum

Diencephalon

- Thalamus
- Ventriculus tertius
- Tractus opticus
- Infundibulum

b

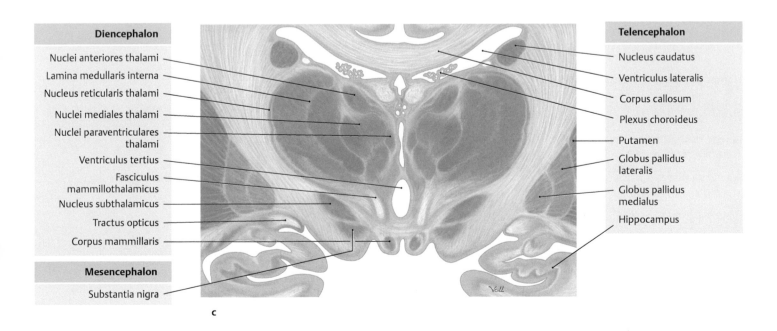

Diencephalon

- Nuclei anteriores thalami
- Lamina medullaris interna
- Nucleus reticularis thalami
- Nuclei mediales thalami
- Nuclei paraventriculares thalami
- Ventriculus tertius
- Fasciculus mammillothalamicus
- Nucleus subthalamicus
- Tractus opticus
- Corpus mammillaris

Mesencephalon

- Substantia nigra

Telencephalon

- Nucleus caudatus
- Ventriculus lateralis
- Corpus callosum
- Plexus choroideus
- Putamen
- Globus pallidus lateralis
- Globus pallidus medialus
- Hippocampus

c

7.4 Thalamus: Thalamic Nuclei

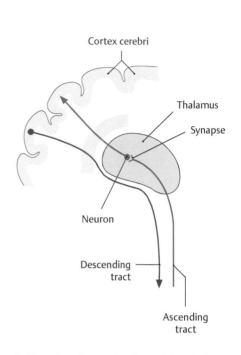

Cortex cerebri

Thalamus

Synapse

Neuron

Descending tract

Ascending tract

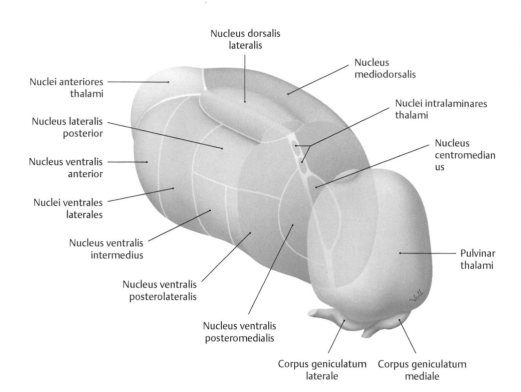

Nucleus dorsalis lateralis

Nuclei anteriores thalami

Nucleus lateralis posterior

Nucleus ventralis anterior

Nuclei ventrales laterales

Nucleus ventralis intermedius

Nucleus ventralis posterolateralis

Nucleus ventralis posteromedialis

Nucleus mediodorsalis

Nuclei intralaminares thalami

Nucleus centromedianus

Pulvinar thalami

Corpus geniculatum laterale

Corpus geniculatum mediale

A Functional organization of the thalamus

Almost all of the sensory pathways are relayed via the thalamus and project to the cortex cerebri (see **G**, radiatio thalami). Consequently, a lesion of the thalamus or its cortical projection fibers caused by a stroke or other disease leads to sensory disturbances. Although a diffuse kind of sensory perception may take place at the thalamic level (especially pain perception), cortical processing (by the telencephalon) is necessary in order to transform unconscious perception into conscious perception. The olfactory system is an exception to this rule, although its bulbus olfactorius is still an extension of the telencephalon.

Note: Major descending motor tracts from the cortex cerebri generally bypass the thalamus.

B Spatial arrangement of the thalamic nuclear groups

Left thalamus viewed from the lateral and occipital aspect, slightly rotated relative to the views on p. 340. The thalamus is a collection of approximately 120 nuclei that process sensory information. They are broadly classified as specific or nonspecific:

- Specific nuclei and the fibers arising from them (radiatio thalami, see **G**) have direct connections with specific areas of the *cortex cerebri*. The specific thalamic nuclei are subdivided into four groups:

- Nuclei anteriores (yellow)
- Nuclei mediales (red)
- Nuclei ventrales thalami and nuclei dorsales thalami (green)
- Nuclei posteriores thalami (blue)

The nuclei posteriores thalami are in contact with the the corpora geniculata medialia and lateralis. Located beneath the pulvinar thalami, these two nuclear bodies contain the *nuclei corporum geniculatorum medialis and lateralis,* and are collectively called the *metathalamus.* Like the pulvinar thalami, they belong to the category of specific thalamic nuclei.

- *Nonspecific nuclei* have no direct connections with the cortex cerebri. Part of a general arousal system, they are connected directly to the truncus encephali. The only nonspecific nuclei shown in this diagram (orange, see **F** for further details) are the nucleus centromedianus and the nuclei intralaminares thalami.

C Nomenclature of the thalamic nuclei

Name	Alternative name	Properties
Specific thalamic nuclei (cortically dependent)	Palliothalamus	Project to the cortex cerebri (pallium)
Nonspecific thalamic nuclei (cortically independent)	Truncothalamus	Project to the truncus encephali, diencephalon, and corpus striatum
Integration nuclei		Project to other nuclei within the thalamus (classified as nonspecific thalamic nuclei)
Intralaminar nuclei		Nuclei in the substantia alba of the lamina medullaris medialis (classified as nonspecific thalamic nuclei)

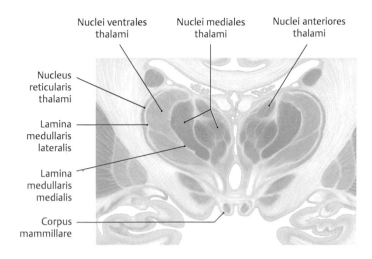

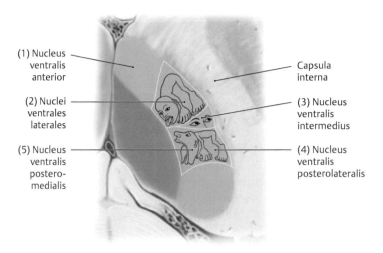

D Division of the thalamic nuclei by the laminae medullares

Coronal section at the level of the corpora mammillaria. Several groups of thalamic nuclei are grossly separated into larger nuclear complexes by fibrous sheets called laminae medullares. The following laminae are shown in the diagram:

- Lamina medullaris medialis between the nuclei mediales thalami and nuclei ventrales thalami
- Lamina medullaris lateralis between the nuclei ventrales thalami and the nucleus reticularis thalami

E Somatotopic organization of the specific thalamic nuclei

Transverse section. The specific thalamic nuclei (defined in **B, C**) are topographically arranged according to their functional relation to specific regions of the body. Afferent fibers from the medulla spinalis, truncus encephali, and cerebellum are localized to specific areas of the thalamus, where the corresponding thalamic nuclei are clustered. This pattern of somatotopic arrangement, a recurring theme in neural organization, is here illustrated for the nuclei ventrales thalami (green in **B, D, E**). Axons from the crossed pedunculus cerebellaris superior terminate in the nuclei ventrales laterales of the thalamus (**2**); information on body position, coordination and muscle tone travels by this pathway to the motor cortex, which also shows a pattern of somatotopic organization (see **B**, p. 457). The *lateral* part of the nuclei ventrales laterales relays impulses from the trunk and limbs, while the *medial* part relays impulses from the head. The nucleus ventralis intermedius (**3**) receives afferent input from the nuclei vestibulares concerning the coordination of gaze toward the ipsilateral side. The large sensory pathways of the medulla spinalis (the tracts of the funiculus posterior) are relayed to the nuclei cuneatus and gracilis, which send their axons through the lemniscus medialis to terminate in the nucleus ventralis posterolateralis (**4**), while the trigeminal sensory pathways from the head terminate in the nucleus ventralis posteriomedialis (**5**, lemniscus trigeminalis, see p. 545). Topographical localization according to function is a basic principle of neural organization.

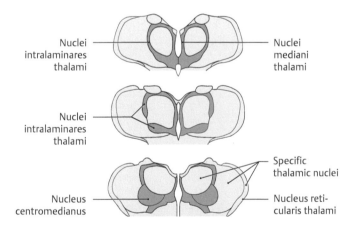

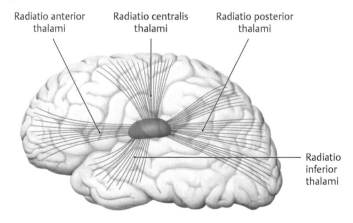

F Nonspecific thalamic nuclei

Coronal sections presented in an oral-to-caudal series. The nonspecific thalamic nuclei project to the truncus encephali, to other nuclei in the diencephalon (including other thalamic nuclei), and to the corpus striatum. They have no direct connections with the cortex cerebri, acting only indirectly on the cortex. The medial *nonspecific* thalamic nuclei are subdivided into two groups:

- Nuclei of the central thalamic substantia grisea (nuclei mediani thalami): small groups of cells distributed along the wall of the ventriculus tertius
- Nuclei intralaminares thalami, located in the lamina medullaris medialis. The largest nucleus of this group is the nucleus centromedianus.

The lateral *specific* thalamic nucleus shown in the diagram is the nucleus reticularis thalami, which is situated lateral to the other specific thalamic nuclei. The nucleus reticularis is the source of the electrical impulses recorded in an electroencephalogram (EEG).

G Radiationes thalami

Ventricularis lateralis of the left hemispherium. The axons of the specific thalamic nuclei (so called because their fibers project to specific cortical areas) are collected into tracts that form the radiationes thalami. The arrangement of the fibers shows that the specific thalamic nuclei have connections with all areas of the cortex. The radiatio anterior thalami projects to the lobus frontalis, the radiatio centralis thalami to the lobus parietalis, the radiatio posterior thalami to the lobus occipitalis, and the radiatio inferior thalami to the lobus temporalis.

345

7.5 Thalamus: Projections of the Thalamic Nuclei

A Nuclei ventrales thalami: afferent and efferent connections

The nucleus ventralis posterolateralis (VPL) and nucleus ventralis posteromedialis (VPM) are the major thalamic relay centers for somatosensory information.

- The *lemniscus medialis* ends in the *VPL*. It contains sensory fibers for position sense, vibration, pressure, discrimination, and touch that are relayed from the nucleus gracilis and nucleus cuneatus.
- Pain and temperature fibers from the trunk and limbs travel through the *tractus spinothalamicus lateralis* to lateral portions of the *VPL*. These sensations are relayed from this nucleus to the somatosensory cortex.
- Pain and temperature information from the head region is conveyed by the *trigeminal system* to the *VPM*. As in the VPL, they synapse with third-order thalamic neurons that project to the gyrus postcentralis (somatosensory cortex).

A *lesion of the VPL* leads to contralateral disturbances of superficial and deep sensation with dysesthesia and an abnormal feeling of heaviness in the limbs (lesion of the lemniscus medialis). Because the pain fibers of the tractus spinothalamicus lateralis terminate in the basal portions of the VPL, lesions in that region may additionally cause severe pain ("thalamic pain"). The **nuclei ventrales laterales** (VL) project to somatomotor cortical areas (6aα and 6aβ). The VL nuclei form a feedback loop with the motor areas of the cortex, and so lesions of these nuclei are characterized by motor deficits.

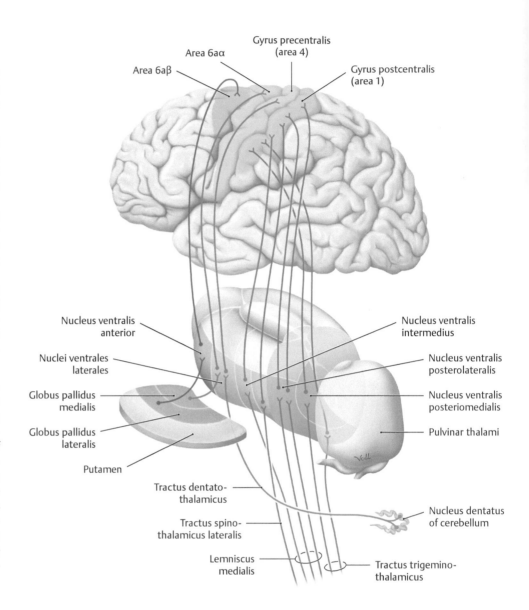

B Nuclei anteriores thalami and nucleus centromedianus: afferent and efferent connections

The nuclei anteriores thalami receives *afferent fibers* from the corpus mammillare by way of the fasciculus mammillothalamicus (bundle of Vicq-d'Azyr). The anterior nucleus establishes both afferent and efferent connections with the gyrus cinguli of the telencephalon. The largest nonspecific thalamic nucleus is the nucleus centromedianus, which is one of the nuclei intralaminares thalami. It receives *afferent fibers* from the cerebellum, formatio reticularis, and globus pallidus medialis. Its *efferent fibers* project to the caput of the nucleus caudatus and the putamen. The nucleus centromedianus is an important component of the **a**scending **r**eticular **a**ctivation **s**ystem (ARAS, arousal system). Essential for maintaining the waking state, the ARAS begins in the formatio reticularis of the truncus encephali and is relayed in the nucleus centromedianus.

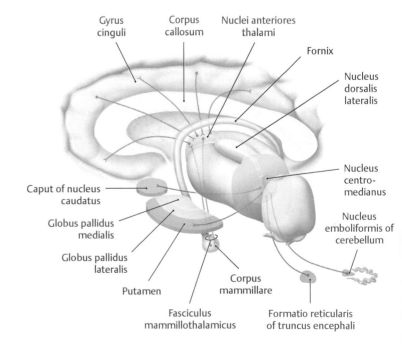

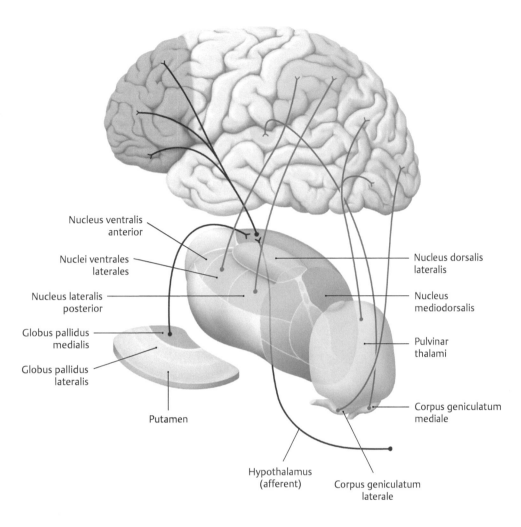

Nucleus ventralis anterior

Nuclei ventrales laterales

Nucleus lateralis posterior

Globus pallidus medialis

Globus pallidus lateralis

Putamen

Nucleus dorsalis lateralis

Nucleus mediodorsalis

Pulvinar thalami

Corpus geniculatum mediale

Hypothalamus (afferent)

Corpus geniculatum laterale

C Nuclei mediales, posteriores, and lateralales thalami: afferent and efferent connections

The **nuclei mediales thalami** receive their afferent input from nuclei ventrales and intralaminares thalami (not shown), the hypothalamus, the mesencephalon, and the globus pallidus. Their efferent fibers project to the lobus frontalis and premotor cortex, and afferent fibers from these regions return to the nuclei. The destruction of these tracts leads to *frontal lobe syndrome,* which is characterized by a loss of self-control (episodes of childish jocularity alternating with suspicion and petulance). The **nuclei posteriores thalami** are formed by the pulvinar thalami, which is the largest nuclear complex of the thalamus. The pulvinar receives afferent fibers from other thalamic nuclei, particularly the nuclei intralaminares (not shown). Its efferent fibers terminate in the association areas of the lobi parietalis and occipitalis, which have reciprocal connections with the pulvinar. The corpus geniculatum laterale (part of the visual pathway) projects to the visual cortex, while the corpus geniculatum mediale (part of the auditory pathway) projects to the auditory cortex. The **nuclei laterales thalami** consist of the nucleus dorsalis lateralis and nucleus lateralis posterior. They represent the dorsal portion of the ventrolateral group (nuclei ventrales) and receive their input from other thalamic nuclei (hence the term "integration nuclei," see p. 344). Their efferent fibers terminate in the lobus parietalis of the brain.

D Synopsis of some clinically important connections of the specific thalamic nuclei

The specific thalamic nuclei project to the cortex cerebri. The table below lists the origins of the tracts that terminate in the nuclei, the nuclei themselves, and the sites to which their afferent fibers project.

Thalamic afferents (structures that project *to* the thalamus)	Thalamic nucleus (abbreviation)	Thalamic efferents (structures *to which* the thalamus projects)
Corpus mammillare (fasciculus mammillothalamicus)	Nuclei anteriores thalami (AN)	Gyrus cinguli (limbic system)
Cerebellum, nucleus ruber	Nuclei ventrales laterales (VL)	Premotor cortex (areae 6aα and 6aβ)
Funiculus posterior, funiculus lateralis (somatosensory input, limbs, trunk)	Nucleus ventralis posterolateralis (VPL)	Gyrus postcentralis (= somatosensory cortex) (see **A**)
Tractus trigeminothalamicus (somatosensory input, head)	Nucleus ventralis posteriomedialis (VPM)	Gyrus postcentralis (= somatosensory cortex) (see **A**)
Brachium colliculi inferioris (part of the auditory pathway)	Corpus geniculatum mediale (MGB)	Gyri temporales transversi (auditory cortex)
Tractus opticus (part of the visual pathway)	Corpus geniculatum laterale (LGB)	Striate area (visual cortex)

7.6 Hypothalamus

A Location of the hypothalamus

Coronal section. The hypothalamus is the lowest level of the diencephalon, situated below the thalamus. It is the only externally visible portion of the diencephalon (see **D**, p. 331). Located on either side of the ventriculus tertius, its size is most clearly appreciated in a midsagittal section that bisects the ventriculus tertius (see **Ba**).

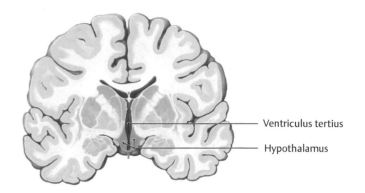

— Ventriculus tertius

— Hypothalamus

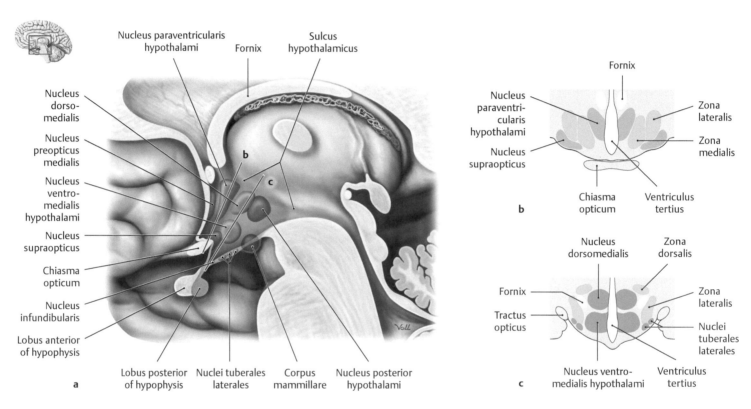

B Nuclei in the right hypothalamus

a Midsagittal section of the right hemispherium viewed from the medial side. **b, c** Coronal sections. The hypothalamus is a small nuclear complex located ventral to the thalamus and separated from it by the sulcus hypothalamicus. Despite its small size, the hypothalamus is the command center for all autonomic functions in the body. The Terminologia Anatomica lists over 30 hypothalamic nuclei located in the lateral wall and floor of the ventriculus tertius. Only a few of the larger, more clinically important nuclei are mentioned in this unit. Three groups of nuclei are listed below in a rostral-to-caudal sequence, and their functions are briefly described:

- The anterior (rostral) group of nuclei (green) synthesizes the hormones released from the lobus posterior of the hypophysis, and consists of the
  - nucleus preopticus,
  - nucleus paraventricularis hypothalami, and
  - nucleus supraopticus.
- The middle (tuberal) group of nuclei (blue) controls hormone release from the lobus anterior of the hypophysis, and consists of the
  - nucleus dorsomedialis,

- nucleus ventromedialis hypothalami, and
- nuclei tuberales laterales.
- The posterior (mammillary) group of nuclei (red) activates the sympathetic nervous system when stimulated. It consists of the
  - nucleus posterior hypothalami and
  - nuclei mammillares located in the corpora mammillaria.

The coronal section (**c**) shows the further subdivision of the hypothalamus by the fornix into zonae lateralis and medialis. The three nuclear groups described above are part of the zona *medialis*, whereas the nuclei in the zona *lateralis* are not subdivided into specific groups (e.g., the zona lateralis takes the place of a nucleus; the course of the fornix is described on p. 321). Bilateral lesions of the corpora mammillaria and their nuclei are manifested by the *Korsakoff syndrome*, which is frequently associated with alcoholism (cause: vitamin B$_1$ [thiamine] deficiency). The memory impairment that occurs in this syndrome mainly affects short-term memory, and the patient may fill in the memory gaps with fabricated information. A major neuropathological finding is the presence of hemorrhages in the corpora mammillaria, which are sectioned at autopsy to confirm the diagnosis.

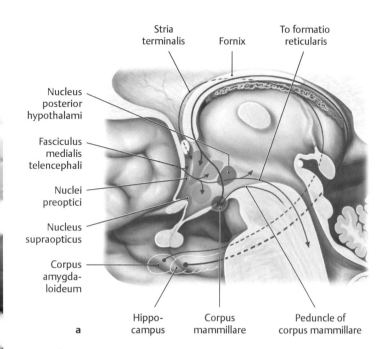

a

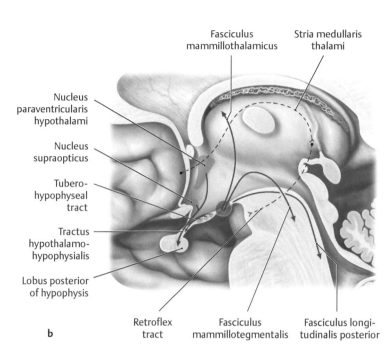

b

C Important afferent and efferent connections of the hypothalamus

Midsagittal section of the right hemisphere viewed from the medial side. Because the hypothalamus coordinates all the autonomic functions in the body, it establishes afferent (blue) and efferent (red) connections with many brain regions. The following are particularly important:

a Afferent connections (to the hypothalamus):
- The fornix conveys afferent fibers from the hippocampus; it is an important fiber tract of the limbic system.
- The fasciculus medialis telencephali transmits afferent fibers from the olfactory areas to the nuclei preoptici.
- The stria terminalis conveys afferent fibers from the corpus amygdaloideum.
- The peduncle of the corpora mammillaria transmits visceral afferent fibers and impulses from erogenous zones (papilla mammaria, genitalia).

b Efferent connections (from the hypothalamus):
- The fasciculus longitudinalis posterior passes to the truncus encephali where it is relayed several times before reaching the parasympathetic nuclei.
- The fasciculus mammillotegmentalis distributes efferent fibers to the tegmentum of the mesencephalon; these are then relayed to the formatio reticularis. The fibers of this tract mediate the exchange of autonomic information between the hypothalamus, nuclei nervorum cranialium, and medulla spinalis.
- The fasciculus mammillothalamicus (bundle of Vicq d'Azyr) conveys efferent fibers to the nuclei anteriores thalami, which are connected to the gyrus cinguli. This is part of the limbic system (see p. 492).
- The tractus hypothalamohypophysialis and tuberohypophyseal tract are efferent tracts to the hypophysis (see p. 350 f).

D Functions of the hypothalamus

The hypothalamus is the coordinating center of the autonomic nervous system. There is no specific sympathetic or parasympathatic control center. Certain functions can be assigned to specific regions or nuclei in the hypothalamus, and these relationships are outlined in the table. Not all of the regions or nuclei listed in the table are shown in the drawings.

Region or nucleus	Function
Anterior preoptic region	Maintains constant body temperature; **Lesion:** central hypothermia
Posterior region	Responds to temperature changes, e.g., sweating; **Lesion:** hypothermia
Midanterior and posterior regions	Activate sympathetic nervous system
Paraventricular and anterior regions	Activate parasympathetic nervous system
Nuclei supraopticus and paraventricularis hypothalami	Regulate water balance; **Lesion:** Diabetes insipidus, also lack of thirst response resulting in hyponatremia
Nucleus anterior hypothalami • Medial part • Lateral part	Regulate appetite and food intake • **Lesion:** Obesity • **Lesion:** Anorexia and emaciation

7.7 Glandula Pituitaria (Hypophysis)

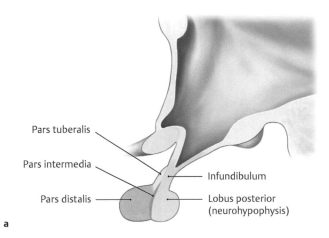

a

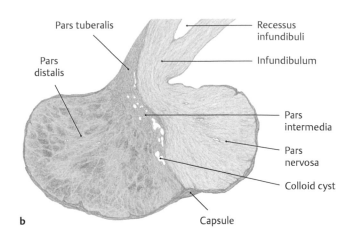

b

A Divisions of the glandula pituitaria
Midsagittal sections: **a** Schematic representation. **b** Histological appearance. The gl. pituitaria (hypophysis) consists of two lobes:

- Lobus anterior (adenohypophysis), which is a hormone-producing and releasing part (see **D** and **E**), and
- Lobus posterior (neurohypophysis), which is a hormone-releasing part for hormones produced in the hypothalamus.

While the lobus posterior hypophysis is an extension of the diencephalon, the lobus anterior hypophysis is derived from the epithelium of the roof of the pharynx. The two lobes establish contact during embryonic development. The pituitary stalk (infundibulum) attaches both lobes of the gland to the hypothalamus. The hypophysis is surrounded by a fibrous capsule and lies in the *sella turcica* over the sinus sphenoidalis, which provides a route of surgical access to pituitary tumors.

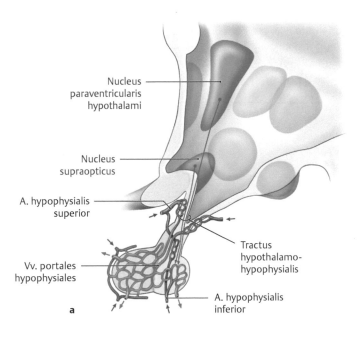

a

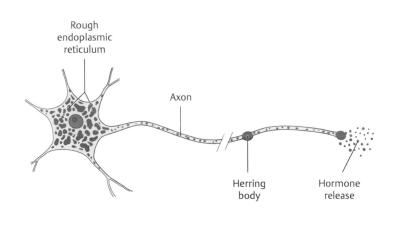

b

B Connections of the hypothalamic nuclei to the lobus posterior of the hypophysis
a Hypothalamic-(neuro)pituitary axis. **b** Neurosecretory neuron in the hypothalamic nucleus.
Pituitary hormones are not synthesized in the *lobus posterior hypophysis* (neurohypophysis) but in neurons located in the nucleus paraventricularis hypothalami and nucleus supraopticus of the hypothalamus. They are then transported by axons of the tractus hypothalamohypophysialis to the neurohypophysis, where they are released as needed. Terminals of the nuclei paraventricularis hypothalami and supraopticus release two hormones in the lobus posterior hypophysis:

- **Oxytocin** from the neurons of the nucleus paraventricularis hypothalami
- **Antidiuretic hormone** (ADH) or **vasopressin** from the neurons of the nucleus supraopticus

The axons from both nuclei pass through the infundibulum to the lobus posterior of the hypophysis. The peptide hormones are stored in vesicles (aggregated into large "Herring bodies") in the cell bodies of the neurosecretory neurons and are carried to the lobus posterior by anterograde axoplasmic transport.

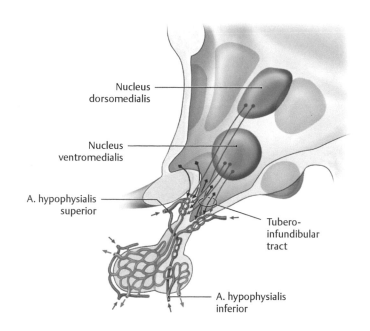

Nucleus dorsomedialis

Nucleus ventromedialis

A. hypophysialis superior

Tubero-infundibular tract

A. hypophysialis inferior

C Hypophyseal portal circulation and connections of the hypothalamic nuclei to the lobus anterior hypophysis

The aa. hypophysiales superiores from each side of the body form a vascular plexus around the infundibulum (pituitary stalk). The axons from neurons of the hypothalamic nuclei (dark red and dark blue arrows) terminate at this plexus and secrete hormones that have been produced in smaller (parvocellular) neurons of the hypothalamus. The secreted hypothalamic hormones are of two types:

- Releasing factors which stimulate hormone release from cells of the lobus anterior hypophysis
- Inhibiting factors which inhibit the hormonal release from these cells

These hormones are carried by the vv. portales hypophysiales (named after the portal circulation of the liver) to capillaries in the lobus anterior, establishing communication between the hypothalamus and endocrine cells of the adenohypophysis.

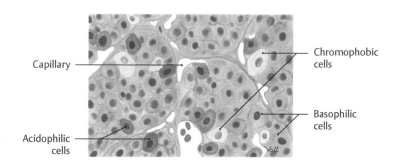

Capillary

Chromophobic cells

Basophilic cells

Acidophilic cells

D Histology of the lobus anterior hypophysis

Three types of cells can be distinguished in the lobus anterior hypophysis using classic histologic methods: acidophilic cells, basophilic cells, and chromophobic cells. The latter have already released their hormones, and are therefore negative in immunohistochemical tests that specifically detect peptide hormones; they are not listed in **E**. The acidophilic (a) cells secrete hormones that act directly on target cells (non-glandotropic hormones) while the basophilic (b) cells stimulate subordinate endocrine cells (glandotropic hormones).

E Hormones of the lobus anterior hypophysis (adenohypophysis)

Hormones and synonyms	Cell designation*	Hormone actions
Somatotropin (STH) Growth hormone (GH) Somatotropic hormone	Somatotropic (a)	Stimulates longitudinal growth; acts on carbohydrate and lipid metabolism
Prolactin (PRL or LTH) Luteotropic hormone Mammotropic hormone	Mammotropic (a)	Stimulates lactation and proliferation of glandular breast tissue
Follitropin (FSH) Follicle-stimulating hormone	Gonadotropic (b)	Acts on the gonads; stimulates follicular maturation, spermatogenesis, estrogen production, expression of lutropin receptors and proliferation of granulosa cells
Lutropin (LH) Interstitial cell stimulating hormone - ICSH Luteinizing hormone	Gonadotropic (b)	Triggers ovulation; stimulates proliferation of follicular epithelial cells, production of testosterone in interstitial Leydig cells of the testis, and synthesis of progesterone; has general anabolic activity
Thyrotropin (TSH) Thyroid stimulating hormone Thyrotropic hormone	Thyrotropic (b)	Stimulates thyroid gland activity; increases O_2 consumption and protein synthesis; influences carbohydrate and lipid metabolism
Corticotropin (ACTH) Adrenocorticotropic hormone	Adrenotropic (b)	Stimulates hormone production in adrenal cortex; influences water and electrolyte balance; acts on carbohydrate formation in liver
Alpha/beta **Melanotropin (MSH)**	Melanotropic (b)	Aids in melanin formation and skin pigmentation; protects against UV radiation**

* Cells are classified as either acidophilic (a) or basophilic (b).
** In humans, melanotropin serves as a neurotransmitter in various brain regions.

7.8 Epithalamus and Subthalamus

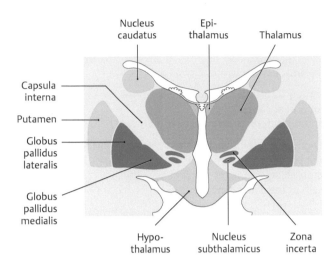

A Location of the epithalamus and subthalamus
Coronal section. The appropriateness of the term "epithalamus" can be appreciated in this plane of section, which shows the epithalamus riding upon the thalamus (epi = "upon"). The **epithalamus** (green) consists of the following structures:

- Gl. pinealis (epiphysis), see **B**.
- Habenulae with the nuclei habenulares, see **D**.
- Commissura habenularum, see **C**.
- Stria medullaris thalami, see **D**.
- Commissura epithalamica (commissura posterior), see **Ca**.

The region of the **subthalamus** (orange), formerly called the ventral thalamus, initially lies directly below the thalamus, but during embryonic development is displaced laterally into the telencephalon by fibers of the capsula interna, forming the *globus pallidus* (see **D**, p. 339). The subthalamus contains nuclei of the medial motor system (motor zones of the diencephalon), and has connections with the motor nuclei of the tegmentum mesencephali. In fact, the subthalamus can be considered the cranial extension of the tegmentum.

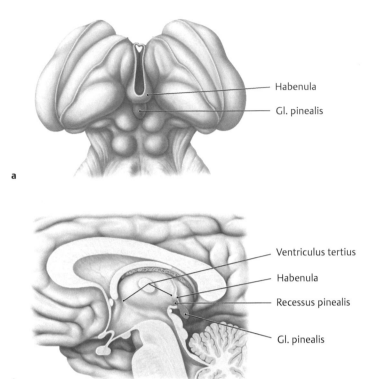

B Location of the glandula pinealis
a Posterior view. **b** Midsagittal section of the right hemispherium viewed from the medial side.
The gl. pinealis resembles a pine cone when viewed from behind. It is connected to the diencephalon by the habenula, which contains both afferent and efferent tracts. Its topographical relationship to the ventriculus tertius is seen particularly well in midsagittal section (recessus pinealis). In reptiles, the calvaria over the gl. pinealis is thinned so that it is receptive to light stimuli. This is not the case in humans, although retinal afferents still communicate with the gl. pinealis through relay stations in the hypothalamus and the ganglion cervicale superius (sympathicum), helping to regulate circadian rhythms.

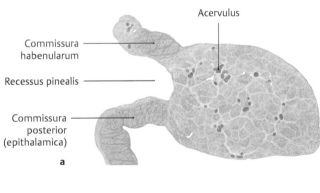

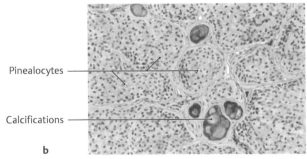

C Structure of the glandula pinealis
a Gross midsagittal tissue section. **b** Histological section.

- **a** In the gross tissue section, the commissura habenularum can be identified at the rostral end of the gl. pinealis. Below it is the commissura posterior (epithalamica). Between the two commissurae is the CSF-filled recessus pinealis of the ventriculus tertius. Calcifications (corpora arenacea, "brain sand") are frequently present and may be visible on radiographs; they have no pathological significance.
- **b** The histological section demonstrates the specific cells of the gl. pinealis, the *pinealocytes*, which are embedded in a connective-tissue stroma and are surrounded by astrocytes. The pinealocytes produce *melatonin*, which plays a role in the regulation of circadian rhythms; it may be taken prophylactically, for example, to moderate the effects of jet lag. If the gl. pinealis ceases to function during childhood, the individual may undergo precocious puberty given that the gl. pinealis has significant, mostly inhibitory, effects on various endocrine systems.

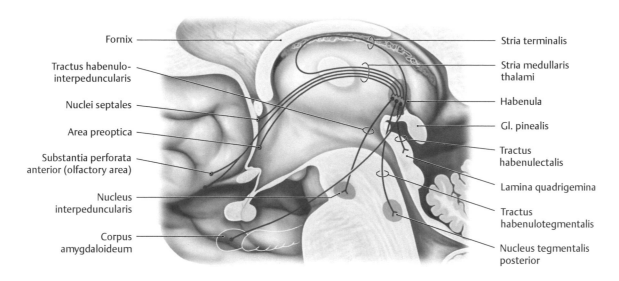

Fornix
Tractus habenulo-interpeduncularis
Nuclei septales
Area preoptica
Substantia perforata anterior (olfactory area)
Nucleus interpeduncularis
Corpus amygdaloideum

Stria terminalis
Stria medullaris thalami
Habenula
Gl. pinealis
Tractus habenulectalis
Lamina quadrigemina
Tractus habenulotegmentalis
Nucleus tegmentalis posterior

D Nuclei habenulares and their fiber connections
Midsagittal section of the right hemispherium viewed from the medial side. The habenula ("reins") and their nuclei function as a relay station for afferent olfactory impulses. After their relay in the nuclei habenulares, their efferent fibers are distributed to the nuclei salivatorii and motores (mastication) in the truncus encephali.

Afferent connections (blue): Afferent impulses from the substantia perforata anterior (olfactory area), nuclei septales, and area preoptica are transmitted by the stria medullaris to the nuclei habenulares. These nuclei also receive impulses from the corpus amygdaloideum via the stria terminalis.

Efferent connections (red): Efferent fibers from the nuclei habenulares are projected to the mesencephalon along three tracts:

*   Habenulotectal tract: terminates in the tectum mesencephali, the lamina quadrigemina, supplying it with olfactory impulses.
*   Habenulotegmental tract: terminates in the nucleus tegmentalis posterior, establishing connections with the fasciculus longitudinalis posterior and with the nuclei salivatorii and motor cranial nerve nuclei. (The smell of food stimulates salivation and gastric acid secretion: e.g., Pavlovian response).
*   Tractus habenulointerpeduncularis: terminates in the nucleus interpeduncularis, which then connects with the formatio reticularis.

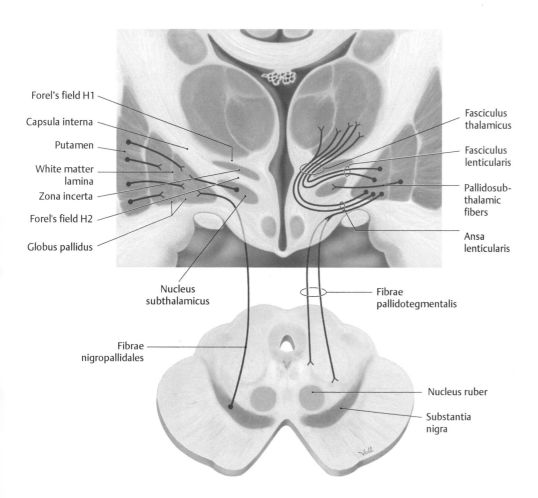

Forel's field H1
Capsula interna
Putamen
White matter lamina
Zona incerta
Forel's field H2
Globus pallidus
Nucleus subthalamicus
Fibrae nigropallidales

Fasciculus thalamicus
Fasciculus lenticularis
Pallidosub-thalamic fibers
Ansa lenticularis
Fibrae pallidotegmentalis
Nucleus ruber
Substantia nigra

E Subthalamic nuclei with their afferent (blue) and efferent (red) connections
The principal nucleus of the subthalamus is the *globus pallidus*, which is displaced laterally during development into the telencephalon by the internal capsule. A lamina of white divides the globus pallidus into a medial (internal) and lateral (external) segment. Certain small nuclei are exempt from this migration and remain near the midline: these are the *zona incerta* and *subthalamic nucleus*. The subthalamic nucleus, substantia nigra, and putamen send afferent fibers to the globus pallidus. The globus pallidus in turn distributes efferent fibers to these regions and also to the thalamus through a tract called the fasciculus lenticularis. Functionally, these nuclei are classified as portions of the nuclei basales. Lesions of these nuclei lead to a movement disorder called contralateral hemiballismus (the functional role of the subthalamus is described on p. 458 f).

8.1 Brainstem (Truncus Encephali), Organization and External Structure

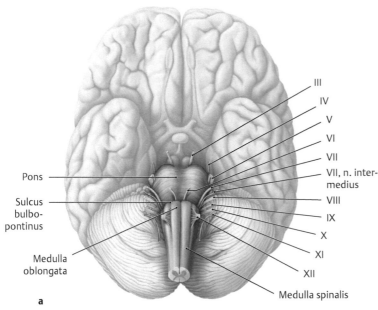

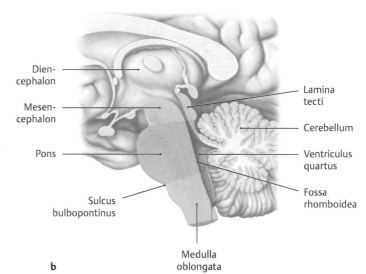

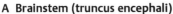

a

b

A Brainstem (truncus encephali)

a View of the intact brain from below; **b** Midsagittal section, left lateral view.

Compared to the telencephalon, the truncus encephali is so small that its parts become visible only in midsagittal section (**b**). Features of the truncus encephali:

- Part of the brain that is most connected to the PNS.
- It is only at the truncus encephali that the ventricular system (via the ventriculus quartus) and the spatium subarachnoideum are connected (see **A**, p. 312 and **C**, p. 315).
- The truncus encephali is connected to the medulla spinalis.
- The cerebellum is situated on the dorsal aspect of the truncus encephali which conects it to the other parts of the CNS (see **A** and **B**, p. 370).

The purely topographical demarcation of zones in the truncus encephali from cranial to caudal is based on its external, macroscopic structure. The mesencephalon begins immediately at the diencephalon and extends to the cranial transverse gyrus of the pons which at its caudal end is separated from the medulla oblongata by the sulcus bulbopontinus. The truncus encephali extends to the point of exit of the first n. spinalis after which the medulla spinalis begins. The external structure of the truncus encephali does not match its internal structure. Here,

nuclear columns of nn. craniales are located, which developmentally follow a specific arrangement pattern, which applies to the entire truncus encephali (see p. 114). Also purely topographical criteria are used to subdivide each truncus encephali section into four parts (see **B**). Regarding of the many functions of the truncus encephali, the internal structure can be roughly divided into the following:

- Nuclear regions (collection of neuron cell bodies), in which the wiring takes place—roughly divided into nuclei, of nn. craniales and nuclei that are not associated with nn. craniales (e.g., nucleus ruber and substantia nigra, both part of the motor system, and nuclei of the formatio reticularis, which maintains autonomic functions)
- Since the truncus encephali is located between diencephalon and medulla spinalis, axons, which are bundled together in tracts, pass through it. All communication between the medulla spinalis and the more rostral regions of the brain diencephalon passes though these tracts within the truncus encephali. Depending on the flow of information, a distinction is drawn between ascending (afferent, to the telencephalon) and descending (efferent, away from the telencephalon) tracts.

Note: Since so many nuclei and tracts lie so closely together in the truncus encephali, even small lesions, for example, in case of bleeding truncus encephali stroke can cause severe damage.

B Overview of the brainstem

Topographical organization
- *Craniocaudal direction:*
  - Mesencephalon (midbrain)
  - Pons
  - Medulla oblongata
- *Anteroposterior direction:*
  - Base (mesencephalon: pedunculi cerebri; pons: basal part; medulla oblongata: pyramids)
  - Tegmentum (present as such in all three parts)
  - Section of ventricular system (aqueductus cerebri, ventriculus quartus, canalis centralis)
  - Tectum ("roof"; present only in the mesencephalon; lamina quadrigemina)
- The cerebellum adjoins the truncus encephali dorsally.

Functional organization
- *Truncus encephali as "control center"*
  - nuclei for nn. craniales III–XII (divided into four longitudinal nuclear columns)
  - coordination center for motor control (nucleus ruber, substantia nigra)
  - formatio reticularis (motor function; respiration; blood circulation; autonomic functions)
  - nuclei pontis (connected to the cerebellum)
  - nuclei of the funiculus posterior (termination point of sensory pathways)
  - interconnection of auditory and visual stimuli (lamina tecti)
- *Truncus encephali as "thoroughfare"*
  - toward and away from the brain: descending (motor) and ascending (sensory) tracts
  - toward and away from the cerebellum: connection of medulla spinalis, truncus encephali, diencephalon and telencephalon (via pons and thalamus) with cerebellum
  - away from the cerebellum: descending autonomic tracts

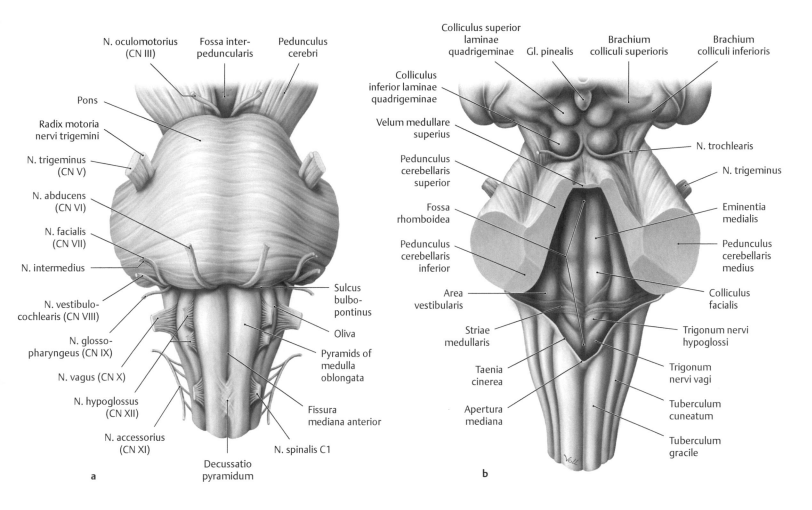

a

- N. oculomotorius (CN III)
- Fossa inter-peduncularis
- Pedunculus cerebri
- Pons
- Radix motoria nervi trigemini
- N. trigeminus (CN V)
- N. abducens (CN VI)
- N. facialis (CN VII)
- N. intermedius
- N. vestibulo-cochlearis (CN VIII)
- N. glosso-pharyngeus (CN IX)
- N. vagus (CN X)
- N. hypoglossus (CN XII)
- N. accessorius (CN XI)
- Decussatio pyramidum
- Sulcus bulbo-pontinus
- Oliva
- Pyramids of medulla oblongata
- Fissura mediana anterior
- N. spinalis C1

b

- Colliculus superior laminae quadrigeminae
- Gl. pinealis
- Brachium colliculi superioris
- Brachium colliculi inferioris
- Colliculus inferior laminae quadrigeminae
- Velum medullare superius
- Pedunculus cerebellaris superior
- Fossa rhomboidea
- Pedunculus cerebellaris inferior
- Area vestibularis
- Striae medullaris
- Taenia cinerea
- Apertura mediana
- N. trochlearis
- N. trigeminus
- Eminentia medialis
- Pedunculus cerebellaris medius
- Colliculus facialis
- Trigonum nervi hypoglossi
- Trigonum nervi vagi
- Tuberculum cuneatum
- Tuberculum gracile

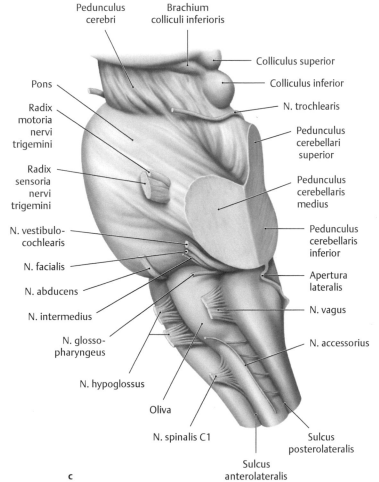

c

- Pedunculus cerebri
- Brachium colliculi inferioris
- Pons
- Radix motoria nervi trigemini
- Radix sensoria nervi trigemini
- N. vestibulo-cochlearis
- N. facialis
- N. abducens
- N. intermedius
- N. glosso-pharyngeus
- N. hypoglossus
- Oliva
- N. spinalis C1
- Colliculus superior
- Colliculus inferior
- N. trochlearis
- Pedunculus cerebellari superior
- Pedunculus cerebellaris medius
- Pedunculus cerebellaris inferior
- Apertura lateralis
- N. vagus
- N. accessorius
- Sulcus posterolateralis
- Sulcus anterolateralis

C Truncus encephali: external structure

a Ventral view. The ventral view is dominated by the pons (a small bridge, which appears to traverse the truncus encephali oriented lengthwise) and the attachment points of nn. craniales III and V–XII (IV is the only n. cranialis to emerge dorsally, see **b**). Cranial to the pons lie the crura cerebri, which contain descending motor pathways. A part of these fibers extend to the pyramides of the the medulla oblongata and most of them cross over in the decussatio pyramidum. The oliva, located lateral to the pyramis, contains a large motor nuclear group, the nuclei olivares.
Note: The medulla spinalis begins at the root of the first n. spinali. Therefore, the decussatio pyramidum lies very close to the border.

b Dorsal view. What is striking is the view of the diamond-shaped ven-triculus quartus, the floor of which is outlined by several n. cranialis nuclei. Located cranially is the tectum mesencephali with the lam-ina tecti, from which the n. cranialis IV emerges. The lamina tecti contains four colliculi (lamina quadrigemina). The colliculi superiores are integrative centers related to visual information and the colliculi inferiores are relay stations of the auditory pathway. The brachium ("arm") of the colliculus superior and the brachium of the colliculus inferior connect these colliculi with their corresponding thalamic nuclei. Lateral to the ventriculus quartus, as a topographic connec-tion between cerebellum and truncus encephali, are three paired pedunculi cerebellares: the superior, medius, and inferior.

c Lateral view from left. Very clearly displayed in this view is the fact that the ventral curvature of the pons extends into the pedunculus cerebellaris medius, which connects the pons with the cerebellum. The nuclei necessary for this cross-wiring lie within the pons (nuclei pontis). The n. trigeminus (n. cranialis V) emerges directly from the pons. Immediately caudal to the pons the left oliva is visible.

355

8.2 Truncus Encephali: Nuclei Nervi Craniales, Nucleus Ruber, and Substantia Nigra

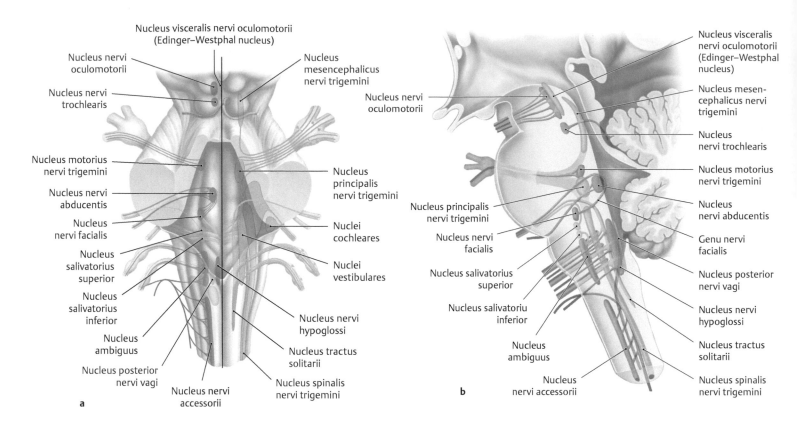

A Nuclei nervi craniales in the truncus encephali

a Posterior view with the cerebellum removed, exposing the fossa rhomboidea; **b** Midsagittal section of the right half of the truncus encephali viewed from the left side.

The diagrams show the nuclei themselves and the course of the nerves (to save space, the nuclei vestibulares and cochleares are not shown).

The arrangement of the nuclei nervorum cranialium is easier to understand when we divide them into functional nuclear columns. The *motor nuclei*, which give rise to the efferent fibers, are shown on the left side

of diagram a, and the *sensory nuclei*, where the afferent fibers terminate, are shown on the right side. The nuclei are shown from the side in **b**. The arrangement of these nuclei can be derived from the arrangement of the nuclei in the medulla spinalis (see p. 114). The function and connections of some of these nn. craniales can be clinically evaluated by testing the *brainstem reflexes* (whose relay centers are located in the truncus encephali). These reflexes are important in the evaluation of comatose patients. A prime example is the pupillary reflexes, which are further described on p. 481.

B Overview of the nuclei of nn. craniales III—XII

Motor nuclei: give rise to efferent (motor) fibers, left in **Aa**	Sensory nuclei: where afferent (sensory) fibers terminate, right in **Aa**
Somatic efferent or somatic motor nuclei (red): – Nucleus nervi oculomotorii (CN III) – Nucleus nervi trochlearis (CN IV) – Nucleus nervi abducentis (CN VI) – Nucleus nervi accessorii (CN XI) – Nucleus nervi hypoglossi (CN XII) **Visceral efferent (visceral motor) nuclei:** • *Nuclei associated with the parasympathetic nervous system (light blue):* – Nucleus visceralis nervi oculomotorii (Edinger–Westphal nucleus) (CN III) – Nucleus salivatorius superior (n. facialis, CN VII) – Nucleus salivatorius inferior (n. glossopharyngeus, CN IX) – Nucleus posterior nervi vagi (CN X) • *Nuclei of the branchial arch nerves (dark blue):* – Nucleus motorius nervi trigemini (CN V) – Nucleus nervi facialis (CN VII) – Nucleus ambiguus (n. glossopharyngeus, CN IX; n. vagus, CN X; n. accessorius, CN XI, cranial root is in fact considered now part of CN X)	**Somatic afferent (somatic or main sensory) and vestibulocochlear nuclei (yellow):** *Sensory nuclei associated with the n. trigeminus (CN V):* – Nucleus mesencephalicus nervi trigemini (special feature: pseudounipolar ganglion cells ("displaced sensory ganglion"), provide direct sensory innervation for mm. masticatorii) – Nucleus principalis nervi trigemini – Nucleus spinalis nervi trigemini *Nuclei of the n. vestibulocochlearis (CN VIII):* • Nuclei vestibulares: – Nucleus vestibularis medialis – Nucleus vestibularis lateralis – Nucleus vestibularis superior – Nucleus vestibularis inferior • Nuclei cochleares: – Nucleus cochlearis anterior – Nucleus cochlearis posterior **Visceral afferent (visceral sensory) nuclei (green):** • Nucleus tractus solitarii (nuclear complex): • Superior part: – Special visceral afferents (taste) from nn. facialis (CN VII), glossopharyngeus (CN IX), and vagus (CN X) • Inferior part: – General visceral afferents from nn. glossopharyngeus (CN IX) and vagus (CN X)

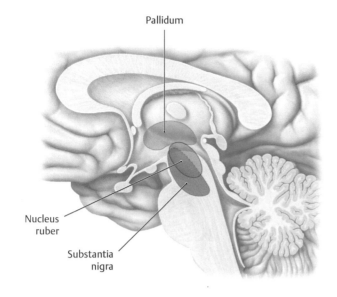

Pallidum

Nucleus ruber

Substantia nigra

C Location of the substantia nigra and nucleus ruber in the mesencephalon

Both of these nuclei, like the nuclei nervi craniales, are well-defined structures that belong functionally to the *extrapyramidal motor* system. Anatomically, the substantia nigra is part of the pedunculi cerebri and therefore is not located in the tegmentum of the mesencephalon (see **A**, p. 362). Owing to their high respective contents of melanin and iron, the substantia nigra and nucleus ruber appear brown and red, respectively, in sections of fresh brain tissue. Both nuclei extend into the diencephalon and are connected to its nuclei by fiber tracts (see **E**).

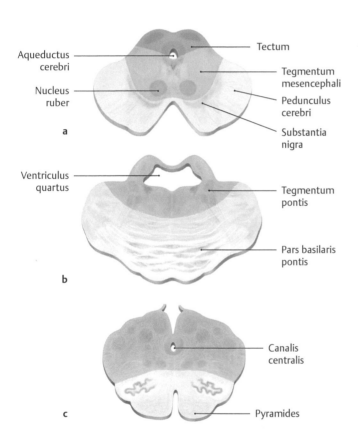

Aqueductus cerebri — Tectum

Nucleus ruber — Tegmentum mesencephali

— Pedunculus cerebri

— Substantia nigra

a

Ventriculus quartus — Tegmentum pontis

— Pars basilaris pontis

b

— Canalis centralis

— Pyramides

c

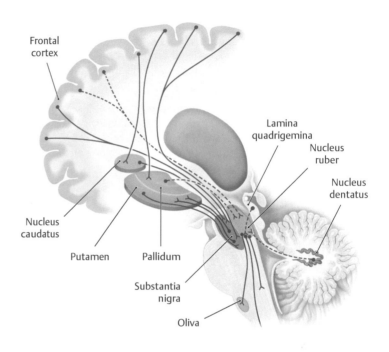

Frontal cortex

Lamina quadrigemina

Nucleus ruber

Nucleus dentatus

Nucleus caudatus

Putamen   Pallidum

Substantia nigra

Oliva

E Afferent (blue) and efferent (red) connections of the nucleus ruber and substantia nigra

These two nuclei are important relay stations in the motor system. The *nucleus ruber* consists of a larger *neorubrum* and a smaller *paleorubrum*. It receives afferent axons from the nucleus dentatus (tractus dentatorubralis), colliculi superiores (tractus tectorubralis), inner pallidum (tractus pallidorubralis), and cortex cerebri (fibrae corticorubrales).

The nucleus ruber sends its axons to the oliva (tractus rubroolivaris and fibrae reticuloolivare, part of the tractus tegmentalis centralis) and to the medulla spinalis (tractus rubrospinalis). It coordinates muscle tone, body position, and gait. A lesion of the nucleus ruber produces resting tremor, abnormal muscle tone (tested as involuntary muscular resistance of the joints in the relaxed patient), and choreoathetosis (involuntary writhing movements, usually involving the distal parts of the limbs).

The **substantia nigra** consists of a *pars compacta* (dark, contains melanin) and a *pars reticularis* (reddish, contains iron; for simplicity, the entire substantia nigra appears dark in the drawing). Most of its axons project diffusely to other brain areas and are not collected into tracts. Some axons from the nucleus caudatus and putamen (fibrae striatonigrales), and precentral cortex (fibrae corticonigrales) terminate in the substantia nigra.

D Cross-sectional structure of the truncus encephali at different levels

Transverse sections through the **a** mesencephalon, **b** pons, and **c** medulla oblongata, viewed from above.

A feature common to all three sections is the dorsally situated tegmentum ("hood," medium gray), the phylogenetically old part of the truncus encephali. The tegmentum of the adult brain contains the brainstem nuclei. Anterior to the tegmentum are the large ascending and descending tracts that run to and from the telencephalon. This region is called the pedunculus cerebri (crus cerebri) in the mesencephalon, the basilar part (base) of the pons at the pontine level, and the pyramidea in the medulla oblongata. The tegmentum is covered dorsally by the tectum (= "roof") only in the region of the mesencephalon. In the mature brain pictured here, this structure forms the lamina quadrigemina containing the colliculi superior and inferior ("little hills"), shown faintly in **Da**. The truncus encephali is covered by the cerebellum at the level of the medulla oblongata and pons and therefore lacks a tectal covering at those levels.

357

8.3 Truncus Encephali: Reticular Formation (Formatio Reticularis)

A Definition, demarcation, and organization

The *formatio reticularis (RF)* is a phylogenetically old, morphologically ill-defined collection of numerous small nuclei in the *tegmentum* of the truncus encephali. These nuclei serve entirely different functions. The morphological term *"formatio reticularis"* incorrectly implies a homogeneity when in fact it represents different centers. Thus, it would be better to refer to them as *nuclei reticulares*, which morpologically are difficult to distinguish from one another. The nuclei reticulares use different neurotransmitters to serve their different functions. Considering these facts, the formatio reticularis can be classified as follows:

- Cytoarchitectonics (morphological classification) takes into account the shape and architecture of the nuclei reticulares (see **C**).
- Transmitter architectonics (chemical classification) takes into account the type of neurotransmitters used by the cells (see **C**).
- The classification based on functional centers (physiological classification) covers the functions associated with the nuclei (see **B**).

Note: Nuclei nervorum cranialium, which are mainly located in the tegmentum of the truncus encephali (but are usually very well defined morphologically) are not part of the RF but are functionally closely linked with it. Neither the nuclear regions of the "nucleus ruber" or "substantia nigra" located in the tegmentum of the mesencephalon nor the nuclei pontis are part of the RF.

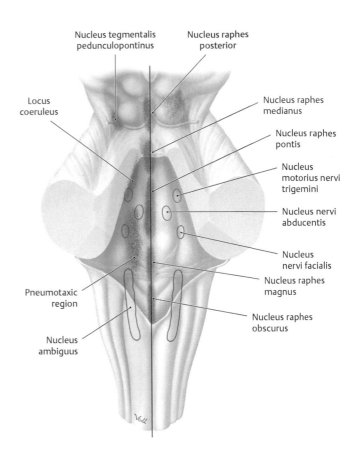

C Cyto- and transmitter architectonics

Dorsal view of the truncus encephali after the cerebellum has been removed; left hemisphere: cytoarchitectonics; right hemisphere: transmitter architectonics. With the help of cytoarchitectonics, the nuclei reticulares can be divided already in the RF on both sides into three longitudinal zones each:

- *lateral zone* with small-cell nuclei (parvocellular zone),
- *medial zone* with large-cell nuclei (magnocellular zone)
- *median zone* (it lies on both sides of the midline = raphe of the truncus encephali; the large-cell nuclei located in this zone are thus also referred to as "raphe nuclei").

The axons of the medial and median zone, after a long course, reach other nuclei of the CNS either in cranial direction up to the telencephalon or in caudal direction down to the sacral spinal region. These two zones are mostly responsible for connecting the RF with other regions of the CNS. They are thus called "effectory." However, the axons of the lateral zone largely remain inside the truncus encephali, connecting individual portions of the RF with one another or interconnecting with nuclei nervorum cranialium in the truncus encephali. They are thus also referred to as "association areas." Some nuclei have been labeled as examples.

Note: The division into three longitudinal zones is not equally visible in all portions of the truncus encephali. It is best visible in the medulla oblongata. As a reference point, the nuclei nervorum cranialium (they are not part of the RF, see introduction), which are closely interconnected with the RF, have also been marked.

Transmitter architectonics can help identify areas in which neurons with a specific transmitter predominate. Catecholamines (adrenaline, noradrenaline, dopamine) as well as serotonin and acetylcholine are examples shown here.

Note: Nuclei raphes (median zone), which send their axons to the limbic system (modulation of moods and feelings) use serotonin as a transmitter. Pharmacologically, influencing the effect of serotonin is said to effectively modulate emotions.

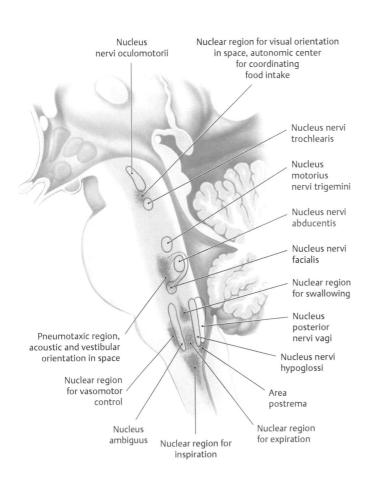

B Functional centers

Left lateral view of the truncus encephali bisected. Displayed is the position of functional centers as well as the position of functionally relevant nuclei nervorum cranialium. For further details of the functional centers see **D**.

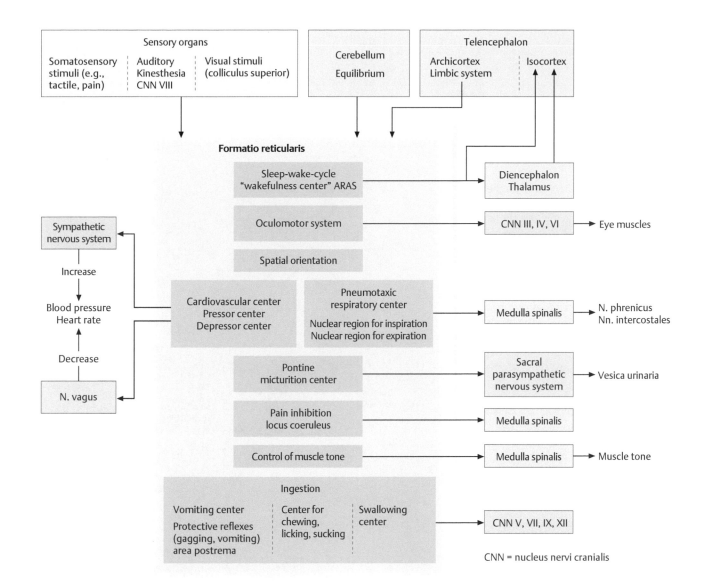

CNN = nucleus nervi cranialis

D Overview of the functions of the formatio reticularis
A distinction is drawn between the following functional relationships of the formatio reticularis with other centers in the CNS:

- **Afferents to the** formatio reticularis: These originate from nuclei of almost all sensory organs, the telencephalon, diencephalon as well as the cerebellum and medulla spinalis. They carry auditory, visual and tactile impulses and to a special degree, pain sensation, but also carry information regarding muscle relaxation, equilibrium, blood pressure, oxygen saturation, and parameters of ingestion.
- **Efferents of the** formatio reticularis: These extend to the telencephalon and diencephalon but also to the motor nuclei of the nn. craniales and the medulla spinalis. These efferents have very different effects:

- regulating sleep-wake transitions and level of alertness of the telencephalon (so-called *"ARAS"*: **A**scending **R**eticular **A**ctivitating **S**ystem),
- regulating eye movement,
- "vital" functions such as regulating blood pressure and respiration,
- functions of ingestion such as licking, sucking and chewing,
- protective reflexes such as gagging and vomiting,
- control of micturition,
- regulating muscle tone in the medulla spinalis, and
- pain inhibition in the medulla spinalis.

E Branching pattern of a neuron in the formatio reticularis of the rat truncus encephali (after Scheibel)
Midsagittal section viewed from the left side. Neurons can be selectively visualized with the silver-impregnation (Golgi) staining method. The axon of the neuron shown here divides into an ascending branch, which comes into contact with the diencephalic nuclei (shown in brown) and a descending branch, which establishes connections with nuclei nervi craniales (green) in the pons and medulla oblongata. This extensive arborization allows neurons of the formatio reticularis to have widespread effects on multiple brain regions.

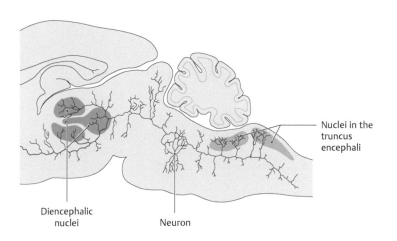

Nuclei in the truncus encephali

Diencephalic nuclei

Neuron

8.4 Brainstem: Descending and Ascending Tracts

A Descending tracts in the truncus encephali

a Midsagittal section viewed from the left side. **b** Posterior view with the cerebellum removed.

The descending tracts shown here begin in the telencephalon and terminate partly in the truncus encephali but mostly in the medulla spinalis. The most prominent tract that descends through the truncus encephali, the *corticospinal tract*, terminates in the medulla spinalis. Its axons arise from large pyramidal neurons of the primary motor cortex and terminate on or near alphamotor neurons in the cornu anterius of the medulla spinalis. Most of the axons cross to the opposite side (decussate) at the level of the pyramides. The fibers in this part of the tractus pyramidalis that descend through the brainstem are called *fibrae corticospinales*. Those fibers in the tractus pyramidalis that terminate in the truncus encephali are called *fibrae corticonucleares*. Corticonuclear axons connect the motor cortex to the nuclei motorii trunci encephali of the nn. craniales.

Note: Direct cortical projections to the nuclei trunci encephali are predominantly

- *bilateral* for
  - the nucleus motorius nervi trigemini (CN V)
  - neurons in the nucleus nervi facialis (CN VII) that innervate muscles in the forehead
  - nucleus ambiguus (CN X)
- *contralateral (crossed)* for
  - the nucleus nervi abducentis (CN VI)
  - neurons in the nucleus nervi facialis (CN VII) that innervate muscles in the lower face
  - the nucleus nervi hypoglossi (CN XII)
- *ipsilateral* for
  - neurons in the nucleus nervi accessorii (CN XI) that innervate the m. sternocleidomastoideus

The pattern of corticonuclear innervation is important in the diagnosis of different lesions, particularly involving the facial nerve (CN VII; see **D**, p. 124). The *fasciculus longitudinalis medialis* is a tractus in trunci encephali containing both ascending and descending fibers that interconnects the nuclei of the truncus encephali (for its function see **C**, p. 483).

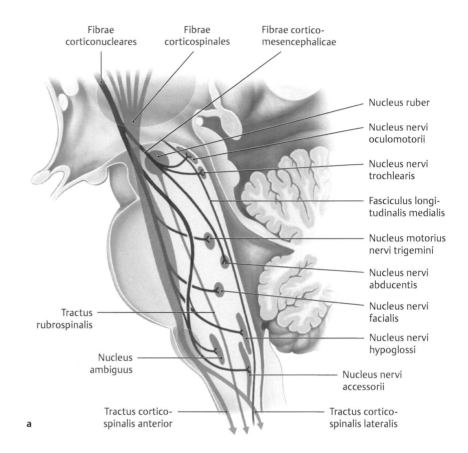

Fibrae corticonucleares — Fibrae corticospinales — Fibrae cortico-mesencephalicae — Nucleus ruber — Nucleus nervi oculomotorii — Nucleus nervi trochlearis — Fasciculus longitudinalis medialis — Nucleus motorius nervi trigemini — Nucleus nervi abducentis — Nucleus nervi facialis — Nucleus nervi hypoglossi — Tractus rubrospinalis — Nucleus ambiguus — Nucleus nervi accessorii — Tractus corticospinalis anterior — Tractus corticospinalis lateralis

a

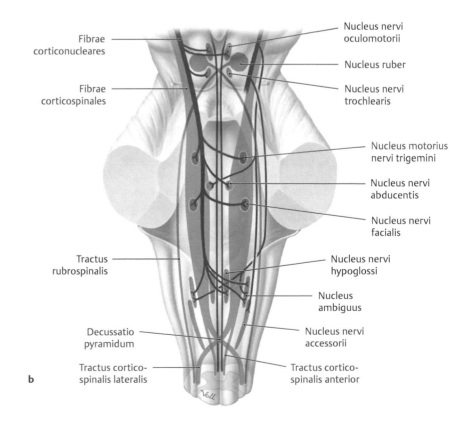

Fibrae corticonucleares — Fibrae corticospinales — Nucleus nervi oculomotorii — Nucleus ruber — Nucleus nervi trochlearis — Nucleus motorius nervi trigemini — Nucleus nervi abducentis — Nucleus nervi facialis — Tractus rubrospinalis — Nucleus nervi hypoglossi — Nucleus ambiguus — Decussatio pyramidum — Nucleus nervi accessorii — Tractus corticospinalis lateralis — Tractus corticospinalis anterior

b

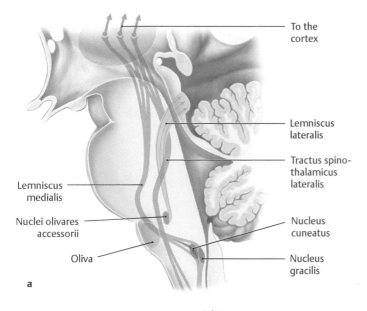

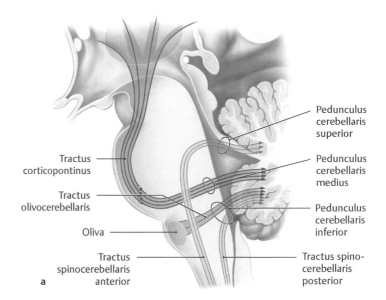

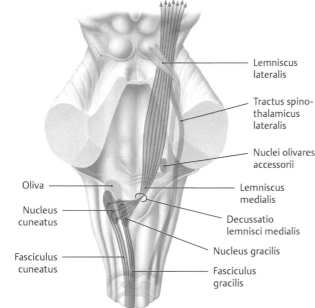

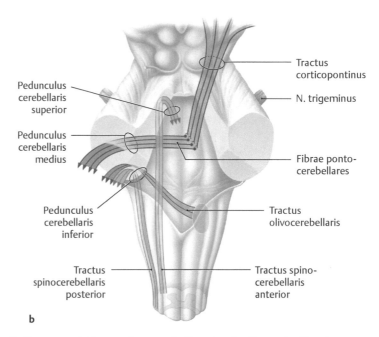

B Courses of ascending tracts through the truncus encephali

a Left lateral view; **b** Posterior view.

Two major ascending medulla spinalis tracts, the tractus spinothalamicus lateralis and funiculus posterior carry somatosensory information from the medulla spinalis to the thalamus (diencephalon, see pp. 344 and 346). Two of the ribbon-like tracts are recongnizable in the truncus encephali (see p. 545), the lemniscus medialis and the lemniscus lateralis:

- The lemniscus medialis consists of axons of the second neurons with the cell bodies in the nuclei gracilis and cuneatus. Afferents to these nuclei come from the fasciculus gracilis or fasciculus cuneatus (e.g., pressure, vibration). Tractus spinothalamicus axons (pain, temperature) join the lemniscus medialis before approaching the thalamus.
- The lemniscus lateralis contains axons from the nuclei cochleares and other stations on the auditory pathway that ascend to the colliculus inferior of the lamina quadrigemina.

The tractus spinothalamicus anterior is not shown because its location in the brainstem is disputed. The tractus spinothalamicus anterior together with the tractus spinothalamicus lateralis is sometimes referred to as the lemniscus spinalis.

C Courses of the major cerebellar tracts through the truncus encephali

a Midsagittal section viewed from the left side; **b** Posterior view (cerebellum has been removed).

The cerebellum is involved in the coordination of fine motor movements and the regulation of muscle tone. Its tracts are composed of ascending (blue) and descending (red) pathways. They enter the cerebellum through the three pedunculi cerebellares (superior, medius, and inferior).

- **Pedunculus cerebellaris superior:** Most of the efferent tracts from the nuclei cerebelli run through the pedunculus cerebellaris superior (see p. 370). The only afferent tract entering the cerebellum through the pedunculus cerebellaris superior is the tractus spinocerebellaris anterior.
- **Pedunculus cerebellaris medius:** Contains only afferent fibers to the cerebellum. They belong to a pathway that originates in the different lobes (tractus corticopontinus). The axons of the tractus corticopontinus synapse with neurons in the nuclei pontis and the axons of these neurons form the fibrae pontocerebellares that cross over and run within the opposite pedunculus cerebellaris medius to the contralateral cerebellum.
- **Pedunculus cerebellaris inferior:** It is mainly afferent to the cerebellum. The Tractus spinocerebellaris posterior, the fibrae cuneocerebellares, and the tractus olivocerebellaris enter the cerebellum through the pedunculus cerebellaris inferior.

The diagram shows the course and location of the distinct cerebellar tracts.

361

8.5 Mesencephalon and Pons, Transverse Section

A Transverse section through the mesencephalon (midbrain)

Superior view.

Nuclei: The most rostral n. cranialis nucleus is the relatively small *nucleus nervi oculomotorii* (see **B**, p. 356 and p. 114). In the same transverse section plan the *nucleus mesencephalicus nervi trigemini* is also present; other trigeminal nuclei can be identified in sections at caudal levels (see **C**). Unique in the CNS, the nucleus mesencephalicus nervi trigemini contains displaced pseudounipolar sensory neurons, closely related to the PNS neurons of the ganglion trigeminale (both populations are derived embryologically from the crista neuralis). The peripheral processes of these mesencephalic neurons are proprioceptors in the mm. masticatorii. The *nucleus colliculi superioris* is part of the visual system. The *nucleus ruber* and *substantia nigra* are involved in coordination of motor activity. The nucleus ruber and all of the nuclei nervorum cranialium are located in the tegmentum of the mesencephalon, the colliculus superior is in the tectum (roof) of the mesencephalon, and the substantia nigra is in the pedunculus cerebri (see **C**, p. 356). Different parts of the formatio reticularis, a diffuse

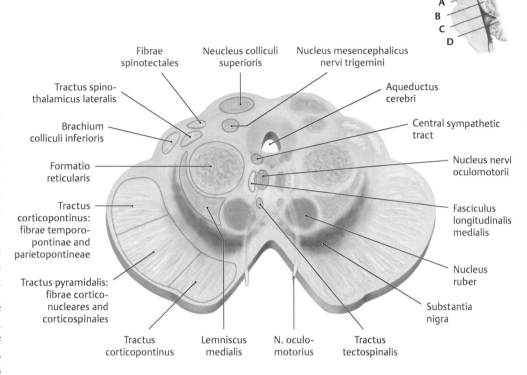

aggregation of nuclear groups, are visible here and in sections below.

Tracts: The tracts at this level run anterior to the nuclear regions. Prominent descending tracts seen at this level include the tractus pyramidalis and the fibrae corticonucleares. Ascending tracts visible at this level include the tractus spinothalamicus lateralis and the lemniscus medialis, both of which terminate in the thalamus.

B Transverse section through the upper pons

Nuclei: The only nucleus nervi cranialis appearing in this plane of section is the nucleus mesencephalicus nervi trigemini. It can be seen that the fibers from the nucleus nervi trochlearis (CN IV) cross to the opposite side (decussate) while still within the truncus encephali

Tracts: The ascending and descending tract systems are the same as in **A** and **C**. The tractus pyramidalis appears less compact at this level compared with the previous section due to the presence of intermingled nuclei pontis. This section cuts the tracts (mostly efferent) that exit the cerebellum through the pedunculus cerebellaris superior. The lemniscus lateralis at the dorsal surface of the section is part of the auditory pathway. The relatively large fasciculus longitudinalis *medialis* extends from the mesencephalon (see **A**) into the medulla spinalis. It interconnects the truncus encephali nuclei and contains a variety of fibers that enter and emerge at various levels (*"highway of the brainstem nuclei"*). The smaller fasciculus longitudinalis posterior connects

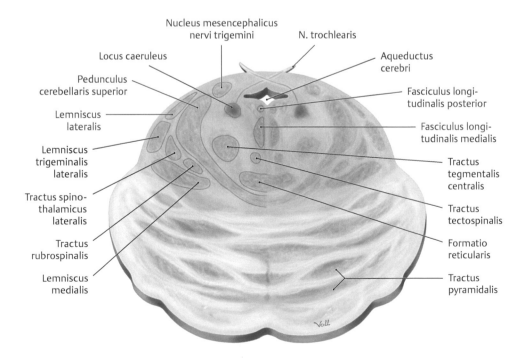

hypothalamic nuclei with the parasympathetic nuclei nervorum cranialium. The size and location of the nuclei of the formatio reticularis, which here are shown graphically within a compact area, vary with the plane of the section. This diagram indicates only the approximate location of the formatio reticularis, and other smaller nuclei and fibers may be found within these regions.

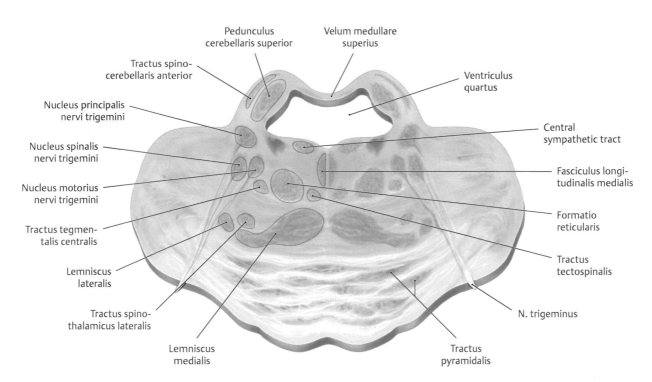

Pedunculus cerebellaris superior
Velum medullare superius
Tractus spino- cerebellaris anterior
Nucleus principalis nervi trigemini
Nucleus spinalis nervi trigemini
Nucleus motorius nervi trigemini
Tractus tegmen- talis centralis
Lemniscus lateralis
Tractus spino- thalamicus lateralis
Lemniscus medialis
Ventriculus quartus
Central sympathetic tract
Fasciculus longi- tudinalis medialis
Formatio reticularis
Tractus tectospinalis
N. trigeminus
Tractus pyramidalis

C Transverse section through the midportion of the pons
Nuclei: The n. trigeminus leaves the truncus encephali at the midlevel of the pons, its various nuclei dominating the tegmentum pontis. The *nucleus principalis nervi trigemini* relays afferents for touch and discrimination, while its *nucleus spinalis* relays pain and temperature fibers. The nucleus motorius nervi trigemini contains the motor neurons for the mm. masticatorii.

Tracts: This section cuts the tractus spinocerebellaris anterior, which passes to the cerebellum, immediately dorsal to the pons.
CSF space: At this level the aqueductus cerebri has given way to the ventriculus quartus, which appears in cross-section. It is covered dorsally by the velum medullare superius.

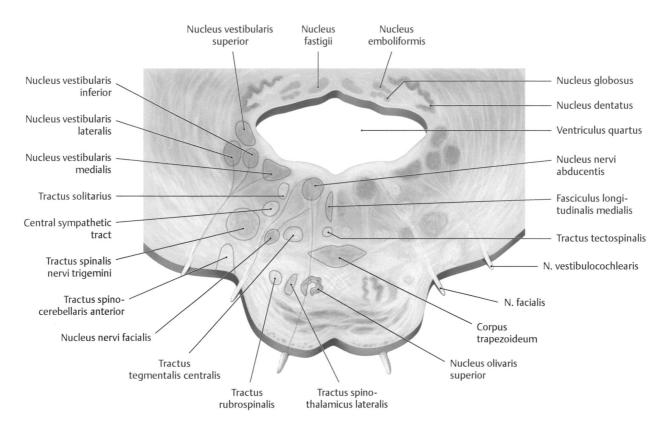

Nucleus vestibularis superior
Nucleus fastigii
Nucleus emboliformis
Nucleus vestibularis inferior
Nucleus vestibularis lateralis
Nucleus vestibularis medialis
Tractus solitarius
Central sympathetic tract
Tractus spinalis nervi trigemini
Tractus spino- cerebellaris anterior
Nucleus nervi facialis
Tractus tegmentalis centralis
Tractus rubrospinalis
Tractus spino- thalamicus lateralis
Nucleus globosus
Nucleus dentatus
Ventriculus quartus
Nucleus nervi abducentis
Fasciculus longi- tudinalis medialis
Tractus tectospinalis
N. vestibulocochlearis
N. facialis
Corpus trapezoideum
Nucleus olivaris superior

D Transverse section through the lower pons
Nuclei: The lower pons contains a number of nuclei nervorum cranialium including the nuclei vestibulares and cochleares and nucleus nervi abducentis, and the nucleus nervi facialis. The fossa rhomboidea is covered dorsally by the cerebellum, whose nuclei also appear in this section—the nuclei fastigii, emboliformis, globosus, and dentatus.

Tracts: The corpus trapezoideum with its subnuclei is an important relay station and crossing point in the auditory pathway (see p. 484). The tractus tegmentalis centralis is an important pathway in the motor system.

8.6 Medulla Oblongata, Transverse Section

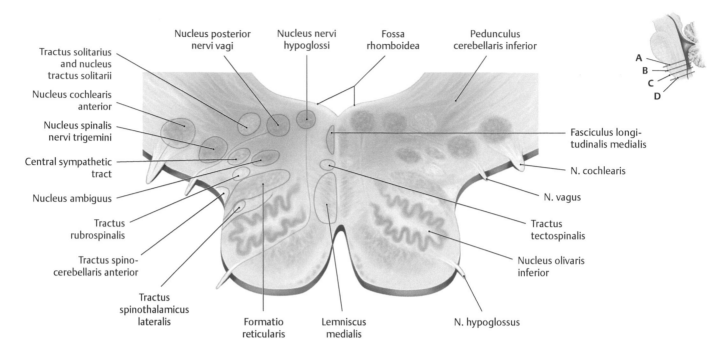

Nucleus posterior nervi vagi

Nucleus nervi hypoglossi

Fossa rhomboidea

Pedunculus cerebellaris inferior

Tractus solitarius and nucleus tractus solitarii

Nucleus cochlearis anterior

Nucleus spinalis nervi trigemini

Central sympathetic tract

Nucleus ambiguus

Tractus rubrospinalis

Tractus spino-cerebellaris anterior

Tractus spinothalamicus lateralis

Formatio reticularis

Lemniscus medialis

N. hypoglossus

Fasciculus longitudinalis medialis

N. cochlearis

N. vagus

Tractus tectospinalis

Nucleus olivaris inferior

A Transverse section through the upper medulla oblongata

Nuclei: The nuclei of the n. hypoglossus, n. vagus, n. vestibulocochlearis, and the nucleus spinalis nervi trigemini appear in the *dorsal* part of the medulla oblongata. The nucleus olivaris inferior, which belongs to the motor system, is located in the *ventral* part of the medulla oblongata. The formatio reticularis is interposed between the nuclei nervorum cranialium and the nucleus olivaris inferior. It appears in all the transverse sections of this unit.

Tracts: Most of the ascending and descending tracts are the same as in the previous unit. A new structure appearing at this level is the *pedunculus cerebellaris inferior*, through which afferent tracts pass to the cerebellum (see p. 361).

CSF space: The floor of the ventriculus quartus is the fossa rhomboidea, which marks the dorsal boundary of this section.

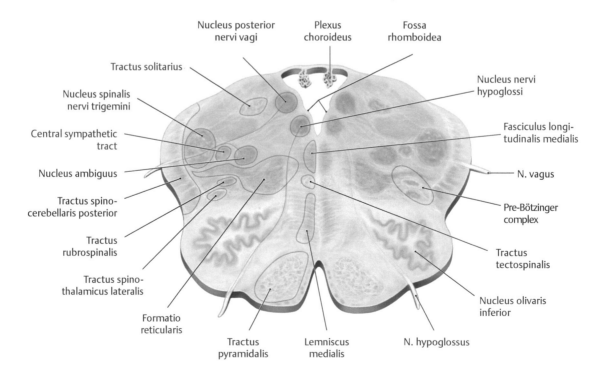

Nucleus posterior nervi vagi

Plexus choroideus

Fossa rhomboidea

Tractus solitarius

Nucleus spinalis nervi trigemini

Central sympathetic tract

Nucleus ambiguus

Tractus spino-cerebellaris posterior

Tractus rubrospinalis

Tractus spino-thalamicus lateralis

Formatio reticularis

Tractus pyramidalis

Lemniscus medialis

N. hypoglossus

Nucleus nervi hypoglossi

Fasciculus longitudinalis medialis

N. vagus

Pre-Bötzinger complex

Tractus tectospinalis

Nucleus olivaris inferior

B Transverse section just above the middle of the medulla oblongata

Nuclei: Of the nuclei nervorum cranialium, only those of the nn. hypoglossus, vagus, et trigeminus remain in the pars posterior tegmenti. The section passes through the nucleus olivaris inferior anterioras well as the pre-Bötzinger complex. It consists of a sparse array of small, lipofuscin-rich neurons that form an integral part of the respiratory network and thus of the mammalian respiratory impulse in the medulla oblongata.

Tracts: The ascending and descending tracts are the same as in the previous unit. The lemniscus medialis is formed by decussated axons originating in the nuclei gracilis and cuneatus (see p. 404). The tractus solitarius carries the gustatory fibers of nervi craniales VII, IX, and X. Dorsolateral to it is the *nucleus tractus solitarii* (not shown). The *tractus pyramidalis* again appears as a compact structure at this level due to the absence of interspersed nuclei and decussating fibers.

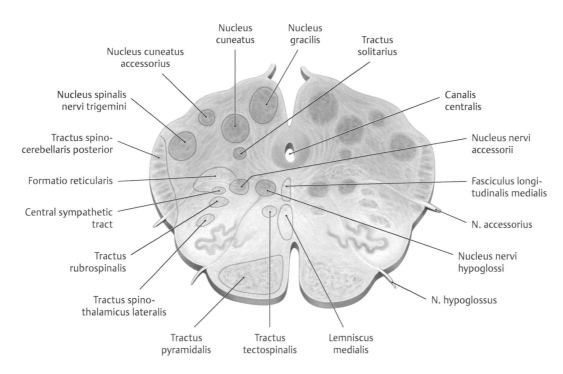

Labels for section C diagram:
Nucleus cuneatus accessorius
Nucleus cuneatus
Nucleus gracilis
Tractus solitarius
Nucleus spinalis nervi trigemini
Canalis centralis
Tractus spino-cerebellaris posterior
Nucleus nervi accessorii
Formatio reticularis
Fasciculus longitudinalis medialis
Central sympathetic tract
N. accessorius
Tractus rubrospinalis
Nucleus nervi hypoglossi
Tractus spino-thalamicus lateralis
N. hypoglossus
Tractus pyramidalis
Tractus tectospinalis
Lemniscus medialis

C Transverse section just below the middle of the medulla oblongata
Nuclei: The nuclei of the hypoglossus and vagus nn. as well as the nucleus spinalis nervi trigemini appear at this level. The irregular outline of the nucleus olivaris inferior is still just visible in the ventral medulla. The nuclei that relay signals from the funiculus posterior—the nucleus cuneatus and nucleus gracilis—appear prominently in the dorsal part of the section. The axons that arise from these nuclei decussate and form the lemniscus medialis (see above).
Tracts: The ascending and descending tracts correspond to those in the previous diagrams. The fossa rhomboidea, which is the floor of the ventriculus quartus, has narrowed substantially at this level to become the canalis centralis.

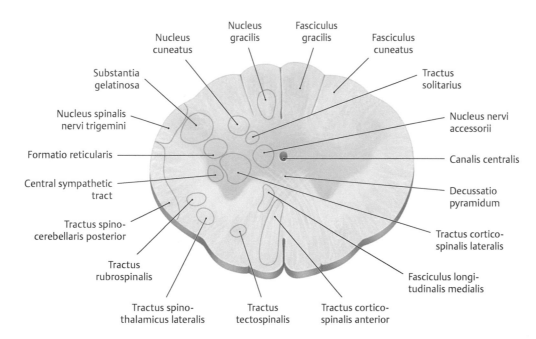

Labels for section D diagram:
Nucleus cuneatus
Nucleus gracilis
Fasciculus gracilis
Fasciculus cuneatus
Substantia gelatinosa
Tractus solitarius
Nucleus spinalis nervi trigemini
Nucleus nervi accessorii
Formatio reticularis
Canalis centralis
Central sympathetic tract
Decussatio pyramidum
Tractus spino-cerebellaris posterior
Tractus cortico-spinalis lateralis
Tractus rubrospinalis
Fasciculus longitudinalis medialis
Tractus spino-thalamicus lateralis
Tractus tectospinalis
Tractus cortico-spinalis anterior

D Transverse section through the lower medulla oblongata
The medulla oblongata is continuous with the medulla spinalis at this level, showing no distinct transition.
Nuclei: The nuclei nervorum cranialium visible at this level are the spinal part of the nucleus spinalis nervi trigemini and the nucleus nervi accessorii. This section passes through the caudal end of the nuclei in the nucleus cuneatus and nucleus gracilis, which are a relay station for the funiculus posterior.

Tracts: The ascending and descending tracts correspond to those in the previous diagrams of this unit. The section passes through the decussatio pyramidum, and we can now distinguish the tractus corticospinalis anterior (uncrossed) from the tractus corticospinalis lateralis (crossed; see pp. 409 and 461).
CSF space: This section passes through a portion of the canalis centralis, which is markedly smaller at this level than in **C**. It may even be obliterated at some sites, but this has no clinical significance.

365

9.1 Cerebellum, External Structure

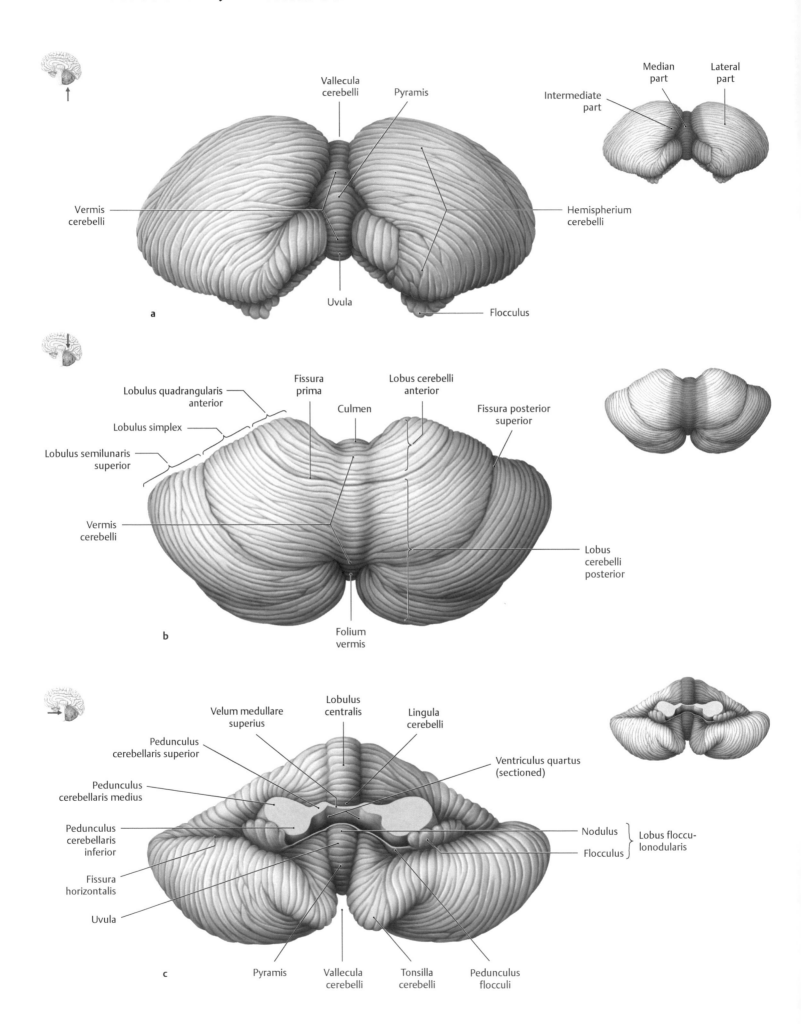

a

Vallecula cerebelli

Pyramis

Median part

Intermediate part

Lateral part

Vermis cerebelli

Hemispherium cerebelli

Uvula

Flocculus

b

Lobulus quadrangularis anterior

Fissura prima

Lobus cerebelli anterior

Culmen

Fissura posterior superior

Lobulus simplex

Lobulus semilunaris superior

Vermis cerebelli

Lobus cerebelli posterior

Folium vermis

c

Velum medullare superius

Lobulus centralis

Lingula cerebelli

Pedunculus cerebellaris superior

Pedunculus cerebellaris medius

Ventriculus quartus (sectioned)

Pedunculus cerebellaris inferior

Nodulus

Lobus flocculonodularis

Flocculus

Fissura horizontalis

Uvula

Pyramis

Vallecula cerebelli

Tonsilla cerebelli

Pedunculus flocculi

A Isolated cerebellum

a Inferior view, **b** superior view, **c** anterior view. Cerebellum with the pedunculi cerebellares detached from the truncus encephali.

Functionally, the cerebellum is part of the motor system. However, it does not trigger any conscious movements but is responsible for unconscious coordination and fine-tuning of movements (see **B**, p. 372). Just like the telencephalon, the cerebellum consists of two hemispheria. The two hemispheria cerebellares are largely separated from one another but connected by commissural tracts of axons. Between hemispheria cerebellares lies an unpaired, worm-shaped structure—the vermis cerebelli. It is a portion of the cerebellum which exhibits the same structure as the hemispheria. Unlike the telencephalon, where all gyri and sulci are individually named, the cerebellar folia and fissurae are not. However, similar to the gyri and sulci, their role is also to increase the surface area of the cortex. Cerebellar fissurae further subdivide the cerebellum into lobi. In particular:

- The fissura prima separates the lobus cerebelli anterior from the lobus cerebelli posterior (see **b**).
- The fissura posterolateralis separates the lobus cerebelli posterior from the lobus flocculonodularis (see **B**).

Other, less important fissurae have no clinical or functional significance and are not described here. Besides these anatomical divisions, the parts of the cerebellum can also be distinguished according to phylogenetic and functional criteria (see **B**, p. 372). The cerebellum is connected to the truncus encephali via the three pairs of pedunculi cerebellares (pedunculi cerebellares superior, medius, and inferior [see **c**]). The pedunculi cerebellares are not equal in size. They contain the afferent and efferent tracts that connect the cerebellum with other parts of the CNS. The truncus encephali shows the analogous sections of the pedunculi cerebellares (see **C, b** and **c**, p. 355). The velum medullare superius stretches between the two pedunculi cerebellares superiores and forms part of the roof of the ventriculus quartus (see **c**). The tonsillae cerebellares protrude downward near the midline on each side, almost to the foramen magnum at the base of the skull (not shown). Increased intracranial pressure may cause the tonsillae cerebellares to herniate into the foramen magnum, impinging upon vital centers in the truncus encephali and posing a threat to life (see **D**, p. 309). Functionally, the medial part of the cerebellum (red) is distinguished from the intermediate part (pale red) and lateral part (gray). This functional classification does not conform to the anatomically defined lobar boundaries. Each of these parts projects to a specific cerebellar nucleus (see p. 368).

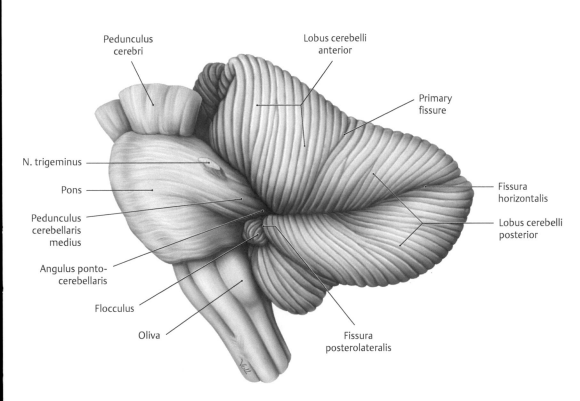

Pedunculus cerebri

Lobus cerebelli anterior

N. trigeminus

Primary fissure

Pons

Pedunculus cerebellaris medius

Fissura horizontalis

Angulus ponto-cerebellaris

Lobus cerebelli posterior

Flocculus

Oliva

Fissura posterolateralis

B Cerebellum on the truncus encephali

Left lateral view. For the truncus encephali and cerebellum, which overlies the dorsal aspect of the truncus encephali, the same terms of location and direction are used. In the lateral view, only the hemispheria cerebelli and the flocculus are visible as well as the pedunculus cerebelli medius along with its origin in the pons. At the angle formed at the junction of the pons and cerebellum (the angulus pontocerebellaris), nn. craniales VII and VIII emerge from the truncus encephali (not shown here, see **Ca**, p. 355). Occasionally, the n. vestibulocochlearis (n. cranialis VIII) develops an acoustic neuroma (more correctly, a vestibular schwannoma). Based on their localization, these tumors are referred to as angulus pontocerebellaris tumors (see **D**, p. 151). Due to the damage to n. cranialis VIII, affected patients mainly suffer from impaired hearing and balance.

C Synopsis of cerebellar classifications

Phylogenetic classification	Anatomical classification	Functional classification based on the origin of afferents
• Archicerebellum	• Lobus flocculonodularis	• Vestibulocerebellum: maintenance of equilibrium
• Paleocerebellum	• Lobus cerebelli anterior • Portions of the vermis • Medial portions of the lobus posterior	• Spinocerebellum: regulation of muscle tone
• Neocerebellum	• Lateral portions of the lobus posterior	• Pontocerebellum (= cerebrocerebellum): skilled movements

9.2 Cerebellum, Internal Structure

A Cerebellum: Positional relationship and cut surface

Midsagittal section, left lateral view. The cerebellum extends along almost the entire dorsal surface of the truncus encephali and abuts the tectum of the mesencephalon in the rostral direction and the medulla oblongata in the caudal direction. Its vela medullaria superius and inferius form the roof of the fourth ventricle (ventriculus quartus). The lingula cerebelli overlies the velum medullare superius and the velum medullare inferius lies below the nodulus. Such a midsagittal section shows only the part of the medially located unpaired vermis cerebelli. The laterally located hemispheria cerebelli remain intact. The fissura prima (that slants superiorly and dorsally) separates the lobi anterior and posterior, which, due to their lateral position, are not visible here (see **C**, p. 368). The (deep) nuclei cerebelli, which are located in the substantia alba of the cerebellum, are barely visible on midsagittal sections. A slightly dorsocaudal-oblique view displays all the nuclei cerebelli (see **B**).

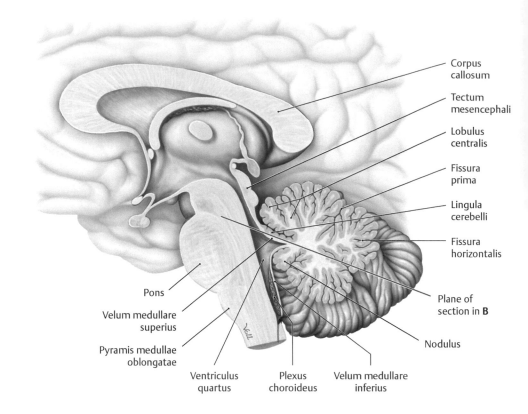

B Nuclei cerebelli

Section through the pedunculi cerebellares superiores (plane of section shown in **A**), viewed from behind. Deep within the cerebellar substantia alba are four pairs of nuclei that contain most of the *efferent* neurons of the cerebellum:

- Nucleus fastigii (green)
- Nucleus emboliformis (blue)
- Nuclei globosi (blue)
- Nucleus dentatus (pink).

The cortical regions have been color-coded to match their corresponding nuclei. The nucleus dentatus nucleus is the largest of the nuclei cerebelli and extends into the hemispheria cerebelli. The nuclei cerebelli receive projections from Purkinje cells in the cortex cerebelli (cf. p. 366). While the *efferent fibers* of the cerebellum can be assigned rather easily to anatomical structures, this is not true of the afferent fibers. Their sources are examined on p. 372.

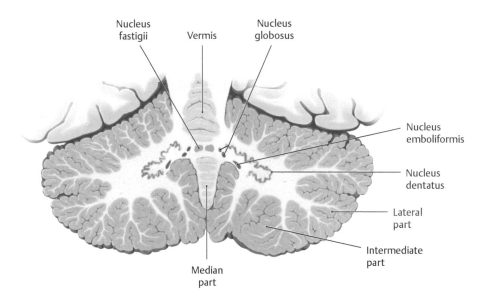

C Nuclei cerebelli and the regions of the cortex from which they receive projections (cf. p. 371)

Cerebellar nucleus	Synonyms	Regions of the cortex cerebelli that send axons to the nucleus
Nucleus dentatus	Nucleus lateralis cerebelli	Lateral part (lateral portions of the hemispheria cerebelli)
Nucleus emboliformis	Nucleus interpositus anterior	Intermediate part (medial portions of the hemispheria cerebelli)
Nuclei globosi	Nucleus interpositus posterior	Intermediate part (medial portions of the hemispheria cerebelli)
Nucleus fastigii	Nucleus medialis cerebelli	Median part (vermis cerebelli)

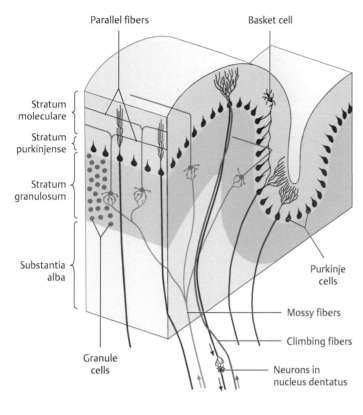

Parallel fibers

Basket cell

Stratum moleculare

Stratum purkinjense

Stratum granulosum

Substantia alba

Purkinje cells

Mossy fibers

Climbing fibers

Granule cells

Neurons in nucleus dentatus

D Cortex cerebelli

The cortex cerebelli consists of three layers:

- Stratum moleculare: outer layer; contains *parallel fibers*, which are the axons of granule cells (blue) from the stratum granulosum. They run parallel to the cerebellar folia and terminate in the stratum moleculare, where they synapse on the dendrites of the Purkinje cells. This layer also contains axons from the oliva and its accessory nuclei (*climbing fibers*) and a small number of inhibitory interneurons (*basket and stellate neurons*).
- Stratum purkinjense: contains the cell bodies of *Purkinje cells* (purple).
- Stratum granulosum: contains mostly *granule cells* (blue), as well as *mossy* and *climbing fibers* (green and pink, respectively), and *Golgi cells* (not shown; the cell types are viewed in **F**).

The substantia alba of the cerebellum is located under the stratum granulare.
Note: The Purkinje cells are the only efferent cells of the cortex cerebelli and project to the nuclei cerebelli and nuclei vestibulares.

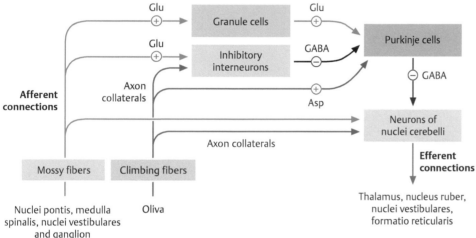

Glu

Granule cells

Glu

Glu

Inhibitory interneurons

GABA

Purkinje cells

GABA

Axon collaterals

Asp

Afferent connections

Mossy fibers

Climbing fibers

Neurons of nuclei cerebelli

Axon collaterals

Efferent connections

Nuclei pontis, medulla spinalis, nuclei vestibulares and ganglion

Oliva

Thalamus, nucleus ruber, nuclei vestibulares, formatio reticularis

E Synaptic circuitry of the cerebellum

(after Bähr and Frotscher)

Afferents on the left, efferents on the right. The cerebellum comprises 10% of the mass of the brain, but slightly more than 50% of its neurons. This is in indication of the complexity of the motor circuitry in the cerebellum. The **afferents** reach the cerebellum via climbing fibers and mossy fibers: The mossy fibers end in the dendritic tree of Purkinje cells, where they release their excitatory transmitter aspartic acid (ASP; see **D**). Their axon collaterals extend to inhibitory intermediate neurons and especially to the neurons of the cerebellar nuclei. The mossy fibers branch out and give off numerous axon collaterals. Some of the mossy fibers form synapses on the dendrites of the granule cells whose neurotransmitter glutamate has an excitatory effect on Purkinje cells. Another part of the mossy

fibers ends at inhibitory intermediate neurons, which inhibit Purkinje cells by means of their inhibitory neurotransmitter GABA. The mossy fibers also send axon collaterals to the cerebellum which are important for function. As mentioned above, the **efferents** of the cerebellum are localized in the cerebellum. Their neurons send basically efferent, excitatory impulses to the periphery. Impulses from the cerebellum are specifically inhibited by the Purkinje cells, which also contain the inhibitory neurotransmitter GABA, as well as by the adjacent nuclei vestibulares. This ensures a coordinated sequence of movements. When the Purkinje cells themselves are inhibited by inhibitory intermediate neurons (see black arrow), the impulses from the cerebellum are transmitted without inhibition so that the motion sequences are impaired (see p. 373).

F Principal neurons and fiber types in the cortex cerebelli

Name	Definition
Climbing fibers	Axons of neurons in the oliva and its associated nuclei
Mossy fibers	Axons of neurons in the nuclei pontis, the medulla spinalis, and nuclei vestibulares (fibrae pontocerebellares, tractus spinocerebellares, and vestibular tracts)
Parallel fibers (see **D**)	Axons of granule cells
Granule cells	Interneurons of the cortex cerebelli
Purkinje cells	The only efferent cells of the cortex cerebelli; exert an inhibitory effect

9.3 Cerebellar Peduncles and Tracts

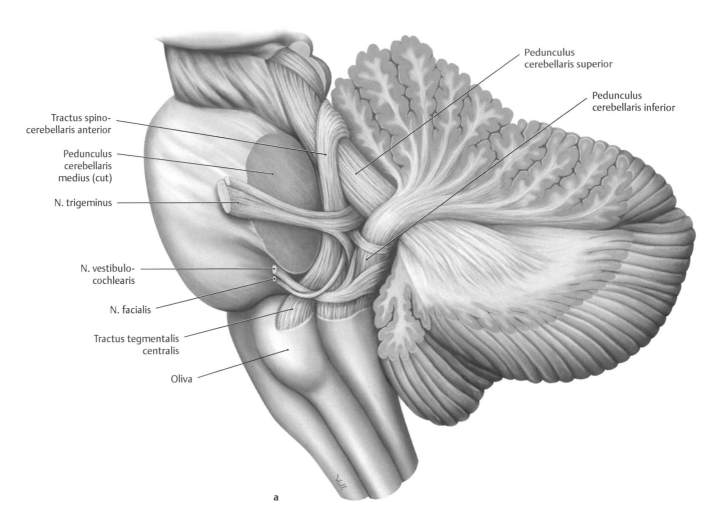

Pedunculus cerebellaris superior

Pedunculus cerebellaris inferior

Tractus spino-cerebellaris anterior

Pedunculus cerebellaris medius (cut)

N. trigeminus

N. vestibulo-cochlearis

N. facialis

Tractus tegmentalis centralis

Oliva

a

A Pedunculi cerebellares

a Left lateral view with the upper portion of the cerebellum and lateral portions of the pons removed. This dissection, which has been prepared to show fiber structure, clearly shows the course of the cerebellar tracts. The size of the pedunculi cerebellares, and thus the mass of entering and emerging axons, is substantial and reflects the extensive neural connections in the cerebellum (see p. 369). The cerebellum requires these numerous connections because it is an integrating center for the coordination of fine movements. In particular, it contains and processes vestibular and proprioceptive afferents and it modulates motor nuclei in other brain regions and in the medulla spinalis. The principal afferent and efferent connections of the cerebellum are reviewed in **B**.

b Left lateral view. Here the cerebellum has been sharply detached from its pedunculi to demonstrate the complementary cut surface of the pedunculi on the truncus encephali (compare with **Ac**, p. 366).

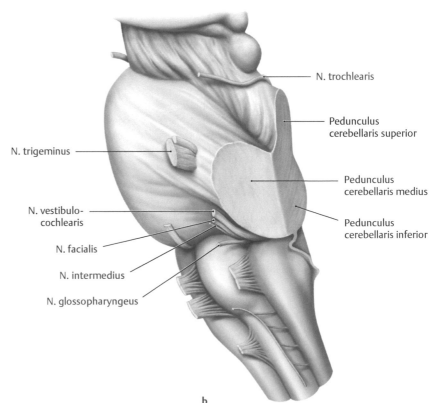

N. trochlearis

Pedunculus cerebellaris superior

N. trigeminus

Pedunculus cerebellaris medius

Pedunculus cerebellaris inferior

N. vestibulo-cochlearis

N. facialis

N. intermedius

N. glossopharyngeus

b

B Synopsis of the pedunculi cerebellares and their tracts

Tracts made up of afferent and efferent axons enter or leave the cerebellum through the pedunculi cerebellares. The afferent axons originate in the medulla spinalis, vestibular organs, oliva and pons, while the efferent axons originate in the nuclei cerebelli (see p. 368). The representation of the body in the cerebellum, unlike in the cerebrum, is ipsilateral. Ascending cerebellar pathways thus either are uncrossed or cross (decussate) twice in order to reach the same side. Compare the synopsis of the distinct tract systems (p. 445).

Cerebellar peduncle and constituent parts*	Origin**	Site of Termination
Pedunculus cerebelli anterior: contains mostly efferent tracts from the nuclei cerebelli. Some tracts cross in the decussation of the pedunculi cerebellares superiores, then divide into a *descending* part (to the pons) and an *ascending* part (to the mesencephalon and thalamus).		
Descending parts (**e**)	Nuclei fastigii and globosi	Formatio reticularis and nuclei vestibulares (projection is mostly *contralateral*)
Ascending parts (**e**)	Nucleus dentatus	Nucleus ruber and thalamus (both *contralateral*)
Tractus spinocerebellaris anterior (**a**)	Secondary neurons in intermediate gray matter, lumbosacral medulla spinalis. Relay proprioception stimuli related to lower limbs and trunk (muscle spindles, tendon receptors, etc.) received from the ganglion sensorium nervi spinalis. Fibers cross locally and then re-cross in the pons to return to the ipsilateral side.	Vermis cerebelli and intermediate part of lobus cerebelli anterior (*ipsilateral*; terminates as mossy fibers)
Pedunculus cerebellaris medius: contains only afferent tracts.		
Fibrae pontocerebellares (**a**)	Nuclei pontis. Relay cerebropontine to pontocerebellar projections (source of 90% of the axons in pedunculus cerebelli medius).	Lateral regions of lobi cerebelli posterior and anterior (*contralateral* to the origin of these fibers in pons; terminate as mossy fibers; branches to nucleus dentatus, also contralateral to the origin in pons)
Pedunculus cerebellaris inferior: contains both afferent and efferent tracts.		
Tractus spinocerebellaris posterior (**a**)	Clarke's nucleus/column. Relays proprioception and cutaneous sensation from the lower limb. Contains large axons with high conduction velocity.	Vermis cerebelli and nearby lobus cerebelli anterior, pyramis, and nearby lobus cerebelli posterior (*ipsilateral*; terminates as mossy fibers)
Fibrae cuneocerebellares (**a**)	Nucleus cuneatus and nucleus cuneatus accessorius. Relays proprioception (external cuneate nucleus) and cutaneous sensation (nucleus cuneatus) from the upper limb, with fast transmission, functionally corresponding to the tractus spinocerebellaris posterior.	Posterior part of lobus cerebelli anterior (*ipsilateral*; terminates as mossy fibers)
Tractus olivocerebellaris (**a**)	Complexus olivaris inferior. Nuclei olivares inferiores receive numerous inputs from sensory and motor systems, including a large contralateral projection from the cerebellum itself (nucleus dentatus, see below).	Stratum moleculare of cortex cerebelli (*contralateral*, terminates as *climbing* fibers)
Tractus vestibulocerebellaris (**a**)	Canales semicirculares (ganglion vestibulare) and nuclei vestibulares. Transmits balance and body position/motion information either directly (vestibular axons via n. vestibulocochlearis [CN VIII], *ipsilateral*) or via synaptic relay in nuclei vestibulares (*bilateral*).	Nodule, flocculus, lobus cerebelli anterior, and vermis cerebelli (*bilateral*, see left; terminates as *mossy* fibers)
Fibrae trigeminocerebellares (**a**)	Nuclei nervi trigemini in the truncus encephali. Relay proprioception and cutaneous sensation from the head.	Rostral part of lobus cerebelli posterior (*ipsilateral*; terminate as mossy fibers)
Fibrae cerebelloolivares (**e**)	Nucleus dentatus	Oliva (*contralateral*)

* Subentries for constituent parts are classified as efferent (**e**) or afferent (**a**).
** In the case of afferents, the type of afferent is listed along with the site of origin.

9.4 Cerebellum, Simplified Functional Anatomy and Lesions

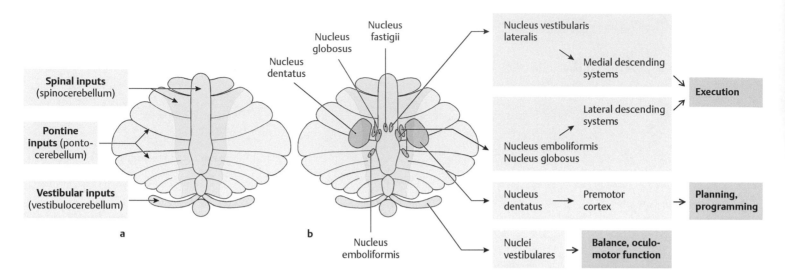

A Simplified functional anatomy of the cerebellum
(after Klinke and Silbernagl)

Two-dimensional representation of the cerebellum. The left side illustrates the afferent information from the periphery, which the cerebellum involved in voluntary motor movement requires; and the cerebellar functions divided based on the origin of its afferents (vestibulocerebellum, spinocerebellum and pontocerebellum, see p. 367 as well as **B**). The afferents are not segregated by externally visible anatomical boundaries. After the afferent information has been processed, the cortex cerebelli sends efferent impulses to the nuclei cerebelli, the eventual cerebellar efferents (shown on the right side).

- The nucleus fastigii and nucleus vestibularis lateralis coordinate the activity of skeletal muscles and thus movement via the medial descending systems; nuclei emboliformis and globosus via the lateral descending systems (see p. 410).
- The nucleus dentatus projects to the cortex cerebri and thus exerts influences on the planning and programming of movements.
- Efferents from the vestibulocerebellum control balance and oculomotor functions.

Visual inputs have not been considered here.

B Synopsis of cerebellar classifications and their relationships to motor deficits
Some cerebellar lesions cause subtle cognitive deficits that cannot be explained simply as a loss of muscle coordination.

Functional classification	Phylogenetic classification	Anatomical classification	Deficit symptoms
• Vestibulocerebellum	• Archicerebellum	• Lobus flocculonodularis	• Truncal, stance, and gait ataxia • Vertigo • Nystagmus • Vomiting
• Spinocerebellum	• Paleocerebellum	• Lobus anterior, parts of vermis cerebelli; lobus posterior, medial parts	• Ataxia, chiefly affecting the lower limb • Oculomotor dysfunction • Speech disorder (asynergy of speech muscles)
• Pontocerebellum (= cerebrocerebellum)	• Neocerebellum	• Lobus posterior, hemispheria	• Dysmetria and hypermetria (positive rebound) • Intention tremor • Nystagmus • Decreased muscle tone

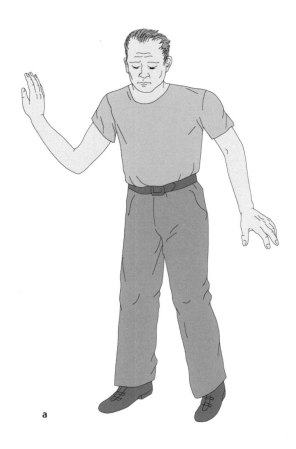

a

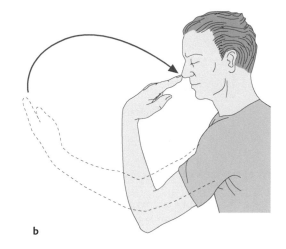

b

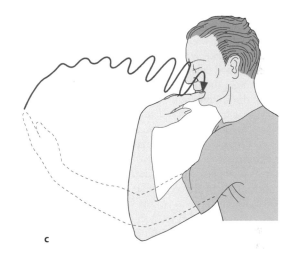

c

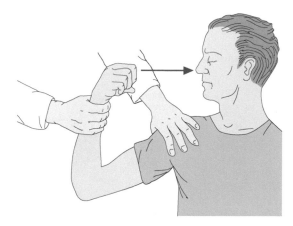

d

C Cerebellar lesions

Cerebellar lesions may remain clinically silent for some time because other brain regions can functionally compensate for them with reasonable effectiveness. Exceptions are direct lesions of the efferent nuclei cerebelli, which cannot be clinically compensated.

Cerebellar symptoms:

Asynergy	Lack of coordination among different muscle groups, especially in the performance of fine movements.
Ataxia	Uncoordinated sequence of movements. Truncal ataxia (patient cannot sit quietly upright) is distinguished from stance and gait ataxia (impaired limb movements, such as an unsteady gait as in inebriation). The patient stands with the legs spread apart and places his hand on the wall for stability (**a**).
Decreased muscle tone	Ipsilateral muscle weakness and rapid fatigability (asthenia).
Intention tremor	Involuntary, rhythmical wavering movement of the hand when a purposeful movement is attempted, as in the finger-nose test: normal test (**b**), test indicating a cerebellar lesion (**c**).
Rebound phenomenon	The patient, with eyes closed, is told to move the arm against a resistance from the examiner (**d**). When the examiner suddenly releases the arm, it forcefully "rebounds" toward the patient (hypermetria).

10.1 Arteries of the Brain: Blood Supply and the Circle of Willis

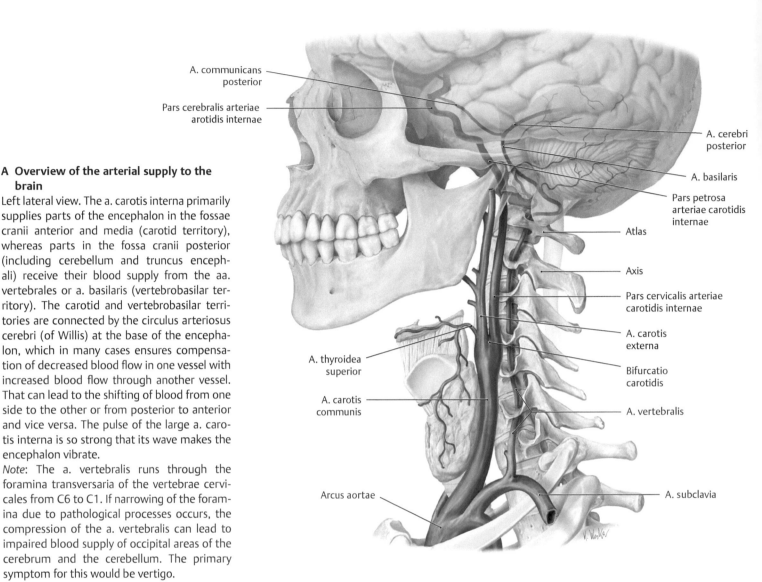

A Overview of the arterial supply to the brain

Left lateral view. The a. carotis interna primarily supplies parts of the encephalon in the fossae cranii anterior and media (carotid territory), whereas parts in the fossa cranii posterior (including cerebellum and truncus encephali) receive their blood supply from the aa. vertebrales or a. basilaris (vertebrobasilar territory). The carotid and vertebrobasilar territories are connected by the circulus arteriosus cerebri (of Willis) at the base of the encephalon, which in many cases ensures compensation of decreased blood flow in one vessel with increased blood flow through another vessel. That can lead to the shifting of blood from one side to the other or from posterior to anterior and vice versa. The pulse of the large a. carotis interna is so strong that its wave makes the encephalon vibrate.

Note: The a. vertebralis runs through the foramina transversaria of the vertebrae cervicales from C6 to C1. If narrowing of the foramina due to pathological processes occurs, the compression of the a. vertebralis can lead to impaired blood supply of occipital areas of the cerebrum and the cerebellum. The primary symptom for this would be vertigo.

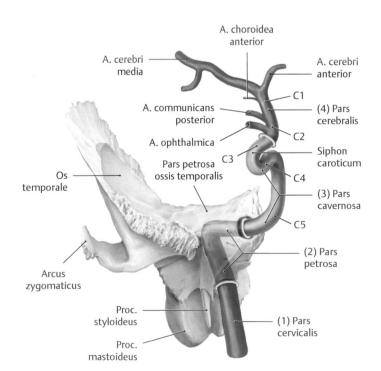

B The four anatomical divisions of the arteria carotis interna

Anterior view of the left a. carotis interna. The a. carotis interna consists of four topographically distinct parts between the bifurcatio carotidis (see **A**) and the point where it divides into the aa. cerebri anterior and media. The parts (separated in the figure by white disks) are as follows:

(1) Pars cervicalis (red): located in the spatium lateropharyngeum.
(2) Pars petrosa (yellow): located in the canalis caroticus of the pars petrosa ossis temporalis.
(3) Pars cavernosa (green): follows an S-shaped curve in the sinus cavernosus.
(4) Pars cerebralis (purple): located in the cisterna chiasmatica of the spatium subarachnoideum.

Except for the pars cervicalis which generally does not give off branches, all the other parts of the a. carotis interna give off numerous branches (see p. 96). The *intracranial* parts of the a. carotis interna are subdivided into five segments (C1–C5) based on clinical criteria:

- C1–C2: the supraclinoid segments, located within the pars cerebralis. C1 and C2 lie above the proc. clinoideus anterior of the ala minor of the os sphenoidale.
- C3–C5: the infraclinoid segments, located within the sinus cavernosus

The segments C2–C4 form the siphon caroticum.

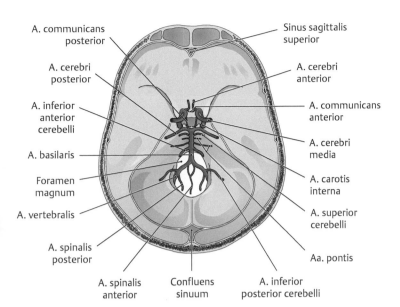

A. communicans posterior
Sinus sagittalis superior
A. cerebri posterior
A. cerebri anterior
A. inferior anterior cerebelli
A. communicans anterior
A. basilaris
A. cerebri media
Foramen magnum
A. carotis interna
A. vertebralis
A. superior cerebelli
A. spinalis posterior
Aa. pontis
A. spinalis anterior
Confluens sinuum
A. inferior posterior cerebelli

C Projection of the circle of Willis (circulus arteriosus cerebri) onto the basis cranii
Superior view. The two aa. vertebrales enter the skull through the foramen magnum and unite behind the clivus to form the unpaired a. basilaris. This vessel then divides into the two aa. cerebri posteriores (additional vessels that normally contribute to the circulus arteriosus cerebri are shown in **D**).
Note: Each a. cerebri media (MCA) is the direct continuation of the a. carotis interna on that side. Clots ejected by the left heart will frequently embolize to the MCA territory.

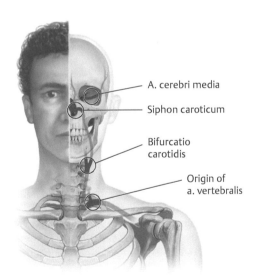

A. cerebri media
Siphon caroticum
Bifurcatio carotidis
Origin of a. vertebralis

E Stenoses and occlusions of arteries supplying the encephalon
Atherosclerotic lesions in older patients may cause the narrowing (stenosis) or complete obstruction (occlusion) of arteries that supply the encephalon. Stenoses most commonly occur at arterial bifurcations, and the sites of predilection are shown. Isolated stenoses that develop gradually may be compensated for by collateral vessels. When stenoses occur simultaneously at multiple sites, the circulus arteriosus cerebri cannot compensate for the diminished blood supply, and cerebral blood flow becomes impaired (varying degrees of cerebral ischemia, see p. 392).
Note: The damage is manifested clinically in the encephalon, but the cause is located in the vessels that supply the encephalon. Because stenoses are treatable, their diagnosis has major therapeutic implications.

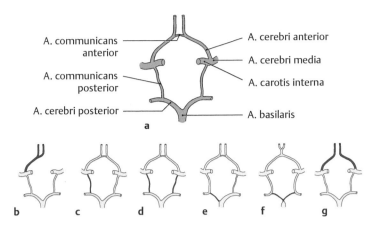

A. communicans anterior
A. cerebri anterior
A. cerebri media
A. communicans posterior
A. carotis interna
A. cerebri posterior
A. basilaris
a
b   c   d   e   f   g

D Variants of the circle of Willis (circulus arteriosus cerebri) (after Lippert and Pabst)
The vascular connections within the circulus arteriosus cerebri are subject to considerable variation. As a rule, the segmental hypoplasias shown here do not significantly alter the normal functions of the arterial ring.

a In most cases, the circle of Willis is formed by the following arteries: the anterior, middle, and posterior cerebral arteries; the anterior and posterior communicating arteries; the internal carotid arteries; and the basilar artery.
b Both anterior aa. cerebri anteriores may arise from one a. carotis interna (10% of cases).
c The a. communicans posterior may be absent or hypoplastic on one side (10% of cases).
d The a. communicans posterior may be absent or hypoplastic on both sides (10% of cases).
e The a. cerebri posterior may arise from the a. carotis interna on one side (10% of cases).
f The a. cerebri posterior may arise from the a. carotis interna both sides (5% of cases).
g The a. communicans anterior may be absent (1% of cases).

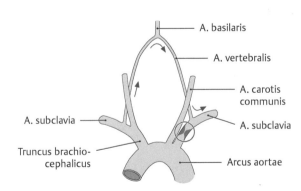

A. basilaris
A. vertebralis
A. carotis communis
A. subclavia
A. subclavia
Truncus brachio-cephalicus
Arcus aortae

F Anatomical basis of subclavian steal syndrome
"Subclavian steal" usually results from stenosis of the left a. subclavia (red circle) located proximal to the origin of the a. vertebralis. This syndrome involves a stealing of blood from the *a. vertebralis* by the a. subclavia. When the left arm is exercised, as during yard work, insufficient blood may be supplied to the arm to accommodate the increased muscular effort (the patient complains of muscle weakness). As a result, blood is "stolen" from the a. vertebralis circulation and there is a reversal of blood flow in the a. vertebralis on the *affected* side (arrows). This leads to deficient blood flow in the a. basilaris and may deprive the encephalon of blood, producing a feeling of lightheadedness.

10.2 Arteries of the Cerebrum

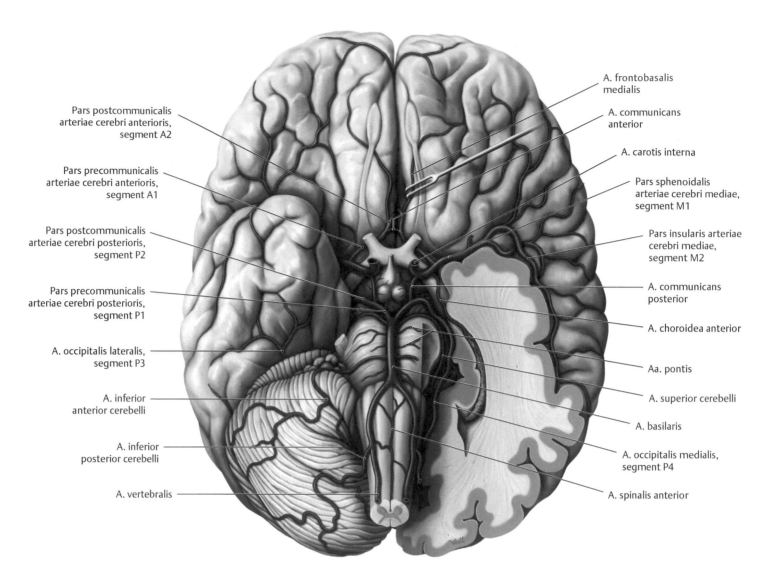

Pars postcommunicalis arteriae cerebri anterioris, segment A2

Pars precommunicalis arteriae cerebri anterioris, segment A1

Pars postcommunicalis arteriae cerebri posterioris, segment P2

Pars precommunicalis arteriae cerebri posterioris, segment P1

A. occipitalis lateralis, segment P3

A. inferior anterior cerebelli

A. inferior posterior cerebelli

A. vertebralis

A. frontobasalis medialis

A. communicans anterior

A. carotis interna

Pars sphenoidalis arteriae cerebri mediae, segment M1

Pars insularis arteriae cerebri mediae, segment M2

A. communicans posterior

A. choroidea anterior

Aa. pontis

A. superior cerebelli

A. basilaris

A. occipitalis medialis, segment P4

A. spinalis anterior

A Arteries at the base of the brain

As this view shows, most of the arteries that supply the brain enter the cerebrum from its basal aspect. The cerebellum and lobus temporalis have been removed on the left side to display the course of the a. cerebri posterior. Note the three principal arteries of the cerebrum, the aa. cerebri anterior, media, et posterior. The first two arteries are branches of the a. carotis interna; the latter artery arises from the flow tract of the aa. vertebrales (see p. 374 f).

The aa. vertebrales also distribute branches to the medulla spinalis, truncus encephali, and cerebellum (a. spinalis anterior, aa. spinales

posteriores, a. superior cerebelli, et aa. inferiores posterior et anterior cerebelli). Immediately after its origin, the a. cerebri anterior courses around the corpus callosum to supply the medial aspect of the brain with blood. As a result, practically the only visible portion of the post-communicating part of the a. cerebri anterior in this view of the underside of the brain is its branch, the a. frontobasalis medialis.

Note: If one of the main vessels of the arterial circle rupture due to a defect in the vascular wall (aneurysm, see **B**, p. 391), blood flows directly into the subarachnoid space resulting in subarachnoid hemorrhage.

B Segments of the arteriae cerebri anterior, media, and posterior

Artery	Parts	Segments
A. cerebri anterior	• Pars precommunicalis • Pars postcommunicalis	• A1 = segment proximal to the a. communicans anterior • A2 = segment distal to the a. communicans anterior
A. cerebri media (MCA)	• Pars sphenoidalis • Pars insularis	• M1 = pars sphenoidalis (pars horizontalis) • M2 = pars insularis
A. cerebri posterior	• Pars precommunicalis • Pars postcommunicalis	• P1 = segment between the a. basilaris bifurcation and a. communicans posterior • P2 = segment between the a. communicans posterior and rr. temporales anteriores • P3 = a. occipitalis lateralis • P4 = a. occipitalis medialis

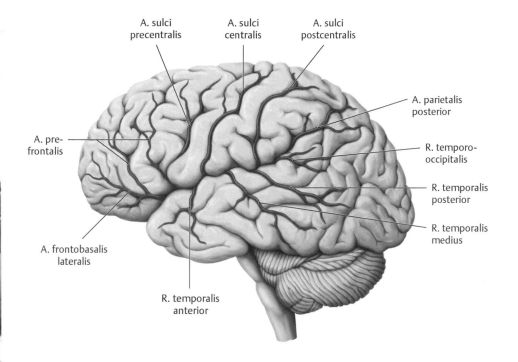

A. sulci precentralis

A. sulci centralis

A. sulci postcentralis

A. parietalis posterior

A. prefrontalis

R. temporooccipitalis

R. temporalis posterior

R. temporalis medius

A. frontobasalis lateralis

R. temporalis anterior

C Terminal branches of the arteria cerebri media on the lateral hemispherium cerebri

Left lateral view. Most of the blood vessels on the lateral surface of the encephalon are terminal branches of the a. cerebri media (MCA). They can be subdivided into two main groups:

- Rr. terminales inferiores (rr. corticales inferiores): supply the lobus temporalis cortex
- Rr. terminales superiores (rr. corticales superiores): supply the lobi frontalis and cortex lobi parietales.

Deeper structures supplied by these branches are not shown in the diagram (see p. 378).

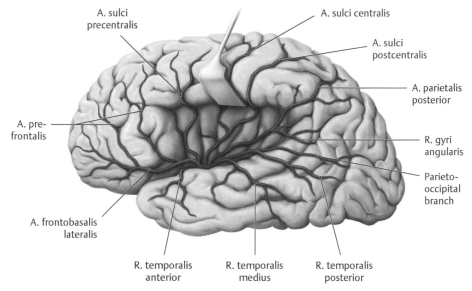

A. sulci precentralis

A. sulci centralis

A. sulci postcentralis

A. prefrontalis

A. parietalis posterior

R. gyri angularis

Parietooccipital branch

A. frontobasalis lateralis

R. temporalis anterior

R. temporalis medius

R. temporalis posterior

D Course of the arteria cerebri media in the interior of the sulcus lateralis

Left lateral view. On its way to the lateral surface of the hemispherium cerebri, the a. cerebri media first courses on the base of the encephalon; this is the pars sphenoidalis of the MCA. It then continues through the sulcus lateralis along the insula, which is the sunken portion of the cortex cerebri. When the lobi temporalis and parietalis are spread apart with a retractor, as shown here, we can see the arteries of the insula (which receive their blood from the pars insularis of the a. cerebri media; see **A**). When viewed in an angiogram, the branches of the pars insularis of the MCA resemble the arms of a candelabrum, giving rise to the term "candelabrum artery" for that arterial segment.

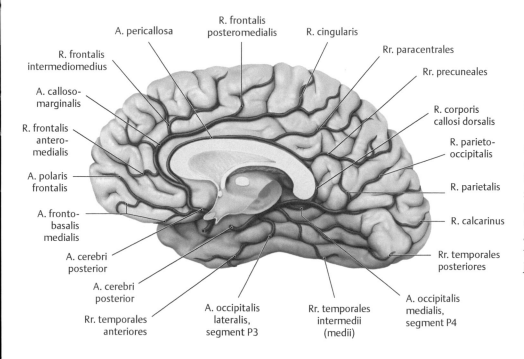

R. frontalis posteromedialis

A. pericallosa

R. cingularis

Rr. paracentrales

R. frontalis intermediomedius

Rr. precuneales

A. callosomarginalis

R. corporis callosi dorsalis

R. frontalis anteromedialis

R. parietooccipitalis

A. polaris frontalis

R. parietalis

A. frontobasalis medialis

R. calcarinus

A. cerebri posterior

Rr. temporales posteriores

A. cerebri posterior

A. occipitalis medialis, segment P4

Rr. temporales anteriores

A. occipitalis lateralis, segment P3

Rr. temporales intermedii (medii)

E Branches of the arteriae cerebri anterior and posterior on the medial surface of the cerebrum

Right hemispherium cerebri viewed from the medial side, with the left hemispherium cerebri and truncus encephali removed. The medial surface of the encephalon is supplied by branches of the aa. cerebri anterior and posterior. While the *a. cerebri anterior* arises from the a. carotis interna, the *a. cerebri posterior* arises from the a. basilaris (which is formed by the junction of the left and right aa. vertebrales).

10.3 Arteries of the Cerebrum, Distribution

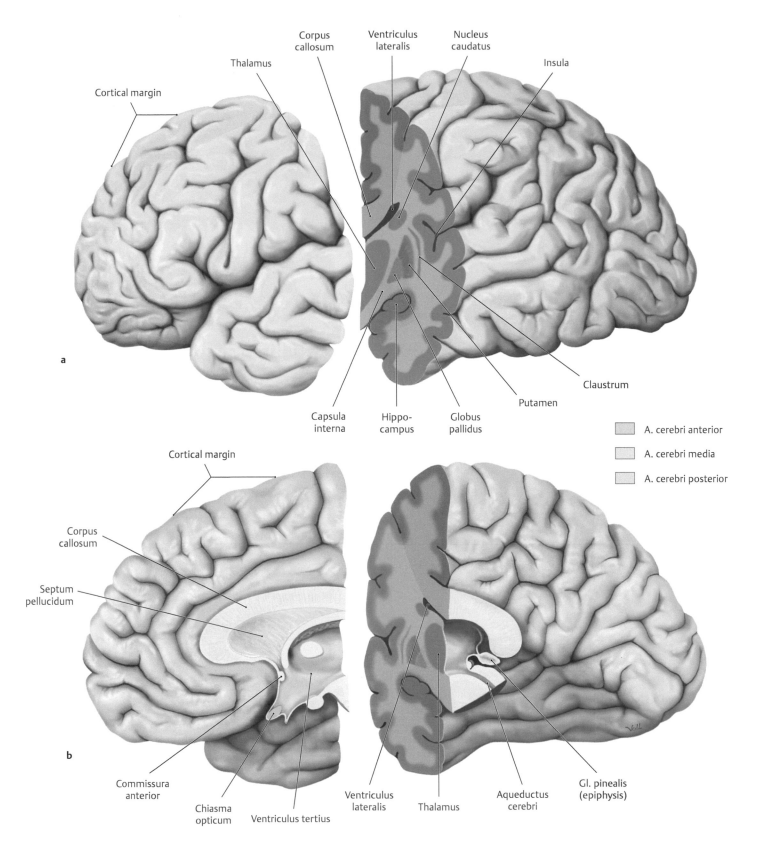

Corpus callosum

Ventriculus lateralis

Nucleus caudatus

Thalamus

Insula

Cortical margin

a

Claustrum

Putamen

Capsula interna

Hippo-campus

Globus pallidus

A. cerebri anterior

A. cerebri media

A. cerebri posterior

Cortical margin

Corpus callosum

Septum pellucidum

b

Commissura anterior

Chiasma opticum

Ventriculus tertius

Ventriculus lateralis

Thalamus

Aqueductus cerebri

Gl. pinealis (epiphysis)

A Distribution areas of the main cerebral arteries
a Lateral view of the left hemispherium cerebri; **b** Medial view of the right hemispherium cerebri. Most of the lateral surface of the brain is supplied by the a. cerebri *media* (green), whose branches ascend to the cortex from the depths of the insula. The branches of the a. cerebri *anterior* supply the polus frontalis of the brain and the cortical areas near the cortical margin (red and pink). The a. cerebri *posterior* supplies the polus occipitalis and lower portions of the lobus temporalis (blue). The central substantiae grisea and alba have a complex blood supply (yellow) that includes the a. choroidea anterior. The aa. cerebri anterior and posterior supply most of the medial surface of the encephalon.

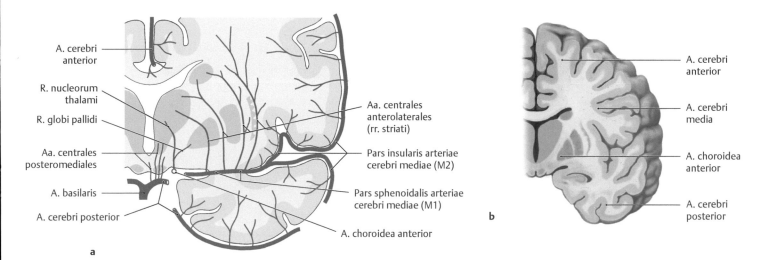

a

b

B Distribution of the three main cerebral arteries in transverse and coronal sections

a, b Coronal sections at the level of the corpora mammillaria. **c** Transverse section at the level of the capsula interna. The capsula interna, nuclei basales, and thalamus derive most of their blood supply from perforating branches of the following vessels at the base of the brain:

- A. choroidea anterior (from the a. carotis interna)
- Aa. centrales anterolaterales (rr. striati) with their terminal branches (from the a. cerebri media)
- Aa. centrales posteromediales (from the a. cerebri posterior)
- Perforating branches (from the a. communicans posterior)

The capsula interna, which is traversed by the tractus pyramidalis and other structures, receives most of its blood supply from the a. cerebri media (crus anterius and genu capsulae internae) and from the a. choroidea anterior (crus posterius). If these vessels become occluded, the tractus pyramidalis and other structures will be interrupted, causing paralysis on the contralateral side of the body (stroke: central paralysis, see **C** on p. 393).

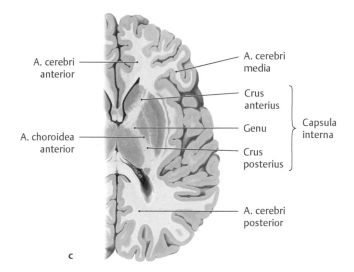

c

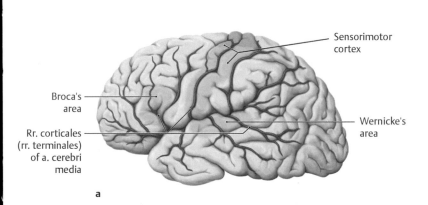

a

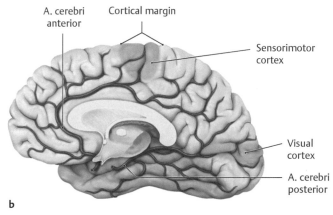

b

C Functional centers on the surface of the cerebrum

a Left lateral view of the telencephalon; regions supplied by branches of the a. cerebri media are shaded green; **b** Medial view of the right hemispherium cerebri; regions supplied by the a. cerebri anterior are shaded red; regions supplied by the branches of the a. cerebri posterior are shaded blue.

Specific functions can be assigned to well-defined areas of the telencephalon. These areas are supplied by branches of the three main cerebral arteries:

- The sensorimotor cortex e.g. of branches of a. cerebri media (gyri precentralis and postcentralis, see **a**) and of branches of the a. cerebri anterior (the superior margin of the hemispherium cerebri, see **b**);

- Broca's area and Wernicke's areas (motor and sensory speech centers) e.g., by branches of the a. cerebri media (see **a**);
- Visual cortex by branches of the a. cerebri posterior (see **b**).

Certain disorders or deficits are indicative of arterial occlusion in a certain territory. A failure, deficit, or outage of the speech center suggests an occlusion of the a. cerebri media, hemianopsia suggests an occlusion of the a. cerebri posterior, and paralysis and sensory disturbances in the lower limbs suggest an occlusion of the a. cerebri anterior (cf. p. 393).

379

10.4 Arteries of the Truncus Encephali and Cerebellum

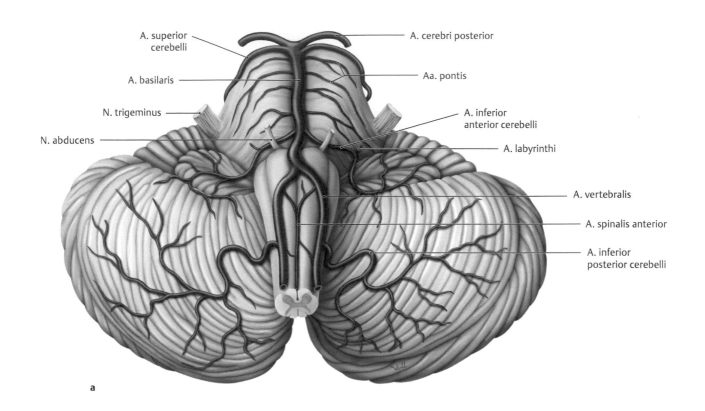

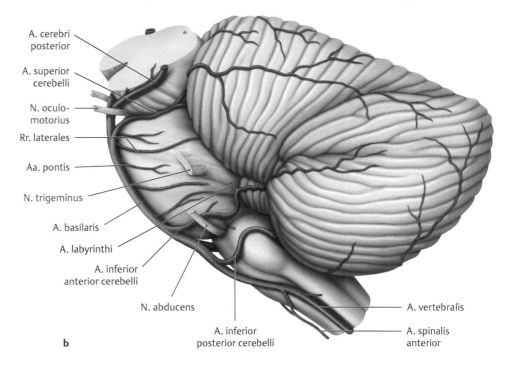

A Arteries of the truncus encephali and cerebellum

a Basal view; **b** Left lateral view.

The truncus encephali and cerebellum are supplied by the aa. basilaris and cerebelli (see below). Because the a. basilaris is formed by the union of the two aa. vertebrales, blood supplied by the a. basilaris is said to come from the *vertebrobasilar complex* (or *system*). The vessels that supply the **truncus encephali** (mesencephalon, pons, and medulla oblongata) arise either directly from the a. basilaris (e.g., the aa. pontis) and aa. vertebrales or from their branches. The branches are classified by their sites of entry and distribution as medial, mediolateral, or lateral. Decreased perfusion in or occlusion of these vessels leads to transient or permanent impairment of blood flow (brainstem syndrome) and may produce a great variety of clinical symptoms, given the many nuclei and tract systems that exist in the truncus encephali. The **medulla spinalis**, receives a portion of its blood supply from the a. spinalis anterior (see **b**), which arises from the a. vertebralis (see p. 404). The **cerebellum** is supplied by three large arteries:

- A. inferior posterior cerebelli (PICA), the largest branch of the a. vertebralis. This vessel is usually referred to by its acronym, PICA.
- A. inferior anterior cerebelli (AICA), the first major branch of the a. basilaris
- A. superior cerebelli (SCA), the last major branch of the a. basilaris before it divides into the aa. cerebri posteriores

Note the a. labyrinthi which supplies the auris interna (see also **D**, p. 157) usually arises from the a. inferior anterior cerebelli, as pictured here, although it may also spring directly from the a. basilaris. Impaired blood flow in the a. labyrinthi leads to an acute loss of hearing (sudden sensorineural hearing loss), frequently accompanied by tinnitus (see **D**, p. 151).

B Distribution of the arteries of the truncus encephali and cerebellum in midsagittal section (after Bähr and Frotscher)
All of the brain sections shown here and below are supplied by the vertebrobasilar complex. The transverse sections are presented in a caudal-to-cranial series corresponding to the direction of the vertebrobasilar blood supply.

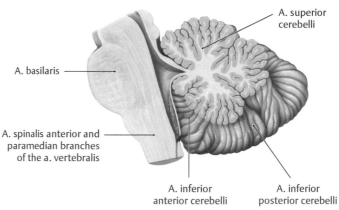

A. superior cerebelli

A. basilaris

A. spinalis anterior and paramedian branches of the a. vertebralis

A. inferior anterior cerebelli

A. inferior posterior cerebelli

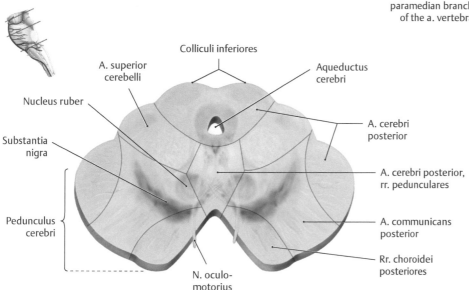

Colliculi inferiores

A. superior cerebelli

Aqueductus cerebri

Nucleus ruber

Substantia nigra

A. cerebri posterior

A. cerebri posterior, rr. pedunculares

Pedunculus cerebri

A. communicans posterior

Rr. choroidei posteriores

N. oculomotorius

C Distribution of the arteries of the mesencephalon in transverse section
Besides branches from the a. superior cerebelli, the mesencephalon is supplied chiefly by branches of the a. cerebri posterior and a. communicans posterior.

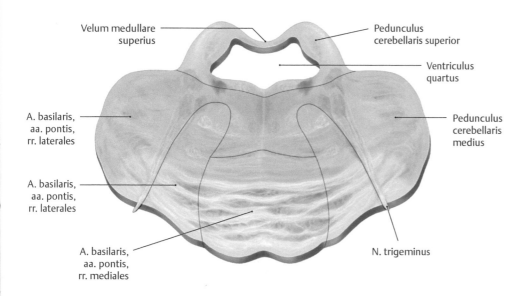

Velum medullare superius

Pedunculus cerebellaris superior

Ventriculus quartus

A. basilaris, aa. pontis, rr. laterales

Pedunculus cerebellaris medius

A. basilaris, aa. pontis, rr. laterales

D Distribution of the arteries of the pons in transverse section
The pons derives its blood supply from short and long branches of the a. basilaris.

A. basilaris, aa. pontis, rr. mediales

N. trigeminus

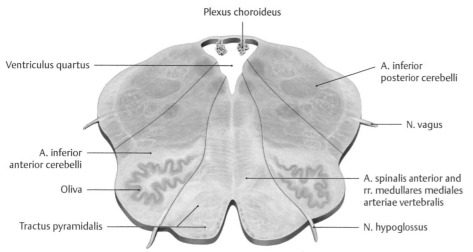

Plexus choroideus

Ventriculus quartus

A. inferior posterior cerebelli

N. vagus

A. inferior anterior cerebelli

Oliva

A. spinalis anterior and rr. medullares mediales arteriae vertebralis

Tractus pyramidalis

N. hypoglossus

E Distribution of the arteries of the medulla oblongata in transverse section
The medulla oblongata is supplied by branches of the a. spinalis anterior, a. inferior posterior cerebelli (both arising from the a. vertebralis), as well as the a. inferior anterior cerebelli (first large branch of the a. basilaris).

10.5 Dural Sinuses (Sinus Durae Matris), Overview

A Relationship of the principal sinus durae matris to the skull

Oblique posterior view from the right side (encephalon removed and tentorium windowed on the right side). Sinus durae matris are located either in the attached or free margins of the dural folds. The falx cerebri has a dural venous sinus on both edges. The larger venous sinuses are those attached to the inside of the cranial bone (e.g., sinus sagittalis superior, transversus, sigmoideus). The wall of the venous sinus is stiff, consisting only of dura mater and an endothelial lining. The absence of muscle in the sinus wall prevents sinus durae matris from contracting if injured and, unlike veins, don't contribute to the control of bleeding. Bleeding from a sinus durae matris caused by cranial injury can be life-threatening. Sinus durae matris collect blood from the encephalon, cavitas orbitalis, and calvaria. Since sinus durae matris do not have valves, the direction of blood flow depends on the position of the head. When a person is lying down or holding the head upright, the sinus durae matris convey blood to the vv. jugulares internae which are located on both sides at the deepest point of the fossa cranii posterior. The system of sinus durae matris is divided into an upper group and a lower group:

- **Upper group:** sinus sagittales superior and inferior, sinus rectus, sinus occipitalis, sinus transversus, sinus sigmoideus, and the confluens sinuum
- **Lower group:** sinus cavernosus with sinus intercavernosi anterior and posterior, sinus sphenoparietalis, sinus petrosi superior and inferior

The upper and lower groups of sinus durae matris communicate with the plexus venosi vertebrales through the sinus marginalis at the inlet to the foramen magnum and through the plexus basilaris on the clivus (see **C**).

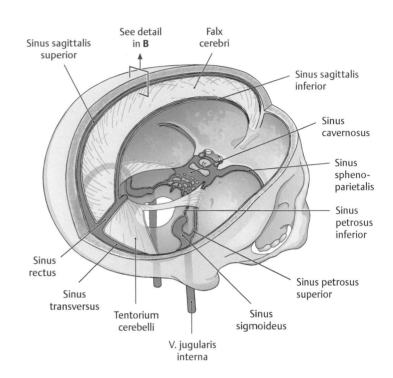

B Structure of a sinus durae matris, shown here for the sinus sagittalis superior

Transverse section, occipital view (detail from **A**). The sinus wall is composed of endothelium and tough, collagenous dural connective tissue with a periosteal and meningeal layer. Between the two layers is the sinus lumen.

Note the lacunae laterales, where the granulationes arachnoideae open into the venous system. Vv. superficiales cerebri (vv. superiores cerebri, bridging veins, see pp. 306 and 308) open into the sinus itself along with vv. diploicae from the adjacent cranial bone. The sinus also receives vv. emissariae—valveless veins that establish connections among the sinuses, the vv. diploicae, and the extracranial veins of the scalp.

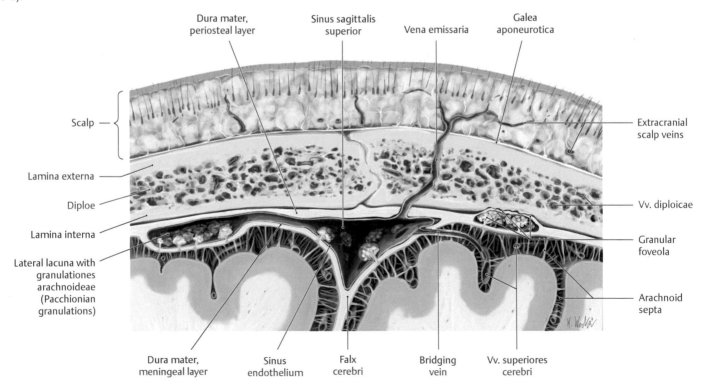

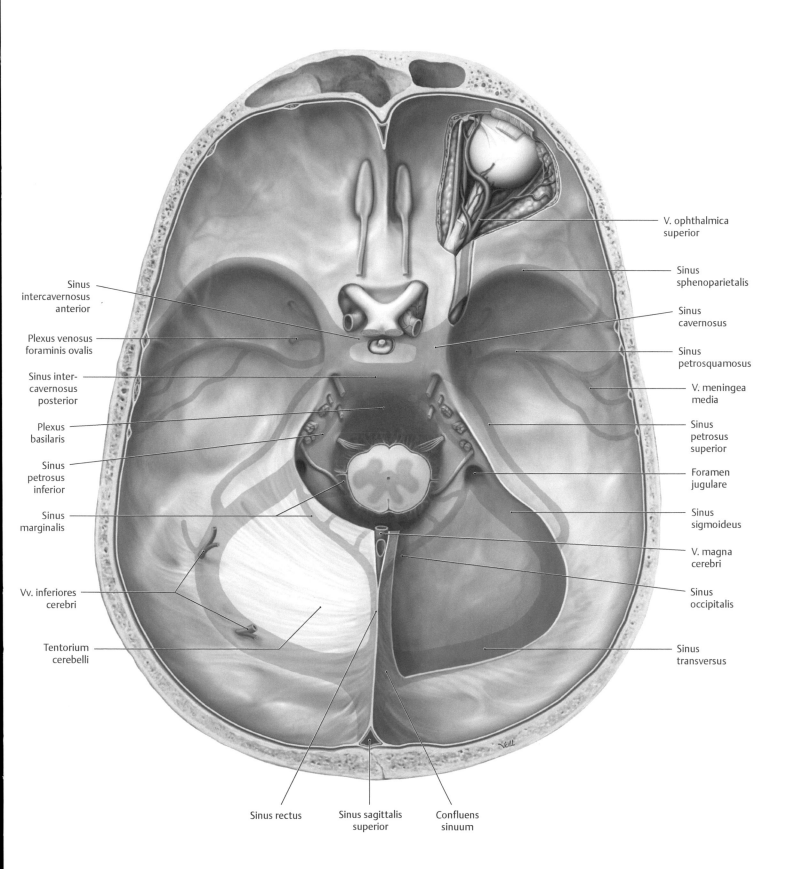

Sinus intercavernosus anterior

Plexus venosus foraminis ovalis

Sinus inter-cavernosus posterior

Plexus basilaris

Sinus petrosus inferior

Sinus marginalis

Vv. inferiores cerebri

Tentorium cerebelli

V. ophthalmica superior

Sinus sphenoparietalis

Sinus cavernosus

Sinus petrosquamosus

V. meningea media

Sinus petrosus superior

Foramen jugulare

Sinus sigmoideus

V. magna cerebri

Sinus occipitalis

Sinus transversus

Sinus rectus

Sinus sagittalis superior

Confluens sinuum

C Sinus durae matris at the basis cranii

Transverse section at the level of the tentorium cerebelli, viewed from above (encephalon removed, orbital roof and tentorium windowed on the right side). The sinus cavernosus forms a ring around the sella turcica, its left and right parts being interconnected at the front and behind by a sinus intercavernosus anterior and posterior. Behind the sinus intercavernosus posterior, on the clivus, is the plexus basilaris. This plexus also contributes to the drainage of the sinus cavernosus.

10.6 Sinus Durae Matris: Tributaries and Accessory Draining Vessels

A Sinus durae matris tributaries from the venae cerebri (after Rauber and Kopsch)
Right lateral view. Venous blood collected deep within the encephalon drains to the sinus durae matris through *vv. superficiales* and profundae cerebri (see p. 386). The red arrows in the diagram show the principal directions of venous blood flow in the major sinuses. Because of the numerous anastomoses, the isolated occlusion of even a complete sinus segment may produce no clinical symptoms.

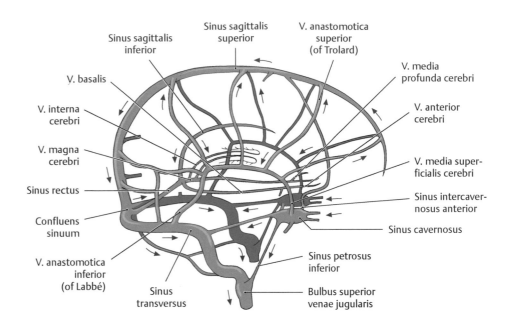

B Accessory drainage pathways of the sinus durae matris
Right lateral view. The sinus durae matris have many accessory drainage pathways besides their principal drainage into the two vv. jugulares internae. The connections between the sinus durae matris and extracranial veins mainly serve to equalize pressure and regulate temperature. These anastomoses are of clinical interest because their normal direction of blood flow may reverse (no venous valves), allowing blood from extracranial veins to reflux into the sinus durae matris. This mechanism may give rise to sinus infections that lead, in turn, to vascular occlusion

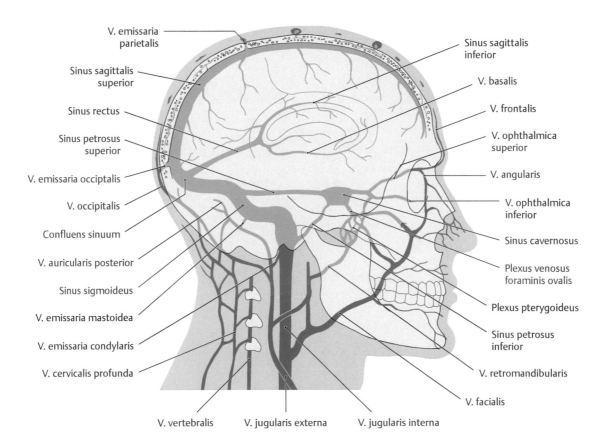

(*venous sinus thrombosis*). The most important accessory drainage vessels include the following:

- Vv. emissariae (vv. diploicae and superior scalp veins), see **C**
- V. ophthalmica superior (vv. angularis and facialis)
- Plexus venosus foraminis ovalis (plexus pterygoideus, v. retromandibularis)
- Sinus marginalis and plexus basilaris (plexus venosi vertebrales interni and externi), see **C**

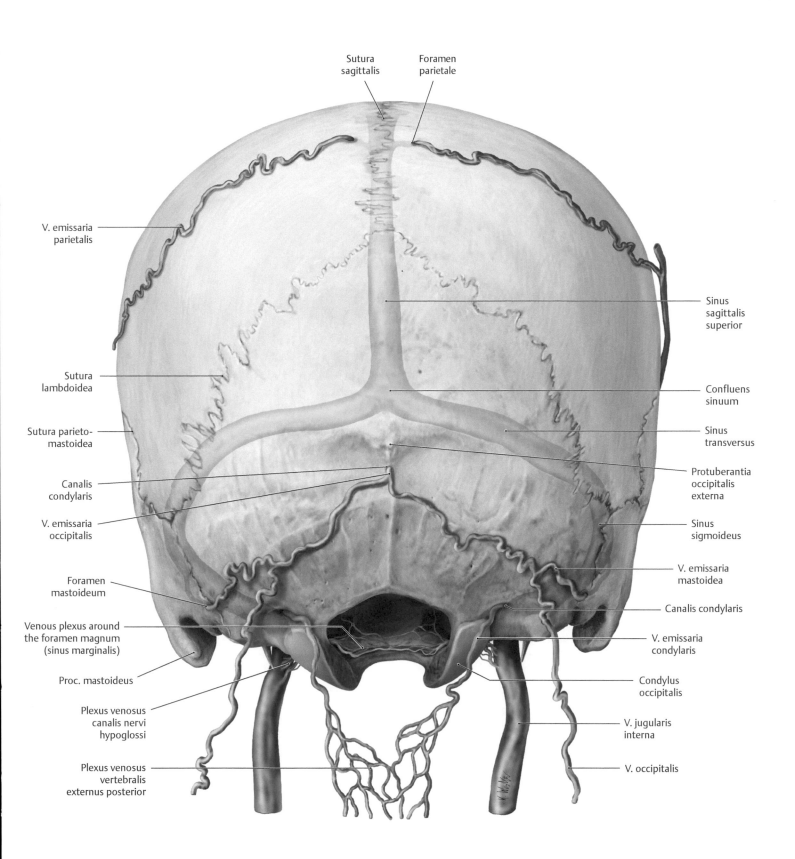

Sutura
sagittalis

Foramen
parietale

V. emissaria
parietalis

Sinus
sagittalis
superior

Sutura
lambdoidea

Confluens
sinuum

Sutura parieto-
mastoidea

Sinus
transversus

Canalis
condylaris

Protuberantia
occipitalis
externa

V. emissaria
occipitalis

Sinus
sigmoideus

V. emissaria
mastoidea

Foramen
mastoideum

Canalis condylaris

Venous plexus around
the foramen magnum
(sinus marginalis)

V. emissaria
condylaris

Proc. mastoideus

Condylus
occipitalis

Plexus venosus
canalis nervi
hypoglossi

V. jugularis
interna

Plexus venosus
vertebralis
externus posterior

V. occipitalis

C Venae emissariae occipitales

Vv. emissariae establish a direct connection between the intracranial sinus durae matris and extracranial veins. They run through small cranial openings such as the foramina parietale and mastoideum. Vv. emissariae are of clinical interest because they create a potential route by which bacteria from the scalp may spread to the dura mater and sinus durae matris.

10.7 Veins of the Brain: Superficial and Deep Veins

Because the veins of the encephalon do not run parallel to the arteries, marked differences are noted between the regions of arterial supply and venous drainage. While all of the cerebral arteries enter the encephalon at its base, venous blood is drained from the entire surface of the encephalon, including the base, and also from the interior of the encephalon by two groups of veins: the *vv. superficiales cerebri* and the *vv. profundae cerebri*. The vv. superficiales cerebri drain blood from the cortex cerebri and substantia alba directly into the sinus durae matris. The vv. profundae cerebri drain blood from the deeper portions of the substantia alba, nuclei basales, corpus callosum, and diencephalon into the v. magna cerebri, which enters the sinus rectus. The two venous regions (those of the superficial and deep veins) are interconnected by numerous intracerebral anastomoses (see **D**).

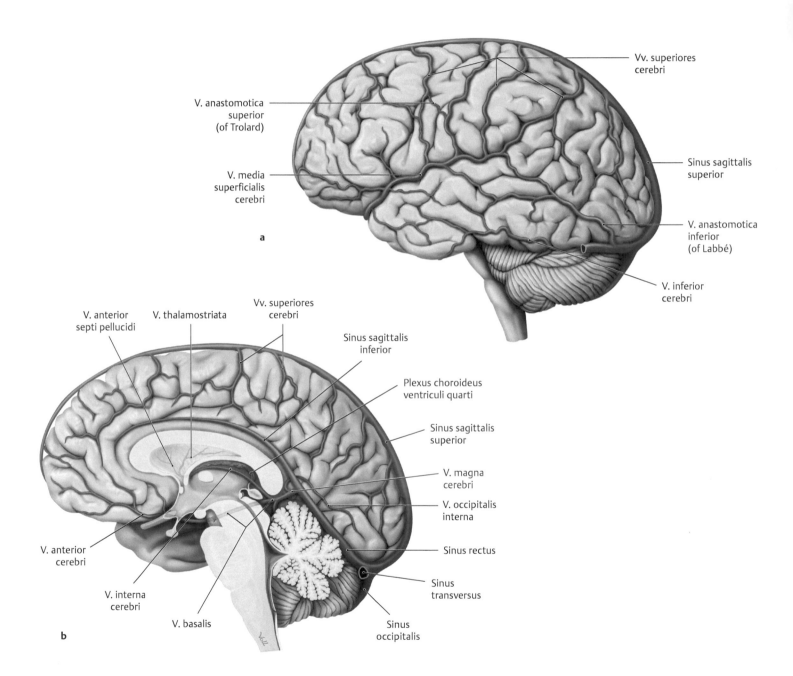

A Superficial veins of the brain (venae superficiales cerebri)
Left lateral view (**a**) and medial view (**b**).
a, b The vv. superficiales cerebri drain blood from the short cortical veins and long medullary veins in the substantia alba (see **D**) into the sinus durae matris. (The vv. profundae cerebri are described in **C**, p. 389.) Their course is extremely variable, and veins in the spatium subarachnoideum do not follow arteries, gyri, or sulci. Consequently, only the most important of these vessels are named here. Just before terminating in the sinus durae matris, the veins leave the spatium subarachnoideum and run a short subdural course between the dura mater and arachnoidea mater. These short subdural venous segments are called bridging veins. The bridging veins have great clinical importance because they may be ruptured by head trauma, resulting in a subdural hematoma (see p. 390).

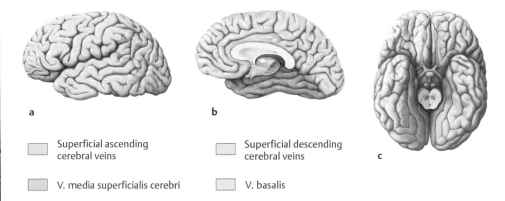

a **b**

c

☐ Superficial ascending cerebral veins

☐ V. media superficialis cerebri

☐ Superficial descending cerebral veins

☐ V. basalis

B Regions drained by the venae superficiales cerebri

a Left lateral view, **b** view of the medial surface of the right hemispherium, **c** basal view.
The veins on the lateral surface of the encephalon are classified by their direction of drainage as ascending (draining into the sinus sagittalis superior) or descending (draining into the sinus transversus). The v. media superficialis cerebri drains into both the sinus cavernosus and transversus (see **A**, p. 384).

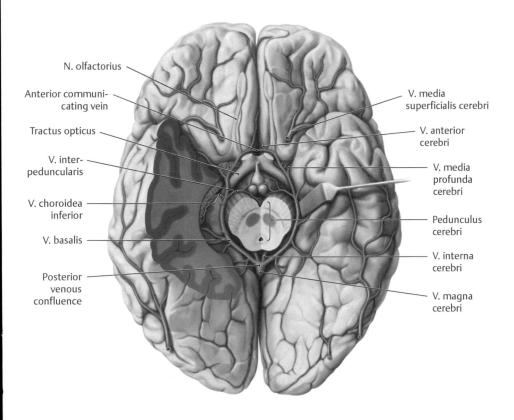

N. olfactorius
Anterior communicating vein
Tractus opticus
V. interpeduncularis
V. choroidea inferior
V. basalis
Posterior venous confluence

V. media superficialis cerebri
V. anterior cerebri
V. media profunda cerebri
Pedunculus cerebri
V. interna cerebri
V. magna cerebri

C Basal cerebral venous system

The basal cerebral venous system drains blood from both vv. superficiales and profundae cerebri. A venous circle formed by the vv. basales (of Rosenthal, see below) exists at the base of the encephalon, analogous to the circulus arteriosus cerebri of Willis. The v. basalis is formed in the substantia perforata anterior by the union of the vv. anteriores cerebri and v. media profunda cerebri. Following the course of the tractus opticus, the v. basalis runs posteriorly around the pedunculus cerebri and unites with the v. basalis from the opposite side on the dorsal aspect of the mesencephalon. The two vv. internae cerebri also terminate at this venous junction, the posterior venous confluence. This junction gives rise to the midline v. magna cerebri, which enters the sinus rectus. The v. basalis receives tributaries from deep brain regions in its course (e.g., veins from the thalamus and hypothalamus, plexus choroideus of the cornu inferius, etc.). The two vv. anteriores cerebri are interconnected by the v. communicans anterior, creating a closed, ring-shaped drainage system.

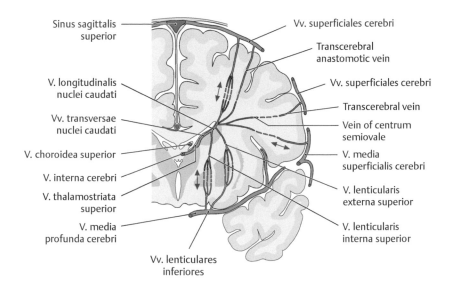

Sinus sagittalis superior
V. longitudinalis nuclei caudati
Vv. transversae nuclei caudati
V. choroidea superior
V. interna cerebri
V. thalamostriata superior
V. media profunda cerebri

Vv. lenticulares inferiores

Vv. superficiales cerebri
Transcerebral anastomotic vein
Vv. superficiales cerebri
Transcerebral vein
Vein of centrum semiovale
V. media superficialis cerebri
V. lenticularis externa superior
V. lenticularis interna superior

D Anastomoses between the venae superficiales and profundae cerebri

Transverse section through the left hemispherium, anterior view. The vv. superficiales cerebri communicate with the vv. profundae cerebri through the anastomoses shown here (see p. 388). Flow reversal (double arrows) may occur in the boundary zones between two territories.

10.8 Veins of the Truncus Encephali and Cerebellum: Deep Veins

A Venae profundae cerebri

Multiplanar transverse section (combining multiple transverse planes) with a superior view of the opened ventriculi laterales. The lobi temporales and occipitales and tentorium cerebelli have been removed on the left side to demonstrate the upper surface of the cerebellum and the vv. superiores cerebelli. On the lateral walls of the cornua anteriora of both ventriculi laterales, the v. thalamostriata superior runs toward the foramen interventriculare in the groove between the thalamus and nucleus caudatus. After receiving the v. anterior septi pellucidi and the v. choroidea superior, it forms the v. interna cerebri and passes through the foramen interventriculare along the roof of the diencephalon toward the lamina quadrigemina, which contains the colliculi superior and inferior. There it unites with the v. interna cerebri of the opposite side, and the vv. basales to form the posterior venous confluence, which gives rise to the v. magna cerebri.

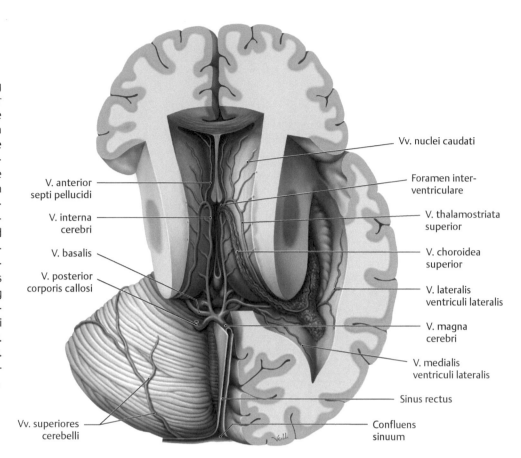

B Venae cerebelli

Posterior view. Like the other veins of the brain, the vv. cerebelli are distributed independently of the aa. cerebelli. Larger trunks cross over gyri and sulci, running mainly in the sagittal direction. A *medial* and a *lateral* group can be distinguished based on their gross topographical anatomy. The medial group of vv. cerebelli drains the vermis and adjacent portions of the cerebellar hemispheria (v. precentralis cerebelli, vv. superior and inferior vermis) and the medial portions of the vv. superiores and inferiores cerebelli. The *lateral* group (v. petrosa and lateral portions of the vv. superiores and inferiores cerebelli) drains most of the two hemispheria cerebelli. All of the cerebellar veins anastomose with one another; their outflow is exclusively infratentorial (i.e., below the tentorium cerebelli).

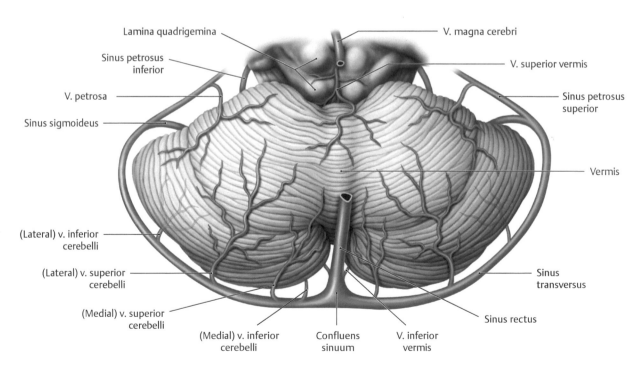

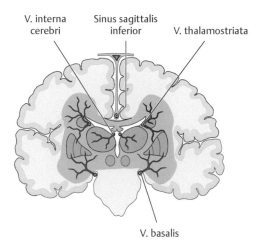

V. interna cerebri — Sinus sagittalis inferior — V. thalamostriata

V. basalis

C Region drained by the venae profundae cerebri

Coronal section. Three principal venous segments can be identified in each hemispherium:

- V. thalamostriata
- V. interna cerebri
- V. basalis

The region drained by the vv. profundae cerebri encompasses large portions of the base of the cerebrum, the nuclei basales, the capsula interna, the plexus choroidei of the ventriculi laterales and tertius, the corpus callosum, and portions of the diencephalon and mesencephalon.

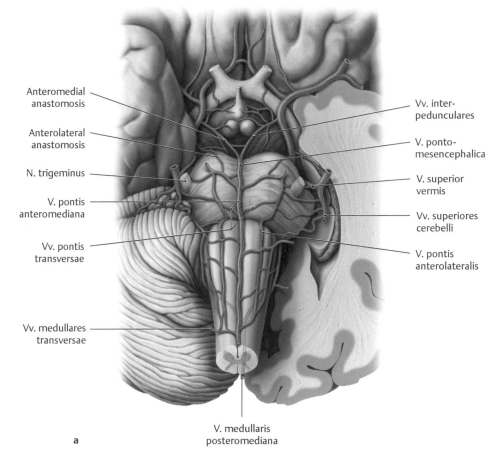

Anteromedial anastomosis — Anterolateral anastomosis — N. trigeminus — V. pontis anteromediana — Vv. pontis transversae — Vv. medullares transversae — V. medullaris posteromediana — Vv. interpedunculares — V. pontomesencephalica — V. superior vermis — Vv. superiores cerebelli — V. pontis anterolateralis

a

D Veins of the truncus encephali

a Anterior view of the truncus encephali in situ (the cerebellum and part of the lobus occipitalis have been removed on the left side). **b** Posterior view of the isolated truncus encephali with the cerebellum removed.

The veins of the truncus encephali are a continuation of the veins of the medulla spinalis and connect them with the basal veins of the encephalon. As on the medulla spinalis, the veins on the lower part of the truncus encephali form a venous plexus consisting of a powerfully developed *longitudinal* system and a more branched transverse system. The veins of the medulla oblongata, pons, and cerebellum make up the infratentorial venous system. Various anastomoses (e.g., anteromedial and lateral) exist at the boundary between the infra- and supratentorial systems.

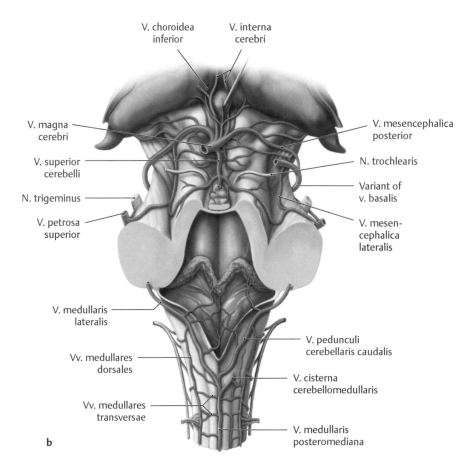

V. choroidea inferior — V. interna cerebri — V. magna cerebri — V. superior cerebelli — N. trigeminus — V. petrosa superior — V. medullaris lateralis — Vv. medullares dorsales — Vv. medullares transversae — V. mesencephalica posterior — N. trochlearis — Variant of v. basalis — V. mesencephalica lateralis — V. pedunculi cerebellaris caudalis — V. cisterna cerebellomedullaris — V. medullaris posteromediana

b

389

10.9 Blood Vessels of the Brain: Intracranial Hemorrhage

Intracranial hemorrhages may be extracerebral (see **A**) or intracerebral (see **C**).

A Extracerebral hemorrhages

Extracerebral hemorrhages are defined as bleeding between the calvaria and encephalon. Because the bony calvaria is immobile, the developing hematoma exerts pressure on the soft encephalon. Depending on the source of the hemorrhage (arterial or venous), this may produce a rapidly or slowly developing incompressible mass with a rise of intracranial pressure that may damage not only the encephalon tissue at the bleeding site but also in more remote encephalon areas. Three types of intracranial hemorrhage can be distinguished based on their relationship to the dura mater:

a Epidural hematoma (epidural = above the dura). This type generally develops after a head injury involving a skull fracture. The bleeding most commonly occurs from a ruptured a. meningea media (due to the close proximity of the a. meningea media to the calvaria, a sharp bone fragment may lacerate the artery). The hematoma forms between the calvaria and the periosteal layer of the dura mater. Pressure from the hematoma separates the dura from the calvaria and displaces the brain. Typically there is an initial transient loss of consciousness caused by the impact, followed 1–5 hours later by a second decline in the level of consciousness, this time due to compression of the brain by the arterial hemorrhage. The interval between the first and second loss of consciousness is called the *lucid interval* (occurs in approximately 30–40% of all epidural hematomas). Detection of the hemorrhage (CT scanning of the head) and prompt evacuation of the hematoma are life-saving.

b Subdural hematoma (subdural = below the dura). Trauma to the head causes the rupture of a *bridging vein* (see p. 308) that bleeds between the dura mater and arachnoidea. The bleeding occurs into a potential "subdural space," which exists only when extravasated blood has dissected the arachnoidea mater from the dura (the spaces are described in **C**, p. 311). Because the bleeding source is venous, the increased intracranial pressure and mass effect develop more slowly than with an arterial epidural hemorrhage. Consequently, a subdural hematoma may develop *chronically* over a period of weeks, even after a relatively mild head injury.

c Subarachnoid hemorrhage is an arterial bleed caused by the rupture of an aneurysm (abnormal outpouching) of an artery at the base of the encephalon (see **B**). It is typically caused by a brief, sudden rise in blood pressure, like that produced by a sudden rise of intra-abdominal pressure (straining at stool or urine, lifting a heavy object, etc.). Because the hemorrhage is into the CSF-filled spatium subarachnoideum, blood can be detected in the liquor cerebrospinalis by means of lumbar puncture. The cardinal symptom of a subarachnoid hemorrhage is a sudden, excruciating headache accompanied by a stiff neck caused by meningeal irritation.

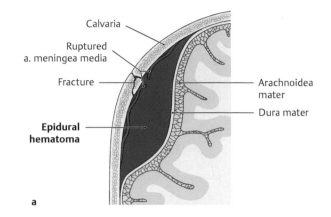

Calvaria
Ruptured a. meningea media
Fracture
Arachnoidea mater
Dura mater
Epidural hematoma

a

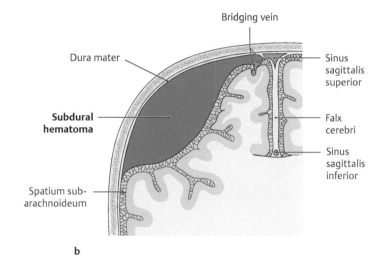

Bridging vein
Dura mater
Sinus sagittalis superior
Subdural hematoma
Falx cerebri
Sinus sagittalis inferior
Spatium sub-arachnoideum

b

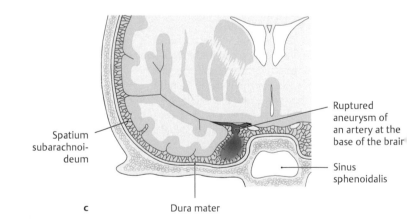

Spatium subarachnoideum
Ruptured aneurysm of an artery at the base of the brain
Sinus sphenoidalis

c   Dura mater

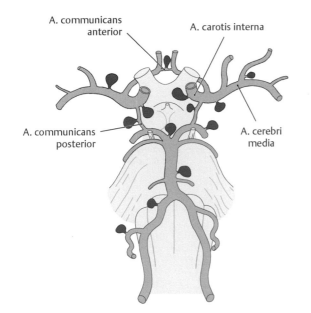

B Sites of berry aneurysms at the base of the encephalon
(after Bähr and Frotscher)
The rupture of congenital or acquired arterial aneurysms at the base of the encephalon is the most frequent cause of subarachnoid hemorrhage and accounts for approximately 5% of all strokes. These are abnormal saccular dilations of the circulus arteriosus cerebri and are especially common at the site of branching. When one of these thin-walled aneurysms ruptures, arterial blood escapes into the spatium subarachnoideum. The most common site is the junction between the aa. cerebri anteriores and communicantes anteriores (1); the second most likely site is the branching of the a. communicans posterior from the a. carotis interna (2).

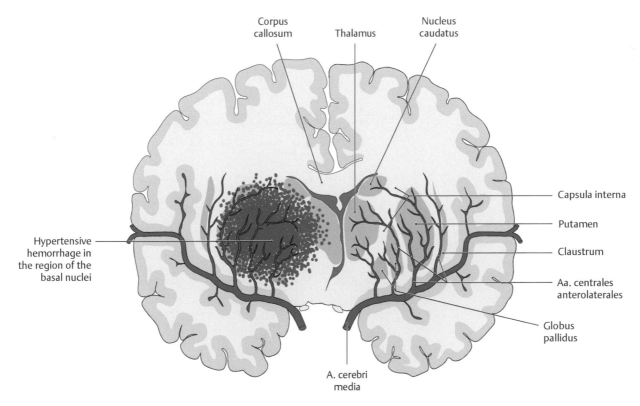

C Intracerebral hemorrhage
Coronal section through the corpora mammillaria. Unlike the intracranial extracerebral hemorrhages (see **A**), intracerebral hemorrhage involves bleeding directly into the substance of the brain. Because the soft brain tissue offers very little resistance, a massive hemorrhage can develop which, in contrast to extracerebral bleeding, cannot be controlled by surgical hemostasis. The most frequent cause of intracerebral hemorrhage (hemorrhagic stroke) is high blood pressure. The hemorrhage produces a cerebral infarction with a central (dark red) area of necrosis surrounded by a lighter halo. This halo is known as a penumbra (Latin *paene* "almost" and *umbra* "shadow") and is readily distinguishable from the central necrotic area on MRI. The penumbra is an area of relative oxygen deficiency. As a result, there is an initial total loss of

function in the affected area of the brain. In contrast to the irreversibly destroyed brain tissue in the area of necrosis, the ischemic tissue in the penumbra can recover in certain cases. The most common sites of vascular rupture are what are known as the "stroke arteries," the aa. centrales anterolaterales in the region of the capsula interna. Because the tractus pyramidalis passes through the capsula interna (see **E**, p. 335), there is a loss of tractus pyramidalis function below the lesion. This is manifested clinically by spastic paralysis of the limbs on the opposite side to the injury (as the tractus pyramidales cross below the level of the lesion). Aside from massive hemorrhages, smaller bleeds may occur in the territories of the three main aa. cerebri, producing a typical clinical presentation.

10.10 Blood Vessels of the Brain: Cerebrovascular Disease

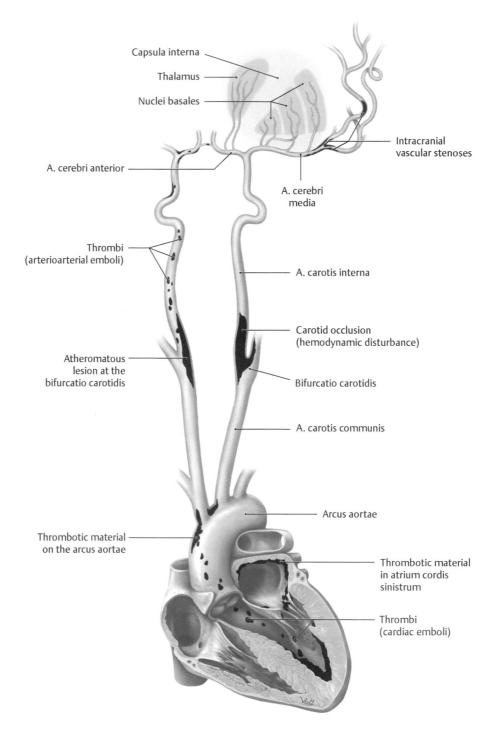

Capsula interna

Thalamus

Nuclei basales

Intracranial vascular stenoses

A. cerebri anterior

A. cerebri media

Thrombi (arterioarterial emboli)

A. carotis interna

Carotid occlusion (hemodynamic disturbance)

Atheromatous lesion at the bifurcatio carotidis

Bifurcatio carotidis

A. carotis communis

Arcus aortae

Thrombotic material on the arcus aortae

Thrombotic material in atrium cordis sinistrum

Thrombi (cardiac emboli)

A Frequent causes of cerebrovascular disease
(after Mumenthaler)

Disturbances of cerebral blood flow that deprive the brain of oxygen (cerebral ischemia) are the most frequent cause of central neurological deficits. The most serious complication is stroke: the vast majority of all strokes are caused by cerebral *ischemic* disease. Stroke has become the third leading cause of death in western industrialized countries (approximately 700,000 strokes occur in the United States each year). Cerebral ischemia is caused by a prolonged diminution or interruption of blood flow and involves *the distribution area of the a. carotis interna* in up to 90% of cases. Much less commonly, cerebral ischemia is caused by an obstruction of venous outflow due to cerebral venous thrombosis (see **B**). A decrease of arterial blood flow in the carotid system most commonly results from an embolic or local thrombotic occlusion. Most emboli originate from atheromatous lesions at the bifurcatio carotidis (arterioarterial emboli) or from the expulsion of thrombotic material from the ventriculus sinister (cardiac emboli). Blood clots (thrombi) may be dislodged from the heart as a result of valvular disease or atrial fibrillation. This produces emboli that may be carried by the bloodstream to the encephalon, where they may cause the functional occlusion of an artery supplying the encephalon. The most common example of this involves all of the distribution region of the a. cerebri media, which is a direct continuation of the a. carotis interna.

Right   Left

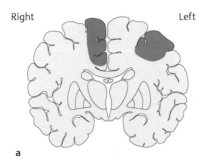

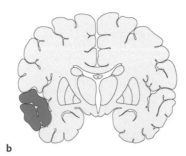

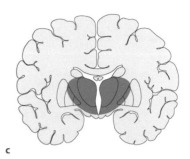

a   b   c

B Cerebral venous thrombosis

Coronal section, anterior view. The vv. cerebri, like the aa. cerebri, serve specific territories (see pp. 386 and 388). Though much less common than decreased arterial flow, the obstruction of venous outflow is an important potential cause of ischemia and infarction. With a thrombotic occlusion, for example, the quantity of blood and thus the venous pressure are increased in the tributary region of the occluded vein. This causes a drop in the capillary pressure gradient, with an increased extravasation of fluid from the capillary bed into the encephalon tissue (edema). There is a concomitant reduction of arterial inflow into the affected region, depriving it of oxygen. The occlusion of specific cerebral veins (e.g., due to cerebral venous thrombosis) leads to brain infarctions at characteristic locations:

a Venae superiores cerebri: Thrombosis and infarction in the areas drained by the

- Medial vv. superiores cerebri (right, *symptoms*: contralateral lower limb weakness)
- Posterior vv. superiores cerebri (left, *symptoms*: contralateral hemiparesis)

Motor aphasia occurs if the infarction involves the motor speech center in the dominant hemispherium.

b Venae inferiores cerebri: Thrombosis of the right vv. inferiores cerebri leads to infarction of the right lobus temporalis (*symptoms*: sensory aphasia, contralateral hemianopia).

c Venae internae cerebri: Bilateral thrombosis leads to a symmetrical infarction affecting the thalamus and nuclei basales. This is characterized by a rapid deterioration of consciousness ranging to coma.

Because the sinus durae matris have extensive anastomoses, a limited occlusion affecting part of a sinus often does not cause pronounced clinical symptoms, unlike the venous thromboses described here (see p. 384).

Vascular territory	Neurological symptoms	
A. cerebri anterior	Paralysis of lower limb (with or without hemisensory deficit)	Vesica urinaria dysfunction
A. cerebri media	Hemiparesis (with or without hemisensory deficit) mainly affecting the arm and face (Wernicke-Mann type)	Aphasia
A. cerebri posterior	Hemisensory losses	Hemianopia

C Cardinal symptoms of occlusion of the three main cerebral arteries (after Masuhr and Neumann)

When the *a. cerebri anterior, media,* or *posterior* becomes occluded, characteristic functional deficits occur in the oxygen-deprived encephalon areas supplied by the occluded vessel (see p. 368). In many cases the affected artery can be identified based on the associated neurological deficit:

- Vesicula urinaria weakness (cortical bladder center) and paralysis of the lower limb (with or without hemisensory deficit, predominantly affecting the leg) on the side opposite the occlusion (see motor and sensory homunculi, pp. 447 and 457) indicate an infarction in the territory of the **a. cerebri anterior**.
- Contralateral hemiplegia affecting the arm and face more than the leg indicates an infarction in the territory of the **a. cerebri media**. If the dominant hemispherium is affected, aphasia also occurs (the patient cannot name objects, for example).
- Visual disturbances affecting the contralateral visual field (contralateral homonymous hemianopsia) may signify an infarction in the territory of the **a. cerebri posterior**, because the structures supplied by this artery include the visual cortex in the sulcus calcarinus of the lobus occipitalis. If branches to the thalamus are also affected, the patient may also exhibit a contralateral hemisensory deficit because the afferent sensory fibers have already crossed below the thalamus.

The extent of the infarction depends partly on whether the occlusion is proximal or distal. Generally a proximal occlusion will cause a much more extensive infarction than a distal occlusion. MCA infarctions are the most common because the a. cerebri media is essentially a direct continuation of the a. carotis interna.

393

11.1 Spinal Cord (Medulla Spinalis): Segmental Organization

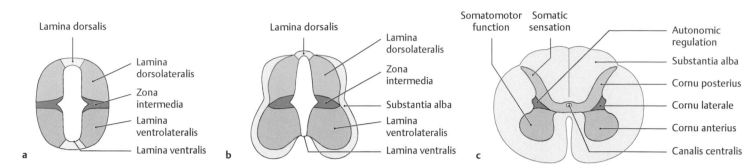

a Lamina dorsalis, Lamina dorsolateralis, Zona intermedia, Lamina ventrolateralis, Lamina ventralis

b Lamina dorsalis, Lamina dorsolateralis, Zona intermedia, Substantia alba, Lamina ventrolateralis, Lamina ventralis

c Somatomotor function, Somatic sensation, Autonomic regulation, Substantia alba, Cornu posterius, Cornu laterale, Cornu anterius, Canalis centralis

A Embryological development of the medulla spinalis
Cross-section through the tubus neuralis at the level where the medulla spinalis eventually develops; cranial view.
a Early neural tube; **b** Intermediate stage; **c** Adult medulla spinalis.
The development of the medulla spinalis has already been explained on p. 263. More than any other part of the CNS, knowledge of the embryological development of the medulla spinalis facilitates the understanding of its structure and function after birth. This is why its developement will be briefly reviewed and highlighted.

- The medulla spinalis as a part of the CNS derives from the tubus neuralis. A cross-section through the early tubus neuralis (**a**) shows a central fluid filled (liquor cerebrospinalis) lumen, which is surrounded by so-called "plates":
  – the unpaired laminae ventralis and dorsalis as well as
  – the paired laminae ventrolaterales and dorsolaterales.

Between laminae ventrolateralis and dorsolateralis lies an intermediate zone (zona intermedia). Numerous neurons develop In the laminae ventrolateralis and dorsolateralis plate as well as in the zona

intermedia. They form the **gray matter (substantia grisea)** as a result of which these areas enlarge and increasingly constrict the lumen leading to the formation of the canalis centralis of the medulla spinalis (**c**), which may become even obstructed in some regions. In the adult medulla spinalis, the three columnae griseae are referred to as cornua anterius, laterale, and posterius.

- The processes (axons) emerging from neurons or the axons arriving from other neurons form the **white matter (substantia alba)**, which topographically can be divided into three columns (funiculi) and functionally into numerous tracts (see p. 396). The substantia alba surrounds the substantia grisea.

Morphologically, the substantia grisea which is surrounded by substantia grisea on all sides, is considered a nucleus or nuclear group. Each of the three cornua can be assigned one main function according to their neurons: cornu anterius: somatomotor function; cornu posterius: somatic sensation; cornu laterale: control of the autonomic functions of organs.

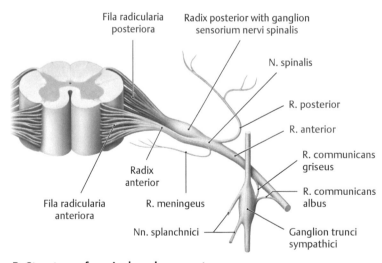

Fila radicularia posteriora, Radix posterior with ganglion sensorium nervi spinalis, N. spinalis, R. posterior, R. anterior, R. communicans griseus, R. communicans albus, Ganglion trunci sympathici, Nn. splanchnici, R. meningeus, Radix anterior, Fila radicularia anteriora

B Structure of a spinal cord segment
Anteriosuperior view of a spinal cord segment as well as a n. spinalis.
The medulla spinalis is a continuous structure located in the canalis vertebralis. A segmental functional or morphological distinction is not precisely identifiable. The medulla spinalis as part of the CNS is continuously connected with the PNS via fila radicularia. These fila radicularia are groups of axons, which

- exit the medulla spinalis on its anterior aspect (typically axons of motor neurons, which terminate in a target organ or ganglion autonomicum) or
- enter the medulla spinalis on its posterior aspect (typically axons of sensory neurons, which carry information from a receptor).

The columna vertebralis consist of segments—corresponding to the indivdual vertebrae—which means that the canalis vertebralis itself is divided (see **C**). It virtually determines a segmental arrangement of the continuous medulla spinalis. It is only at the openings between individual vertebrae—at the foramina intervertebralia—that the fila radicularia that form the nn. spinales can either enter or exit the canalis vertebralis. They don't do that individually but in bundles in form of a **root (radix)**:

- The fila radicularia anteriora form a radix anterior.
- The fila radicularia posteriora form a radix posterior.

Both radices merge to form the **spinal nerve (n. spinalis)**. The fila radicularia, radices, and medulla spinalis are parts of the PNS. Functionally, a spinal cord segment is based on a longitudinal division of the medulla spinalis, which contains the cell bodies of motor neurons that form precisely one radix anterior. Each spinal segment (which is a continous part of the CNS) is therefore connected with a n. spinalis (which is a discontinous part of the PNS).
Note: The radix posterior is not "involved" in the functional definition because the fibers entering the medulla spinalis through the radix posterior don't always end on neurons located at the same level of the medulla spinalis (i.e., in certain cases they will end in the medulla oblongata). Since the n. spinalis consists of (motor) radix anterior and (sensory) radix posterior, it has mixed functions. The only exception among the nn. spinales: the n. spinalis from the C1 segment does not have a radix posterior (thus there are no fila radicularia posteriora): it is exclusively motor. For all other nn. spinales, it could be said that in morphological terms, a segment of the medulla spinalis is the part where the fila radicularia, which merge to form a n. spinalis, enter or exit the medulla spinalis.

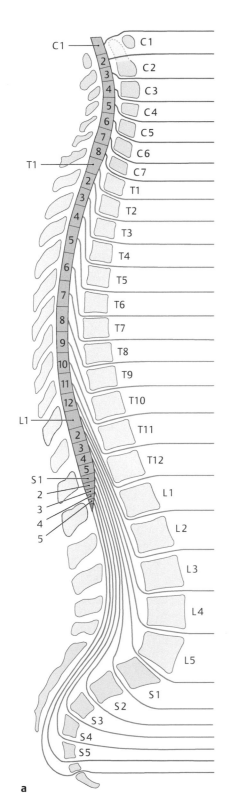

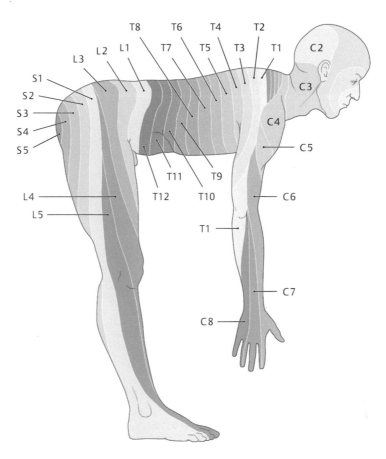

D Simplified schematic representation of the segmental innervation of the skin
(after Mumenthaler)

Distribution of the dermatomes on the body. Sensory innervation of the skin correlates with the radices sensoriae (radices posteriores) of the nn. spinales in **D**. Every spinal cord segment (except for C1, see below) innervates a particular skin area (dermatome). From a clinical standpoint, it is important to know the precise correlation of dermatomes with medulla spinalis segments so that the level of a spinal cord lesion can be determined based on the location of the affected dermatome. For example, a lesion of the radix nervi spinalis C8 is characterized by a loss of sensation on the ulnar (small-finger) side of the hand.

Note: There is no C1 dermatome because there is no radix posterior. Proprioceptive fibers from the short neck muscles in the n. suboccipitalis course via the plexus cervicalis posterior into the radix posterior of C2.

Spinal cord segment	Corpus vertebrae	Processus spinosus
C8	Inferior margin of C6, superior margin of C7	C6
T6	T5	T4
T12	T10	T9
L5	T11	T10
S1	T12	T12

C Relation between spinal cord segments and vertebral bodies in adults

a Midsagittal section of the columna vertebralis, viewed from the right side; **b** Spinal cord segments (selected).

A spinal cord segment is named after the foramen intervertebrale from which "its" n. spinalis emerges. In the fetus, a segment, foramen intervertebrale, and n. spinalis are still located almost at the same level. Since the columna vertebralis grows faster and longer than the medulla spinalis, the lower vertebrae and thus the foramina intervertebralia grow farther apart in relation to the medulla spinalis. Radices anteriores and posteriores, which have to cover comparatively long distances from their segment to their corresponding foramen intervertebrale and run in the canalis vertebralis in caudal direction as the cauda equina (horse tail). Topographically, the lowest spinal cord segment (Coccygeal 1) is located at the level of the corpus vertebrae L1. Knowledge of these topographical relationships is important when intending to perform a lumbar puncture (see **C, E**, p. 419). For reference, some segments have been summarized in **b**.

Note: The n. spinalis C1 emerges between the os occipitale and the first cervical vertebra (atlas), the n. spinalis C8 emerges between the seventh cervical vertebra and first thoracic vertebra. That is why there are seven cervical vertebrae but eight cervical nn. spinales (and eight cervical segments). Starting with the T1, all nn. spinales emerge below "their" corresponding vertebrae. Thus, injuries below the L1 vertebra don't damage the medulla spinalis but affect the radices anteriores and posterior roots (cauda equina syndrome).

11.2 Medulla Spinalis: Organization of Spinal Cord Segments

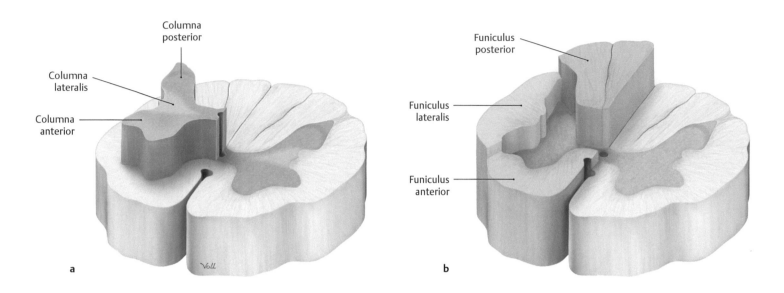

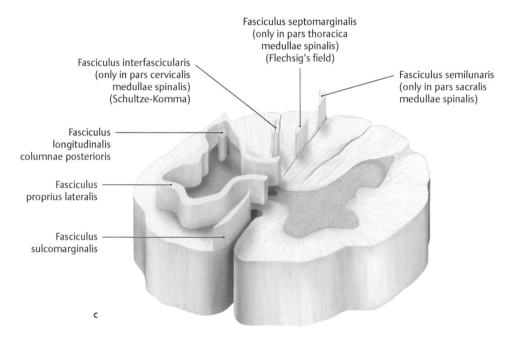

A Substantiae grisea and alba of the medulla spinalis

Three-dimensional representation of the medulla spinalis, oblique anterior view from upper left.

a Substantia grisea; **b** Substantia alba: the funiculi; **c** Substantia alba: fasciculi proprii.

The typical cross-sectional view of the medulla spinalis simplifies the fact that the functional arrangement of neurons occurs in columns (called nuclear columns) (see **A**, p. 398). Thus, the representation of the substantia grisea in three columnae (**a**), columnae anterior, lateralis, and posterior, the cross-section of which shows the respective cornu, is more than a topographic aspect. For the functional understanding of muscles through nuclear columns on one hand (see p. 388) and for knowledge about the function of fasciculi proprii (see **c**) on the other hand, the concept of the columnae is essential. With reference to the definition of a segment (see **B**, p. 394), the columna anterior is the place where all motor neurons that form the radix anterior are located. The columnae lateralis and posterior contain autonomic and sensory neurons as has already been mentioned in **A** p. 394 in connection with the respective

cornua. The substantia alba consists of tracts. They can generally be distinguished based on their destination:

b Tracts that run through the medulla spinalis—p.r.n after interconnecting inside the medulla spinalis—and permit communication with other parts of the CNS. With respect to the medulla spinalis's extrinsic circuits, the substantia alba is divided into three funiculi: anterior, lateralis, and posterior.

c Tracts that interconnect neurons in the columnae inside the medulla spinalis and are responsible for the "intrinsic circuits" of the medulla spinalis. The axons of these tracts belong to interneurons that are arranged around the substantia grisea. The intrinsic circuit is organized as fasciculi proprii, typically located adjacent to the gray matter. These fibers can also run horizontally and interconnect neurons of one level (not shown here).

In both circuits, the tracts can be ascending or descending. In the extrinsic circuits, ascending tracts are sensory while descending tracts are motor.

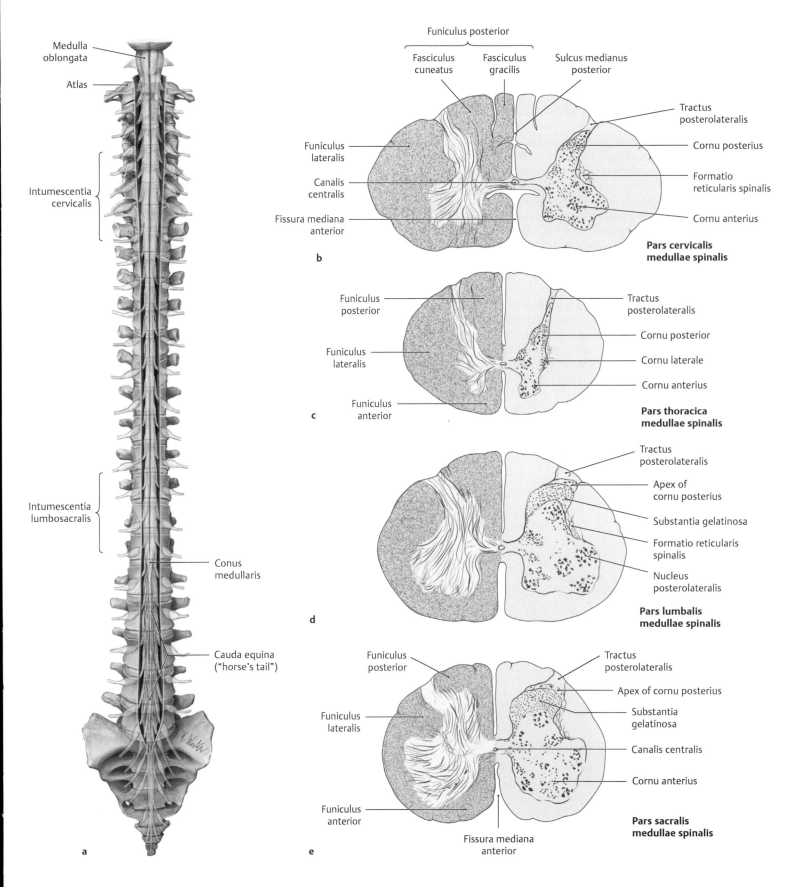

Medulla oblongata

Atlas

Intumescentia cervicalis

Intumescentia lumbosacralis

Conus medullaris

Cauda equina ("horse's tail")

a

Funiculus posterior

Fasciculus cuneatus — Fasciculus gracilis — Sulcus medianus posterior

Funiculus lateralis

Canalis centralis

Fissura mediana anterior

b

Tractus posterolateralis

Cornu posterius

Formatio reticularis spinalis

Cornu anterius

Pars cervicalis medullae spinalis

Funiculus posterior

Funiculus lateralis

Funiculus anterior

c

Tractus posterolateralis

Cornu posterior

Cornu laterale

Cornu anterius

Pars thoracica medullae spinalis

Tractus posterolateralis

Apex of cornu posterius

Substantia gelatinosa

Formatio reticularis spinalis

Nucleus posterolateralis

Pars lumbalis medullae spinalis

d

Funiculus posterior

Funiculus lateralis

Funiculus anterior

Fissura mediana anterior

e

Tractus posterolateralis

Apex of cornu posterius

Substantia gelatinosa

Canalis centralis

Cornu anterius

Pars sacralis medullae spinalis

B Position of the medulla spinalis in the dural sac
a Anterior view with the corpora vertebrarum partially removed to display the anterior aspect of the medulla spinalis. The transverse sections (**b–e**) depict fiber tracts (left side, myelin stain) and neuron cell bodies (right side, Nissl stain) at different levels of the medulla spinalis. The areas of the intumescentiae cervicalis and lumbosacaralis have been demarcated (**a**). In these areas, which provide innervation to the limbs, the gray matter is significantly expanded.

11.3 Medulla Spinalis: Internal Divisions of the Substantia Grisea

A Organizational principles of the columna anterior of the medulla spinalis

Motor neurons that innervate specific muscles are arranged into vertical columns in the cornu anterius (ventral) of the substantia grisea of the medulla spinalis. Analogous to the truncus encephali motor nuclei, these columns can themselves be called nuclei, and are arranged in a somatotopic fashion (see **B** for a mapping of these nuclei to their target muscles). The motor columns innervating the trunk have a relatively simple arrangement that follows the linear segmental organization of nn. spinales and dermatomes. The intumescentiae cervicalis and lumbrosacralis, which innervate the limbs, have a more complex pattern of innervation than the trunk muscles: during the migratory processes of embryonic development, muscle precursors "carry" their original innervation with them, generating a motor column that sends its axons through multiple radices nervorum from multiple spinal cord levels. The muscles innervated by such a column are accordingly called *multisegmental muscles* (see **B**, p. 390). Muscles whose motor neurons are situated entirely within one segment are referred to as *indicator muscles*; testing the function of indicator muscles is valuable in clinical assessment.

Note: Although one muscle may be innervated by axons from multiple spinal segments, those axons arise from a *single* motor column.

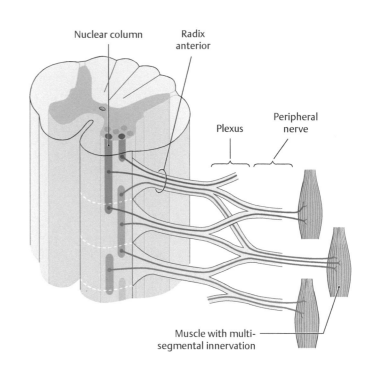

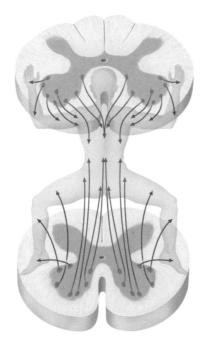

a

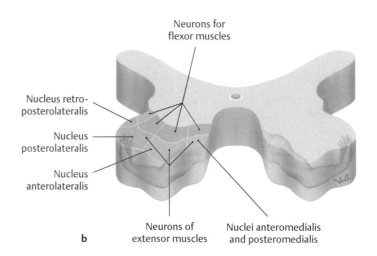

b

B Somatotopic organization of nuclear columns of the cornu anterius (after Bossy)

a Common pattern of organization in the medulla spinalis. More medial nuclear columns of the cornu anterius innervate muscles close to the midline, while more lateral nuclear columns tend to innervate muscles outside the trunk.

b Intumescentia cervicalis. The same pattern of medial-to-lateral organization exists (see **a**) with medial nuclei innervating axial muscles

and lateral nuclei innervating muscles at the extremities. However, there is also an anterior-to-posterior segregation of motor columns. Neurons serving extensor muscles (shades of blue) are found in the most anterior parts of the cornu anterius, while those serving flexor muscles (shades of pink) are found in the more posterior regions. These nuclei are further divided into the following:

- Nuclei anteromedialis and posteromedialis: innervate nuchal, back, intercostal, and abdominal muscles
- Nucleus anterolateralis: innervates shoulder girdle and upper arm muscles
- Nucleus posterolateralis: innervates forearm muscles
- Nucleus retroposterolateralis: innervates small muscles of the fingers.

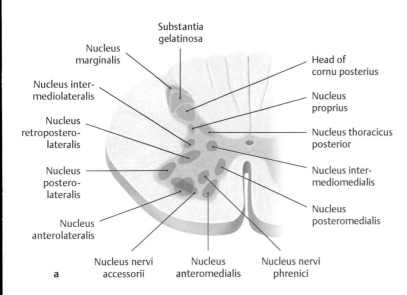

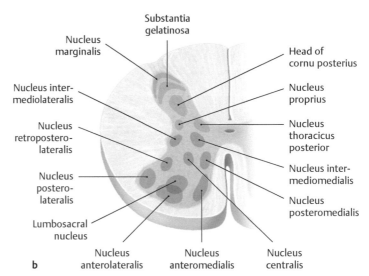

a — Cervical cord

b — Lumbar cord

C Cell groups in the substantia grisea of the medulla spinalis
a Cervical cord; **b** Lumbar cord. The neurons in the substantia grisea of the medulla spinalis are classified in cell groups (nuclei) according to their shape and position. When one excludes the neurons not involved in local information processing, the cornu anterius essentially contains the somatoefferent motor neurons. As a result, the cornu anterius is significantly larger than the cornu posterius, which essentially contains the projection neurons of the ascending pathways. As the positions of the nuclear groups can vary in the different sections, the illustration shows the cervical and lumbar part of the medulla spinalis. A few cell columns are specific to the respective segment of the medulla spinalis. For example, the nucleus for the n. phrenicus is found only in the cervical part. The sacral part of the medulla spinalis (not shown here) contains a small nucleus (on average 625 neurons), nucleus X after Onuf, on the anterior aspect of lamina IX (see **D**) at the level of (S1)-S2-S3. This nucleus contains the motor neurons of the pudendal nerve, which are responsible for urinary and fecal continence (external sphincters for the anus and urethra) and for orgasm (ischiocavernosus and bulbocavernosus).

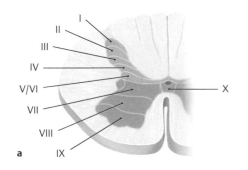

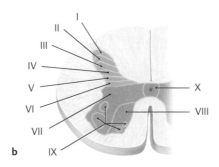

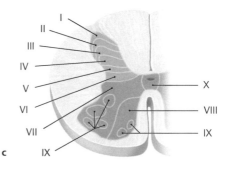

a — Pars cervicalis

b — Pars thoracica

c — Pars lumbalis

D Classification of the nuclei in layers after Rexed
a Pars cervicalis; **b** Pars thoracica; **c** Pars lumbalis. The complex organization of the CNS means that there are different ways to classify the substantia grisea. Aside from the division described above, the substantia grisea can also be divided into cytoarchitectural layers (laminae I–X) after Rexed. This laminar architecture is especially well defined in the cornu posterius; in the cornu anterius, the arrangement of the laminae resembles that of the nuclei (see **C**). The site at which the sensory axons of the ganglia sensoria nervorum spinalium end is often specified as the lamina after Rexed. This figure can serve as a reference.

E Substantia grisea neurons of the medulla spinalis

Root cells

Neurons whose axons exit from the radix anterior. These are further differentiated as follows:
- Somatomotor root cells (extend to the skeletal muscles; α and γ motor neurons)
- Visceral motor root cells (extending to the viscera)

Intrinsic neurons
Neurons whose axons do not leave the CNS. These are further differentiated as follows:
- *Projection neurons*: Intrinsic neurons in the columna posterior whose axons leave the substantia grisea and extend in the substantia alba as ascending pathways to higher centers. They represent the second sensory neuron; the first lies in the ganglion sensorium nervi spinalis (see p. 403). Because their axons terminate in higher centers, they are referred to collectively as projection neurons (analogously to the descending projection neurons).

- *Interneurons*: Neurons distributed throughout the substantia grisea whose axons do not leave the gray matter. These are further differentiated as follows:
- Relay cells: Neurons whose axons terminate within one side on a single segment level (see **C**, S. 401)
- Commissural cells: Neurons whose axons extend in the commissura (alba) to the opposite side (see **C**, S. 401)
- Associative cells: Neurons whose axons interconnect various segments on one side; intersegmental correlation system (see **C**, S. 401)
- Renshaw cells: Neurons which are stimulated by axon collaterals of the excitatory alpha motor neuron. They then release and inhibitory neurotransmitter that acts in a retrograde manner on the stimulating alpha motor neuron (retrograde inhibition; see **D**, p. 401).

11.4 Medulla Spinalis: Reflex Arcs and Intrinsic Circuits

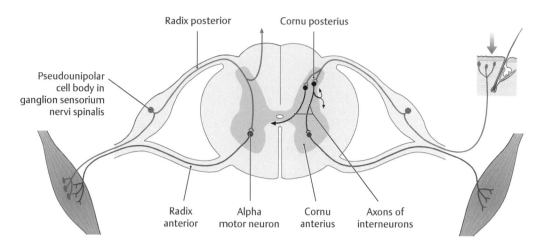

Radix posterior · Cornu posterius

Pseudounipolar cell body in ganglion sensorium nervi spinalis

Radix anterior · Alpha motor neuron · Cornu anterius · Axons of interneurons

A Integrative function of the substantia grisea of the medulla spinalis: Reflexes

Afferent nerves are shown in blue, efferent nerves in red. Black indicates neurons of the spinal reflex circuit.

The substantia grisea of the medulla spinalis supports muscular function at the unconscious (reflex) level, holding the body upright during stance and enabling us to walk and run without conscious control. To perform this coordinating function, the neurons of the substantia grisea must receive information from the muscles and their surroundings; this information enters the cornu posterius of the medulla spinalis via the axons of neurons in the ganglia sensoria nervorum spinalium (see p. 436). Two types of reflex exist:

- **Monosynaptic reflex** (left): intrinsic reflex in which information from the periphery (e.g., on muscle length and stretch) comes from the muscle itself. Receptors in the muscle transmit signals to alpha motor neurons via neurons whose cell bodies are in the ganglia sensoria nervorum spinalium. These afferent neurons release excitatory neurotransmitters which cause the alpha motor neurons to stimulate muscle contraction (see **D**).
- **Polysynaptic reflex** (right): reflex mediated by receptors in the skin or other sites *outside* the muscle. These receptors act via *interneurons* (see **C**) to stimulate muscular contraction.

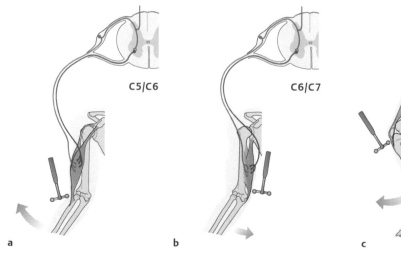

C5/C6 · C6/C7

a · b

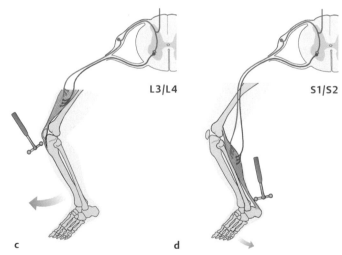

L3/L4 · S1/S2

c · d

B Clinically important monosynaptic reflexes

a Biceps reflex; **b** Triceps reflex; **c** Patellar reflex (quadriceps reflex); **d** Achilles tendon reflex.

The drawings show the muscles, the trigger points for eliciting the reflexes, the nerves involved in the reflexes (afferent nerves in blue, efferent nerves in red), and the corresponding spinal cord segments.

The principal monosynaptic reflexes should be tested in every physical examination. Each reflex is elicited by briskly tapping the appropriate

tendon with a reflex hammer to stretch the muscle. If the muscle contracts in response to this stretch, the reflex arc is intact. Although each test involves just one muscle and one peripheral nerve supplying the muscle, the innervation involves several spinal cord segments (multisegmental muscles, see **A**, p. 398). The right and left sides should always be compared in clinical reflex testing because this is the only way to recognize a *unilateral* increase, decrease, or other abnormality.

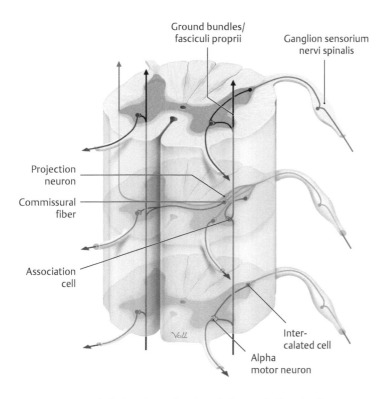

Ground bundles/
fasciculi proprii

Ganglion sensorium
nervi spinalis

Projection
neuron

Commissural
fiber

Association
cell

Inter-
calated cell

Alpha
motor neuron

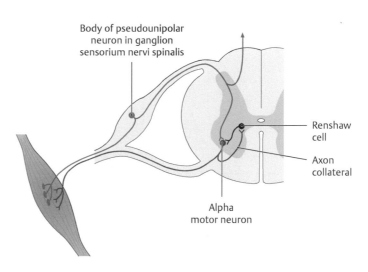

Body of pseudounipolar
neuron in ganglion
sensorium nervi spinalis

Renshaw
cell

Axon
collateral

Alpha
motor neuron

C Components of the intrinsic circuits of the medulla spinalis

Afferent neurons are shown in blue, efferent neurons in red. The neurons of the spinal reflex circuits are shown in black. Polysynaptic reflexes often must be coordinated at the spinal cord level by multiple segments. Interneurons, some of whose axons show a T-shaped branching pattern, convey the afferent signals to higher and lower segments along crossed and uncrossed pathways (types of interneurons are described in **E**, p. 399). These chains of interneurons, which are entirely contained within the medulla spinalis, make up the *intrinsic circuits* of the medulla spinalis. The axons of the neurons in the intrinsic circuits pass to adjacent segments in intrinsic fascicles (fasciculi proprii) located at the edge of the substantia alba (see **A**, p. 396). These fascicles are the conduction apparatus of the intrinsic circuits.

D Effects of the Renshaw cell on the alpha motor neuron

The afferent fibers in a monosynaptic reflex originate in neurons of the ganglia sensoria nervorum spinalium. They terminate on the alpha motor neurons, where they release the excitatory transmitter acetylcholine. In response to this transmitter release, the alpha motor neuron transmits excitatory impulses to the neuromuscular junction (the transmitter is also acetylcholine). The excitatory alpha motor neuron has axon collaterals that enable it to exert a stimulatory effect on an inhibitory interneuron called a Renshaw cell. In response to this stimulation, the Renshaw cell releases the *inhibitory* transmitter glycine. This self-inhibiting mechanism serves to prevent overexcitation of the alpha motor neurons (recurrent inhibition). The clinical importance of the Renshaw cells is dramatically illustrated in patients with tetanus. The tetanus toxin inhibits the release of glycine from the Renshaw cells. Inhibition of the alpha motor neurons fails to occur, and so the patient experiences sustained (tetanic) muscle contractions.

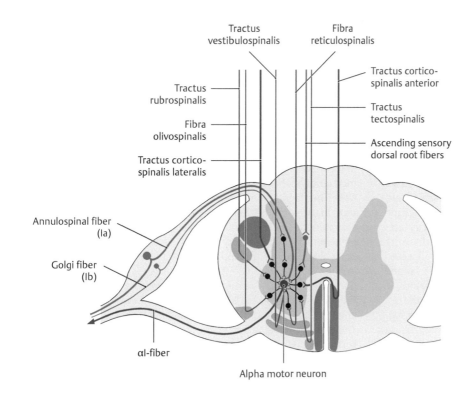

Tractus
vestibulospinalis

Fibra
reticulospinalis

Tractus cortico-
spinalis anterior

Tractus
rubrospinalis

Tractus
tectospinalis

Fibra
olivospinalis

Ascending sensory
dorsal root fibers

Tractus cortico-
spinalis lateralis

Annulospinal fiber
(Ia)

Golgi fiber
(Ib)

αI-fiber

Alpha motor neuron

E Effects of long tracts on the alpha motor neuron

The alpha motor neuron not only receives afferent fibers from the medulla spinalis itself, but is also strongly modulated by fibers from long tracts that originate in the encephalon. Most of these fibers have an inhibitory effect on the alpha motor neuron. If these effects are abolished due to a complete cord lesion above the alpha motor neuron, for example, the disproportionately strong influence of the spinal intrinsic circuits will lead to spastic paralysis (see p. 461).

11.5 Ascending Tracts of the Medulla Spinalis: Tractus Spinothalamici

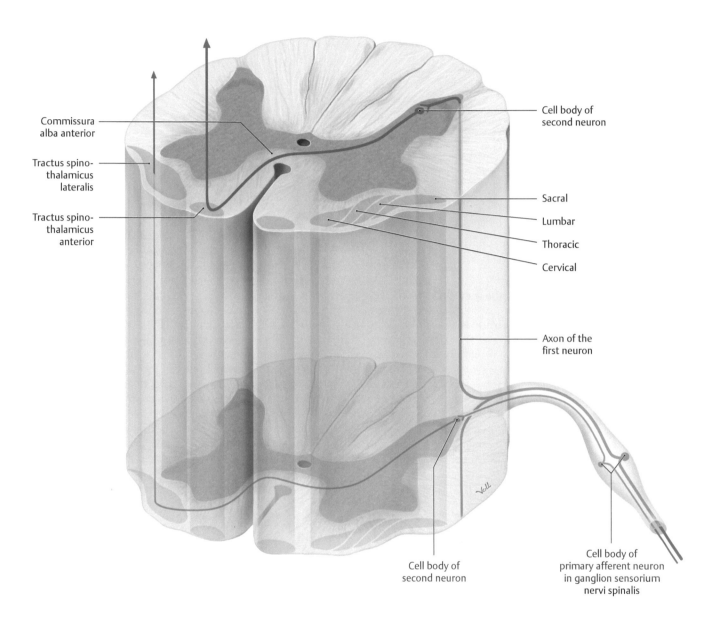

Commissura alba anterior

Tractus spino-thalamicus lateralis

Tractus spino-thalamicus anterior

Cell body of second neuron

Sacral

Lumbar

Thoracic

Cervical

Axon of the first neuron

Cell body of second neuron

Cell body of primary afferent neuron in ganglion sensorium nervi spinalis

A Course of the tractus spinothalamici anterior and lateralis in a transverse section of the medulla spinalis

The axons of the tractus spinothalamicus anterior run in the funiculus anterior of the medulla spinalis, while those of the tractus spinothalamicus lateralis run in both the funiculi anterior and lateralis. (These two tracts are sometimes referred to collectively as the *anterolateral system*.) The tractus spinothalamicus anterior is the pathway for crude touch and pressure sensation, while the tractus spinothalamicus lateralis conveys pain, temperature, tickle, itch, and sexual sensation. The cell bodies of the primary afferent neurons for both tracts are located in the ganglia sensoria nervorum spinalium. Both tracts contain second neurons that crossed in the commissura alba anterior. The somatotopic organization of the tractus spinothalamicus lateralis is shown on the left side of the diagram. Starting dorsally and moving clockwise, we successively encounter the sacral, lumbar, thoracic, and cervical fibers. In older terminology a distinction is sometimes drawn between *epicritic* and *protopathic* sensation. According to this terminology, the tractus

spinothalamici anterior and lateralis are classified as *protopathic pathways* while the tracts of the funiculus posterior are classified as an *epicritic sensory pathway*. Today the original classification has been dropped because it does not correspond well to the assignment of sensory modalities of anatomically defined tracts.

Note: The tractus spinothalamicus is formed by fibers that cross (decussate) in the commissura alba anterior but is not part of the commissura alba anterior. The commissura alba anterior, just like the commissura alba posterior (not represented here), is a true commissure, in which fibers cross between the right and left halves of the medulla spinalis. The commissura alba anterior is not to be confused with the commissura anterior, which is also a true commissure. However, the latter is not located in the medulla spinalis but in the telencephalon where it connects the left and right lobi temporales as well as the left and right olfactory nuclei. The commissura alba posterior is not to be confused with the commissura posterior, which is a true commissure located in the diencephalon.

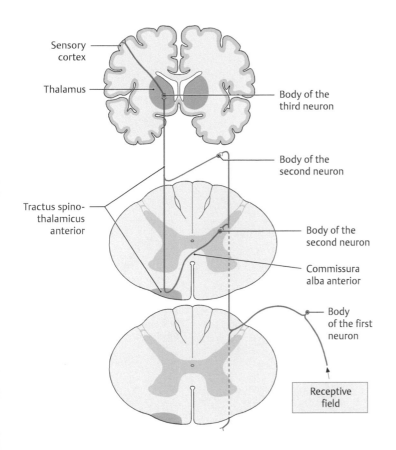

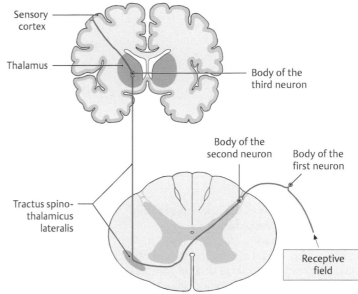

B The tractus spinothalamici and their central connections

a Tractus spinothalamicus anterior; **b** Tractus spinothalamicus lateralis. Both tractus spinothalamici deal with stimuli received from cutaneous receptors but each of them relays information related to different types of sensation:

- The tractus spinothalamicus anterior carries impulses via tactile corpuscles found in the skin as well as hair follicle receptors (mechanoreceptors) through moderately myelinated peripheral neuronal processes (dendritic axons).
- The tractus spinothalamicus lateralis carries information about pain and temperature from the free nerve endings in the skin.

In both tracts, the cell bodies of the first neurons (primary neurons) are located in the ganglia sensoria nervorum spinalium. There are other similarities regarding the further course of the tractus spinothalamici. Both tracts transmit information toward the sensory cortex in the gyrus postcentralis. Thus, the impulses they carry are consciously processed in the encephalon. However, there is one, also clinically significant, difference between the two tracts regarding their pathway:

- In the case of the tractus spinothalamicus anterior:
  - **(a)** The axons of the first neuron initially branch in a T-shaped pattern. After entering the medulla spinalis, they descend 1–2 segment and ascend 2–15 segments. Only then, and not at the level where they enter the spinal cord segment, do they synapse with neurons in the cornu posterius (second neurons). Axons of these second neurons than cross in the commissura alba anterior and ascend in the opposite funiculus anterior.

- In the case of the tractus spinothalamicus lateralis:
  - **(b)** The axons of the first neurons synapse with the second neurons as soon as they enter the substantia grisea of the medulla spinalis, thus on the same level where they enter it! The axons of the second neurons, also, cross the midline in the commissura alba anterior and ascend in the opposite funiculus lateralis. Knowledge about these differences can be significant when evaluating a patient with *Brown-Séquard Syndrome* (see **E**, p. 473).

Both tractus spinothalamici (which in the truncus encephali are also referred to as fibrae spinothalamicae) ascend in the truncus encephali in a composite bundle of tracts, called the lemniscus spinalis, to the nucleus ventralis posterolateralis of the thalamus where they synapse with the third neurons. The axons of the third neurons pass through the capsula interna and reach the fourth neurons in the gyrus postcentralis. *Note:* A lesion to the tractus spinothalamici leads to reduced or complete loss of sensation to different sensory stimuli such as pain, temperature, and crude touch. Since both tracts are hardly separable, an isolated lesion to only one of them is practically never encountered. A lesion affecting the tractus spinothalamici will always result in clinical deficit that is contralateral to the side of the lesion; therefore on the same side with the ganglion sensorium nervi spinalis that contains the bodies of the first neurons of the pathway. Moreover, based on the crossing of the second neurons of these tracts, a lesion of the left first neuron of the same pathway (part of the PNS) or the left second neuron (part of the CNS) before it crosses the midline will result in a deficit on the left side of the patient. A lesion of the right third and fourth neurons (both of them in the CNS) will result in a deficit on the left side of the patient.

11.6 Ascending Tracts of the Medullla Spinalis: Fasciculus Gracilis and Fasciculus Cuneatus

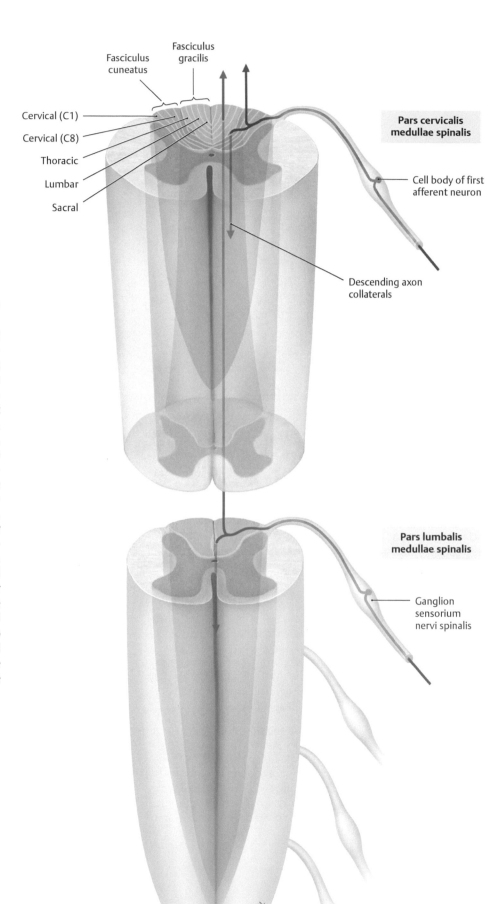

A Ascending axons in the fasciculus gracilis and fasciculus cuneatus

The fasciculus gracilis ("slender fasciculus") and fasciculus cuneatus ("wedge-shaped fasciculus") are the two large ascending tracts in the funiculus posterior. Since these tracts largely run analogous to the tractus spinothalamici and also carry information about conscious perception to the telencephalon, they are depicted immediately thereafter. Both tracts convey fibers for position sense (conscious proprioception) and fine cutaneous sensation (touch, vibration, fine pressure sense, two-point discrimination). The fasciculus gracilis carries fibers from the lower limbs, while the fasciculus cuneatus carries fibers only from the upper limbs and is therefore not present in the medulla spinalis below the T3 level. The cell bodies of the first neuron are located in the ganglion sensorium nervi spinalis. Their fibers are heavily myelinated and therefore conduct impulses rapidly. They pass uncrossed (the level of the decussation is shown in **C**) to the dorsal column nuclei (nuclei gracilis and cuneatus, see **C**). Both nuclei are located in the caudal portion of the medulla oblongata. The fasciculi are somatotopically organized.

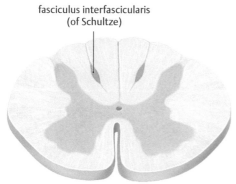

fasciculus interfascicularis
(of Schultze)

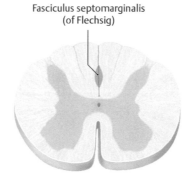

Fasciculus septomarginalis
(of Flechsig)

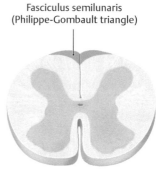

Fasciculus semilunaris
(Philippe-Gombault triangle)

Pars cervicalis medullae spinalis   **Pars thoracica medullae spinalis**   **Pars sacralis medullae spinalis**

B Descending axons

Besides the ascending axons contained in the fasciculus gracilis and fasciculus cuneatus (both shown in **A**), there are also descending axon collaterals that are distributed to lower segments. This pathway takes different shapes at different levels, appearing as the comma tract of Schultze (fasciculus interfascicularis) in the pars cervicalis, the oval area of Flechsig (fasciculus septomarginalis) in the pars thoracica, and the Philippe-Gombault triangle (fasciculus semilunaris) in the pars sacralis. These tracts are concerned with sensorimotor innervation at the spinal cord level and are thus considered part of the intrinsic circuits of the medulla spinalis (see pp. 396 and 400).

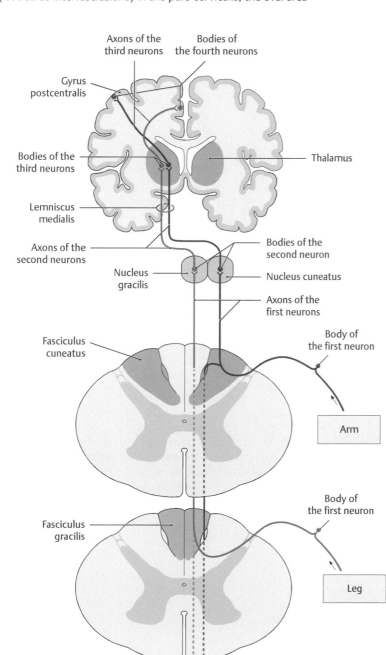

Axons of the third neurons
Bodies of the fourth neurons
Gyrus postcentralis
Thalamus
Bodies of the third neurons
Lemniscus medialis
Axons of the second neurons
Nucleus gracilis
Bodies of the second neuron
Nucleus cuneatus
Axons of the first neurons
Body of the first neuron
Fasciculus cuneatus
Arm
Body of the first neuron
Fasciculus gracilis
Leg

C Fasciculi gracilis and cuneatus and their central connections

- Just like in the case of the tractus spinothalamici (see p. 402 f), the axons of the third neurons of the dorsal columns—lemniscus medialis pathway—terminate in the somatosensory cortex of the telencephalon, the gyrus postcentralis. That means that impulses carried by those tracts are also perceived consciously (conscious proprioception via muscle and tendon receptors as well as perception of vibration via Vater-Pacini corpuscles, fine touch via cutaneous receptors and so on).
- Just like in the case of the tractus spinothalamici, the cell bodies of the first neurons are located in the ganglia sensoria nervorum spinalium.
- The axons of the first neurons ascend uncrossed in the posterior columns to the nuclei gracilis and cuneatus (that contain the cell bodies of the second neurons) located in the caudal part of the medulla oblongata.
- The axons of the second neurons cross the midline and form the lemniscus medialis that ascends through the truncus encephali to the thalamus (where they synapse with the third neurons).

Note: A lesion to the fasciculi gracilis and cuneatus leads to reduced or total loss of fine touch and consious proprioception. The disturbance caused by this lesion is always localized on the side of the body where the cell body of the first neuron (thus the peripheral neuron in the ganglion sensorium nervi spinalis) of the tract is located. This finding is explained by the above mentioned crossing of the axons of the second neuron that occurs in the medulla oblongata (while the second neurons of other sensory pathways are located in the medulla spinalis!). For example, symptoms on the left side of the body are associated with lesions to the first neuron or the body of the second neuron on the left side or lesions to the lemniscus medialis, the third neuron or the gyrus postcentralis on the right side.

11.7 Ascending Tracts of the Medulla Spinalis: Tractus Spinocerebellares

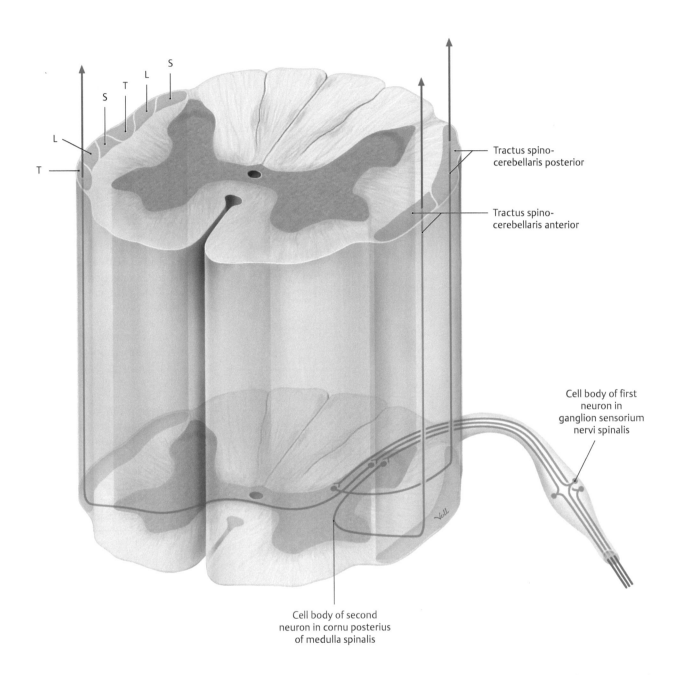

Tractus spino-cerebellaris posterior

Tractus spino-cerebellaris anterior

Cell body of first neuron in ganglion sensorium nervi spinalis

Cell body of second neuron in cornu posterius of medulla spinalis

A Tractus spinocerebellares anterior and posterior
The tractus spinocerebellares are located in the funiculus lateralis of the medulla spinalis and unlike the previously mentioned ascending tracts of the medulla spinalis don't carry their information toward the cortex cerebri (via thalamus) but to the cerebellum. That means that the impulses they carry are not consciously perceived. Their afferent input is involved in the unconscious coordination of motor activities such as running or bike riding (unconscious proprioception). Both tracts have the same somatotopy from ventral to dorsal (represented clockwise on the figure):

- thoracic (T)
- lumbar (L)
- sacral (S)

Fibers with similar function from the cervical region pass through the fasciculus cuneatus to the nucleus cuneatus accessorius and continue as fibrae cuneocerebellares to the cerebellum. However, they do not pass through the tractus spinocerebellaris posterior, which contains no fibers from the pars cervicalis medullae spinalis.

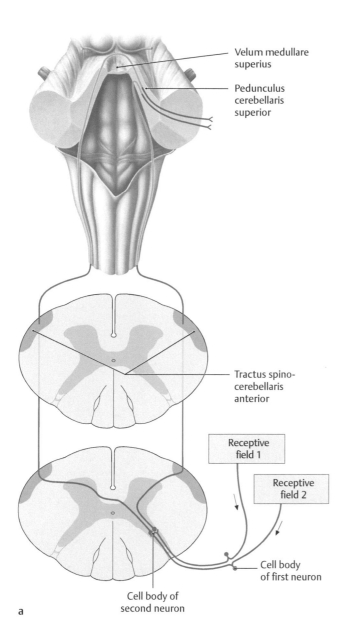

a

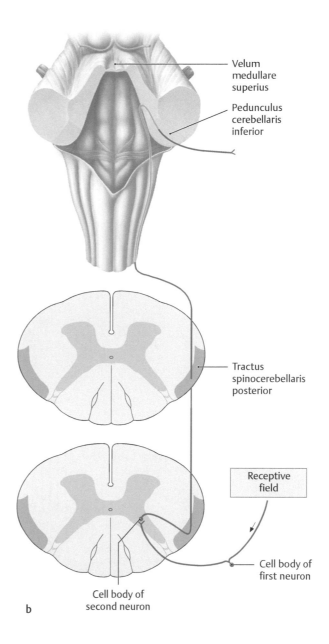

b

B Tractus spinocerebellares anterior and posterior and their central connections

a Tractus cerebellaris anterior; **b** Tractus spinocerebellaris posterior.

- Unlike the previously mentioned ascending tracts, both tractus spinocerebellares end in the cerebellum (no conscious processing of information!) mainly in the vermis, which due to the input from the medulla spinalis is functionally referred to as "*Spinocerebellum.*" However, they reach the cerebellum via different pedunculi cerebellares:

  - the tractus spinocerebellaris anterior via the pedunculus cerebellaris superior
  - the tractus spinocerebellaris posterior via the pedunculus cerebellaris inferior

- Like with all other ascending tracts, the cell bodies of the first neurons of both tracts are located in the ganglia sensoria nervorum spinalium. Their axons are IA fibers, which are rapidly conducting,

myelinated fibers. They convey the information from muscle spindles and tendon receptors to the second neurons, which for both tracts are located in the cornu posterius of the medulla spinalis albeit at different places:

- The second neuron of the tractus spinocerebellaris *anterior* is located in the middle of the cornu posterius.
- The second neuron of the tractus cerebellaris *posterior* is located in the nucleus thoracicus posterior, which extends from C8 to L2.

The axons of the tractus spinocerebellaris *posterior* ascend only ipsilaterally to the cerebellum; the axons of the tractus spinocerebellaris *anterior* however, only partly ascend ipsilaterally. A part of the fibers cross in the medulla spinalis and then run contralaterally to the truncus encephali. These contralateral fibers then cross in the velum medullare superius back to their orignal side and thus reach the same side of the cerebellum as the uncrossed fibers.

11.8 Descending Tracts of the Medulla Spinalis: Tractus Pyramidales (Corticospinales)

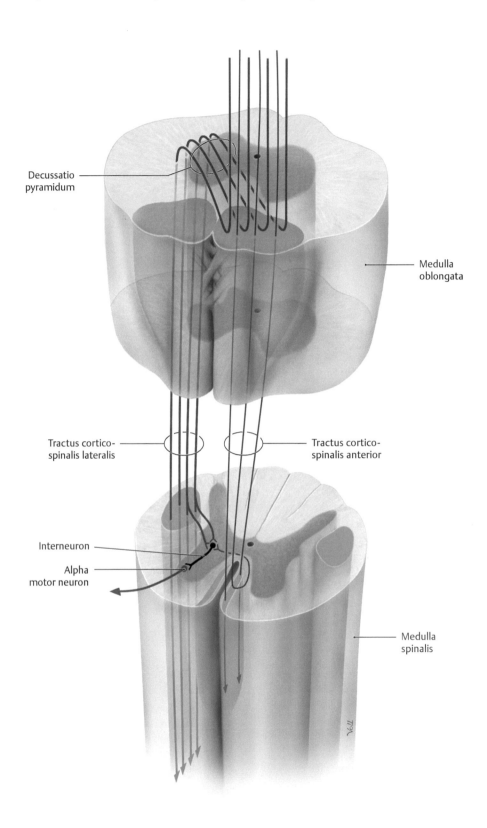

Decussatio pyramidum

Medulla oblongata

Tractus cortico-spinalis lateralis

Tractus cortico-spinalis anterior

Interneuron

Alpha motor neuron

Medulla spinalis

A Course of the tractus corticospinales anterior and lateralis (tractus pyramidales) in the lower medulla oblongata and medulla spinalis

The tractus pyramidalis, which begins in the motor cortex, is the most important pathway for voluntary motor function. Some of its axons,

the *fibrae corticonucleares*, terminate at the nuclei nervorum cranialium while others, the *fibrae corticospinales*, terminate on the motor cornu anterius cells of the medulla spinalis (see **B** for further details). A third group, the *fibrae corticoreticulares*, are distributed to nuclei of the formatio reticularis.

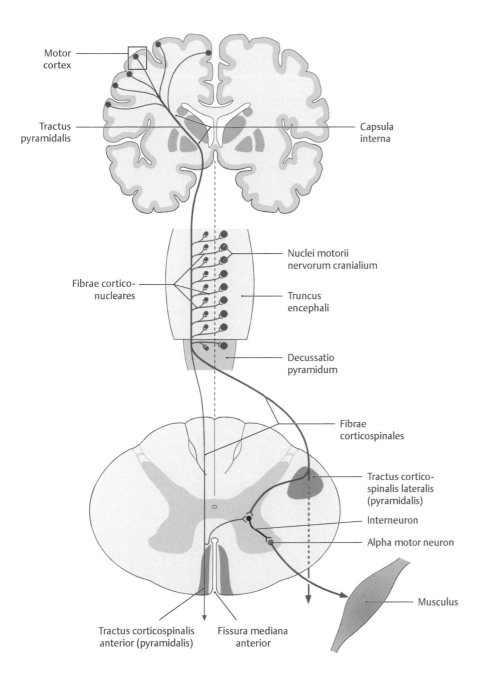

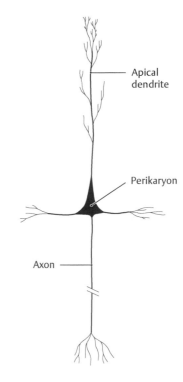

C Silver-impregnation (Golgi) method staining of pyramidal cell

This method produces a silhouette of the stained neurons. The axons of the pyramidal cells form the tractus pyramidalis. Approximately 40% are located in the motor cortex (Brodmann area 4, see p. 328).

B Course of the tractus pyramidalis

- The tractus pyramidalis originates in the motor cortex at the pyramidal cells (large afferent neurons with pyramid-shaped cell bodies, see **C**). The tractus pyramidalis has three components:
  - *Fibrae corticonucleares* for the nuclei nervorum cranialium
  - *Fibrae corticospinales* for the medulla spinalis
  - *Fibrae corticoreticulares* to the formatio reticularis
- All three components pass through the capsula interna from the telencephalon, continuing into the truncus encephali and medulla spinalis.
- In the truncus encephali, the fibrae *corticonucleares* are distributed to the motor nuclei of the nn. craniales.
- The fibrae *corticospinales* descend to the decussatio pyramidum in the lower medulla oblongata, where approximately 80% of them cross to the opposite side. The fibers continue into the medulla spinalis, where they form the tractus corticospinalis lateralis, which has a somatotopic organization: the fibers for the pars sacralis medullae spinalis are the most lateral, while the fibers for the pars cervicalis medullae spinalis are the most medial.

- The remaining 20% of fibrae *corticospinales* continue to descend without crossing, forming the *tractus corticospinalis anterior*, which borders the fissura mediana anterior in a transverse section of the medulla spinalis. The tractus corticospinalis anterior is particularly well developed in the pars cervicalis medullae spinalis, but is not present in the lower partes thoracica, lumbalis, or sacralis medullae spinalis.
- Most fibers of the *tractus corticospinalis anterior* cross at the segmental level to terminate on the same motor neurons as the *tractus corticospinalis lateralis*. The axons of the pyramid cells terminate via intercalated cells on alpha and gamma motor neurons, Renshaw cells, and inhibitory interneurons (not shown).

Lesions of the tractus pyramidalis are discussed on p. 451. Other motor tracts are closely applied to the tractus pyramidalis in the region of the capsula interna and will be described in the next unit. While the tractus pyramidalis controls conscious movement (voluntary motor activity), *supplementary motor tracts* are essential for involuntary muscle processes (e.g., standing, walking, running; see p. 460).

409

11.9 Descending Tracts of the Medulla Spinalis: Extrapyramidal and Autonomic Tracts

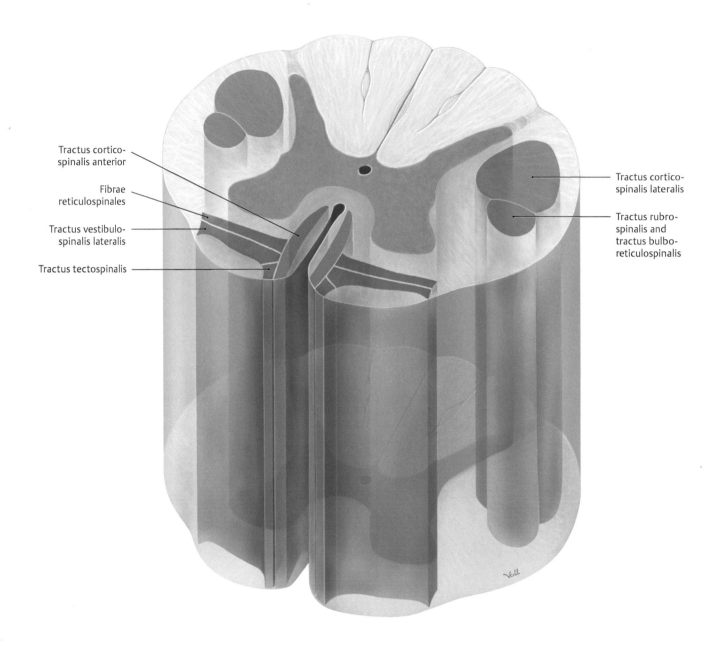

Tractus cortico-spinalis anterior

Fibrae reticulospinales

Tractus vestibulo-spinalis lateralis

Tractus tectospinalis

Tractus cortico-spinalis lateralis

Tractus rubro-spinalis and tractus bulbo-reticulospinalis

A Tracts of the extrapyramidal motor system in the spinal cord
Unlike the pyramidal tract, which controls conscious, voluntary motor activities (e.g., raising a cup to the mouth), the *extra*pyramidal motor system (cerebellum, basal nuclei, and motor nuclei of the brainstem) is necessary for *automatic* and *learned* motor processes (e.g., walking, running, cycling). The division into a pyramidal and extrapyramidal system has proven useful in clinical practice. For central circuitry see **B**. As the tractus pyramidalis and tractus extrapyramidales are closely integrated with one another and course adjacent to each other, injuries generally involve both simultaneously (see p. 394). Isolated lesions of the one system or the other at the spinal cord level are virtually unknown. A recent classification that combines the classic tractus pyramidalis et extrapyramidales differentiates lateral and medial topographic and functional systems. The lateral system includes two tracts: the tractus corticospinalis lateralis (tractus pyramidalis lateralis) and the tractus rubrospinalis. The lateral system projects to the distal musculature of the upper extremity and is responsible for the fine motor function of the hand and arm (in humans the tractus rubrospinalis probably extends only as far as the superior part of the spinalis). The medial system consists of three tracts: the fibrae reticulospinales, the tractus vestibulospinalis lateralis, and the tractus tectospinalis. This system is responsible for motor function in the torso and for postural motor function.

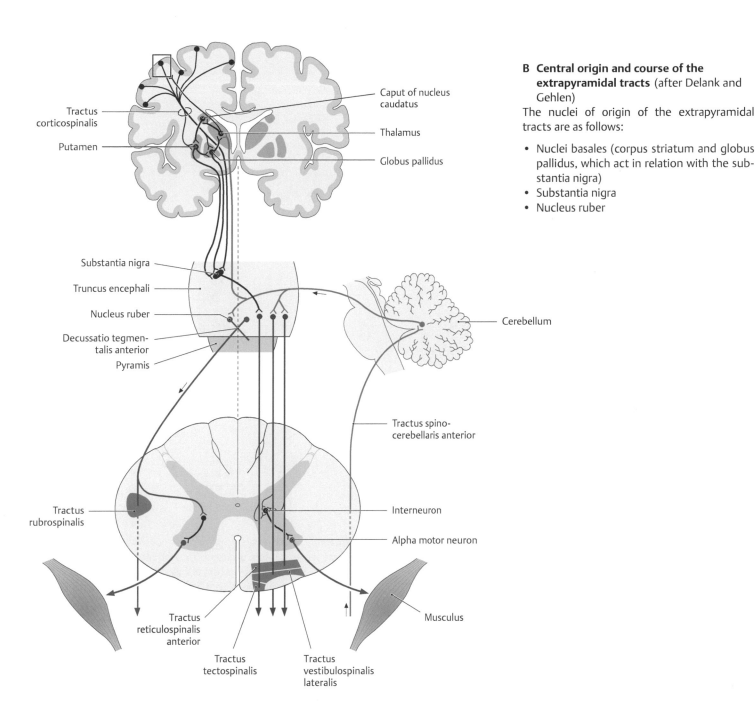

Tractus corticospinalis

Putamen

Caput of nucleus caudatus

Thalamus

Globus pallidus

Substantia nigra

Truncus encephali

Nucleus ruber

Decussatio tegmentalis anterior

Pyramis

Cerebellum

Tractus spinocerebellaris anterior

Tractus rubrospinalis

Interneuron

Alpha motor neuron

Musculus

Tractus reticulospinalis anterior

Tractus tectospinalis

Tractus vestibulospinalis lateralis

B Central origin and course of the extrapyramidal tracts (after Delank and Gehlen)

The nuclei of origin of the extrapyramidal tracts are as follows:

- Nuclei basales (corpus striatum and globus pallidus, which act in relation with the substantia nigra)
- Substantia nigra
- Nucleus ruber

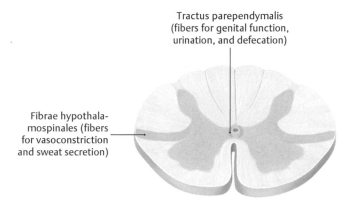

Tractus parependymalis (fibers for genital function, urination, and defecation)

Fibrae hypothalamospinales (fibers for vasoconstriction and sweat secretion)

C Autonomic pathways of the medulla spinalis

Autonomic pathways have a somewhat diffuse arrangement in the medulla spinalis and rarely form closed tract systems. There are two exceptions:

1. The descending central sympathetic tract for vasoconstriction and sweat secretion (fibrae hypothalamospinales) borders the tractus pyramidalis anteriorly and shows the same somatotopic organization as the tractus pyramidalis.
2. The tractus parependymalis runs on both sides of the canalis centralis and contains both ascending and descending fibers. Passing from the medulla spinalis to the hypothalamus, this tract is concerned with urination, defecation, and genital functions.

411

11.10 Tracts of the Medulla Spinalis, Overview

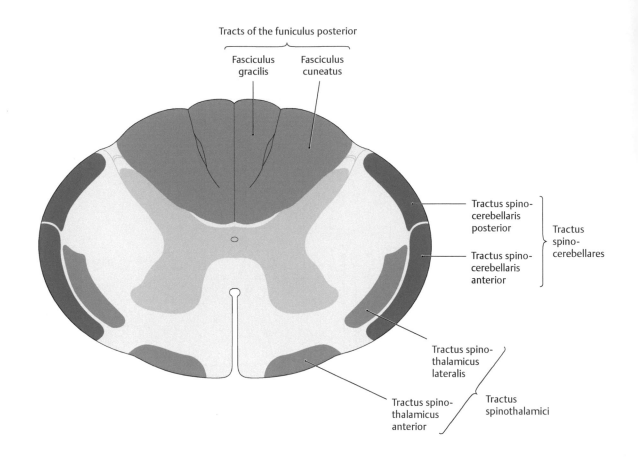

A Ascending tracts in the medulla spinalis

Transverse section through the medulla spinalis. Ascending tracts are afferent (= sensory) pathways that carry information from the trunk and limbs to the brain. The most important ascending tracts and their functions are listed below.

Tractus spinothalamici

– Tractus spinothalamicus anterior (coarse touch sensation)
– Tractus spinothalamicus lateralis (pain and temperature sensation)

Tracts of the funiculus posterior

– Fasciculus gracilis (fine touch sensation, conscious proprioception of the *lower* limb)
– Fasciculus cuneatus (fine touch sensation, conscious proprioception of the *upper* limb).

Tractus spinocerebellares

– Tractus spinocerebellaris anterior (unconscious proprioception to the cerebellum)
– Tractus spinocerebellaris posterior (unconscious proprioception to the cerebellum)

Proprioception involves the perception of limb position in space ("position sense"). It lets us know, for example, that our arm is in front of or behind our chest even when our eyes are closed. The information involved in proprioception is complex. Thus, our position sense tells us where our joints are in relation to one another while our motion sense tells us the speed and direction of joint movements. We also have a "force sense" by which we can perceive the muscular force that is associated with joint movements. Moreover, proprioception takes place on both a conscious (I know that my hand is making a fist in my pants pocket without seeing it) and an unconscious level, enabling us to ride a bicycle and climb stairs without thinking about it. The table on p. 445 gives a comprehensive review of all the ascending tracts.

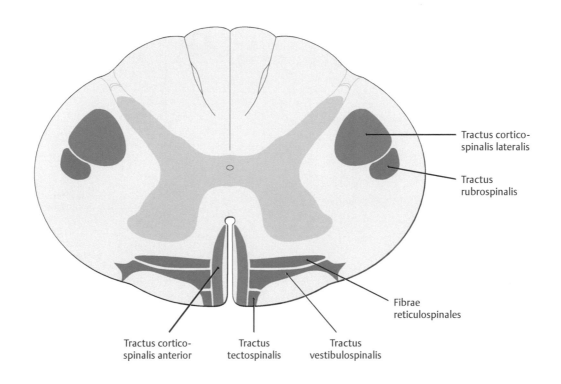

Tractus cortico-
spinalis lateralis

Tractus
rubrospinalis

Fibrae
reticulospinales

Tractus cortico-   Tractus   Tractus
spinalis anterior   tectospinalis   vestibulospinalis

B Descending tracts in the medulla spinalis
Transverse section through the medulla spinalis. The descending tracts of the medulla spinalis are concerned with motor function. They convey information from higher motor centers to the motor neurons in the medulla spinalis. According to a relatively recent classification (not yet fully accepted in clinical medicine), the descending tracts of the medulla spinalis can be divided into two motor systems:

- **Lateral motor system** (concerned with fine, precise motor skills in the hands):
  - Tractus pyramidalis (tractus corticospinalis anterior and lateralis)
  - Tractus rubrospinalis
- **Medial motor system** (innervates medially situated motor neurons controlling trunk movement and stance):
  - Fibrae reticulospinales
  - Tractus tectospinalis
  - Tractus vestibulospinales

Except for the tractus pyramidalis, which may be represented as a monosynaptic pathway in a simplified scheme, it is difficult to offer a simple and direct classification of the motor system because sequences of movements are programmed and coordinated in multiple feedback mechanisms called "motor loops" (see p. 459). There is no point, then, in listing the various tracts in a simplified table. While the tracts can be distinguished rather clearly from one another at the level of the medulla spinalis, their fibers are so intermixed at the higher cortical levels that isolated motor disturbances (unlike sensory disturbances) essentially do not occur at the level of the medulla spinalis.

11.11 Blood Vessels of the Medulla Spinalis: Arteries

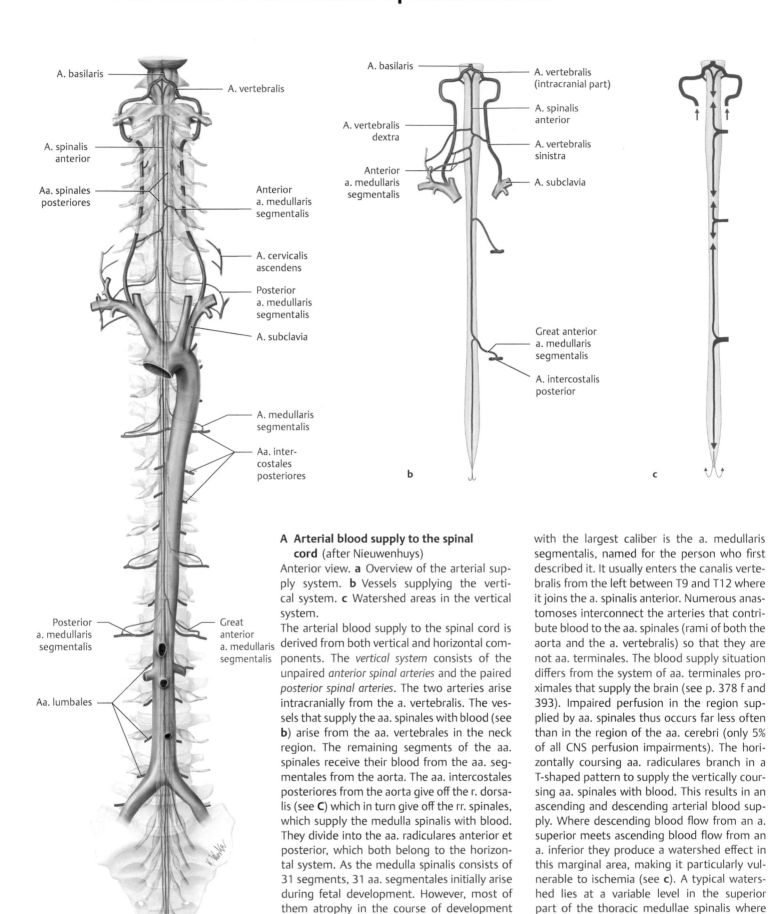

A Arterial blood supply to the spinal cord (after Nieuwenhuys)

Anterior view. **a** Overview of the arterial supply system. **b** Vessels supplying the vertical system. **c** Watershed areas in the vertical system.

The arterial blood supply to the spinal cord is derived from both vertical and horizontal components. The *vertical system* consists of the unpaired *anterior spinal arteries* and the paired *posterior spinal arteries*. The two arteries arise intracranially from the a. vertebralis. The vessels that supply the aa. spinales with blood (see **b**) arise from the aa. vertebrales in the neck region. The remaining segments of the aa. spinales receive their blood from the aa. segmentales from the aorta. The aa. intercostales posteriores from the aorta give off the r. dorsalis (see **C**) which in turn give off the rr. spinales, which supply the medulla spinalis with blood. They divide into the aa. radiculares anterior et posterior, which both belong to the horizontal system. As the medulla spinalis consists of 31 segments, 31 aa. segmentales initially arise during fetal development. However, most of them atrophy in the course of development so that on average only six aa. anteriores and twelve aa. posteriores persist (at individually variable segment levels). The a. segmentalis with the largest caliber is the a. medullaris segmentalis, named for the person who first described it. It usually enters the canalis vertebralis from the left between T9 and T12 where it joins the a. spinalis anterior. Numerous anastomoses interconnect the arteries that contribute blood to the aa. spinales (rami of both the aorta and the a. vertebralis) so that they are not aa. terminales. The blood supply situation differs from the system of aa. terminales proximales that supply the brain (see p. 378 f and 393). Impaired perfusion in the region supplied by aa. spinales thus occurs far less often than in the region of the aa. cerebri (only 5% of all CNS perfusion impairments). The horizontally coursing aa. radiculares branch in a T-shaped pattern to supply the vertically coursing aa. spinales with blood. This results in an ascending and descending arterial blood supply. Where descending blood flow from an a. superior meets ascending blood flow from an a. inferior they produce a watershed effect in this marginal area, making it particularly vulnerable to ischemia (see **c**). A typical watershed lies at a variable level in the superior part of the thoracic medullae spinalis where blood flows from the a. subclavia and aorta meet. This region is particularly vulnerable to infarction.

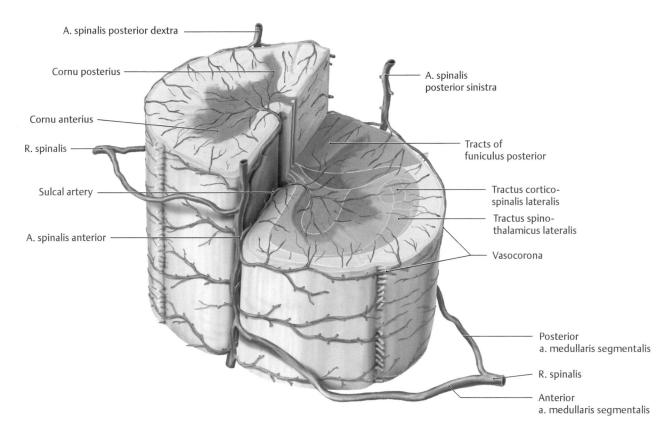

A. spinalis posterior dextra

Cornu posterius

Cornu anterius

R. spinalis

Sulcal artery

A. spinalis anterior

A. spinalis posterior sinistra

Tracts of funiculus posterior

Tractus cortico-spinalis lateralis

Tractus spino-thalamicus lateralis

Vasocorona

Posterior a. medullaris segmentalis

R. spinalis

Anterior a. medullaris segmentalis

B Blood supply to the spinal cord segments

In each spinal cord segment, the *a. spinalis anterior* gives off several (5–9) **sulcal arteries** which course posteriorly in the fissura mediana anterior. Typically, each sulcal artery enters one half of the medulla spinalis, supplying the cornu anterius, base of the cornu posterius, and the funiculi anterior and lateralis (approximately two-thirds of the total area) in that half; the sulcal arteries tend to alternate direction (left or right) to supply both halves of the spinal cord segment. The paired *aa. spinales posteriores* provide the blood supply to the posterior one-third of the cord, including the cornu posterius and funiculus posterior. All three aa. spinales contribute numerous delicate anastomosing **vasocoronae** on the pial surface of the medulla spinalis which in turn send branches into the periphery of the cord. The sulcal arteries are the only end-arteries within the medulla spinalis, and their occlusion may produce clinical symptoms. Occlusion of the a. spinalis anterior at segmental levels may damage the cornu anterius and radices anteriores resulting in flaccid paralysis of the muscles supplied by these segments. If the tractus corticospinalis lateralis in the funiculus lateralis is involved, spastic paralysis will develop below the lesion level. An occlusion of the aa. spinales posteriores in one or more segments will affect the cornu posterius and funiculus posterior leading to disturbances of proprioception, vibration, and pressure sensation.

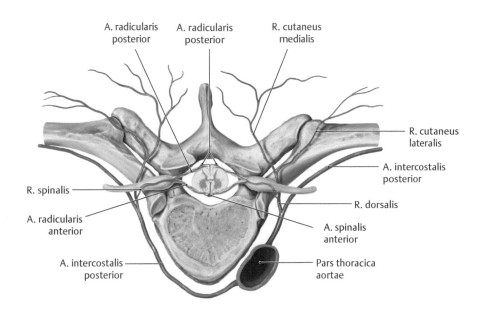

A. radicularis posterior

A. radicularis posterior

R. cutaneus medialis

R. cutaneus lateralis

A. intercostalis posterior

R. dorsalis

A. spinalis anterior

Pars thoracica aortae

R. spinalis

A. radicularis anterior

A. intercostalis posterior

C Blood vessels supplying the medulla spinalis

Thoracic vertebra viewed from above. The rr. spinales arise from the posterior branches of aa. medullares segmentales and divide into an a. radicularis anterior and an a. radicularis posterior. The aa. radiculares supply the radices posteriores and anteriores nervorum spinalium, and peripheral portions of the cornua posteriora and anteriora; they also communicate with the vasocorona. These arteries have a better developed connection with the a. spinalis anterior at some levels and with the aa. spinales posteriores at other levels.

415

11.12 Blood Vessels of the Medulla Spinalis: Veins

A Venous drainage of the medulla spinalis
(after Nieuwenhuys)

Anterior view. Analogous to the arterial supply, the venous drainage of the medulla spinalis consists of a *horizontal system* (venous rings, see **B**) and a vertical system that drains the venous rings. The vertical system is illustrated here. While the arterial blood supply is based on three vessels, the interior of the medulla spinalis drains through venous plexuses into only two unpaired vessels: a v. spinalis anterior and a v. spinalis posterior (see **B**). The v. spinalis *anterior* communicates superiorly with veins of the truncus encephali. Its lower portion enters the filum terminale (a glial filament extending from the conus medullaris to the sacral end of the dural sac, where it is attached). The larger v. spinalis *posterior* communicates with the **radicular veins** at the cervical level and ends at the conus medullaris. The radicular veins connect these veins, which lie within the pia mater, with the plexus venosi vertebrales interni (see **C**). Blood from the cord drains into the **vv. vertebrales**, which open into the vena cava superior. Blood from the pars thoracica medullae spinalis drains into the **vv. intercostales**, which drain into the vena cava superior via the vv. azygos and hemiazygos system. Radicular veins are present at only certain segments, as shown. Their distribution varies among individuals.

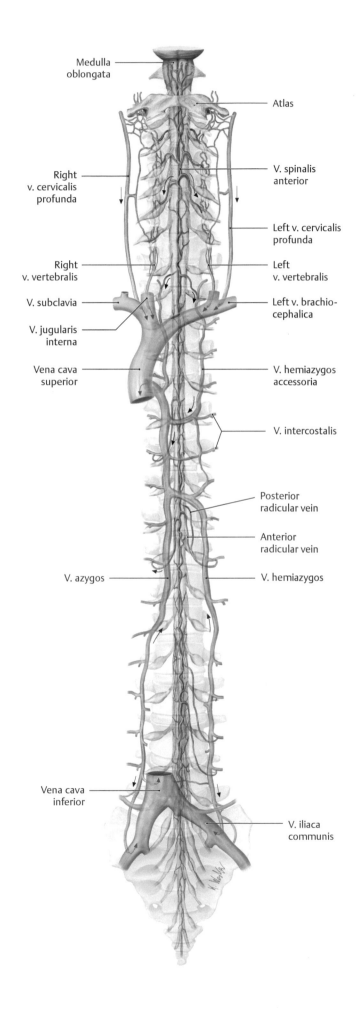

Medulla oblongata

Atlas

Right v. cervicalis profunda

V. spinalis anterior

Left v. cervicalis profunda

Right v. vertebralis

Left v. vertebralis

V. subclavia

Left v. brachiocephalica

V. jugularis interna

Vena cava superior

V. hemiazygos accessoria

V. intercostalis

Posterior radicular vein

Anterior radicular vein

V. azygos

V. hemiazygos

Vena cava inferior

V. iliaca communis

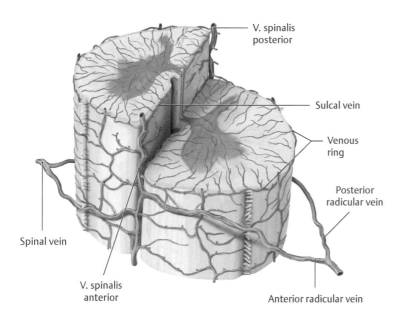

V. spinalis
posterior

Sulcal vein

Venous
ring

Posterior
radicular vein

Spinal vein

V. spinalis
anterior

Anterior radicular vein

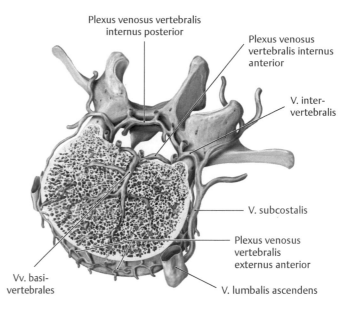

Plexus venosus vertebralis
internus posterior

Plexus venosus
vertebralis internus
anterior

V. inter-
vertebralis

V. subcostalis

Plexus venosus
vertebralis
externus anterior

Vv. basi-
vertebrales

V. lumbalis ascendens

B Venous drainage of a spinal cord segment

Anterior view from upper left. A medulla spinalis segment is drained by the vv. spinales anterior and posterior. These vessels are located within the pia mater and are interconnected by an anastomotic venous ring. Both veins channel blood through the radicular veins to the plexus venosi vertebrales interni (see **C**). Unlike the radicular veins, the veins *inside* the medulla spinalis have no valves. As a result, venous stasis may cause a hazardous rise of pressure in the medulla spinalis. A typical cause of increased intramedullary venous pressure is an arteriovenous fistula, which is an abnormal communication between an artery and vein in the medulla spinalis. Because the pressure in the arteries is higher than in the veins, arterial blood tends to enter the veins of the medulla spinalis through the fistulous connection. The fistula will remain asymptomatic as long as the intramedullary veins maintain an adequate drainage capacity. But if the flow across the fistula outstrips their drainage capacity, the functions of the medulla spinalis will be impaired by the increased pressure. This is manifested clinically by disturbances of gait, spastic paralysis, and sensory disturbances. Untreated, the decompensated fistula will eventually cause a complete functional transection of the medulla spinalis. The treatment of choice is surgical correction of the fistula.

C Plexus venosus vertebralis

Transverse section viewed obliquely from upper left. The veins of the medulla spinalis and its coverings are connected to the plexus venosi vertebrales interni via the radicular veins and vv. spinales. Located in the fatty tissue of the spatium epidurale, this plexus occupies the inner circumference of the canalis vertebralis. The internal plexus is connected to the plexus venosi vertebrales interni by the vv. *inter*vertebrales and *basi*vertebrales. Anastomoses exist between the tributary regions of the vv. spinales anteriores and posteriores. Oblique anastomoses are located in the interior of the medulla spinalis and may extend over several segments (not shown). These connections are particularly important in maintaining a constant intramedullary venous pressure.

D Epidural veins in the partes sacralis and lumbalis canalis vertebralis (after Nieuwenhuys)

Posterior view (canalis vertebralis windowed). The internal veins of the medulla spinalis are valveless up to the point at which they emerge from the dura mater spinalis. The plexus venosus vertebralis internus is connected by other valveless veins (not shown here) to the plexus venosus prostaticus. It is relatively easy for prostatic carcinoma cells to pass along the veins of the plexus venosus prostaticus to the plexus venosus sacralis and destroy the surrounding tissue. For this reason, prostatic carcinoma frequently metastasizes to this region and destroys the surrounding bone, resulting in severe pain.

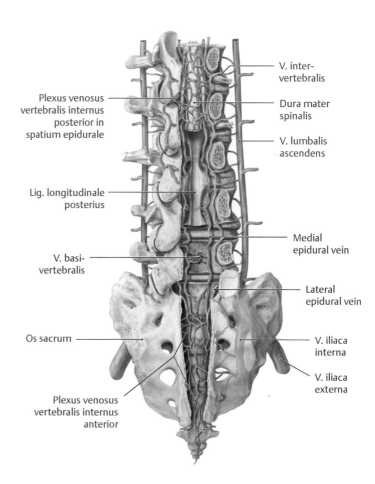

V. inter-
vertebralis

Plexus venosus
vertebralis internus
posterior in
spatium epidurale

Dura mater
spinalis

V. lumbalis
ascendens

Lig. longitudinale
posterius

Medial
epidural vein

V. basi-
vertebralis

Lateral
epidural vein

Os sacrum

V. iliaca
interna

V. iliaca
externa

Plexus venosus
vertebralis internus
anterior

11.13 Medulla Spinalis, Topography

A Medulla spinalis and nervus spinalis in the canalis vertebralis at the level of the C4 vertebra

Transverse section viewed from above. The medulla spinalis occupies the center of the foramen vertebrale and is anchored within the spatium subarachnoideum to the dura mater spinalis by the lig. denticulatum. The root sleeve, an outpouching of the dura mater in the foramen intervertebrale, contains the ganglion sensorium and the radices posterior and anterior of the n. spinalis. The dura mater spinalis is bounded externally by the spatium epidurale, which contains venous plexuses, fat, and connective tissue. The spatium epidurale extends upward as far as the foramen magnum, where the dura becomes fused to the cranial periosteum (see p. 311)

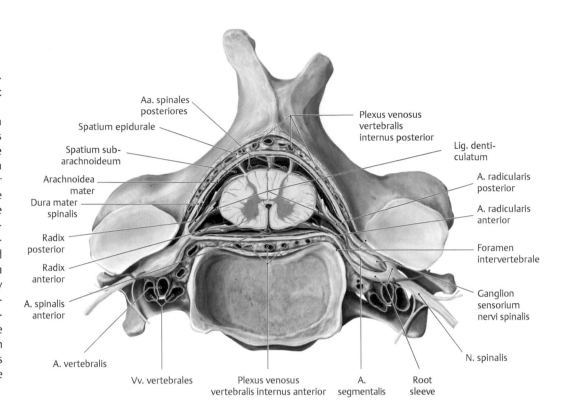

Aa. spinales posteriores
Spatium epidurale
Spatium subarachnoideum
Arachnoidea mater
Dura mater spinalis
Radix posterior
Radix anterior
A. spinalis anterior
A. vertebralis
Vv. vertebrales
Plexus venosus vertebralis internus anterior
A. segmentalis
Root sleeve
Plexus venosus vertebralis internus posterior
Lig. denticulatum
A. radicularis posterior
A. radicularis anterior
Foramen intervertebrale
Ganglion sensorium nervi spinalis
N. spinalis

B Cauda equina at the level of the L2 vertebra

Transverse section viewed from below. The medulla spinalis usually ends at the level of the first lumbar vertebra (L1). The space below the lower end of the medulla spinalis is occupied by the cauda equina and filum terminale in the dural sac (cisterna lumbalis, see p. 311), which ends at the level of the S2 vertebra (see **C** and **D**). The spatium epidurale expands at that level and contains extensive venous plexuses and fatty tissue.

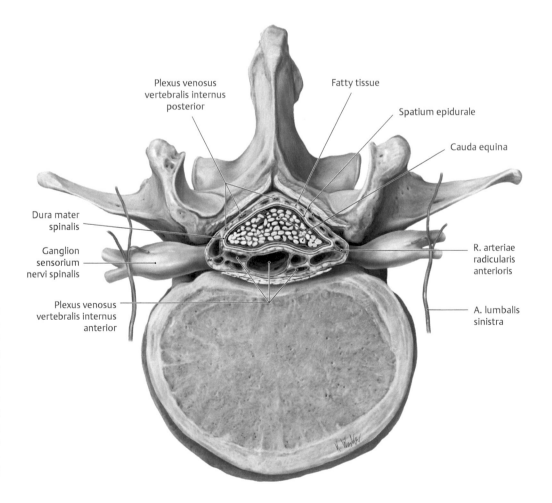

Plexus venosus vertebralis internus posterior
Dura mater spinalis
Ganglion sensorium nervi spinalis
Plexus venosus vertebralis internus anterior
Fatty tissue
Spatium epidurale
Cauda equina
R. arteriae radicularis anterioris
A. lumbalis sinistra

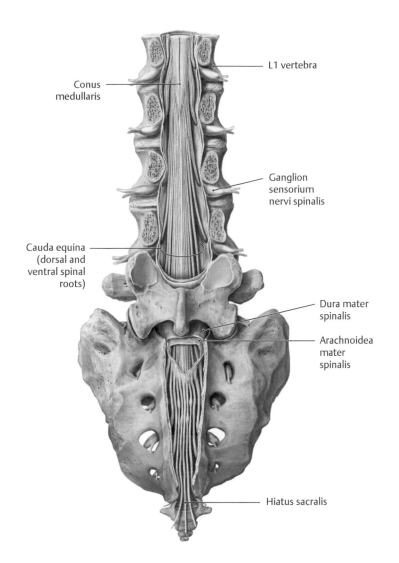

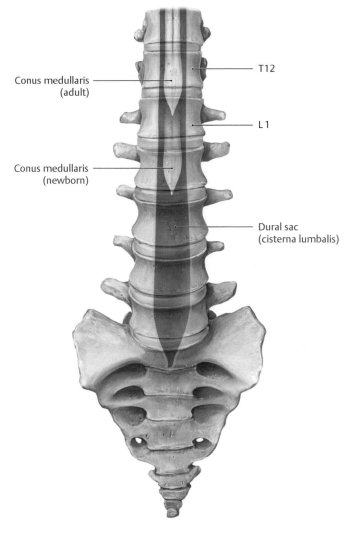

Conus
medullaris

L1 vertebra

Ganglion
sensorium
nervi spinalis

Cauda equina
(dorsal and
ventral spinal
roots)

Dura mater
spinalis

Arachnoidea
mater
spinalis

Hiatus sacralis

Conus medullaris
(adult)

T12

L1

Conus medullaris
(newborn)

Dural sac
(cisterna lumbalis)

C Cauda equina in the canalis vertebralis

Posterior view. The laminae and the dorsal surface of the os sacrum have been partially removed. The medulla spinalis in the adult terminates at approximately the level of the first lumbar vertebra (L1). The radices posterior and anterior nervorum spinalium extending from the lower end of the medulla spinalis (conus medullaris) are known collectively as the cauda equina. During lumbar puncture at this level, a needle introduced into the spatium subarachnoideum (cisterna lumbalis) normally slips past the radices nervorum spinalium without injuring them.

D The medulla spinalis, dural sac, and columna vertebralis at different ages

Anterior view. As an individual grows, the longitudinal growth of the medulla spinalis increasingly lags behind that of the columna vertebralis. At birth the distal end of the medulla spinalis, the conus medullaris, is at the level of the L3 vertebral body (where lumbar puncture is contraindicated). The medulla spinalis of a tall adult ends at the T12/L1 level, while that of a short adult extends to the L2/L3 level. The dural sac always extends into the upper os sacrum. It is important to consider these anatomical relationships during lumbar puncture. It is best to introduce the needle at the L3/L4 interspace.

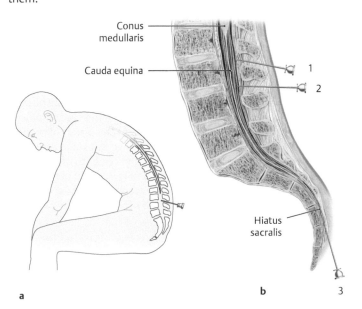

Conus
medullaris

Cauda equina

1

2

Hiatus
sacralis

a

b

3

E Lumbar puncture, epidural anesthesia, and lumbar anesthesia

In preparation for a **lumbar puncture**, the patient bends far forward to separate the procc. spinosi of the lumbar spine. The spinal needle is usually introduced between the procc. spinosi of the L3 and L4 vertebrae. It is advanced through the skin and into the dural sac (cisterna lumbalis) to obtain a liquor cerebrospinalis sample. This procedure has numerous applications, including the diagnosis of meningitis. For **epidural anesthesia**, a catheter is placed in the spatium epidurale without penetrating the dural sac (1). **Lumbar anesthesia** is induced by injecting a local anesthetic solution into the dural sac (2). Another option is to pass the needle into the spatium epidurale through the hiatus sacralis (3).

419

12.1 Coronal Sections: I and II (Frontal)

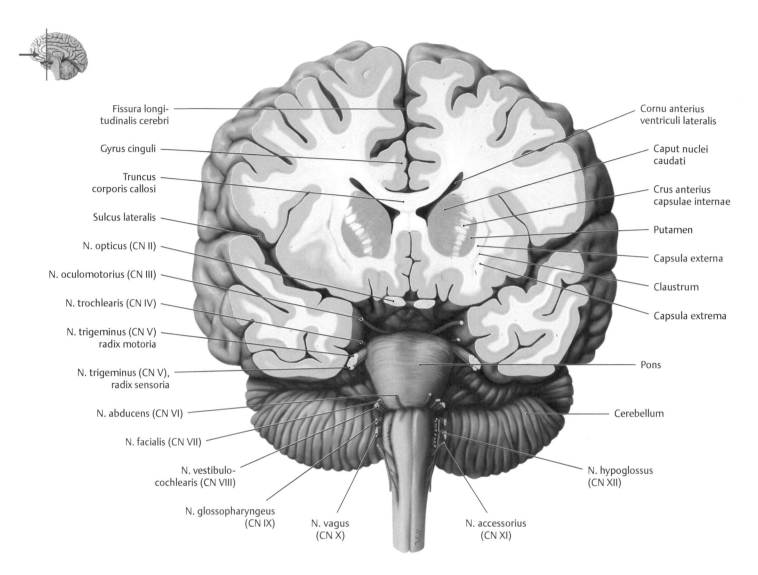

Fissura longi-
tudinalis cerebri

Gyrus cinguli

Truncus
corporis callosi

Sulcus lateralis

N. opticus (CN II)

N. oculomotorius (CN III)

N. trochlearis (CN IV)

N. trigeminus (CN V)
radix motoria

N. trigeminus (CN V),
radix sensoria

N. abducens (CN VI)

N. facialis (CN VII)

N. vestibulo-
cochlearis (CN VIII)

N. glossopharyngeus
(CN IX)

N. vagus
(CN X)

N. accessorius
(CN XI)

Cornu anterius
ventriculi lateralis

Caput nuclei
caudati

Crus anterius
capsulae internae

Putamen

Capsula externa

Claustrum

Capsula extrema

Pons

Cerebellum

N. hypoglossus
(CN XII)

General remarks on sectional brain anatomy

The series of sections (coronal, transverse, and sagittal) in this chapter
The series of sections (coronal, transverse, and sagittal) in this chapter is intended to help the reader gain an appreciation of the three-
dimensional anatomy of the brain. This is necessary for the correct
interpretation of modern sectional imaging modalities (CT and MRI for
the investigation of suspected stroke, encephalon tumors, meningitis,
and trauma). In offering this synoptic perspective, we assume that the
reader has read the previous chapters and has gained at least a general
appreciation of the functional and descriptive anatomy of the encephalon. The legends and especially the small accompanying schematic diagrams are intended to facilitate a three-dimensional understanding of
the two-dimensional sections (the plane of the section in each figure is
indicated by a red line in the small, inset image).

The planes of section have been selected to display the structures of
greatest clinical importance more clearly than can be done in actual
tissue sections, which are not always optimally fixed and preserved.
Because the sections were modeled on specimens taken from different
individuals, some structures will not be found at the same location in
every figure. The structures of the encephalon were assigned to specific ontogenetic regions in previous chapters, and these relationships are
summarized in **B**, p. 443, at the end of this chapter.

Note the relationship of the sectional planes to the Forel axis in the
anterior part of the encephalon and to the Meynert axis in the truncus
encephali region (see **B**, p. 270).

A Coronal section I

The body (trunk) of the *corpus callosum*, which interconnects the two
hemispheria cerebri, is prominently displayed in this coronal section.
Superior to the corpus callosum is the *gyrus cinguli*, which also appears
in subsequent sections. Inferior to the corpus callosum is the *nucleus
caudatus*, which appears particularly large because this section passes
through the widest portion of its caput (see **C**). The nucleus appears different in later sections because it tapers occipitally to a narrow cauda
(see the units that follow). The schematic lateral view (**C**) shows how the
nucleus caudatus is closely applied to the *ventriculus lateralis* and follows
its concavity (shown in green). The nucleus caudatus and the putamen
together form the corpus striatum, whose "striation" is formed by the
crus anterius of the capsula interna, a streak of substantia alba. The putamen still appears quite small at this level because the section passes
only through its anterior tip. It becomes larger as the planes of section
move further occipitally. The structures anterior to this plane consist of
the cortex and substantia alba of the lobus frontalis, both of which are
easily identified. The lobi temporales, which still appear to be separate,
detached structures, join the rest of the telencephalon in more occipital
sectional planes (see **B**).

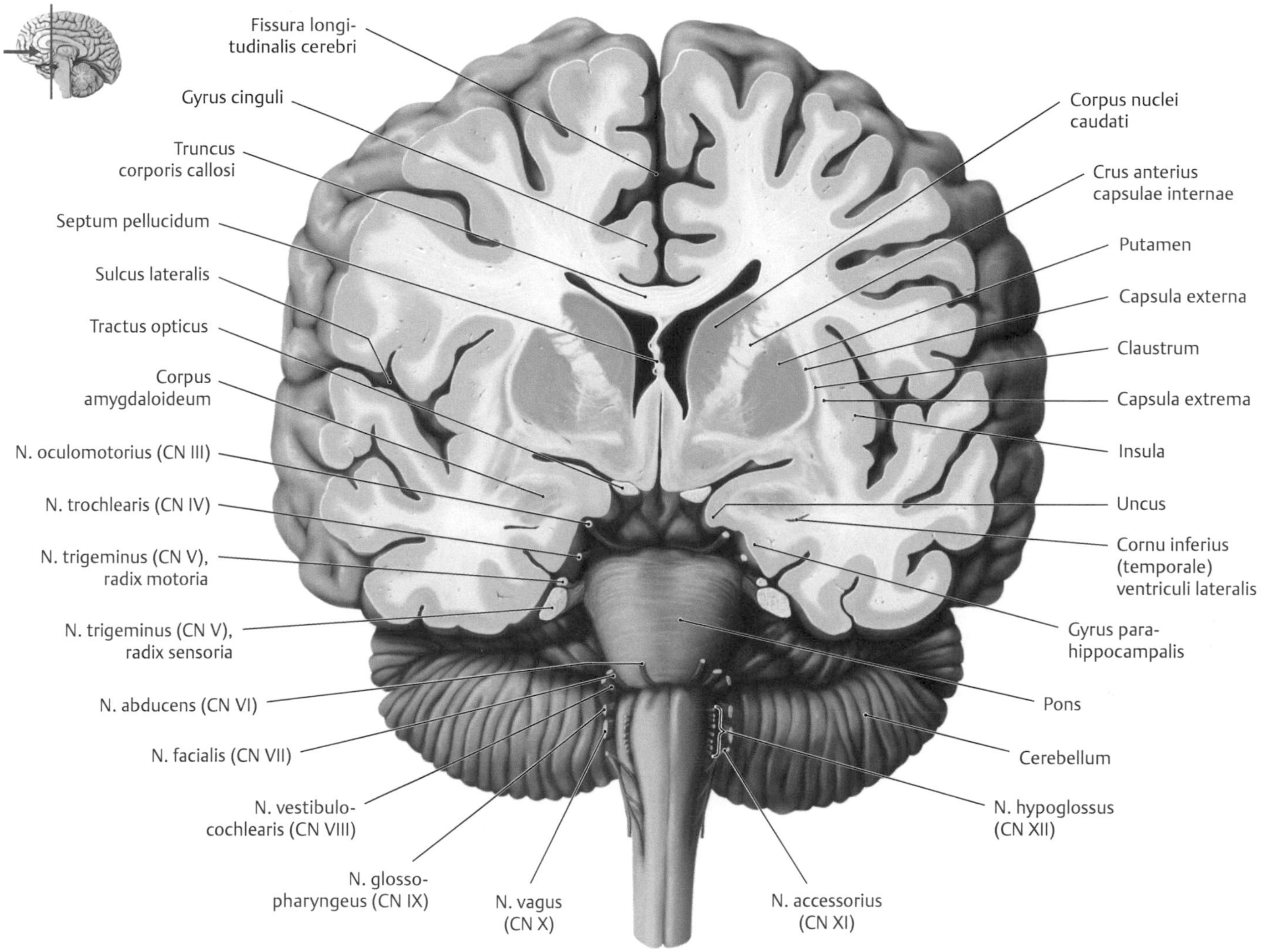
Fissura longitudinalis cerebri
Gyrus cinguli
Truncus corporis callosi
Septum pellucidum
Sulcus lateralis
Tractus opticus
Corpus amygdaloideum
N. oculomotorius (CN III)
N. trochlearis (CN IV)
N. trigeminus (CN V), radix motoria
N. trigeminus (CN V), radix sensoria
N. abducens (CN VI)
N. facialis (CN VII)
N. vestibulocochlearis (CN VIII)
N. glossopharyngeus (CN IX)
N. vagus (CN X)
N. accessorius (CN XI)
N. hypoglossus (CN XII)
Cerebellum
Pons
Gyrus parahippocampalis
Cornu inferius (temporale) ventriculi lateralis
Uncus
Insula
Capsula extrema
Claustrum
Capsula externa
Putamen
Crus anterius capsulae internae
Corpus nuclei caudati

B Coronal section II
This section contains essentially the same structures as in **A**. The plane no longer passes through the *caput* of the nucleus caudatus, instead passing through its slender corpus. The *cornu inferius* (cornu temporale) of the ventriculus lateralis appears as a slitlike structure and also provides a useful landmark: ventral to the cornu inferius is a portion of the *gyrus parahippocampalis*. Superior and medial to the cornu inferius is the *amygdala* (corpus amygdaloideum, visible here for the first time; compare with **D**). The corpus amygdaloideum is bordered by the *uncus*, which is the hook-shaped anterior end of the gyrus parahippocampalis. The capsula interna, which pierces the corpus striatum, appears considerably thicker in this plane than in **A**. The lobus temporalis has merged at this level with the rest of the telencephalon, and the *insular cortex* is clearly visible.

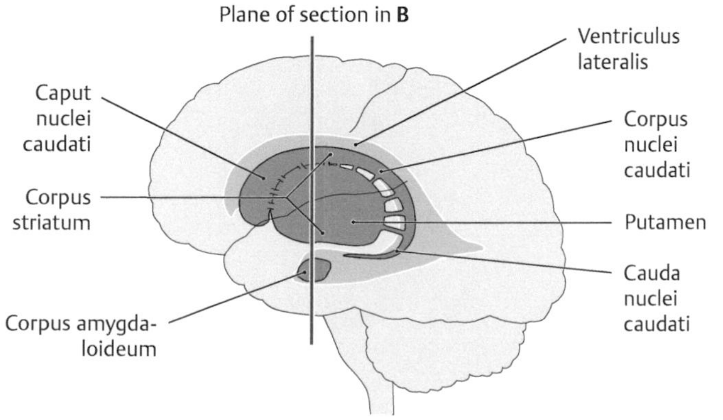
Plane of section in B
Ventriculus lateralis
Caput nuclei caudati
Corpus nuclei caudati
Corpus striatum
Putamen
Cauda nuclei caudati
Corpus amygdaloideum

C Relationship between the caudate nucleus and lateral ventricle
Left lateral view.

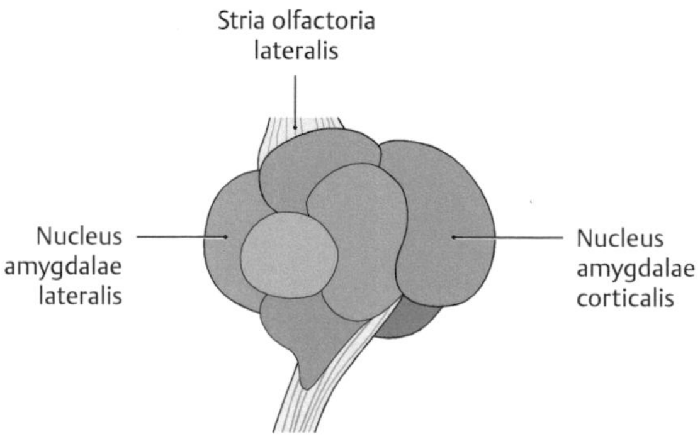
Stria olfactoria lateralis
Nucleus amygdalae lateralis
Nucleus amygdalae corticalis

D Corpus amygdaloideum
Right lateral view.

12.2 Coronal Sections: III and IV

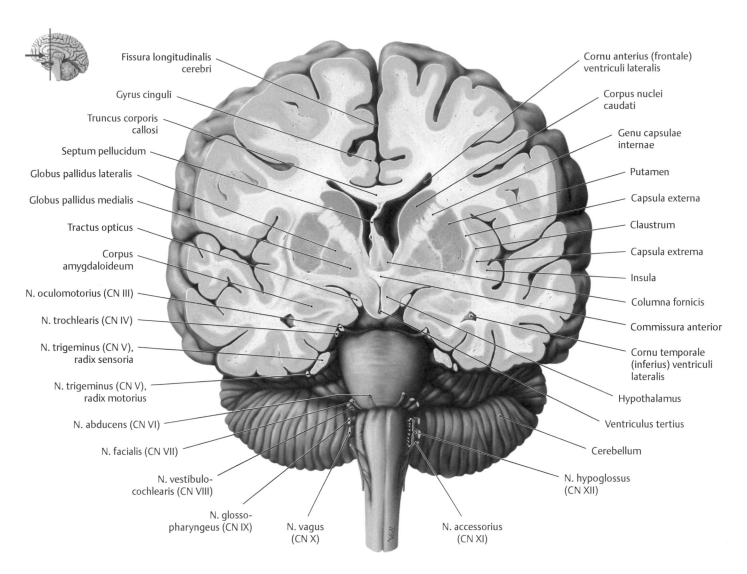

A **Coronal section III**

The cornu inferius (temporale) of the ventriculus lateralis appears somewhat larger in the plane of this section. In the ventricular system, we can now see the floor of the *ventriculus tertius* (see **B**) and the surrounding hypothalamus. The thalamus cannot yet be seen given that it lies slightly above and behind the hypothalamus. The *commissura anterior* appears in this plane as does the *globus pallidus*, which consists of a medial and a lateral segment. The large descending pathway, the fibrae corticospinales, passes through the capsula interna, which has a somatotopic organization. The genu *capsulae internae* transmits axons of the fibrae corticonucleares. The course of these axons is shown schematically in **C** (the fornix appears in **D**).

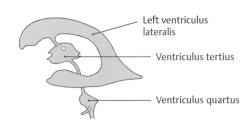

B **Ventricular system**
Left lateral view.

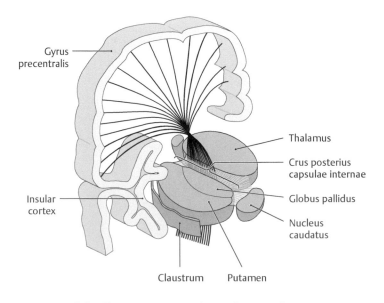

C **Course of the fibrae corticospinales in the capsula interna**
Left anterior view.

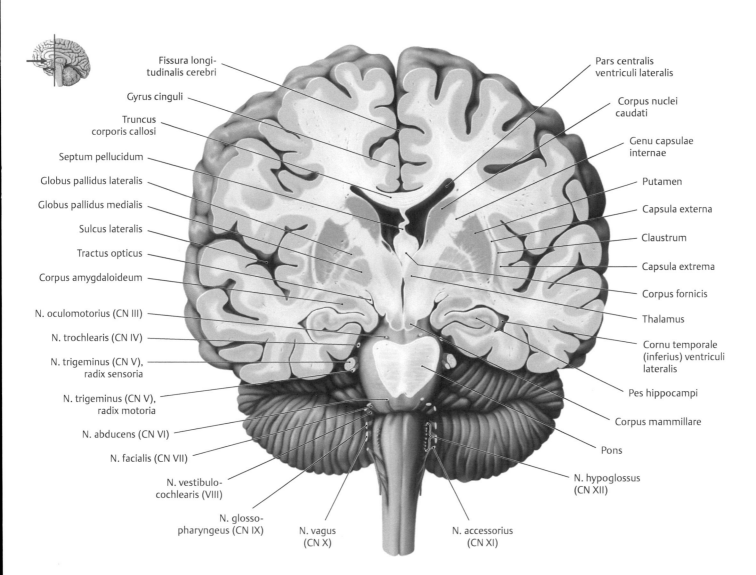

Fissura longi-
tudinalis cerebri

Gyrus cinguli

Truncus
corporis callosi

Septum pellucidum

Globus pallidus lateralis

Globus pallidus medialis

Sulcus lateralis

Tractus opticus

Corpus amygdaloideum

N. oculomotorius (CN III)

N. trochlearis (CN IV)

N. trigeminus (CN V),
radix sensoria

N. trigeminus (CN V),
radix motoria

N. abducens (CN VI)

N. facialis (CN VII)

N. vestibulo-
cochlearis (VIII)

N. glosso-
pharyngeus (CN IX)

N. vagus
(CN X)

N. accessorius
(CN XI)

Pars centralis
ventriculi lateralis

Corpus nuclei
caudati

Genu capsulae
internae

Putamen

Capsula externa

Claustrum

Capsula extrema

Corpus fornicis

Thalamus

Cornu temporale
(inferius) ventriculi
lateralis

Pes hippocampi

Corpus mammillare

Pons

N. hypoglossus
(CN XII)

D Coronal section IV

The division of the globus pallidus into medial and lateral segments can now be seen clearly. This section displays the full width of both the cornu inferior of the ventriculus lateralis and the *claustrum* (believed to be important in the regulation of sexual behavior). While the plane in A passed through the commissura anterior, this more occipital plane slices the corpora mammillaria (see E). Pathological changes in the corpora mammillaria can be found during autopsy of chronic alcoholics. The corpora mammillaria are flanked on each side by the pes *hippocampi*.

An important part of the limbic system, the corpora mammillaria are connected to the hippocampus by the *fornix* (see **F**). Due to the anatomical curvature of the fornix, its *columnae* are visible in more frontal sections (see **A**), while its *crura* appear as widely separated structures in more occipital sections (see **C**, p. 427). The *septum pellucidum* stretches between the fornix and corpus callosum, forming the medial boundary of the ventriculi laterales (see **A** and **D**).

The first structure of the truncus encephali, the pons, can also be identified in this section.

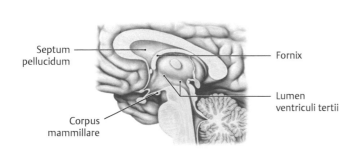

Septum
pellucidum

Fornix

Lumen
ventriculi tertii

Corpus
mammillare

E Midsagittal section through the diencephalon and truncus encephali

Lateral view.

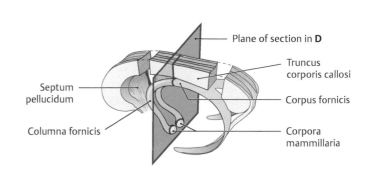

Plane of section in **D**

Truncus
corporis callosi

Corpus fornicis

Corpora
mammillaria

Septum
pellucidum

Columna fornicis

F Corpora mammillaria and fornix

423

12.3 Coronal Sections: V and VI

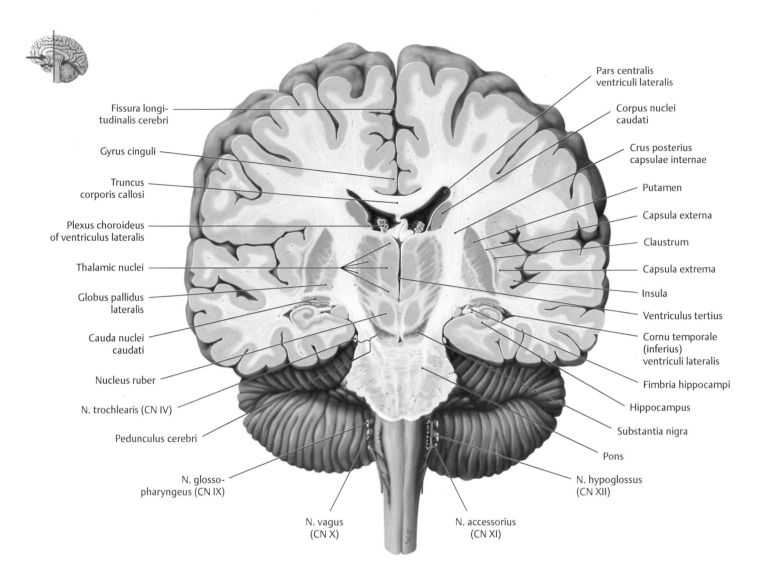

Fissura longi-
tudinalis cerebri

Gyrus cinguli

Truncus
corporis callosi

Plexus choroideus
of ventriculus lateralis

Thalamic nuclei

Globus pallidus
lateralis

Cauda nuclei
caudati

Nucleus ruber

N. trochlearis (CN IV)

Pedunculus cerebri

N. glosso-
pharyngeus (CN IX)

N. vagus
(CN X)

Pars centralis
ventriculi lateralis

Corpus nuclei
caudati

Crus posterius
capsulae internae

Putamen

Capsula externa

Claustrum

Capsula extrema

Insula

Ventriculus tertius

Cornu temporale
(inferius)
ventriculi lateralis

Fimbria hippocampi

Hippocampus

Substantia nigra

Pons

N. hypoglossus
(CN XII)

N. accessorius
(CN XI)

A Coronal section V

The appearance of the central nuclear region has changed markedly. The *nucleus caudatus* is cut twice by the plane of this section. Its corpus borders the body of the ventriculus lateralis, and a small portion of its cauda borders the cornu inferius of the ventricle (see **C** and **E**). Because the caput and corpus of the nucleus caudatus rim the lateral aspect of the cornu anterior (frontale) and the pars centralis of the ventriculus lateralis, the nucleus caudatus has a curved shape similar to that of the ventriculus lateralis (see **C**). Thus, the cauda of the nucleus caudatus is ventral and lateral in relation to its caput and corpus. Panel **E** shows that a coronal section through the cauda of the nucleus caudatus cuts the occipital portions of the *putamen*. A section in a slightly more occipital plane may not contain any part of the nuclei basales at all (see **B**). The pars centralis of the lateral horn has become much narrower due

to the presence of the *thalamus*, showing here several thalamic nuclei. This is the first plane that displays the *plexus choroideus*, which can be seen within the ventriculi laterales. The plexus choroideus extends from the foramen interventriculare (not visible here) into the cornu inferius. Because the foramen lies anterior to the thalamus, the plexus can be seen only in coronal sections that also pass through thalamic structures. Ventral to the thalamus are the *nucleus ruber* and *substantia nigra*; these are important midbrain structures that bulge into the diencephalon and extend almost to the level of the globus pallidus (not visible here; see **B**). The *hippocampus* indents the floor of the cornu temporale, and its fimbria can be seen. This section also shows how the fibrae corticospinales pass through the crus posterius of the capsula interna and continue into the pedunculi cerebri and pons.

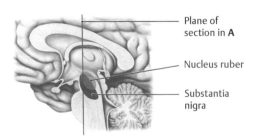

Plane of
section in **A**

Nucleus ruber

Substantia
nigra

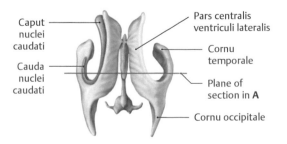

Caput
nuclei
caudati

Cauda
nuclei
caudati

Pars centralis
ventriculi lateralis

Cornu
temporale

Plane of
section in **A**

Cornu occipitale

B Nucleus ruber and substantia nigra
Midsagittal section.

C Ventricular system
Superior view.

Fissura longi-
tudinalis cerebri

Truncus
corporis callosi

Plexus choroideus
of ventriculus lateralis

Crus fornicis

Thalamic nuclei

Cauda nuclei
caudati

Fimbria
hippocampi

Commissura
posterior

Ventriculus tertius

Pedunculus
cerebellaris superior

Pedunculus
cerebellaris medius

Pars centralis
ventriculi lateralis

Corpus nuclei
caudati

Crus posterius
capsulae internae

Insula

Corpus geniculatum
mediale

Corpus geniculatum
laterale

Hippocampus

Plexus choroideus
of ventriculus lateralis

Gyrus dentatus

Lobus cerebelli
anterior

Fissura horizontalis

Flocculus

Medulla
oblongata

D Coronal section VI

The caudal thalamic nuclei are well displayed in this section, bordering the ventriculi laterales from below and the ventriculus tertius from the sides. The putamen lies at a more rostral level and is no longer visible in this plane (see the transverse section on p. 336). This section passes through the crus posterius of the capsula interna (see also **C**, p. 422) and the anterior part of the *commissura posterior* (see **A**, p. 426 and

D p. 427). The *corpora geniculata mediale* and *laterale*, which are components of the auditory and visual pathways respectively, appear as two darker nuclei that flank the thalamus on the right and left sides at the same level as the commissure (see **F**). The crura of the fornix can be seen between the thalamus and corpus callosum. This is the first section that passes through parts of the cerebellum. Here the *pedunculus cerebellaris medius* passes laterally toward the hemispheria cerebelli.

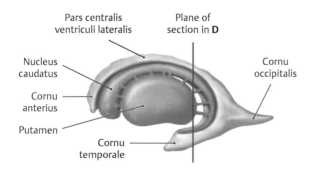

Pars centralis
ventriculi lateralis

Plane of
section in **D**

Nucleus
caudatus

Cornu
occipitalis

Cornu
anterius

Putamen

Cornu
temporale

E Topographical relationship between the nucleus caudatus and ventricular system

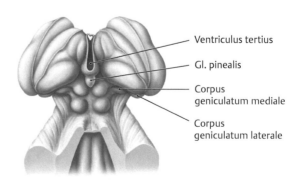

Ventriculus tertius

Gl. pinealis

Corpus
geniculatum mediale

Corpus
geniculatum laterale

F The diencephalon (with corpora geniculata) and truncus encephali

Posterior view.

12.4 Coronal Sections: VII and VIII

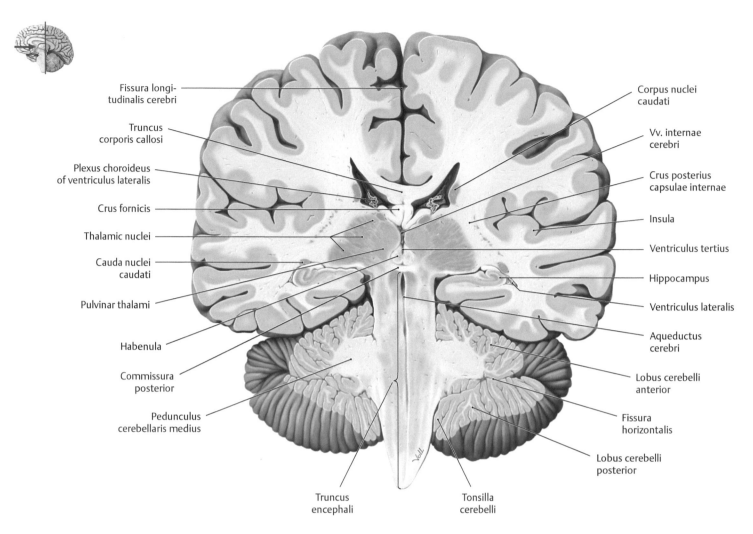

Fissura longi-
tudinalis cerebri

Truncus
corporis callosi

Plexus choroideus
of ventriculus lateralis

Crus fornicis

Thalamic nuclei

Cauda nuclei
caudati

Pulvinar thalami

Habenula

Commissura
posterior

Pedunculus
cerebellaris medius

Corpus nuclei
caudati

Vv. internae
cerebri

Crus posterius
capsulae internae

Insula

Ventriculus tertius

Hippocampus

Ventriculus lateralis

Aqueductus
cerebri

Lobus cerebelli
anterior

Fissura
horizontalis

Lobus cerebelli
posterior

Truncus
encephali

Tonsilla
cerebelli

A Coronal section VII

Among the diencephalic and telencephalic nuclei, we can still identify the thalamus and occipital portions of the nucleus caudatus, which become progressively smaller in the following sections until they finally disappear (see **C** and p. 428). The occipital part of the *hippocampus* can be seen below the medial wall of the ventriculus lateralis. This section cuts the truncus encephali along the *aqueductus cerebri* (see **C**). The cerebellum is connected to the truncus encephali by three substantia alba stalks: the *pedunculus cerebellaris superior* (mainly efferent), *pedunculus cerebellaris medius* (afferent), and pedunculus cerebellaris inferior (afferent and efferent). Because the pedunculus cerebellaris medius

extends further anteriorly than the other two peduncles (note its relationship to the truncus encephali axis), it is the first peduncle to appear in this frontal-to-occipital series of sections (see also **A**, p. 424, and **D**, p. 425). The pedunculus cerebellaris *superior* begins on the posterior side of the pons and thus appears in a later section (see **B**). There are no natural anatomical boundaries between the pedunculi cerebellares medius and inferior, and therefore the latter is not separately labeled in the sections. The superficial veins were removed from the encephalon when this section was prepared, and only the vv. internae cerebri appear in this and the following section.

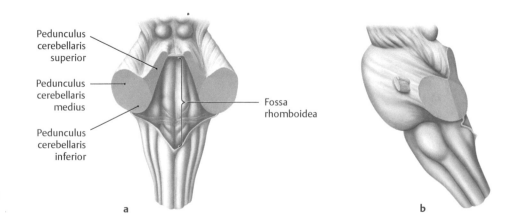

Pedunculus
cerebellaris
superior

Pedunculus
cerebellaris
medius

Pedunculus
cerebellaris
inferior

Fossa
rhomboidea

B Pedunculi cerebellares on the truncus encephali

a Posterior view; **b** Lateral view.

a

b

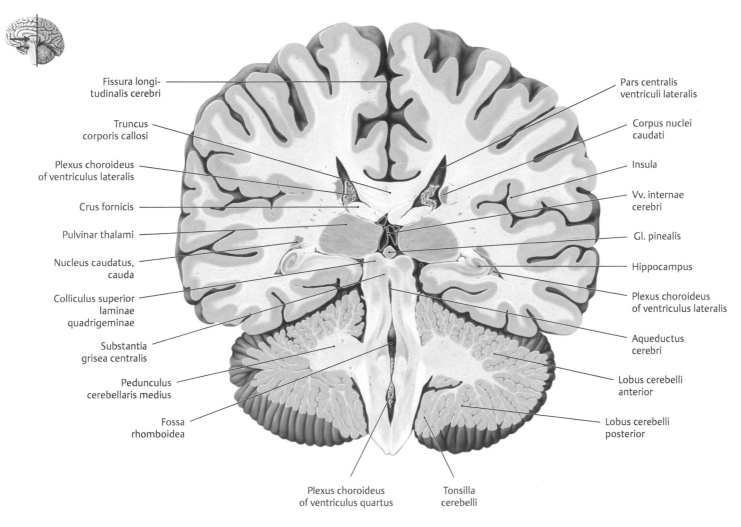

C Coronal section VIII

The thalamic nuclei appear smaller than in previous sections, and more of the cortex cerebelli is seen. This plane passes through part of the aqueductus cerebri. The *fossa rhomboidea*, which forms the floor of the ventriculus quartus, is clearly visible in the dorsal part of the truncus encephali (see **D** and **Ba**). The lamina quadrigemina (lamina tecti) is also visible. Its smaller colliculi *superiores* are particularly well displayed in this section, while the colliculi *inferiores* are more prominent in the next section (see **A**, p. 428). The gl. pinealis is only partially visible because of

its somewhat more occipital location (see **D**); a full cross-section can be seen in **A**, p. 428. The present section shows the division of the paired fornix tract into its two *crura*. The hippocampus here borders on the cornu inferius of the ventriculus lateralis on each side, bulging into its floor from the medial side (see also the previous sections and **E**). The hippocampus is an important component of the limbic system and is one of the first structures to undergo detectable morphological changes in Alzheimer's disease.

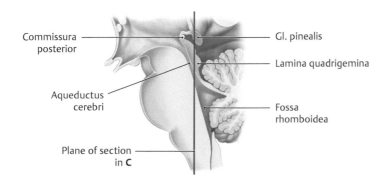

D Midsagittal section through the rhombencephalon, mesencephalon, and diencephalon

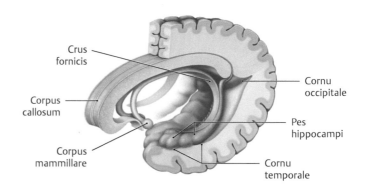

E Hippocampal formation
Left anterior and lateral oblique view.

427

12.5　Coronal Sections: IX and X

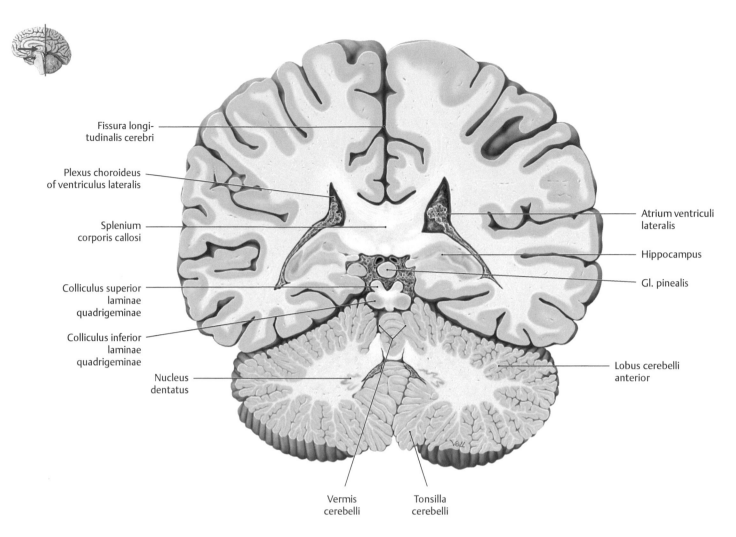

Fissura longi-
tudinalis cerebri

Plexus choroideus
of ventriculus lateralis

Splenium
corporis callosi

Colliculus superior
laminae
quadrigeminae

Colliculus inferior
laminae
quadrigeminae

Nucleus
dentatus

Atrium ventriculi
lateralis

Hippocampus

Gl. pinealis

Lobus cerebelli
anterior

Vermis
cerebelli

Tonsilla
cerebelli

A　Coronal section IX

The gl. pinealis, a control center for circadian rhythms, is here displayed in full cross-section (contrast with the previous section; see also **D**, p. 427). Below it lies the lamina quadrigemina, the dorsal part of the mesencephalon (note its relationship to the truncus encephali axis). The larger colliculi *inferiores* of the lamina quadrigemina are more prominent here than in the previous section (the inclination of the truncus encephali gives them a more posterior location). The colliculi *inferiores* are part of the auditory pathway, while the colliculi *superiores* (more clearly seen in the previous section) are part of the visual pathway. At the level of the cerebellum, the *vermis cerebelli* can be identified as an unpaired midline structure. The only cerebellar nucleus visible at this level is the *nucleus dentatus*, which is surrounded by the cerebellar substantia alba. The other deep nuclei cerebelli are not visible in the plane of this section.

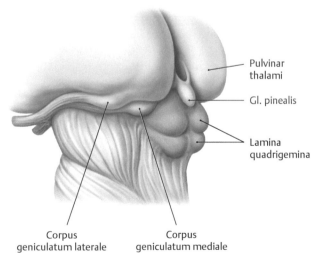

Pulvinar
thalami

Gl. pinealis

Lamina
quadrigemina

Corpus
geniculatum laterale

Corpus
geniculatum mediale

B　Lamina quadrigemina (tectum)
Left posterior oblique view.

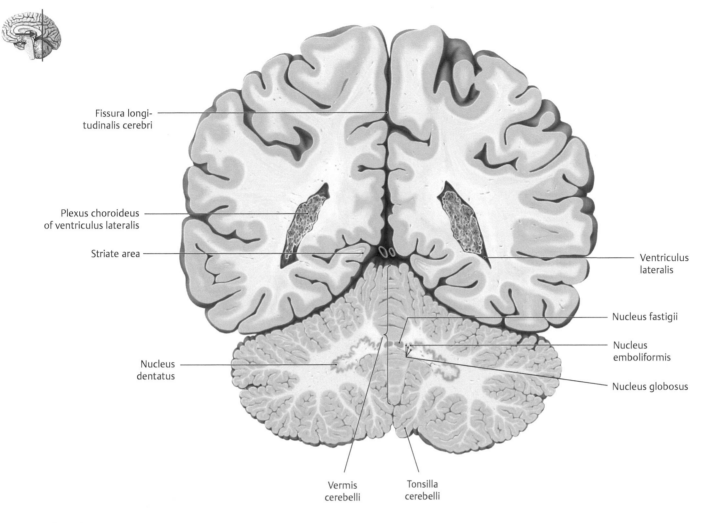

Fissura longi-
tudinalis cerebri

Plexus choroideus
of ventriculus lateralis

Striate area

Nucleus
dentatus

Ventriculus
lateralis

Nucleus fastigii

Nucleus
emboliformis

Nucleus globosus

Vermis
cerebelli

Tonsilla
cerebelli

C Coronal section X

This plane presents the four *nuclei cerebelli*:

- Nucleus dentatus (nucleus lateralis cerebelli)
- Nucleus emboliformis (nucleus interpositus anterior)
- Nucleus globosus (nucleus interpositus posterior)
- Nucleus fastigii (nucleus medialis cerebelli)

The longitudinally cut **vermis cerebelli** presents a larger area here than in the previous section. The **ventriculus quartus** is no longer visible in the plane of this section.

12.6 Coronal Sections: XI and XII (Occipital)

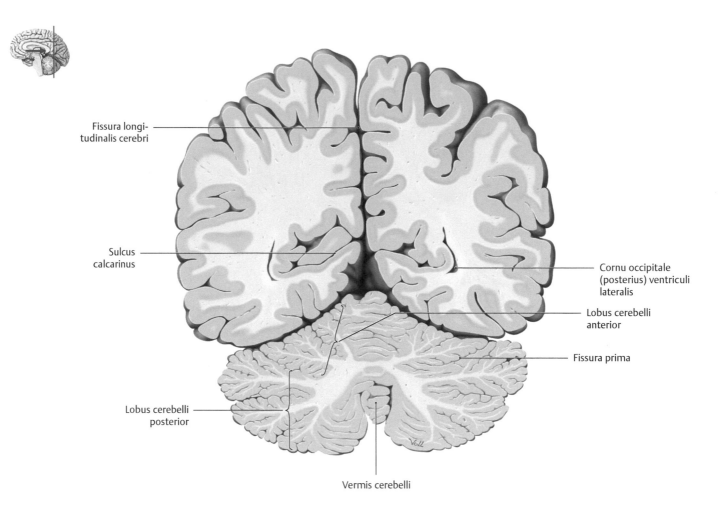

Fissura longi-
tudinalis cerebri

Sulcus
calcarinus

Cornu occipitale
(posterius) ventriculi
lateralis

Lobus cerebelli
anterior

Fissura prima

Lobus cerebelli
posterior

Vermis cerebelli

A Coronal section XI

The plane of this section clearly shows the cornua posteriora (occipitalia) of the ventriculi laterales; these appear only as narrow slits in the next section (see **D**). The section also illustrates once again how the cornu posterius is an extension of the cornu inferius (temporale) (see **B**). Between the cerebellum and the lobus occipitalis of the cerebrum lies the *tentorium cerebelli* (see **C**). The tentorium cerebelli contains the sinus rectus, which passes to the confluens sinuum. It is one of the sinus durae matris that drain blood from the encephalon, beginning at the confluence of the v. magna cerebri and the sinus sagittalis inferior (removed during preparation of the falx cerebri). Because the dura is removed from the encephali in the preparation of most tissue sections, the sinuses enclosed by the dura mater also tend to be removed.

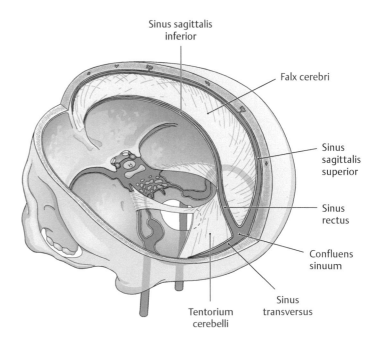

Sinus sagittalis
inferior

Falx cerebri

Sinus
sagittalis
superior

Sinus
rectus

Confluens
sinuum

Sinus
transversus

Tentorium
cerebelli

C The sinus durae matris
Viewed from upper left.

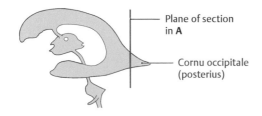

Plane of section
in **A**

Cornu occipitale
(posterius)

B Ventricular system viewed from the left side

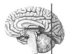

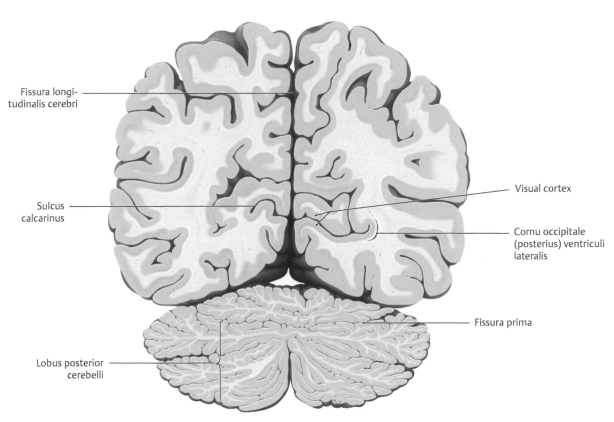

Fissura longi-
tudinalis cerebri

Sulcus
calcarinus

Visual cortex

Cornu occipitale
(posterius) ventriculi
lateralis

Fissura prima

Lobus posterior
cerebelli

D Coronal section XII
In the plane of this section, the cornu posterius (occipitale) of the ventriculus lateralis has dwindled to a narrow slit. The relatively long *sulcus calcarinus* is visible in the lobus occipitalis of the cerebrum, and also appears in several of the preceding sections. It is surrounded by the *striate area* (primary visual cortex, also called area 17 in the Brodmann brain map), the size of which is best appreciated on the medial surface of the brain (see **E**). More occipital sections are not presented in this chapter, as they would show nothing but cortex and subcortical substantia alba.

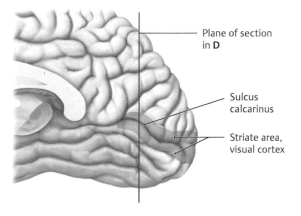

Plane of section
in **D**

Sulcus
calcarinus

Striate area,
visual cortex

E Right striate area (visual cortex)
Medial surface of the right hemisphere, viewed from the left side.

12.7 Transverse Sections: I and II (Cranial)

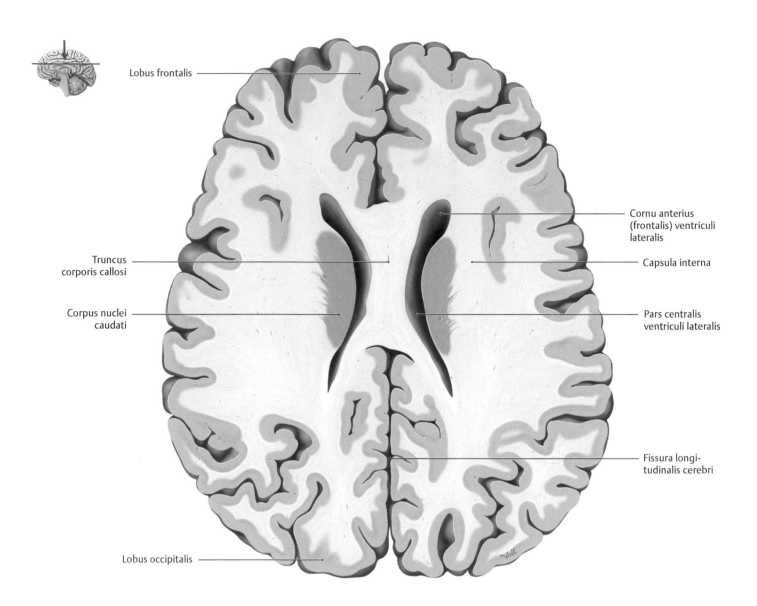

Lobus frontalis

Cornu anterius (frontalis) ventriculi lateralis

Truncus corporis callosi

Capsula interna

Corpus nuclei caudati

Pars centralis ventriculi lateralis

Fissura longitudinalis cerebri

Lobus occipitalis

General remarks on transverse (axial, horizontal) brain sections

The sections in this series are viewed from above and behind the head (position of axes see p. 270); that is, the observer is looking at the surface of the slice as it would typically appear in a brain autopsy or during a neurosurgical operation. Thus, the left side of the encephalon appears on the left side of the drawing. This contrasts with the image orientation in CT and MRI, where encephalon slices are always viewed from below; that is, the left side of the brain appears on the right side of the image.

A Transverse section I

This highest of the transverse brain sections passes through frontal, parietal, and occipital structures of the telencephalon. Each of the two ventriculi laterales is bordered laterally by the corpus of the nucleus caudatus, and medially by the truncus corporis callosi. The corpus callosum transmits fiber tracts which interconnect areas in both hemispheria that serve the same function (commissural tracts). When viewed in crosssection, the corpus callosum appears to be interrupted by the ventriculi and nucleus caudatus, when, in fact, it arches over these structures, forming the roof of the ventriculi laterales. The course of the tracts that pass through the corpus callosum can be appreciated by looking at a coronal section (see **B**).

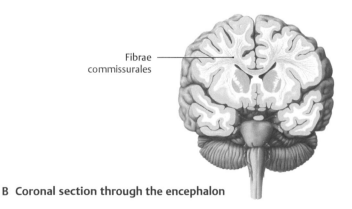

Fibrae commissurales

B Coronal section through the encephalon

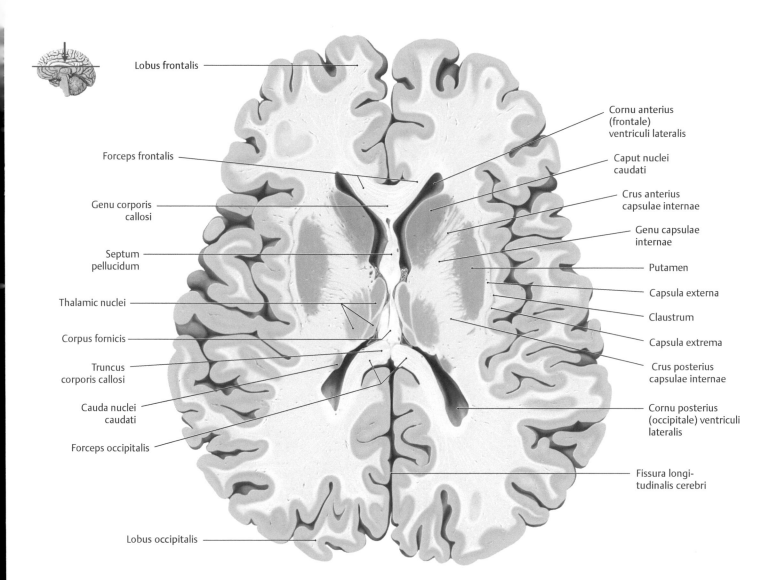

Lobus frontalis

Forceps frontalis

Genu corporis callosi

Septum pellucidum

Thalamic nuclei

Corpus fornicis

Truncus corporis callosi

Cauda nuclei caudati

Forceps occipitalis

Lobus occipitalis

Cornu anterius (frontale) ventriculi lateralis

Caput nuclei caudati

Crus anterius capsulae internae

Genu capsulae internae

Putamen

Capsula externa

Claustrum

Capsula extrema

Crus posterius capsulae internae

Cornu posterius (occipitale) ventriculi lateralis

Fissura longitudinalis cerebri

C Transverse section II

In this section, unlike the previous one, each *ventriculus lateralis* appears divided in two. Because this section is at a lower level, it cuts the cornua anterius and posterius of the ventriculus lateralis separately, missing the pars centralis of the ventriculus (see **D**). It also cuts a broad swath of the *capsula interna* with its genu and crura anterius and posterius. The radiatio optica, which runs in the substantia alba of the lobus occipitalis, is not labeled here because it has no grossly visible anatomical boundaries. The *corpus callosum* also appears divided into two parts: the genu anteriorly and the truncus more posteriorly. This apparent division results from a second curvature of the corpus callosum at its genu ("knee"),

where it is anteriorly convex. The diagram in **E** demonstrates why this section passes successively through the genu of the corpus callosum, the septum pellucidum, the corpus of the fornix, and finally the truncus of the corpus callosum. The septum pellucidum forms the anteromedial wall of both ventriculi laterales. The septum itself contains small nuclei. Sections of the thalamic nuclei (nuclei ventralis lateralis, dorsalis lateralis, and anteriores) are also visible along with the putamen and nucleus caudatus. The caput and cauda of the nucleus caudatus appear separately in the section (see also p. 336). The putamen, nucleus caudatus, and intervening fibers of the capsula interna are collectively called the corpus striatum.

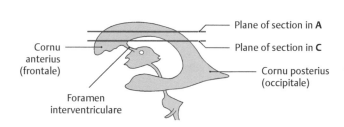

Cornu anterius (frontale)

Foramen interventriculare

Plane of section in **A**

Plane of section in **C**

Cornu posterius (occipitale)

D Lateral view of the ventricular system

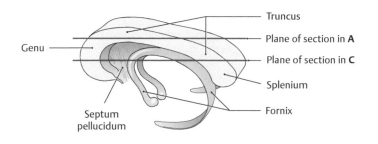

Genu

Septum pellucidum

Truncus

Plane of section in **A**

Plane of section in **C**

Splenium

Fornix

E Corpus callosum and fornix

12.8 Transverse Sections: III and IV

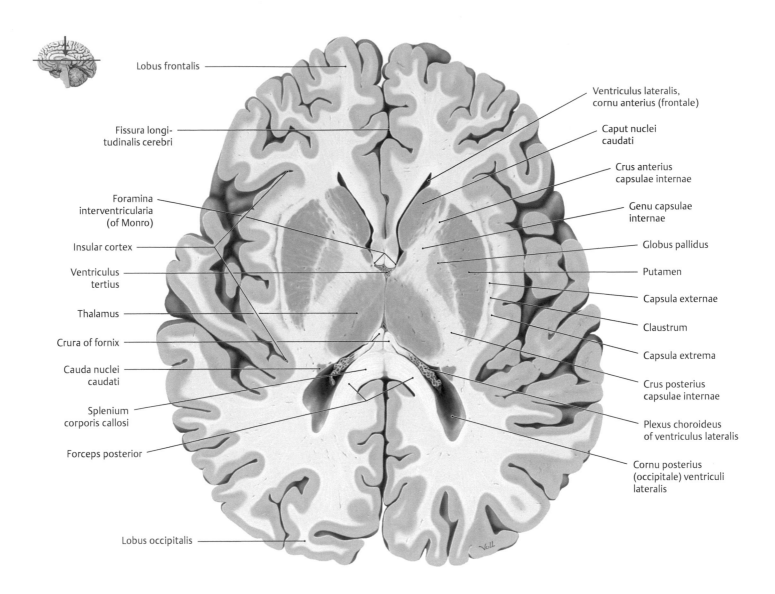

Lobus frontalis

Fissura longitudinalis cerebri

Foramina interventricularia (of Monro)

Insular cortex

Ventriculus tertius

Thalamus

Crura of fornix

Cauda nuclei caudati

Splenium corporis callosi

Forceps posterior

Lobus occipitalis

Ventriculus lateralis, cornu anterius (frontale)

Caput nuclei caudati

Crus anterius capsulae internae

Genu capsulae internae

Globus pallidus

Putamen

Capsula externae

Claustrum

Capsula extrema

Crus posterius capsulae internae

Plexus choroideus of ventriculus lateralis

Cornu posterius (occipitale) ventriculi lateralis

A Transverse section III

The ventriculi laterales communicate with the ventriculus tertius through the *foramina interventricularia* (of Monro). They are located directly anterior to the thalamus (see **D**, p. 433). The nuclei of the telencephalon make up the deep gray matter of the cerebrum. The spatial relationship between the nucleus caudatus and thalamus is illustrated in **B**. The nucleus caudatus is larger frontally, and the thalamus larger occipitally. While the nucleus caudatus and putamen of the motor system belong to the telencephalon, the thalamus of the sensory system belongs to the diencephalon. This transverse section passes through the nucleus caudatus twice due to the anatomical curvature of the nucleus. This is the first transverse section that displays the globus pallidus, part of the motor system. The insular cortex is seen with the *claustrum* medial to it. The *crura of the fornix* are seen as posterior to the thalamus (see also **E**, p. 433). They unite at a slightly higher level to form the *corpus of the fornix*, which lies just below the corpus callosum and was visible in the previous section (see **C**, p. 433). The course of the capsula interna is visible in both this section and the last.

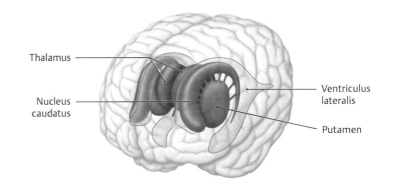

Thalamus

Nucleus caudatus

Ventriculus lateralis

Putamen

B Spatial relationships of the nucleus caudatus, putamen, thalamus, and ventriculi laterales

Left anterior oblique view.

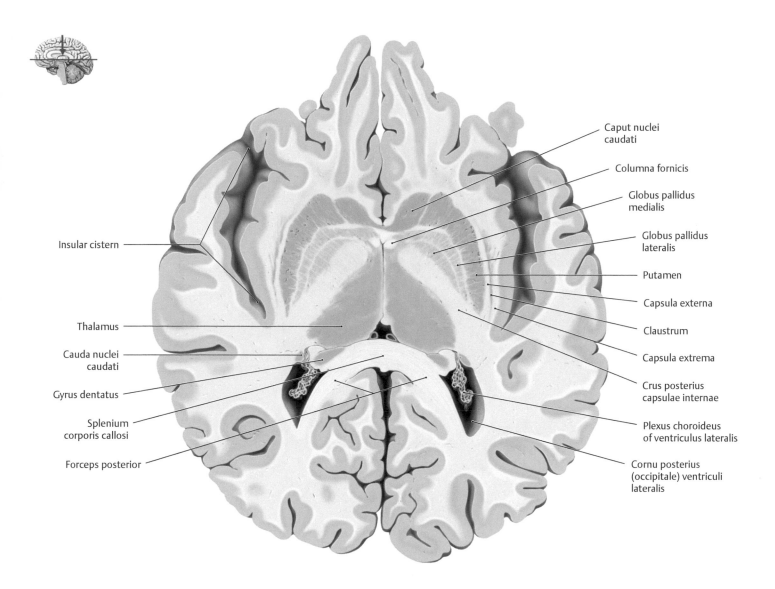

Caput nuclei
caudati

Columna fornicis

Globus pallidus
medialis

Globus pallidus
lateralis

Putamen

Capsula externa

Claustrum

Capsula extrema

Crus posterius
capsulae internae

Plexus choroideus
of ventriculus lateralis

Cornu posterius
(occipitale) ventriculi
lateralis

Insular cistern

Thalamus

Cauda nuclei
caudati

Gyrus dentatus

Splenium
corporis callosi

Forceps posterior

C Transverse section IV
The nuclei shown in the previous section here appear as a roughly circular mass at the center of the brain, surrounded by the substantia grisea of the cortex cerebri, also called the *pallium* ("cloak") for obvious reasons. The plexus choroideus is here visible in both ventriculi laterales. This section cuts the occipital part of the corpus callosum, the *splenium*, as well as the basal portion of the *insular cortex* (see **E**, p. 423). The insula is a cortical region that lies below the surface and is covered by the opercula. The insular cistern should be used as a reference point, for example, when comparing this section to **A** and **D**.

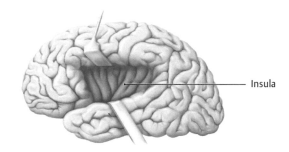

Insula

D Left insular region
Lateral view.

12.9 Transverse Sections: V and VI (Caudal)

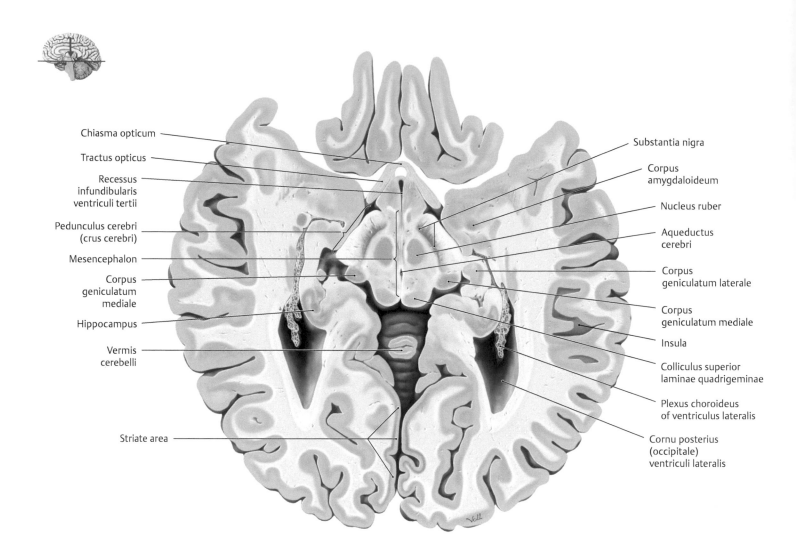

Chiasma opticum

Tractus opticus

Recessus infundibularis ventriculi tertii

Pedunculus cerebri (crus cerebri)

Mesencephalon

Corpus geniculatum mediale

Hippocampus

Vermis cerebelli

Striate area

Substantia nigra

Corpus amygdaloideum

Nucleus ruber

Aqueductus cerebri

Corpus geniculatum laterale

Corpus geniculatum mediale

Insula

Colliculus superior laminae quadrigeminae

Plexus choroideus of ventriculus lateralis

Cornu posterius (occipitale) ventriculi lateralis

A Transverse section V

Structures visible in this section include the aqueductus cerebri, the basal part of the ventriculus tertius (see also **B**, p. 422), and the *optic recess*. While the ventriculus tertius is slitlike at this level, the section cuts a very large area of the ventricular system where it opens into the two cornua posteriora (occipitalia). This is the first transverse section that displays the midbrain (*mesencephalon*), passing through its oral portion (note: terms of location and direction refer to the truncus encephali axis). The pedunculi cerebrales (*crura cerebri*), the substantia nigra, and the *colliculi superiores* of the lamina quadrigemina can also be seen. Visible structures of the *diencephalon* in this plane include the *copora geniculata medialia* and *lateralia* (appearing only on the right side, see **B**) and the *tractus opticus*, which is an extension of the diencephalon. *Note:* Closely adjacent structures in the encephalon may belong to different ontogenetic regions. For example, the corpora geniculata medialia and lateralia are part of the diencephalon, while the colliculi superiores and inferiores (the latter is not visible), which make up the lamina quadrigemina, are part of the mesencephalon. It should be recalled, however, that the corpus geniculatum laterale and colliculus superior are part of the visual pathway while the corpus geniculatum mediale and colliculus inferior are part of the auditory pathway.

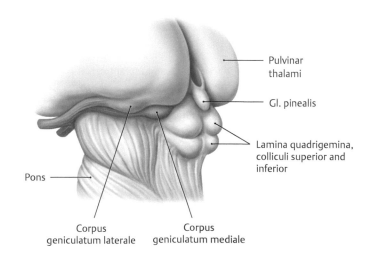

Pulvinar thalami

Gl. pinealis

Lamina quadrigemina, colliculi superior and inferior

Pons

Corpus geniculatum laterale

Corpus geniculatum mediale

B Pons, mesencephalon, and adjacent diencephalon

Left posterior oblique view.

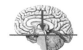

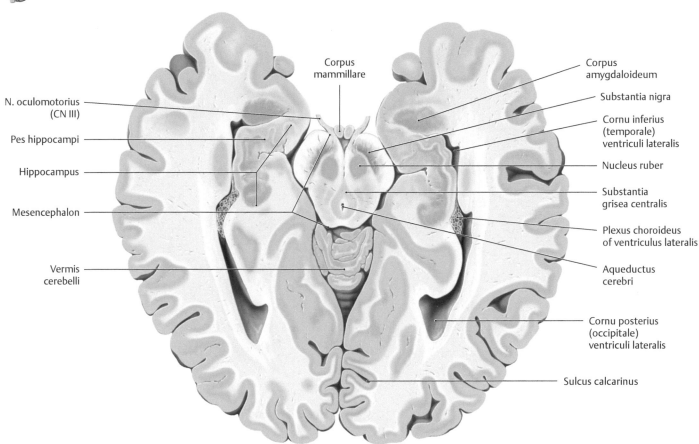

Corpus mammillare

Corpus amygdaloideum

N. oculomotorius (CN III)

Substantia nigra

Pes hippocampi

Cornu inferius (temporale) ventriculi lateralis

Hippocampus

Nucleus ruber

Mesencephalon

Substantia grisea centralis

Plexus choroideus of ventriculus lateralis

Vermis cerebelli

Aqueductus cerebri

Cornu posterius (occipitale) ventriculi lateralis

Sulcus calcarinus

C Transverse section VI

The structures that occupy the largest area at this level are the telencephalon, the medial portions of the mesencephalon, and the cerebellum. The nuclei located on the anteromedian aspect of each lobus temporalis of the telencephalon are the *corpora amygdaloidea*. The lower part of the section cuts the *sulcus calcarinus* with the surrounding visual cortex. This section also passes through the plexus choroideus of the ventriculi laterales, whose *cornua posteriora* and *inferiora* are displayed. Important structures of the *mesencephalon* are the substantia nigra and nucleus ruber, both of which are part of the motor system. The corpora mammillaria are part of the *diencephalon* and are connected by the fornix (not visible in this section) to the hippocampus, which is part of the *telencephalon*. The corpora mammillaria lie in the same horizontal plane as the hippocampus and the same coronal plane as its pes (foot). These relationships result from the curved shape of the fornix (see **D**). More transverse sections at lower levels would supply little additional information on the cerebrum; therefore our series of transverse sections ends here. The truncus encephali structures lying below the mesencephalon are displayed in a separate group of sections (see p. 362 ff).

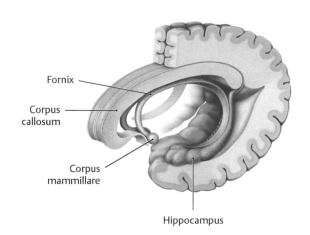

Fornix

Corpus callosum

Corpus mammillare

Hippocampus

D Fornix
Left anterior oblique view.

12.10 Sagittal Sections: I–III (Lateral)

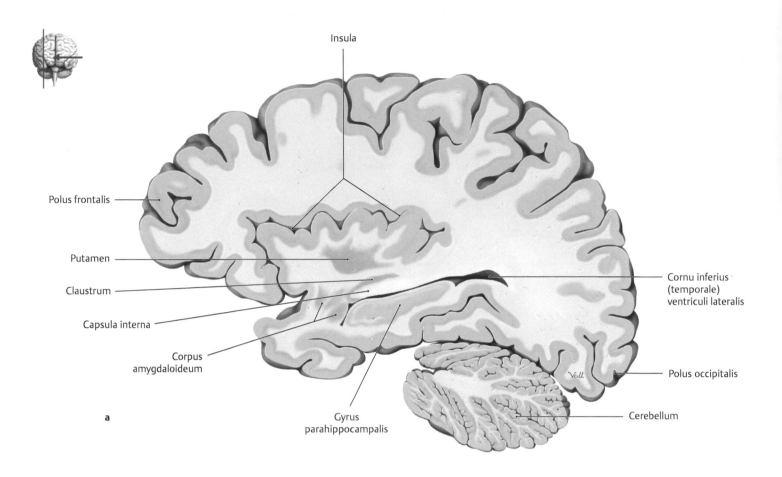

Insula

Polus frontalis

Putamen

Claustrum

Capsula interna

Corpus
amygdaloideum

a

Gyrus
parahippocampalis

Cornu inferius
(temporale)
ventriculi lateralis

Polus occipitalis

Cerebellum

A Sagittal sections I–III

Left lateral view. The plane of section a passes through the *cornu inferius* (*temporale*) of the ventriculus lateralis; the more medially situated *cornu posterius* (*occipitale*) is seen in **b** and **c** (see **C**, p. 424 for relative position of both horns). The *corpus amygdaloideum*, which is directly anterior to the cornu inferius, lies in the same sagittal plane as the gyrus parahippocampalis (**a–c**; see also **C**, p. 437). The capsula interna can also be seen in sections **a–c**; the long ascending and descending tracts pass through this structure. The most lateral section (**a**) offers the only view of the *insular cortex*, a part of the cortex cerebri that has sunk below the surface of the hemispherium (compare with the coronal sections on p. 421 and the following pages). The *putamen*, the most laterally situated among the nuclei basales of the telencephalon (see also **A**, p. 424) is also found in **a**, but appears larger in the more medial sections (**b**, **c**). A portion of the *claustrum* can be seen ventral to the putamen (**a**), although most of the claustrum is lateral to the putamen (see **A**, p. 424) and outside the plane of the section. Section **b** just cuts the cauda of the *nucleus caudatus*, which is situated more laterally than its caput and corpus (see also **C**, p. 424 and **E**, p. 425). The most medial section in this series (**c**) cuts the *sulcus calcarinus* (see p. 440) and the *corpus geniculatum laterale* which lies at the edge of the thalamus. The globus pallidus lateralis can also be seen (**c**): the segments of the *globus pallidus* are actually medial to the putamen (see **D**, p. 423), but can be visualized here due to their concentric arrangement.

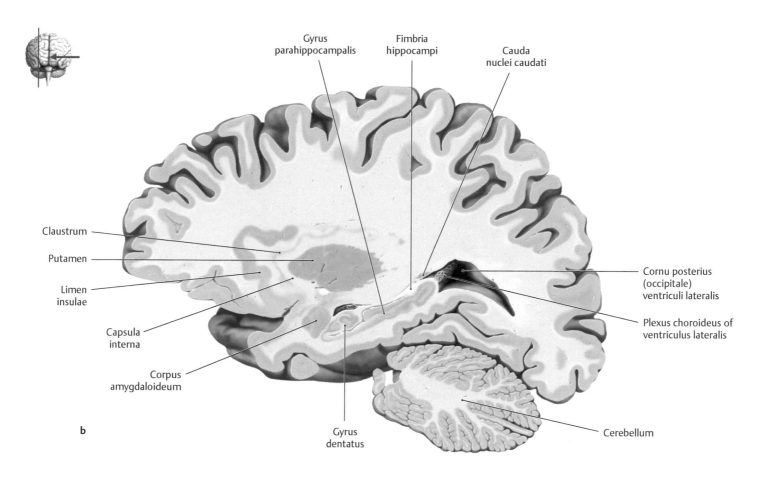

Gyrus parahippocampalis

Fimbria hippocampi

Cauda nuclei caudati

Claustrum

Putamen

Limen insulae

Capsula interna

Corpus amygdaloideum

Cornu posterius (occipitale) ventriculi lateralis

Plexus choroideus of ventriculus lateralis

Gyrus dentatus

Cerebellum

b

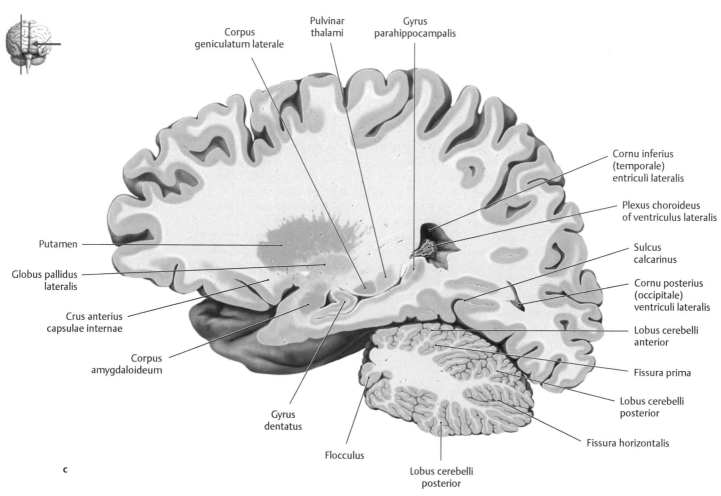

Corpus geniculatum laterale

Pulvinar thalami

Gyrus parahippocampalis

Putamen

Globus pallidus lateralis

Crus anterius capsulae internae

Corpus amygdaloideum

Gyrus dentatus

Flocculus

Lobus cerebelli posterior

Cornu inferius (temporale) entriculi lateralis

Plexus choroideus of ventriculus lateralis

Sulcus calcarinus

Cornu posterius (occipitale) ventriculi lateralis

Lobus cerebelli anterior

Fissura prima

Lobus cerebelli posterior

Fissura horizontalis

c

439

12.11 Sagittal Sections: IV–VI

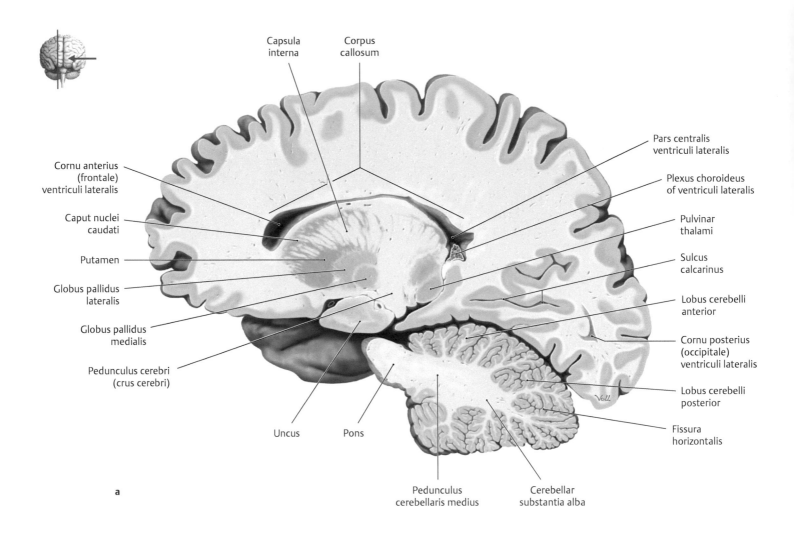

Capsula interna

Corpus callosum

Cornu anterius (frontale) ventriculi lateralis

Caput nuclei caudati

Putamen

Globus pallidus lateralis

Globus pallidus medialis

Pedunculus cerebri (crus cerebri)

Uncus

Pons

Pedunculus cerebellaris medius

Cerebellar substantia alba

Pars centralis ventriculi lateralis

Plexus choroideus of ventriculi lateralis

Pulvinar thalami

Sulcus calcarinus

Lobus cerebelli anterior

Cornu posterius (occipitale) ventriculi lateralis

Lobus cerebelli posterior

Fissura horizontalis

a

A Sagittal sections IV–VI

Left lateral view. The dominant ventricular structures in all three of these sections are the cornu anterius and pars centralis of the *ventriculus lateralis* (the junction with the laterally situated cornu posterius appears only in **a**). The *corpus callosum*, which connects functionally related areas of the two hemispheria cerebri (commissural tracts), can be identified in the cerebral substantia alba although it is not sharply delineated (**a–c**). As the sections move closer to the midline, the putamen grows smaller while the nucleus caudatus becomes increasingly promiment (**a–c**). These two bodies are known collectively as the *corpus striatum*, and their characteristic striations are seen particularly well in a (the substantia alba that separates the substantia grisea streaks of the corpus striatum is the *capsula interna*). The previous sagittal sections showed only the *globus pallidus* lateralis (see p. 439), but the globus pallidus medialis is displayed in both **a** and **b**. As the globus pallidus

disappears and the putamen becomes less prominent, the nuclei of the medially situated thalamus become visible below the ventriculus lateralis (**c**; the subthalamic nuclei include the anterior, posterior, and lateral ventral nuclei of the diencephalon). The location of the thalamus explains why it is sometimes referred to as the *dorsal thalamus*. Section **c** also shows the *substantia nigra* in the mesencephalon (below the diencephalon), the nuclei olivares inferiores in the underlying medulla oblongata, and the *nucleus dentatus* of the cerebellum. The ascending and descending tracts previously visible only in the capsula interna can now be seen in the pons, part of the truncus encephali (**c**, fibrae corticospinales). The only visible portion of the ventriculus quartus, barely sectioned in **c**, is its lateral recess.

The sectioned nucleus accumbens in **c** is an important part of the brain's reward system, which for example controls addictive behavior and can be affected in case of severe depression.

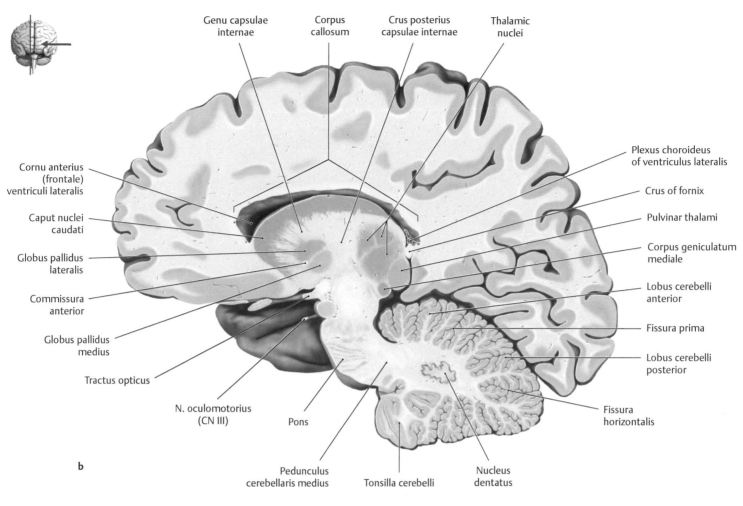

Genu capsulae internae

Corpus callosum

Crus posterius capsulae internae

Thalamic nuclei

Cornu anterius (frontale) ventriculi lateralis

Caput nuclei caudati

Globus pallidus lateralis

Commissura anterior

Globus pallidus medius

Tractus opticus

N. oculomotorius (CN III)

Pons

Pedunculus cerebellaris medius

Tonsilla cerebelli

Nucleus dentatus

Plexus choroideus of ventriculus lateralis

Crus of fornix

Pulvinar thalami

Corpus geniculatum mediale

Lobus cerebelli anterior

Fissura prima

Lobus cerebelli posterior

Fissura horizontalis

b

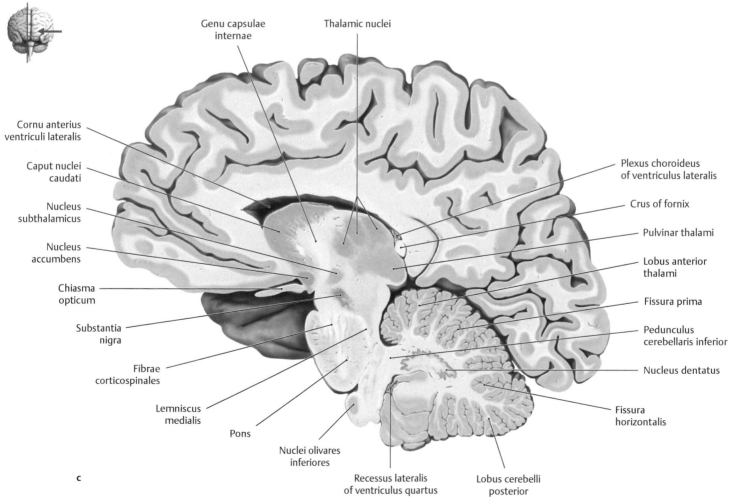

Genu capsulae internae

Thalamic nuclei

Cornu anterius ventriculi lateralis

Caput nuclei caudati

Nucleus subthalamicus

Nucleus accumbens

Chiasma opticum

Substantia nigra

Fibrae corticospinales

Lemniscus medialis

Pons

Nuclei olivares inferiores

Recessus lateralis of ventriculus quartus

Lobus cerebelli posterior

Plexus choroideus of ventriculus lateralis

Crus of fornix

Pulvinar thalami

Lobus anterior thalami

Fissura prima

Pedunculus cerebellaris inferior

Nucleus dentatus

Fissura horizontalis

c

441

12.12 Sagittal Sections: VII and VIII (Medial)

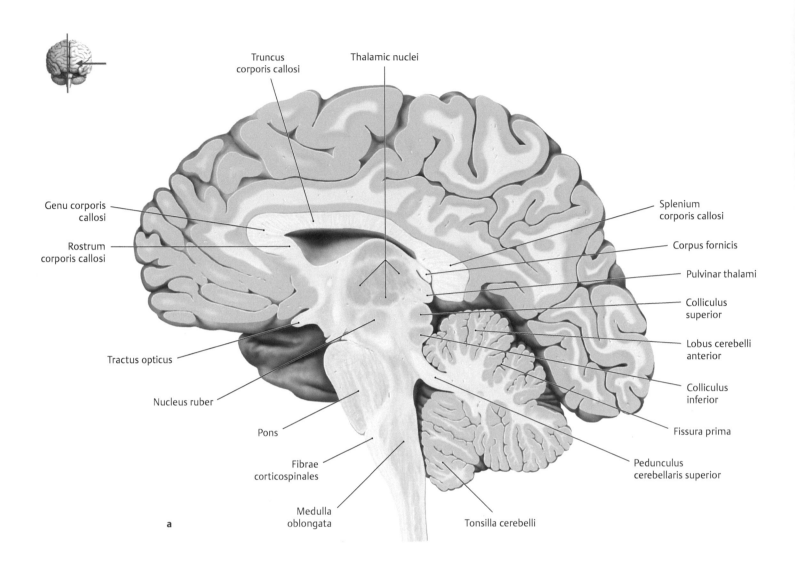

Truncus corporis callosi

Thalamic nuclei

Genu corporis callosi

Rostrum corporis callosi

Tractus opticus

Nucleus ruber

Pons

Fibrae corticospinales

Medulla oblongata

Splenium corporis callosi

Corpus fornicis

Pulvinar thalami

Colliculus superior

Lobus cerebelli anterior

Colliculus inferior

Fissura prima

Pedunculus cerebellaris superior

Tonsilla cerebelli

a

A Sagittal sections VII and VIII

Left lateral view. This section (**a**) is so close to the midline that it passes through the principal paramedian structures: the substantia nigra, the nucleus ruber, and one each of the paired colliculi superior and inferior. The tractus pyramidalis (fibrae corticospinales) runs in front of the oliva in the medulla oblongata. A complete sagittal section of the corpus callosum is displayed, and most of the fornix tract is displayed in longitudinal section (**b**). The cerebellum has reached its maximum extent and forms the roof of the ventriculus quartus (**b**). A portion of the *septum pellucidum*, which stretches between the fornix and corpus callosum, is also displayed.

When the encephalon is removed, the hypophysis, which appears in **b**, remains in the sella turcica; that is, it is always torn from the brain at its stalk when the encephalon is removed.

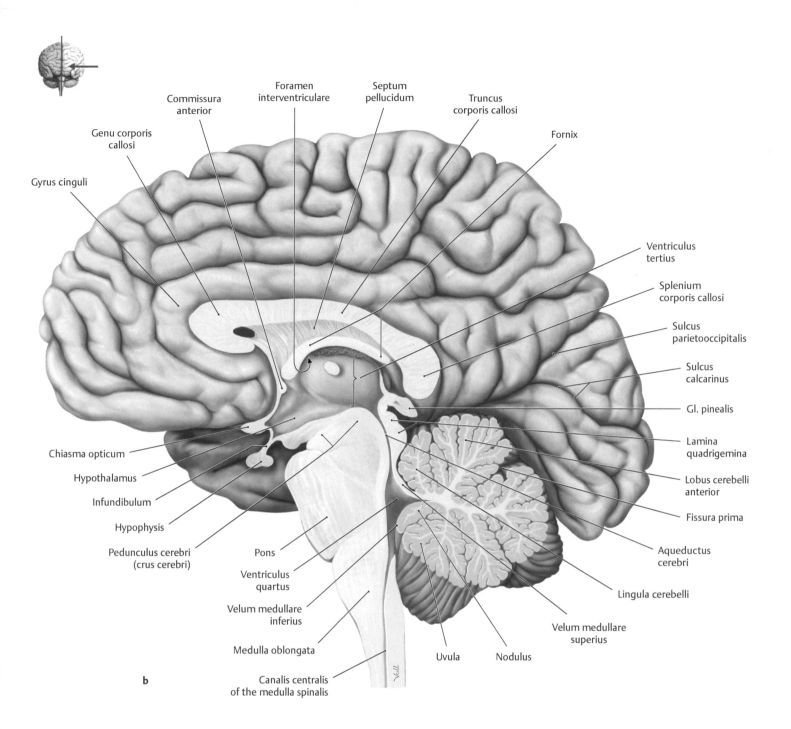

Gyrus cinguli

Genu corporis callosi

Commissura anterior

Foramen interventriculare

Septum pellucidum

Truncus corporis callosi

Fornix

Ventriculus tertius

Splenium corporis callosi

Sulcus parietooccipitalis

Sulcus calcarinus

Gl. pinealis

Lamina quadrigemina

Lobus cerebelli anterior

Fissura prima

Aqueductus cerebri

Lingula cerebelli

Velum medullare superius

Chiasma opticum

Hypothalamus

Infundibulum

Hypophysis

Pedunculus cerebri (crus cerebri)

Pons

Ventriculus quartus

Velum medullare inferius

Medulla oblongata

Uvula

Nodulus

b

Canalis centralis of the medulla spinalis

B Principal structures in the serial sections

The major structures seen in the serial sections are here assigned to their corresponding brain regions. Within each region, the structures are listed from most rostral to most caudal.

Telencephalon (endbrain)
- Capsula externa
- Capsula extrema
- Capsula interna
- Claustrum
- Commissura anterior
- Corpus amygdaloideum
- Corpus callosum
- Fornix
- Globus pallidus
- Gyrus cinguli
- Hippocampus
- Nucleus caudatus
- Putamen
- Septum pellucidum

Diencephalon (interbrain)
- Corpus geniculatum laterale
- Corpus geniculatum media
- Gl. pinealis
- Pulvinar thalami
- Thalamus
- Tractus opticus
- Corpus mammillare

Mesencephalon (midbrain)
- Aqueductus cerebri
- Lamina quadrigemina (lamina tecti)
- Colliculus superior
- Colliculus inferior
- Nucleus ruber
- Substantia nigra
- Pedunculus cerebri (crus cerebri)

13.1 Somatosensory System: Synopsis of the Pathways

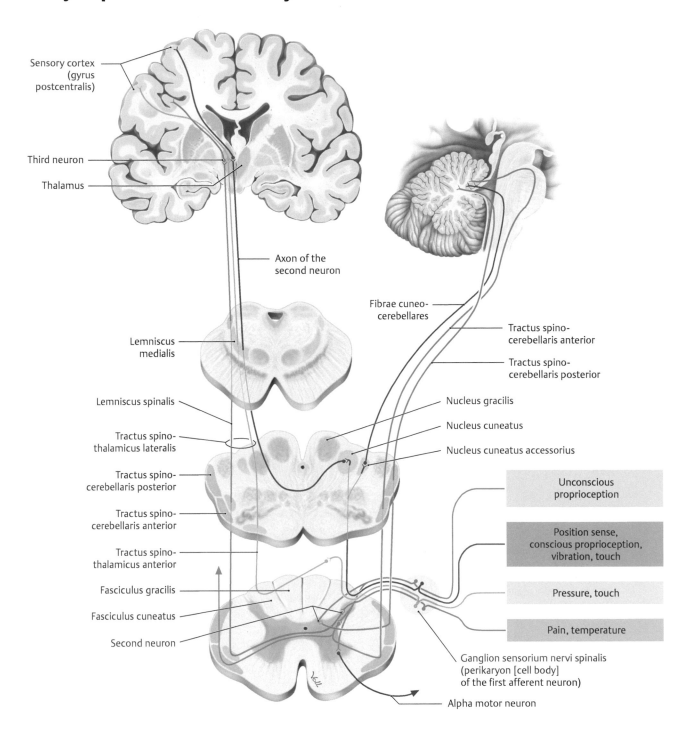

Sensory cortex (gyrus postcentralis)

Third neuron

Thalamus

Axon of the second neuron

Fibrae cuneo-cerebellares

Tractus spino-cerebellaris anterior

Tractus spino-cerebellaris posterior

Lemniscus medialis

Lemniscus spinalis

Nucleus gracilis

Nucleus cuneatus

Tractus spino-thalamicus lateralis

Nucleus cuneatus accessorius

Tractus spino-cerebellaris posterior

Tractus spino-cerebellaris anterior

Unconscious proprioception

Position sense, conscious proprioception, vibration, touch

Tractus spino-thalamicus anterior

Fasciculus gracilis

Pressure, touch

Fasciculus cuneatus

Pain, temperature

Second neuron

Ganglion sensorium nervi spinalis (perikaryon [cell body] of the first afferent neuron)

Alpha motor neuron

A Simplified diagram of the somatosensory pathways of the medulla spinalis

Stimuli generate impulses in various receptors in the periphery of the body which are transmitted to the cerebrum and cerebellum along the sensory (afferent) pathways or tracts shown here (see **B** for details). **Proprioception** is concerned with the perception of the position of the limbs in space (position sense). The types of information involved in proprioception (depth sense) are complex: position sense (the position of the limbs in relation to one another) is distinguished from motion sense (speed and direction of joint movements) and force sense (the muscular force associated with joint movements). We also distinguish between conscious and unconscious proprioception.

- Information on *conscious proprioception* travels in the funiculus posterior of the medulla spinalis (fasciculus gracilis and fasciculus

cuneatus) and is relayed through their nuclei (nucleus gracilis and nucleus cuneatus) to the *thalamus*. From there it is conveyed to the *sensory cortex* (gyrus postcentralis), where the information rises to consciousness ("I know that my left hand is making a fist, even though my eyes are closed").

- *Unconscious proprioception*, which enables us to ride a bicycle and climb stairs without thinking about it, is conveyed by the tractus spinocerebellares to the *cerebellum*, where it remains at the unconscious level.

Sensory information from the head is mediated by the n. trigeminus and is not depicted here (see p. 448).

B Synopsis of somatosensory pathways

The impulses generated by various stimuli in different receptors are transmitted via peripheral nerves to the medulla spinalis. The cell body of the first afferent neuron which is connected with the receptors for all pathways is located in the ganglion sensorium nervi spinalis. The axons from the ganglion pass along various tracts in the medulla spinalis to the second neuron. The axon of the second neuron either passes directly to the cerebellum or reaches the thalamus where it synapses with the third order neurons that project to the cortex cerebri.

Name of pathway	Sensory quality	Receptor	Course in the medulla spinalis	Central course (rostral to the medulla spinalis)
Tractus spinothalamici				
Tractus spinothalamicus anterior	• Crude touch	• Hair follicles • Various skin receptors	The cell body of the second neuron is located in the cornu posterius and may be up to 15 segments above or 2 segments below the entry of the first neuron. Its axons cross in the commissura anterior (see p. 402)	The axons of the second neuron (lemniscus spinalis) terminate in the nucleus ventralis posterolateralis of the thalamus (see **D**, p. 347). There they synapse onto the third neuron, whose axons project to the gyrus postcentralis
Tractus spinothalamicus lateralis	• Pain and temperature	• Mostly free nerve endings	The cell body of the second neuron is in the substantia gelatinosa. Its axon crosses at the same level in the commissura anterior (see p. 402)	The axons of the second neuron (lemniscus spinalis) terminate in the nucleus ventralis posterolateralis of the thalamus, where they synapse with the third neuron, whose axons project to the gyrus postcentralis
Tracts of the funiculus posterior (dorsal column)				
Fasciculus gracilis	• Fine touch • Conscious proprioception of *lower* limb	• Vater-Pacini corpuscles • Muscle and tendon receptors	The axons of the first neuron pass to the nucleus gracilis in the caudal medulla oblongata (second neuron) (see p. 404 and **B**, p. 361)	The axons of the second neuron cross in the truncus encephali and traverse the lemniscus medialis (see **B**, p. 361) to the nucleus ventralis posterolateralis of the thalamus. There they synapse with the third neuron, whose axons project to the gyrus postcentralis
Fasciculus cuneatus	• Fine touch • Conscious proprioception of *upper* limb	• Vater-Pacini corpuscles • Muscle and tendon receptors	The axons of the first neuron pass to the nucleus cuneatus in the caudal medulla oblongata (second neuron) (see p. 404 and **B**, p. 361)	The axons of the second neuron cross in the truncus encephali and travel in the lemniscus medialis (see **B**, p. 361) to the nucleus ventralis posterolateralis of the thalamus. There they synapse with the third neuron, whose axons project to the gyrus postcentralis
Tractus spinocerebellares				
Tractus spinocerebellaris anterior (of Gowers)	• Unconscious crossed and uncrossed extero- and proprioception to the cerebellum	• Muscle spindles • Tendon receptors • Joint receptors • Skin receptors	The second neuron is located in the cornu posterius of the medulla spinalis. The axons of the second neuron run directly to the cerebellum, both crossed and uncrossed, (see p. 406)	The axons of the second neuron pass through the pedunculus cerebellaris superior to the vermis cerebelli (no third neuron) (see also p. 371)
Tractus spinocerebellaris posterior (of Flechsig)	• Unconscious uncrossed extero- and proprioception to the cerebellum	• Muscle spindles • Tendon receptors • Joint receptors • Skin receptors	The second neuron is located in the Clarke column (nucleus thoracicus posterior) in the substantia grisea at the base of the cornu posterius. The axons of the second neuron run directly to the cerebellum without crossing (see p. 406)	The axons of the second neuron pass through the pedunculus cerebellaris inferior to the vermis cerebelli (no third neuron) (see also p. 371)

13.2 Somatosensory System: Stimulus Processing

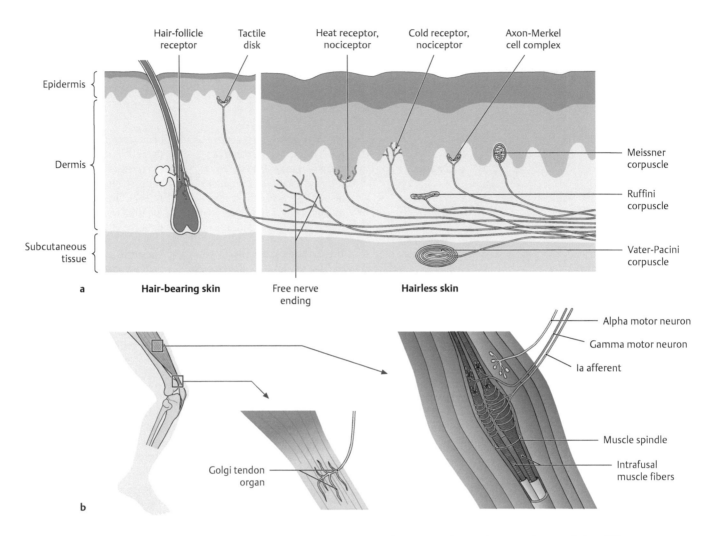

a **Hair-bearing skin**   **Hairless skin**

b

A Receptors of the somatosensory system

a **Skin receptors:** Various types of stimuli generate impulses in different receptors in the periphery of the body (illustrated here in sections through hair-bearing and hairless skin). These impulses are transmitted through peripheral nerves to the medulla spinalis, from which they are relayed and carried by specific tracts to the thalamus and then the somatosensory cortex (see p. 445). Sensory modalities cannot always be uniquely assigned to specific receptors. The figure

does not indicate the prevalence of the different receptor types. Nociceptors (pain receptors), like heat and cold receptors, consist of free nerve endings. Nociceptors make up approximately 50% of all receptors.

b **Joint receptors:** Proprioception encompasses position sense, motion sense, and force sense. Proprioceptors include muscle spindles, tendon sensors, and joint sensors (not shown).

B Receptive field sizes of cortical modules in the upper limb of a primate

Sensory information is processed in cortical "modules" (see **C**, p. 317). This drawing shows the size of the receptive fields supplied by modules. In areas where high resolution of sensory information is not required (e.g., the forearm), one module supplies a large receptive field. In areas that require finer tactile sensation (e.g., the fingers), one module supplies a much smaller receptive field. The size of these fields determines the overall proportions of the sensory homunculus (see **C**). Because one skin area may be innervated by several neurons, many of the receptive fields overlap. Information is transmitted from the receptive field to the cortex by a chain of neurons and their axons. These neurons and axons are located at specific sites in the CNS (topographical principle).

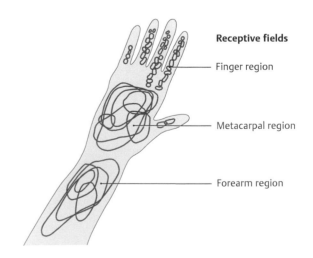

Receptive fields

Finger region

Metacarpal region

Forearm region

C Somatotopic organization of the somatosensory cortex: the sensory homunculus

Anterosuperior view of the right postcentral gyrus.

Sensory information from the medulla spinalis and skull are transmitted to neurons in the posterior thalamus, where they are forwarded. The axons of these neurons pass through the capsula interna (especially the crus posterius) and are projected over a wide area onto the primary somatosensory cortex in the gyrus postcentralis, where the information reaches the conscious level. The gyrus postcentralis has a somatotopic organization, meaning that each body region is represented in a particular cortical area. In this manner, a "sensory image" of the body or "sensory homunculus" is created. The cortical body regions are not proportionate to their actual physical size but are proportionate to their sensitivity and thus their required "circuit density." Highly sensitive areas of the body such as the fingers and head have a correspondingly large cortical representation, whereas less sensitive areas such as the torso have significantly smaller representations.

Note: The gyrus postcentralis always projects the contralateral half of the body so that the right gyrus projects the left half and vice versa. The cortical area of the skull is separated from the rest of the body. In contrast to the "headless" torso, the skull is upright. The jaw and teeth have their own cortical area beneath the head area. The leg and genital are represented on the medial surface of the brain beneath the margin of the mantle.

Descending motor pathways from the motor cortex also course within the capsula interna in addition to the sensory pathways. The close proximity of the sensory and motor pathways explains why damage to the capsula interna (as can occur in a stroke) often simultaneously produces sensory and motor deficits, always on the side opposite the lesion (see motor homunculus, **B**, p. 457).

Note: The continuation of the *gyrus postcentralis* on the medial surface of the brain is known as the *gyrus paracentralis posterior*.

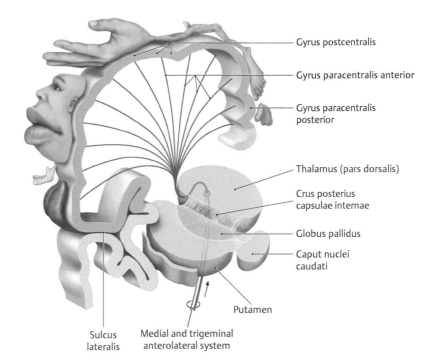

Gyrus postcentralis

Gyrus paracentralis anterior

Gyrus paracentralis posterior

Thalamus (pars dorsalis)

Crus posterius capsulae internae

Globus pallidus

Caput nuclei caudati

Putamen

Sulcus lateralis — Medial and trigeminal anterolateral system

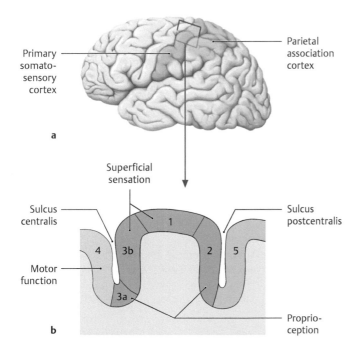

Primary somatosensory cortex

Parietal association cortex

a Left lateral view.

Superficial sensation

Sulcus centralis

Sulcus postcentralis

1

4   3b   2   5

Motor function

3a

Proprioception

b

D Primary somatosensory cortex and parietal association cortex

a Left lateral view. The Brodmann areas are numbered in the sectional view (**b**). The contralateral half of the body is represented in the primary somatosensory cortex (except the perioral region, which is represented bilaterally). This area of the cortex is concerned with somatosensory perception. The parietal association cortex receives information from both sides of the body. Thus, the processing of stimuli becomes increasingly complex in these cortical areas.

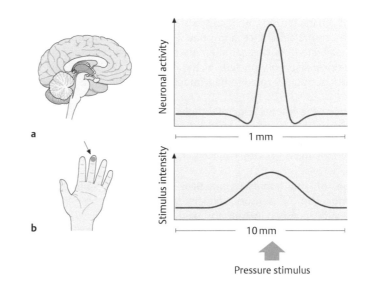

Neuronal activity

a

1 mm

Stimulus intensity

b

10 mm

Pressure stimulus

E Activity of cortical cell columns in the primary somatosensory cortex

a Amplitude of the neuronal response in the primary somatosensory cortex in response to a peripheral pressure stimulus. The intensity of the stimulus is shown in **b**. The diagrams illustrate the principle of sensory information processing in the cortex. When approximately 100 intensity detectors in the fingertip are stimulated by pressure, approximately 10,000 neurons in the corresponding cell column in the primary somatosensory cortex (see columnar organization of the cortex, **C** p. 327) respond to the stimulus. Because the intensity of the peripheral pressure stimulus is maximal at the center and fades toward the edges, it is processed in the cortex accordingly. Cortical processing amplifies the contrast between the greater and lesser stimulus intensities, resulting in a sharper peak (**a**). While the stimulated area on the fingertip measures approximately 100 mm², the information is processed in only a 1-mm² area of the primary somatosensory cortex.

447

13.3 Somatosensory System: Lesions

A Sites of occurrence of lesions in the somatosensory pathways
(after Bähr and Frotscher)

The central portions of the somatosensory pathways may be damaged at various sites from the spinal root to the somatosensory cortex as a result of trauma, tumor mass effect, hemorrhage, or infarction. The signs and symptoms are helpful in determining the location of the lesion. This unit deals strictly with lesions in conscious pathways. The innervation of the trunk and limbs is mediated by the nn. spinales. The innervation of the head is mediated by the n. trigeminus, which has its own nuclei (see below).

Cortical or subcortical lesion (1, 2): A lesion at this level is manifested by paresthesia (tingling) and numbness in the corresponding regions of the trunk and limbs on the *opposite* side of the body. The symptoms may be most pronounced distally because of the large receptive fields on the fingers and the relatively small receptive fields on the trunk (see p. 447). The motor and somatosensory cortex are closely interlinked because fibers in the sensory tracts from the thalamus also terminate in the motor cortex, and because the cortical areas are adjacent (gyri pre- and postcentralis).

Lesions caudal to the thalamus (3): All sensation is abolished in the *contralateral* half of the body (thalamus = "gateway to consciousness"). A partial lesion that spares the pain and temperature pathways **(4)** is characterized by hypesthesia (decreased tactile sensation) on the *contralateral* face and body. Pain and temperature sensation are unaffected. As cortical afferents travel crossed and uncrossed to the principal sensory nucleus of the n. trigeminus, it is possible that epicritic sensitivity could remain intact in a unilateral lesion.

Lesion of the tractus trigeminothalamicus and tractus spinothalamicus lateralis (5): Damage to these pathways in the truncus encephali causes a loss of pain and temperature sensation in the *contralateral* half of the face and body. Other sensory modalities are unaffected.

Lesion of the lemniscus medialis and tractus spinothalamicus anterior (6): All sensory modalities on the *opposite* side of the body are abolished except for pain and temperature. The lemniscus medialis transmits the axons of the second neurons of the tractus spinothalamicus anterior and both tracts of the funiculus posterior. The axons of the second neuron of the tractus spinothalamicus anterior connect to the lemniscus medialis in the medulla oblongata.

Lesion of the nucleus spinalis nervi trigemini, tractus spinalis nervi trigemini, and tractus spinothalamicus lateralis (7): Pain and temperature sensation is abolished on the *ipsilateral* side of the face (uncrossed axons of the first neuron from the ganglion trigeminale) and on the *contralateral* side of the body (axons of the crossed second neuron in the tractus spinothalamicus lateralis).

Lesion of the funiculi posteriores (8): This lesion causes an *ipsilateral* loss of position sense, vibration sense, and two-point discrimination. Because coordinated motor function relies on sensory input that operates in a feedback loop, the lack of sensory input leads to ipsilateral sensory ataxia.

Cornu posterius lesion (9): A circumscribed lesion involving one or a few segments causes an *ipsilateral* loss of pain and temperature sensation in the affected segment(s), because pain and temperature sensation are relayed to the second neuron within the cornu posterius. Other sensory modalities including crude touch are transmitted in the funiculus posterior and relayed to the columna posterior nuclei; hence they are unaffected. The effects of a cornu posterius lesion are called a "dissociated sensory deficit."

Radix posterior lesion (10): This lesion causes *ipsilateral*, radicular sensory disturbances that may range from pain in the corresponding dermatome to a complete loss of sensation. Concomitant involvement of the radix anterior leads to segmental weakness. This clinical situation may be caused by a herniated discus intervertebralis (see p. 463).

Lesions of *unconscious* tractus cerebellares that lead to sensorimotor deficits are not considered here. The volume on *General Anatomy and Musculoskeletal System* may be consulted for information on peripheral sensory nerve lesions.

B Terminology of the lemnisci

Lemniscus (= ribbon) is a purely morphologic term for a sensory pathway in the truncus encephali. There are historical reasons for this term. Structurally, it does not represent a "new" pathway, rather the continuation of an existing pathway under another name. Four lemnisci are distinguished:

- *Lemniscus medialis:* Epicritic somatic sensation of the torso and extremities; it is the continuation of the fasciculus gracilis and fasciculus cuneatus.
- *Lemniscus spinalis:* Protopathic somatic sensation of the torso and extremities; it is the continuation of the tractus spinothalamicus anterior and tractus spinothalamicus lateralis.
- *Lemniscus trigeminalis:* Epicritic and protopathic sensation of the area innervated by the n. trigeminus.
- *Lemniscus lateralis:* Part of the auditory pathway ("specific somatosensitivity"). The lemniscus lateralis is not shown in the figure on p. 449.

The four lemnisci are described in greater detail on p. 539.

Neuroanatomy —— *13. Functional Systems*

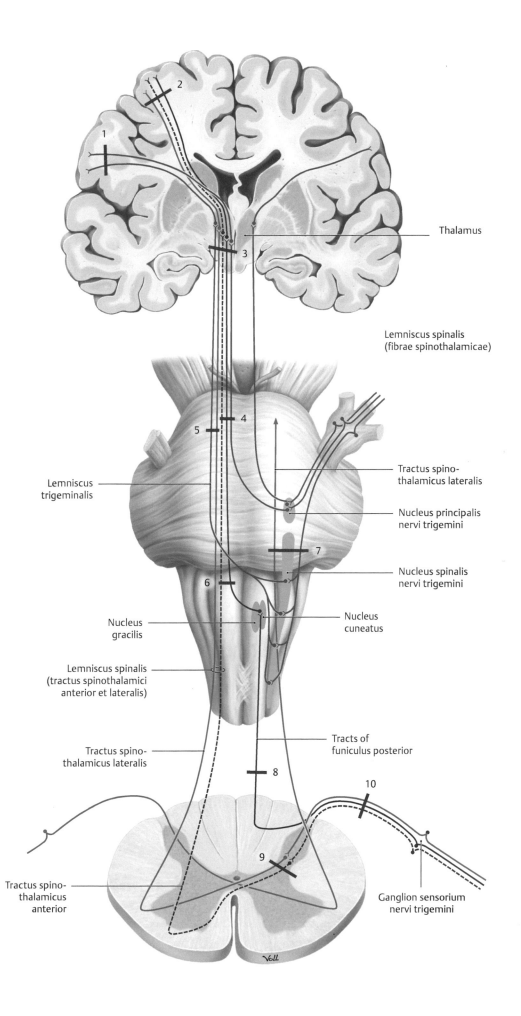

Thalamus

Lemniscus spinalis
(fibrae spinothalamicae)

Lemniscus
trigeminalis

Tractus spino-
thalamicus lateralis

Nucleus principalis
nervi trigemini

Nucleus spinalis
nervi trigemini

Nucleus
cuneatus

Nucleus
gracilis

Lemniscus spinalis
(tractus spinothalamici
anterior et lateralis)

Tracts of
funiculus posterior

Tractus spino-
thalamicus lateralis

Tractus spino-
thalamicus
anterior

Ganglion sensorium
nervi trigemini

13.4 Somatosensory System: Pain Conduction

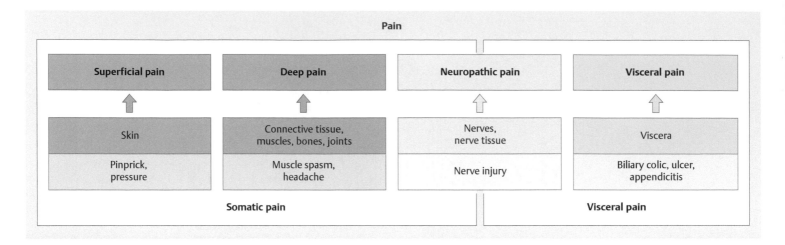

A Synopsis of pain modalities

The International Association for the Study of Pain defines pain as "an unpleasant sensory and emotional experience associated with actual or potential tissue damage, or described in terms of such damage." Pain is classified by its site of origin as *somatic or visceral*. Somatic pain generally originates in the trunk, limbs, or head, while visceral pain originates in the internal organs. *Neuropathic* pain is caused by damage to the nerves themselves. It may involve nerves of the somatic and/or autonomic nervous system. The somatic pain fibers described below travel with the nn. spinales or craniales, while the visceral pain fibers travel with the autonomic nerves (see p. 302).

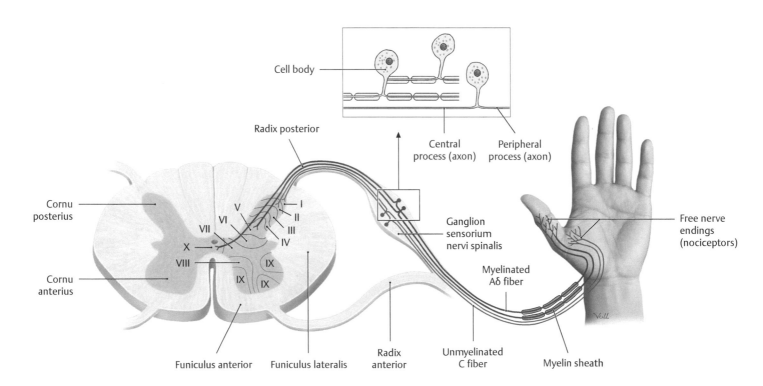

B Peripheral somatic pain conduction (after Lorke)

Somatic pain impulses from the trunk and limbs are conducted by myelinated Aδ fibers (temperature, pain, position) and unmyelinated C fibers (temperature, pain). The cell bodies of these afferent nerve fibers are located in the ganglion sensorium nervi spinalis (pseudounipolar neurons). Their axons terminate in the cornu posterius of the medulla spinalis, chiefly in the Rexed laminae I, II, and IV–VI. The nociceptors, afferent fibers ascend after synapsing in the cornu posterius (see **C**). *Note*: Most somatosensory pain fibers are myelinated, while the viscerosensory fibers are unmyelinated.

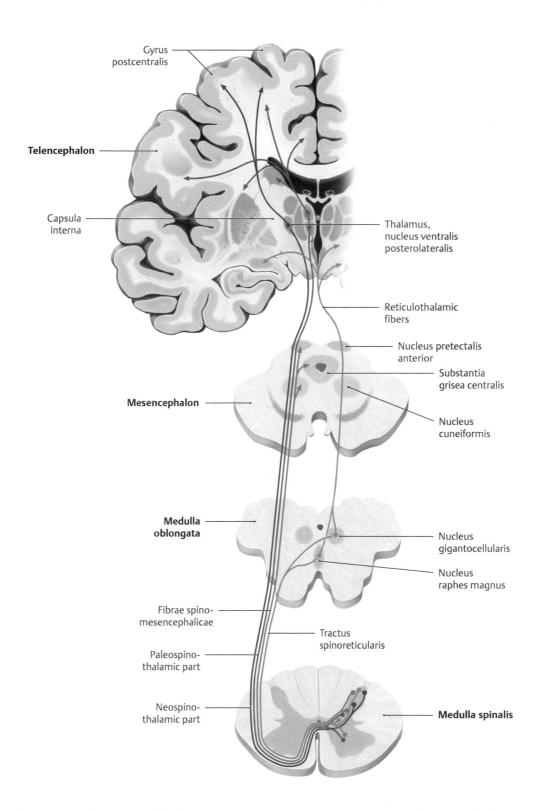

Gyrus postcentralis

Telencephalon

Capsula interna

Thalamus, nucleus ventralis posterolateralis

Reticulothalamic fibers

Nucleus pretectalis anterior

Substantia grisea centralis

Mesencephalon

Nucleus cuneiformis

Medulla oblongata

Nucleus gigantocellularis

Nucleus raphes magnus

Fibrae spino-mesencephalicae

Tractus spinoreticularis

Paleospino-thalamic part

Neospino-thalamic part

Medulla spinalis

C Ascending pain pathways from the trunk and limbs

The axons of the primary afferent neurons for pain sensation in the trunk and limbs terminate on the neurons (shown above) located in the cornu posterius of the medulla spinalis. The tractus spinothalamicus lateralis is subdivided into a neo- and paleospinothalamic part. The second neuron of the *neospinothalamic part* of the pain pathway (red) terminates in the nucleus ventralis posterolateralis of the thalamus. The third neuron projects from there to the primary somatosensory cortex (gyrus postcentralis) of the brain. The second neuron of the *paleospinothalamic tract* (blue) terminates in the nuclei intralaminares and mediales thalami, whose third neuron then projects to a variety of brain regions.

This pain pathway is mainly responsible for the emotional component associated with pain. In addition to these pain pathways that end on the cortex cerebri, there are also pain pathways that end in *subcortical* regions—the fibrae spinomesencephalicae and tractus spinoreticularis. The second neuron of the *fibrae spinomesencephalicae* (green) terminates mainly in the substantia grisea centralis. Other axons terminate in the nucleus cuneiformis or nucleus pretectalis anterior. The second neuron of the *tractus spinoreticularis* (orange) ends in the formatio reticularis, represented here by the nucleus raphes magnus and the nucleus gigantocellularis. Reticulothalamic fibers transmit the pain impulses onward to the medial thalamus, hypothalamus, and limbic system.

451

13.5 Somatosensory System: Pain Pathways in the Head and the Central Analgesic System

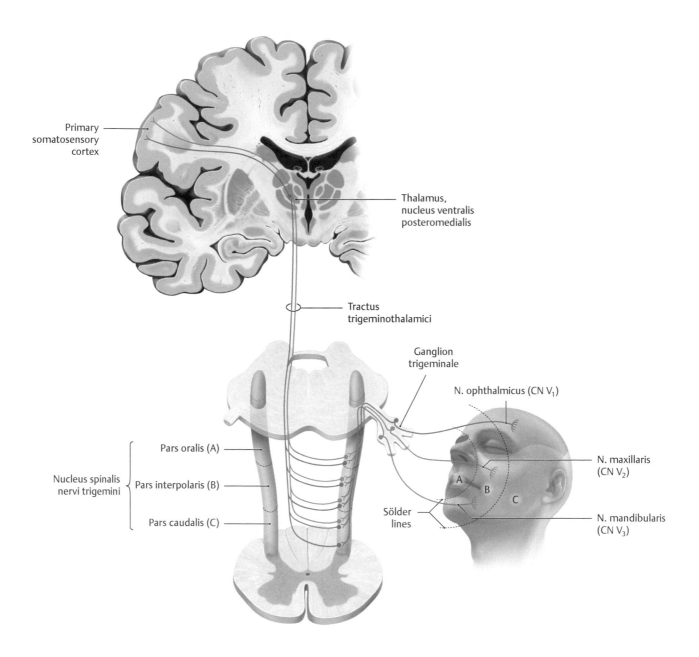

A Pain pathways in the head (after Lorke)

The pain fibers in the head accompany the principal divisions of the n. trigeminus (CN V₁–V₃). The cell bodies of these primary afferent neurons of the pain pathway are located in the ganglion trigeminale. Their axons terminate in the nucleus spinalis nervi trigemini.

Note the somatotopic organization of this nuclear region: The perioral region (**a**) is cranial and the occipital region (**c**) is caudal. Because of this arrangement, central lesions lead to deficits that are distributed along the Sölder lines (see **D**, p. 121).

The axons of the second neurons cross the midline and travel in the tractus trigeminothalamici to the nucleus ventralis posteromedialis and to the nuclei intralaminares thalami on the opposite side, where they terminate. The third (thalamic) neuron of the pain pathway ends in the primary somatosensory cortex. Only the pain fibers of the n. trigeminus are pictured in the diagram. In the n. trigeminus itself, the other sensory fibers run parallel to the pain fibers but terminate in various trigeminal nuclei (see p. 120).

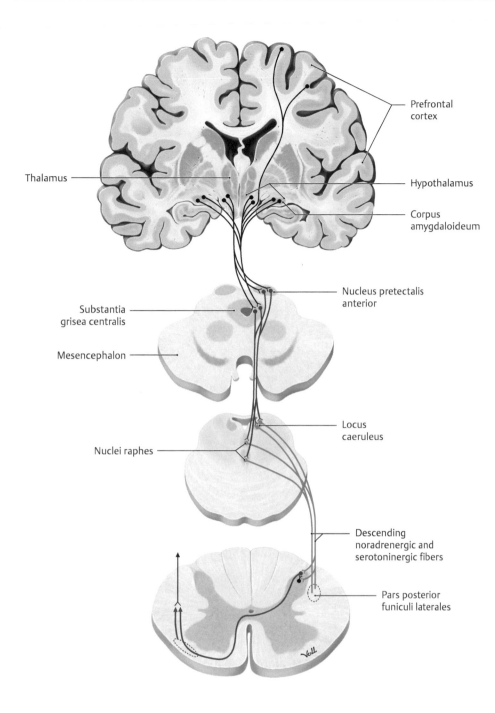

Prefrontal cortex

Thalamus

Hypothalamus

Corpus amygdaloideum

Nucleus pretectalis anterior

Substantia grisea centralis

Mesencephalon

Locus caeruleus

Nuclei raphes

Descending noradrenergic and serotoninergic fibers

Pars posterior funiculi laterales

B Pathways of the central descending analgesic system
(after Lorke)

Besides the ascending pathways that carry pain sensation to the primary somatosensory cortex, there are also descending pathways that have the ability to suppress pain impulses. The central relay station for the descending analgesic (pain-relieving) system is the substantia grisea centralis of the mesencephalon. It is activated by afferent input from the hypothalamus, the prefrontal cortex, and the corpora amygdaloidea (part of the limbic system, not shown). It also receives afferent input from the medulla spinalis (see p. 450). The axons from the excitatory glutaminergic neurons (red) of the substantia grisea centralis terminate on serotoninergic neurons in the nuclei raphes and on noradrenergic neurons in the locus caeruleus (both shown in blue). The axons from both types of neuron descend in the pars posterior funiculi lateralis. They terminate directly or indirectly (via inhibitory neurons) on the analgesic projection neurons (second afferent neuron of the pain pathway), thereby inhibiting the further conduction of pain impulses.

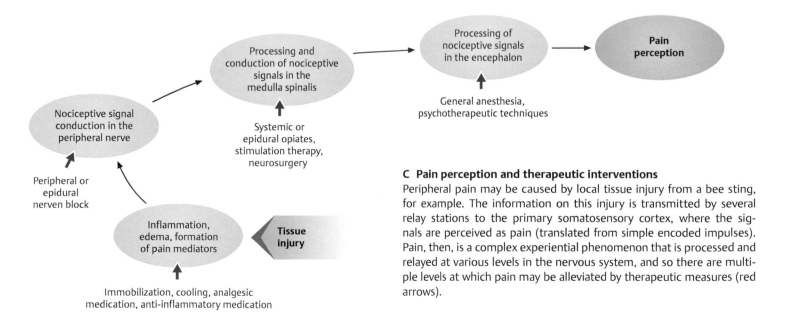

Processing and conduction of nociceptive signals in the medulla spinalis

Processing of nociceptive signals in the encephalon

Pain perception

General anesthesia, psychotherapeutic techniques

Nociceptive signal conduction in the peripheral nerve

Systemic or epidural opiates, stimulation therapy, neurosurgery

Peripheral or epidural nerven block

Inflammation, edema, formation of pain mediators

Tissue injury

Immobilization, cooling, analgesic medication, anti-inflammatory medication

C Pain perception and therapeutic interventions

Peripheral pain may be caused by local tissue injury from a bee sting, for example. The information on this injury is transmitted by several relay stations to the primary somatosensory cortex, where the signals are perceived as pain (translated from simple encoded impulses). Pain, then, is a complex experiential phenomenon that is processed and relayed at various levels in the nervous system, and so there are multiple levels at which pain may be alleviated by therapeutic measures (red arrows).

13.6 Motor System, Overview

A Simplified representation of the anatomical structures involved in a voluntary movement (pyramidal motor system)

(after Klinke and Silbernagl)

The first step in performing a voluntary movement is to plan the movement in the association cerebral cortex (e.g., goal: "I want to pick up my coffee cup"). The hemispheria cerebelli and nuclei basales work in parallel to program the movement and inform the premotor cortex of the result of this planning. The premotor cortex passes the information to the primary motor cortex (M1), which relays the information through the *tractus pyramidalis* to the alpha motor neuron (*pyramidal motor system*). The alpha motor neuron then transmits the information to the skeletal muscle, which transforms the program into a specific voluntary movement. Sensorimotor functions provide important feedback during this process (How far has the movement progressed? How strong is my grip on the cup handle?—different from gripping an eggshell, for example). Although some of the later figures portray the primary motor cortex as the starting point for a voluntary movement, this diagram shows that many motor centers are involved in the execution of a voluntary movement (including the *extrapyramidal motor system*, see **C** and **D**; cerebellum). For practical reasons, however, the discussion commonly begins at the primary motor cortex (M1).

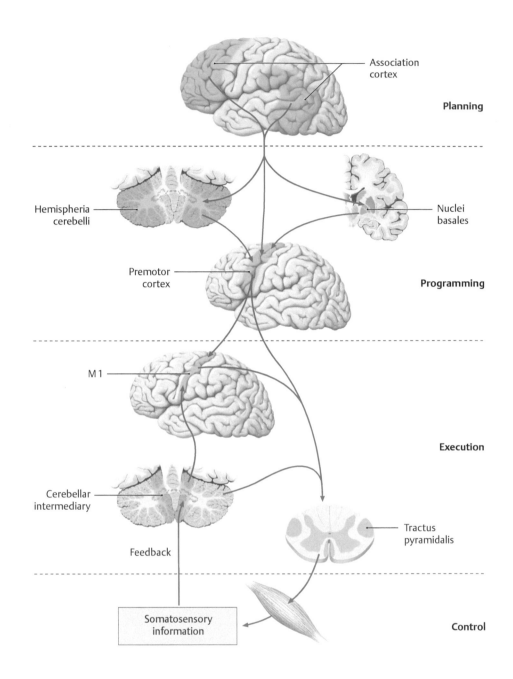

B Cortical areas with motor function: Initiating a movement

Lateral view of the left hemispherium cerebri. The initiation of a voluntary movement (reaching for a coffee cup) results from the interaction of various cortical areas. The *primary motor cortex* (M1, Brodmann area 4) is located in the gyrus precentralis (execution of a movement). The rostrally adjacent area 6 consists of the lateral premotor cortex and medial supplementary motor cortex (initiation of a movement). Fibrae associationis (see p. 334) establish close functional connections with sensory areas 1, 2, and 3 (gyrus postcentralis with primary somatosensory cortex, S1) and with areas 5 and 7 (posterior parietal cortex), which have an associative motor function. These areas provide the cortical representation of space, which is important in precision grasping movements and eye movements.

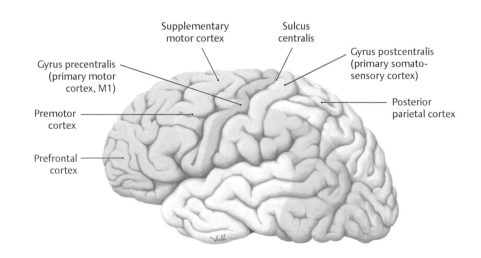

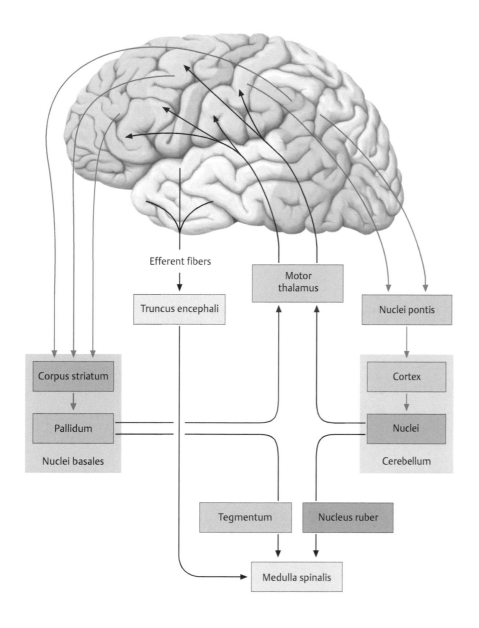

Efferent fibers

Motor thalamus

Truncus encephali

Nuclei pontis

Corpus striatum

Cortex

Pallidum

Nuclei

Nuclei basales

Cerebellum

Tegmentum

Nucleus ruber

Medulla spinalis

C Connections of the cortex with the nuclei basales and cerebellum: Programming of complex movements

The pyramidal motor system (the primary motor cortex and the tractus pyramidalis arising from it) is assisted by the nuclei basales and cerebellum in the planning and programming of complex movements. While afferent fibers of the motor nuclei (green) project directly to the nuclei basales (left) without synapsing, the cerebellum is indirectly controlled via nuclei pontis (right; see **C**, p. 361). The motor thalamus provides a feedback loop for both structures (see p. 459). The efferent fibers of the nuclei basales and cerebellum are distributed to lower structures including the medulla spinalis. The importance of the nuclei basales and cerebellum in voluntary movements can be appreciated by noting the effects of lesions in these structures. While diseases of the nuclei basales impair the initiation and execution of movements (e.g., in Parkinson's disease), cerebellar lesions are characterized by uncoordinated movements (e.g., the reeling movements of inebriation, caused by a temporary toxic insult to the cerebellum).

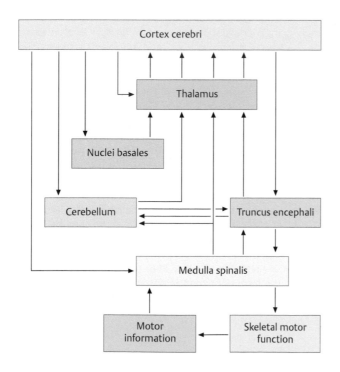

Cortex cerebri

Thalamus

Nuclei basales

Cerebellum

Truncus encephali

Medulla spinalis

Motor information

Skeletal motor function

D Simplified block diagram of the sensorimotor system in the control of movement

Voluntary movements require constant feedback from the periphery (muscle spindles, tendon organs) in order to remain within the desired limits. Because the motor and sensory systems are so closely interrelated functionally, they are often described jointly as the sensorimotor system. The medulla spinalis, truncus encephali, cerebellum, and cortex cerebri are the three control levels of the sensorimotor system. All information from periphery, cerebellum, and the nuclei basales passes through the thalamus on its way to the cortex cerebri. The clinical importance of the sensory system in movement is illustrated by the sensory ataxia that may occur when sensory function is lost (see **D**, p. 471). The oculomotor component of the sensorimotor system is not shown.

13.7 Motor System: Tractus Pyramidalis (Corticospinalis)

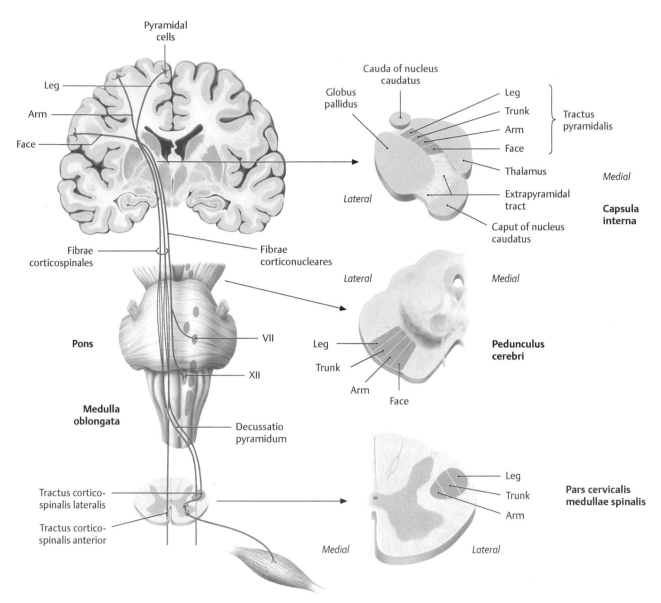

A Course of the tractus pyramidalis (fibrae corticospinales)

The tractus pyramidalis consists of three fiber systems: fibrae corticospinales, fibrae corticonucleares, and fibrae corticoreticulares (the latter are not shown here; they pass to the nucleus gigantocellularis of the formatio reticularis in the truncus encephali and will not be further discussed). These groups of fibers constitute the descending motor pathways from the primary motor cortex. The fibrae corticospinales pass to the motor neurons in the cornu anterius of the medulla spinalis, while the fibrae corticonucleares pass to the motor nuclei of nn. craniales.

Corticospinal fibers: Only a small percentage of the axons of the fibrae corticospinales originate from the large pyramidal neurons in lamina V of the gyrus precentralis (the laminar structure of the motor cortex is shown in **D**). Most of the axons arise from small pyramidal cells and other neurons in laminae V and VI. Other axons originate from adjacent brain regions. All of them descend through the capsula interna. Eighty percent of the fibers *cross the midline* at the level of the medulla oblongata (decussatio pyramidum) and descend in the medulla spinalis as the *tractus corticospinalis lateralis*. The *uncrossed* fibers descend in the cord as the *tractus corticospinalis anterior* and cross later at the segmental level. Most of the axons terminate on intercalated cells whose synapses end on motor neurons.

Note: The basic pattern of somatotopic organization described earlier at the medulla spinalis level is found at all levels of the tractus pyramidalis. This facilitates localization of the lesion in the tractus pyramidalis.

Corticonuclear fibers: The motor nuclei and motor segments of the nn. craniales receive their axons from pyramidal cells in the facial region of the premotor cortex. These fibrae corticonucleares terminate in the contralateral motor nuclei of nn. craniales III–VII and IX–XII in the truncus encephali (the fibers to other truncus encephali nuclei are shown in **C**). Besides this contralateral supply, axons also pass to several n. cranialis nuclei on the same (ipsilateral) side, resulting in a bilateral innervation pattern (not shown here). This dual supply is clinically important in lesions of the n. facialis, for example (upper versus lower face) (see **D**, p. 125).

Notes on the "tractus pyramidalis": Some authors interpret this term as applying strictly to the portion of the tract below the decussatio pyramidum, while other authors apply the term to the entire tract. Most publications, including this atlas, use "tractus pyramidalis" as a collective term for all of the fiber tracts described here. Some authors derive the term not from the decussatio pyramidum but from the giant pyramidal cells (Betz cells) in the cortex cerebri (see **C** and p. 409).

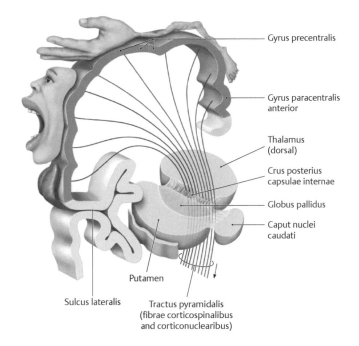

Gyrus precentralis

Gyrus paracentralis anterior

Thalamus (dorsal)

Crus posterius capsulae internae

Globus pallidus

Caput nuclei caudati

Putamen

Sulcus lateralis

Tractus pyramidalis (fibrae corticospinalibus and corticonuclearibus)

B Somatotopic organization of the somatomotor cortex: the motor homunculus

Anterosuperior view of the gyrus precentralis dexter. Axons of neurons of the primary somato*motor* cortex in the gyrus precentralis extend as the tractus pyramidalis to the motor neurons in the truncus encephali and medulla spinalis. The axons pass through the capsula interna (primarily the crus posterius) and course as cortico*nuclear* fibers to the cranial nerves (*nuclei*) or as the tractus corticospinalis anterior or lateralis to the *medulla spinalis*. The gyrus precentralis exhibits *somatotopic organization*. Specific cortical areas control the motor function of specific parts of the body. The result is a "motor representation" of the body, a *Motor homunculus*. Body parts with complex motor function such as the hands or head (facial expression) require a large number of cortical neurons and are represented in large regions on the cortex regardless of their actual physical size. The gyrus precentralis always controls the motor function of the contralateral half of the body. The cortical area of the skull is separated from the rest of the body. In contrast to the "headless" torso, the skull is upright. The leg is represented on the medial surface of the brain beneath the margin of the mantle. A few motor functions *only on the skull* are also represented bilaterally (see **D**, p. 125). Compare this with the illustration of the sensory homunculus on p. 447.

Note: The continuation of the gyrus precentralis on the medial surface of the brain is known as the gyrus paracentralis anterior.

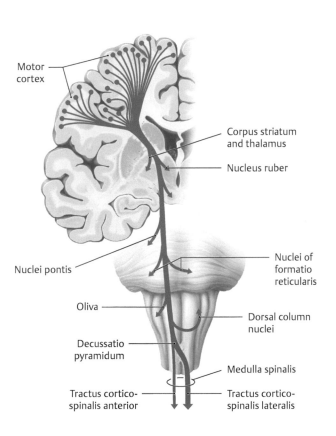

Motor cortex

Corpus striatum and thalamus

Nucleus ruber

Nuclei pontis

Nuclei of formatio reticularis

Oliva

Dorsal column nuclei

Decussatio pyramidum

Medulla spinalis

Tractus cortico-spinalis anterior

Tractus cortico-spinalis lateralis

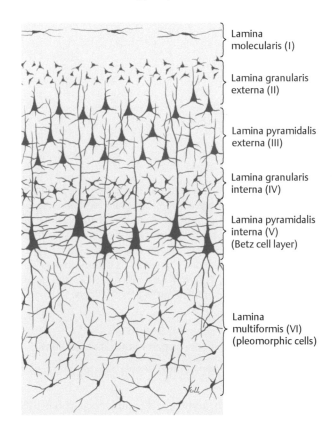

Lamina molecularis (I)

Lamina granularis externa (II)

Lamina pyramidalis externa (III)

Lamina granularis interna (IV)

Lamina pyramidalis interna (V) (Betz cell layer)

Lamina multiformis (VI) (pleomorphic cells)

C Variety of cortical efferent fibers

Anterior view. Besides the fibrae corticospinales and corticonucleares described above, a variety of axons descends from the cortex to various subcortical regions and into the medulla spinalis. The following subcortical regions also receive cortical efferent fibers: the corpus striatum, thalamus, nucleus ruber, nuclei pontis, formatio reticularis, oliva, dorsal column nuclei (these nuclear regions are described on p. 460), and medulla spinalis. The supraspinal efferent fibers listed above consist partially of axon collaterals from tractus pyramidalis neurons and partially of separate axons.

D Laminar structure of the motor cortex (= area 4 in the gyrus precentralis)

The axons from giant pyramidal cells (Betz cells) in lamina V account for only a small percentage (<4%) of the axons that make up the fibrae corticospinales. Small pyramidal cells and other neurons from laminae V and VI contribute the rest. In all, however, only about 40% of the axons of the tractus pyramidalis originate in area 4. The remaining 60% come from neurons in the supplementary motor fields and other cortical areas (see p. 454).

13.8 Motor System: Motor Nuclei

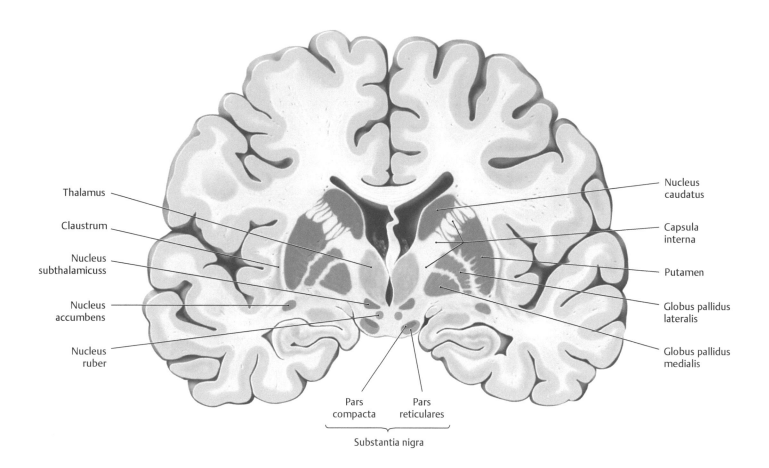

Thalamus

Claustrum

Nucleus subthalamicuss

Nucleus accumbens

Nucleus ruber

Nucleus caudatus

Capsula interna

Putamen

Globus pallidus lateralis

Globus pallidus medialis

Pars compacta   Pars reticulares

Substantia nigra

A Motor nuclei

Coronal section. The nuclei basales (basal ganglia) are subcortical nuclei of the telencephalon that have a role in the planning and execution of movements. They are the central relay station of the extrapyramidal motor system and make up almost all the central substantia grisea of the cerebrum. The only other central substantia grisea structure is the thalamus, which is primarily sensory ("gateway to consciousness") and is involved only secondarily, through feedback mechanisms, in motor sequences. The three largest motor nuclei are as follows:

• Nucleus caudatus
• Putamen
• Globus pallidus (developmentally, part of the diencephalon)

These three nuclei are sometimes known by varying collective designations:

• The *nucleus lentiformis* is formed by the putamen, globus pallidus, and intervening fiber tracts.

• The *corpus striatum* consists of the putamen, nucleus caudatus, and intervening streaks of gray matter. In addition to these three nuclei, there are other nuclei that are considered functional components of the motor system (also shown here).

In a strictly anatomical sense, only the telencephalic structures listed above are constituents of the nuclei basales (basal ganglia). Some textbooks mistakenly include the *nucleus subthalamicus* of the diencephalon (see p. 352) and the *substantia nigra* of the mesencephalon (see p. 357) among the nuclei basales because of their close functional relationship to nuclei. Functional disturbances of the nuclei basales are characterized by movement disorders (e.g., Parkinson's disease).

The nucleus accumbens is part of the reward circuit. For instance, when stimulated, it translates desires into action.

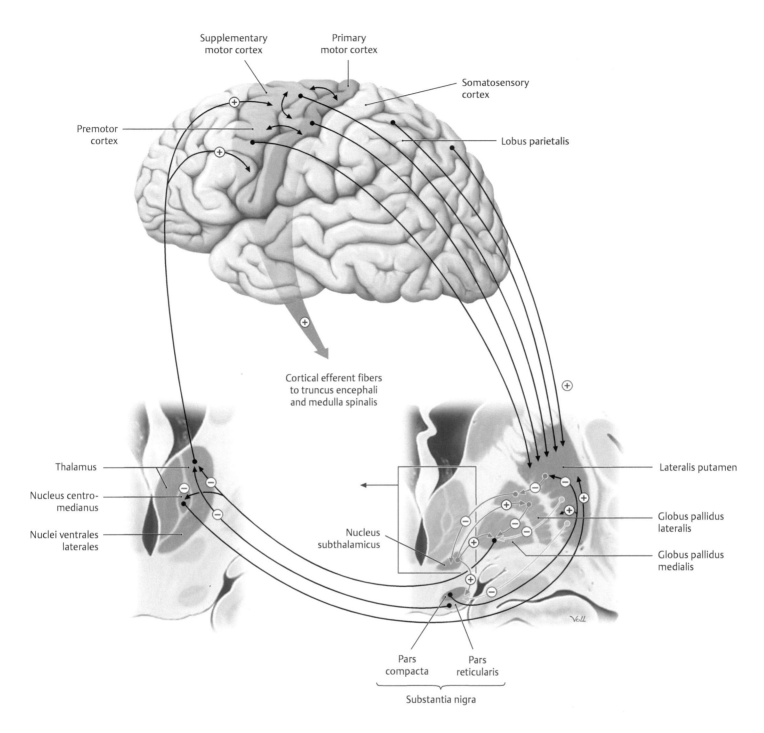

B Flow of information between motor cortical areas and nuclei basales: Motor loop

The nuclei basales are concerned with the controlled, purposeful execution of fine voluntary movements (e.g., picking up an egg without breaking it). They integrate information from the cortex and subcortical regions, which they process in parallel and then return to motor cortical areas via the thalamus (feedback). Neurons from the premotor, primary motor, supplementary motor, and somatosensory cortex and from the lobus parietalis send their axons to the putamen (see p. 337). Initially, there is a direct (yellow) and indirect (green) pathway for relaying the information out of the putamen. Both pathways ultimately lead to the motor cortex by way of the thalamus. In the *direct* pathway (yellow), the neurons of the putamen project to the globus pallidus medialis and to the pars reticularis of the substantia nigra. Both nuclei then return feedback signals to the motor thalamus, which projects back to

motor areas of the cortex. The *indirect* pathway (green) leads from the putamen through the globus pallidus lateralis and nucleus subthalamicus to the globus pallidus medialis, which then projects to the thalamus. An alternate indirect route leads from the nucleus subthalamicus to the pars reticularis of the substantia nigra, which in turn projects to the thalamus. When inhibitory dopaminergic neurons in the pars compacta of the substantia nigra cease to function, the indirect pathway is suppressed and the direct pathway is no longer facilitated. Both effects lead to the increased inhibition of thalamocortical neurons, resulting in decreased movements (*hypokinetic disorder*, e.g., in Parkinson's disease). Conversely, reduced activation of the globus pallidus medialis and the pars reticularis of the substantia nigra leads to increased activation of the thalamocortical neurons, resulting in abnormal spontaneous movements (*hyperkinetic disorder*, e.g., Huntington's disease). The diagram at lower left shows a close-up view of the boxed area (thalamus).

13.9 Motor System: Extrapyramidal Motor System and Lesions

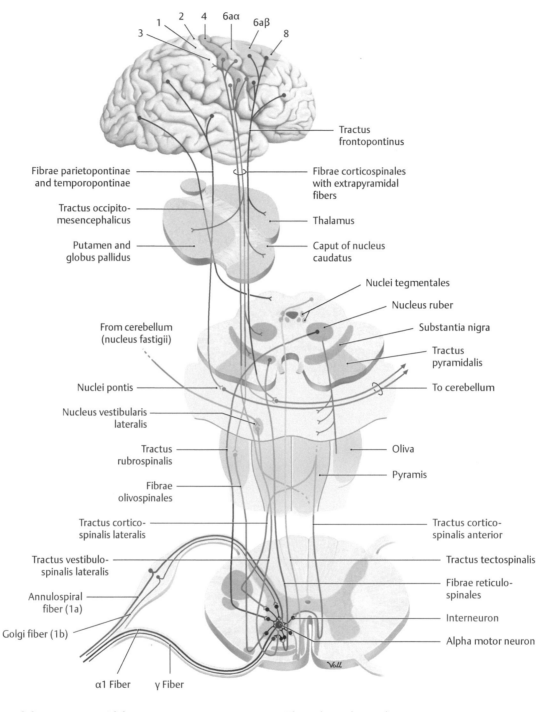

Labels on the figure:

2   4   6aα   6aβ
1   8
3

Tractus frontopontinus

Fibrae parietopontinae and temporopontinae

Fibrae corticospinales with extrapyramidal fibers

Tractus occipito-mesencephalicus

Thalamus

Putamen and globus pallidus

Caput of nucleus caudatus

Nuclei tegmentales

Nucleus ruber

From cerebellum (nucleus fastigii)

Substantia nigra

Tractus pyramidalis

Nuclei pontis

To cerebellum

Nucleus vestibularis lateralis

Tractus rubrospinalis

Oliva

Fibrae olivospinales

Pyramis

Tractus cortico-spinalis lateralis

Tractus cortico-spinalis anterior

Tractus vestibulo-spinalis lateralis

Tractus tectospinalis

Annulospiral fiber (1a)

Fibrae reticulo-spinales

Golgi fiber (1b)

Interneuron

Alpha motor neuron

α1 Fiber   γ Fiber

A Descending tracts of the extrapyramidal motor system

The neurons of origin of the descending tracts of the extrapyramidal motor system* arise from a heterogeneous group of nuclei that includes the nuclei basales (putamen, globus pallidus, and nucleus caudatus), the nucleus ruber, the substantia nigra, and even motor cortical areas (e.g., area 6). The following descending tracts are part of the extrapyramidal motor system:

• Tractus rubrospinalis
• Fibrae olivospinales
• Tractus vestibulospinales
• Tractus reticulospinales
• Tractus tectospinalis

These long descending tracts terminate on interneurons which then form synapses onto alpha and gamma motor neurons, which they control. Besides these long descending motor tracts, the motor neurons additionally receive sensory input (blue). All impulses in these pathways are integrated by the alpha motor neuron and modulate its activity, thereby affecting muscular contractions. The functional integrity of the alpha motor neuron is tested clinically by reflex testing.

* The term "extrapyramidal motor system" has been criticized because its functional and anatomical components are so closely linked to the pyramidal motor system that the distinction seems arbitrary in an anatomical sense — particularly since the system does not include cerebellar tracts that are also involved in the control of motor function.

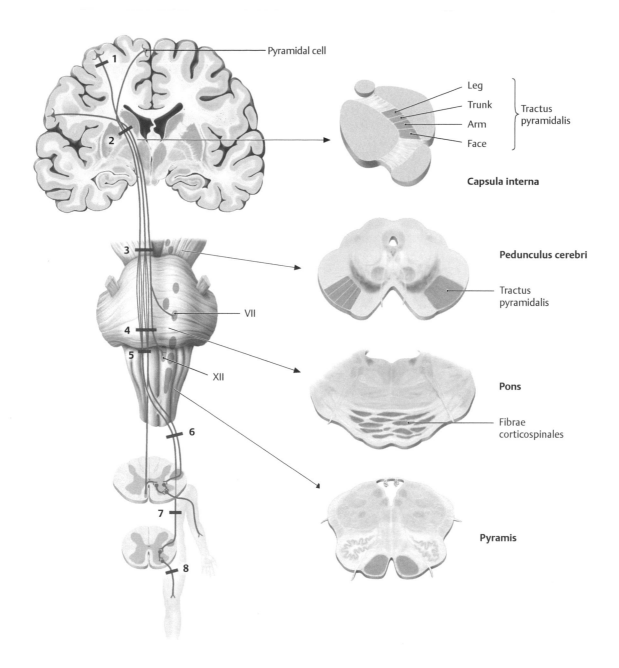

Pyramidal cell

Leg
Trunk } Tractus
Arm   } pyramidalis
Face

Capsula interna

Pedunculus cerebri

Tractus pyramidalis

VII

XII

Pons

Fibrae corticospinales

Pyramis

B Lesions of the central motor pathways and their effects

Lesion near the cortex (1): paralysis of the muscles innervated by the damaged cortical area. Because the face and hand are represented by particularly large areas in the motor cortex (see **B**, p. 457), paralysis often affects primarily the arm and face ("brachiofacial" paralysis). The paralysis invariably affects the side opposite the lesion (due to decussatio pyramidum) and is flaccid and partial *(paresis)* rather than complete because the extrapyramidal fibers are not damaged. If the extrapyramidal fibers were also damaged, the result would be contralateral *complete spastic paralysis* (see below).

Lesion at the level of the capsula interna (2): This leads to chronic, contralateral, spastic hemi*plegia* (complete paralysis) because the lesion affects both the tractus pyramidalis and the extrapyramidal motor pathways,* which mix with tractus pyramidalis fibers in front of the capsula interna. Stroke is a frequent cause of lesions at this level.

Lesion at the level of the pedunculus cerebri (crus cerebri) (3): Contralateral spastic hemi*paresis*.

Lesion at the level of the pons (4): Contralateral hemiparesis or bilateral paresis, depending on the size of the lesion. Because the fibrae corticospinales occupy a larger cross-sectional area in the pons than in the capsula interna, not all of the fibers are damaged in many cases. For example, the fibers for the n. facialis and n. hypoglossus are usually unaffected because of their dorsal location. Damage to the nucleus

nervi abducentis may cause ipsilateral damage to the nucleus trigeminus (not shown).

Lesion at the level of the pyramis (5): Flaccid contralateral paresis occurs because the fibers of the extrapyramidal motor pathways (e.g., tractus rubrospinalis and tractus tectospinalis) are more dorsal than the tractus pyramidalis fibers and are therefore unaffected by an isolated lesion of the pyramis.

Lesion at the level of the medulla spinalis (6, 7): A lesion at the level of the pars cervicalis medullae spinalis (6) leads to ipsilateral spastic hemiplegia because the fibers of the pyramidal and extrapyramidal system are closely interwoven at this level and have already crossed to the opposite side. A lesion at the level of the pars thoracica medullae spinalis (7) leads to spastic paralysis of the ipsilateral leg.

Lesion at the level of the peripheral nerve (8): This lesion damages the axon of the alpha motor neuron, resulting in flaccid paralysis.

---

* Thus, spastic paralysis is actually a sign of extrapyramidal motor damage. This fact was unknown when tractus pyramidalis lesions were first described, however, and it was assumed that a *tractus pyramidalis lesion* led to spastic paralysis. Because this fact has few practical implications, spasticity is still described in some textbooks as the classic sign of a tractus pyramidalis lesion. In most cases it would be better simply to regard spastic paralysis as a form of central paralysis.

461

13.10 Radicular Lesions: Sensory Deficits

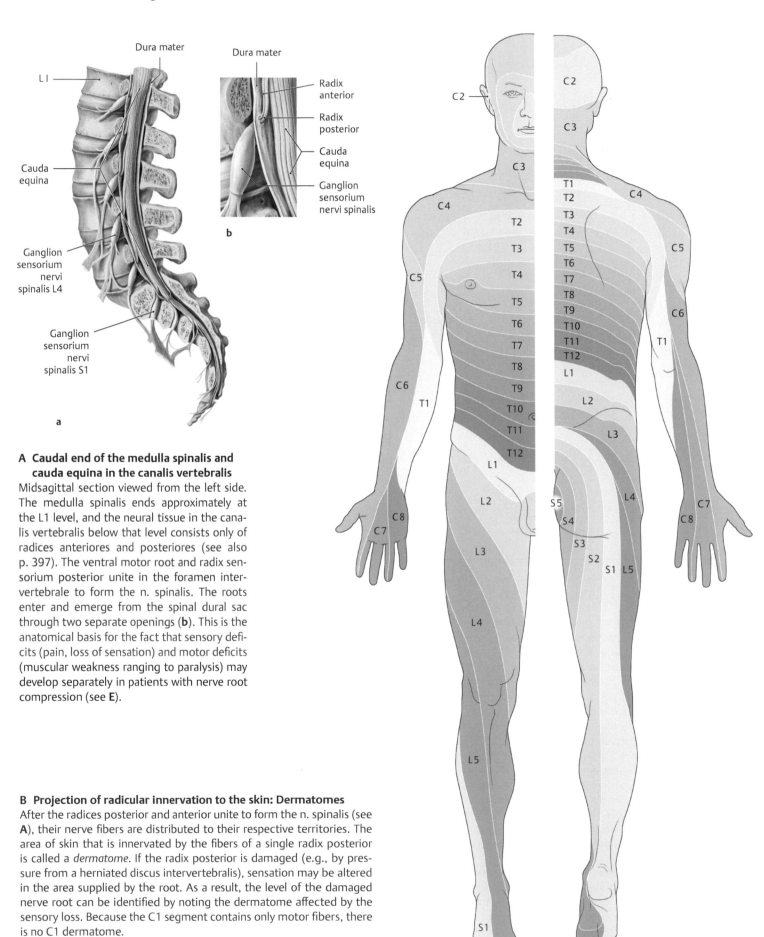

A Caudal end of the medulla spinalis and cauda equina in the canalis vertebralis

Midsagittal section viewed from the left side. The medulla spinalis ends approximately at the L1 level, and the neural tissue in the canalis vertebralis below that level consists only of radices anteriores and posteriores (see also p. 397). The ventral motor root and radix sensorium posterior unite in the foramen intervertebrale to form the n. spinalis. The roots enter and emerge from the spinal dural sac through two separate openings (**b**). This is the anatomical basis for the fact that sensory deficits (pain, loss of sensation) and motor deficits (muscular weakness ranging to paralysis) may develop separately in patients with nerve root compression (see **E**).

B Projection of radicular innervation to the skin: Dermatomes

After the radices posterior and anterior unite to form the n. spinalis (see **A**), their nerve fibers are distributed to their respective territories. The area of skin that is innervated by the fibers of a single radix posterior is called a *dermatome*. If the radix posterior is damaged (e.g., by pressure from a herniated discus intervertebralis), sensation may be altered in the area supplied by the root. As a result, the level of the damaged nerve root can be identified by noting the dermatome affected by the sensory loss. Because the C1 segment contains only motor fibers, there is no C1 dermatome.

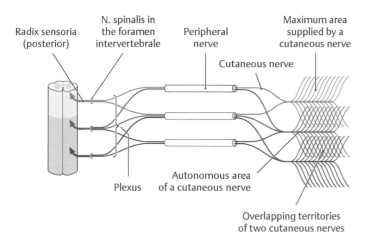

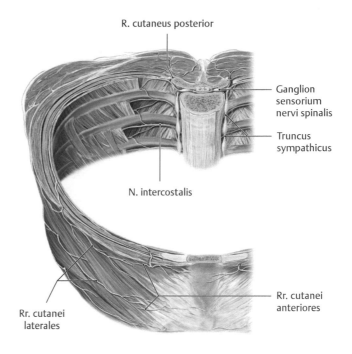

C Location of a radicular lesion

A radicular lesion is located on the radix anterior (motoria) or radix posterior (sensoria) between its site of emergence from the medulla spinalis and the union of both radices to form a n. spinalis. Accordingly, a lesion of the radix anterior leads to motor deficits (see p. 464) while a radix posterior lesion leads to sensory disturbances in the corresponding dermatome. The dermatomes on the limbs are shifted because of migratory processes during embryonic development, but the dermatomes on the trunk retain their segmental pattern of innervation (see **B** and **D**). Due to the overlap between adjacent dermatomes, the sensory loss that results from damage to a dermatome may be smaller than the size of the dermatome as it appears in the diagram. The brain does not "know" the location of the lesion; it processes information as if the lesion were located in the area supplied by the nerve (i.e., in the dermatome).

D Radicular innervation of the trunk

The segmental arrangement of the musculature is preserved in the trunk, and so the trunk retains a segmental (radicular) innervation pattern. Because the nerves in the trunk do not form plexuses, the radicular innervation pattern continues into the peripheral territory of a cutaneous nerve (T 2 – T 12; see **B**). It can be seen that afferent fibers from the truncus sympathicus reach the peripheral nerves distal to the roots. This explains why radicular lesions are usually not associated with autonomic deficits in the affected dermatomes.

E Pressure on radices nervorum spinalium from a herniated lumbar disk of L 4/5

A herniated discus intervertebralis may exert pressure on the radix nervi spinalis or cauda equina. The discus intervertebralis consists of a central gelatinous core (nucleus pulposus) and a peripheral ring of fibrocartilage (anulus fibrosus). When the anulus fibrosus is damaged, material from the nucleus pulposus may be extruded through the anulus defect and impinge upon the root at its entry into the foramen intervertebrale. This is a frequent cause of radicular symptoms, which have two grades of severity:

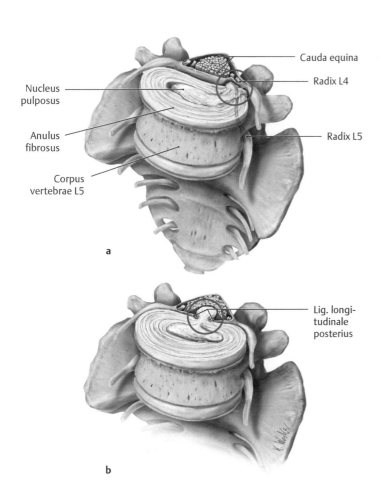

- Irritation of the nerve root in the region of the foramen intervertebrale. This leads to pain in the low back (lumbago), potentially accompanied by pain radiating into the lower limb in the dermatone of the affected root (sciatica).
- A large discus herniation may compress the radix posterior and/or radix anterior nervi spinalis, causing severe pain in addition to sensory deficits and (if the radix anterior is affected) motor deficits.

a **Posterolateral disk herniation** at the L 4/5 level. This damages the L 5 root passing behind the herniated discus but not the descending L 4 root, which has already entered the foramen intervertebrale at that level. As a result, the sensory deficits are manifested in the L 5 dermatome (see **B**). Only a far lateral discus herniation will damage the root that exits at the same level as the affected discus intervertebralis.

b **Posteromedial disk herniation** at the L 4/5 level. The material herniates through the lig. longitudinale posterius and impinges on the cauda equina. Cauda equina syndrome may develop if a lesion in this region compresses multiple roots. The locations of the deficits associated with specific root lesions are described in the next unit.

13.11 Radicular Lesions: Motor Deficits

A Indicator muscles of radicular lesions — limb muscles and diaphragma (after Kunze)

While a lesion of the radices posteriores (sensoriae) leads to sensory disturbances in specific dermatomes (see p. 462 and **C**, p. 463), a lesion of the *radices anteriores (motoriae)* will cause weakness to develop in specific muscles. Just as the affected dermatome indicates the site of the radix sensoria lesion, the affected muscle indicates the level of the damaged medulla spinalis segment or its root. The muscles that are predominantly supplied by a particular medulla spinalis segment are called its *indicator muscles* (analogous to the dermatomes for the radices posteriores). Because indicator muscles are supplied predominantly but, as a rule, not exclusively by a single segment, a lesion in one segment or radix nervi spinalis usually causes weakness (paresis) of the affected muscle rather than complete paralysis (plegia). Slight weakness may also be noted in muscles that receive some innervation from the affected segment but are not principally supplied by it. The indicator muscles in the upper and lower limbs are listed in the tables below. Whereas radix sensoria (posterior) lesions may occur in isolation, radix motoria (anterior) lesions usually occur in association with radix posterior lesions, and therefore the dermatomes are also listed in the tables.

Note: Because the nerves of the trunk are derived directly from the n. spinalis roots without any intervening plexuses, the pattern of segmental innervation in the trunk is identical to the pattern of peripheral innervation.

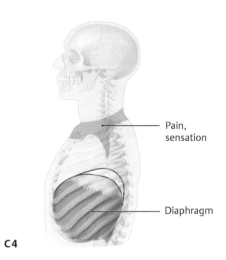

C4

Location of pain or sensory disturbance	Shoulder
Indicator muscle	Diaphragma
Reflexes abolished by a segmental lesion	None

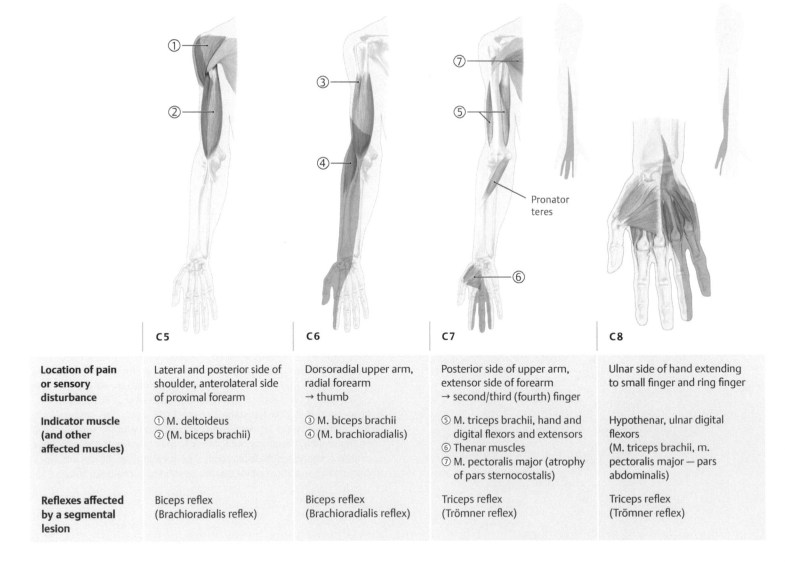

	C5	**C6**	**C7**	**C8**
Location of pain or sensory disturbance	Lateral and posterior side of shoulder, anterolateral side of proximal forearm	Dorsoradial upper arm, radial forearm → thumb	Posterior side of upper arm, extensor side of forearm → second/third (fourth) finger	Ulnar side of hand extending to small finger and ring finger
Indicator muscle (and other affected muscles)	① M. deltoideus ② (M. biceps brachii)	③ M. biceps brachii ④ (M. brachioradialis)	⑤ M. triceps brachii, hand and digital flexors and extensors ⑥ Thenar muscles ⑦ M. pectoralis major (atrophy of pars sternocostalis)	Hypothenar, ulnar digital flexors (M. triceps brachii, m. pectoralis major — pars abdominalis)
Reflexes affected by a segmental lesion	Biceps reflex (Brachioradialis reflex)	Biceps reflex (Brachioradialis reflex)	Triceps reflex (Trömner reflex)	Triceps reflex (Trömner reflex)

Pain, sensation

Diaphragm

Pronator teres

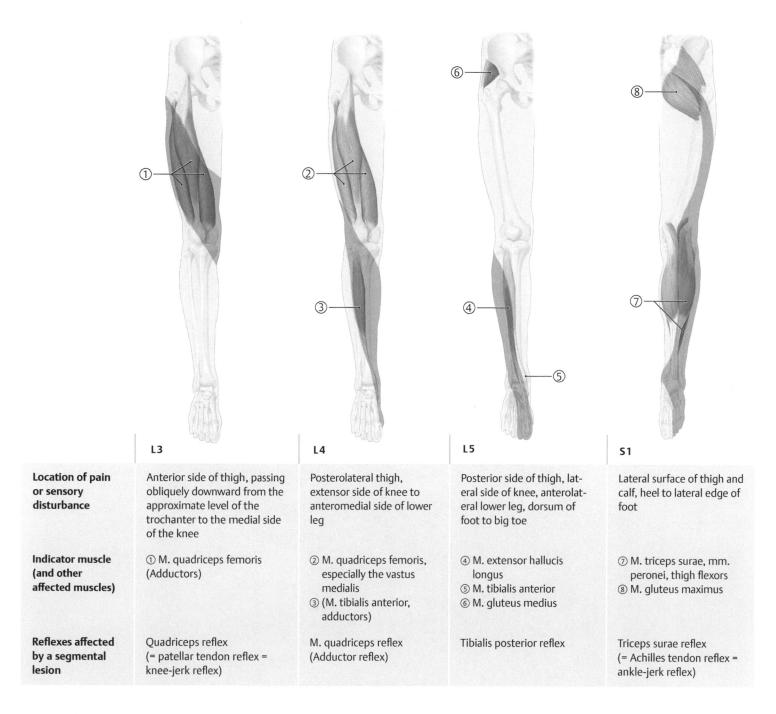

	L3	L4	L5	S1
Location of pain or sensory disturbance	Anterior side of thigh, passing obliquely downward from the approximate level of the trochanter to the medial side of the knee	Posterolateral thigh, extensor side of knee to anteromedial side of lower leg	Posterior side of thigh, lateral side of knee, anterolateral lower leg, dorsum of foot to big toe	Lateral surface of thigh and calf, heel to lateral edge of foot
Indicator muscle (and other affected muscles)	① M. quadriceps femoris (Adductors)	② M. quadriceps femoris, especially the vastus medialis ③ (M. tibialis anterior, adductors)	④ M. extensor hallucis longus ⑤ M. tibialis anterior ⑥ M. gluteus medius	⑦ M. triceps surae, mm. peronei, thigh flexors ⑧ M. gluteus maximus
Reflexes affected by a segmental lesion	Quadriceps reflex (= patellar tendon reflex = knee-jerk reflex)	M. quadriceps reflex (Adductor reflex)	Tibialis posterior reflex	Triceps surae reflex (= Achilles tendon reflex = ankle-jerk reflex)

B Principal indicator muscles of the medulla spinalis segments
The table lists the typical indicator muscles for each cord segment.

Cord segment	Indicator muscle
C4	Diaphragma
C5	M. deltoideus
C6	M. biceps brachii
C7	M. triceps brachii
C8	Hypothenar muscles, m. flexor digitorum profundus on ulnar side
L3	M. quadriceps femoris
L4	M. quadriceps femoris, m. vastus medialis
L5	M. extensor hallucis longus, m. tibialis anterior
S1	M. triceps surae, mm. peronei, m. gluteus maximus

C Clinical manifestations of nerve root irritation

- Pain in the affected dermatome
- Sensory losses in the affected dermatome
- Increased pain during coughing, sneezing, or straining
- Pain fibers more severely affected than other sensory fibers
- Motor deficits in the indicator muscles of the segment
- Reflexes associated with the affected segment are absent or diminished.

13.12 Lesions of the Plexus Brachialis

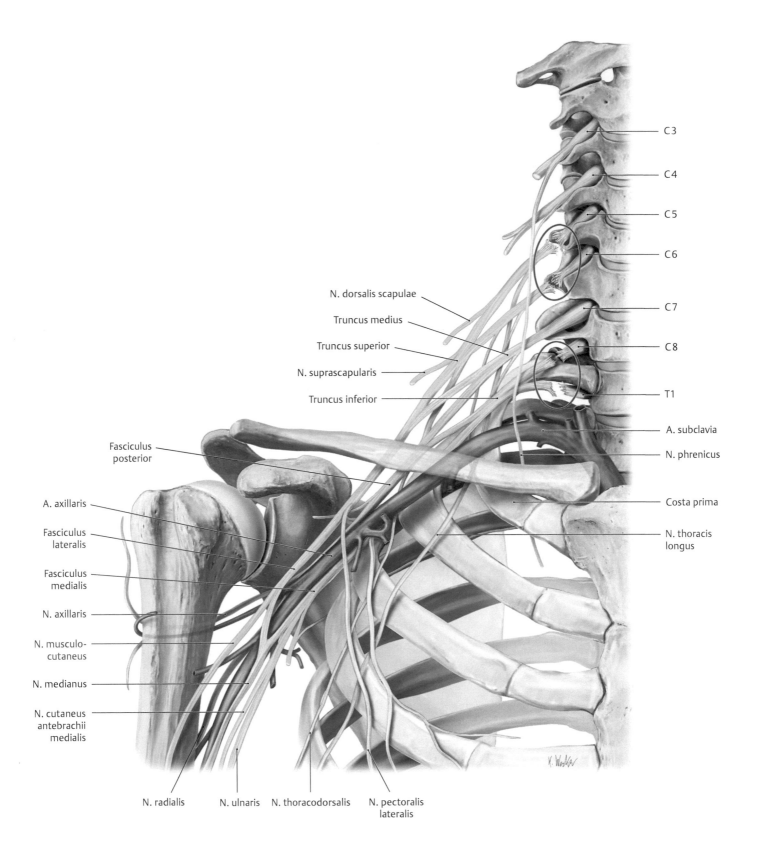

C3
C4
C5
C6
C7
C8
T1

N. dorsalis scapulae
Truncus medius
Truncus superior
N. suprascapularis
Truncus inferior

A. subclavia
N. phrenicus

Fasciculus posterior

Costa prima

A. axillaris

N. thoracis longus

Fasciculus lateralis

Fasciculus medialis

N. axillaris

N. musculo- cutaneus

N. medianus

N. cutaneus antebrachii medialis

N. radialis   N. ulnaris   N. thoracodorsalis   N. pectoralis lateralis

A Plexus brachialis paralysis
Anterior view of the right side. Lesions are circled. By definition, two forms of plexus brachialis paralysis are distinguished: *upper plexus brachialis paralysis*, which is caused by a lesion of the rr. anteriores C5 and C6 (see **C**), and *lower plexus brachialis paralysis*, which is caused by a lesion of the rr. anteriores C8 and T1 (see **D**). C7 forms a "watershed" between the two forms of paralysis and is typically unaffected by either form. A complete lesion of the plexus brachialis may also occur in severe trauma.

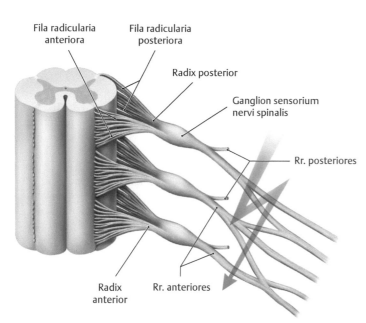

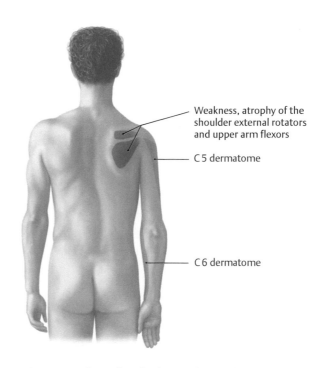

B Site of lesion in plexus brachialis paralysis

A plexus brachialis lesion affects the rr. anteriores of several nn. spinales, which transmit afferent signals to the plexus. Because the rr. anteriores carry both motor and sensory fibers, a plexus brachialis lesion always causes a combination of motor and sensory deficits. The resulting paralysis (see **C**) is always of the flaccid type because of its peripheral nature (lesion of the second motor neuron).

C Example: Upper plexus brachialis paralysis (Erb's palsy)

This condition results from a lesion of the rr. anteriores of the nn. spinales C5 and C6, causing paralysis of the abductors and external rotators of the shoulder joint and of the upper arm flexors and m. supinator. The arm hangs limply at the side (loss of the upper arm flexors), and the palm faces backward (loss of the m. supinator with dominance of the pronators). There may also be partial paralysis of the extensor muscles of the elbow joint and hand. Typical cases present with sensory disturbances on the lateral surface of the upper arm and forearm, but these signs may be absent. A frequent cause of upper plexus brachialis paralysis is obstetric trauma.

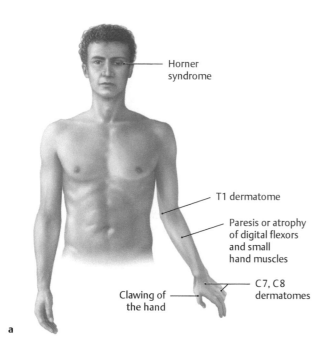

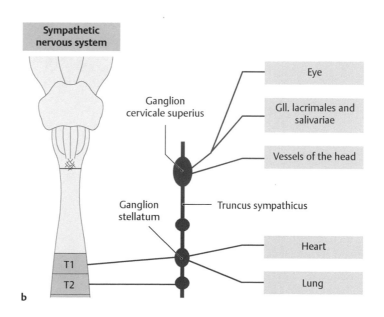

D Example: Lower plexus brachialis paralysis (Dejerine–Klumpke palsy)

This paralysis results from a lesion of the rr. anteriores of the nn. spinales C8 and T1 (see **A**). It affects the hand muscles, the digital flexors, and the flexor muscles in the wrist (claw hand with atrophy of hand muscles, **a**). Sensory disturbances affect the ulnar surfaces of the forearm and hand. Because the sympathetic fibers for the head leave the medulla spinalis at T1 (**b**), the sympathetic innervation of the head is also lost. This is manifested by a *unilateral Horner syndrome*, characterized by miosis (contracted pupilla due to paralysis of the m. dilator pupillae) and narrowing of the rima palpebrarum (not ptosis) due to a loss of sympathetic innervation to the mm. tarsales superior and inferior. The narrowed rima palpebrarum mimics enophthalmos (sinking of the eyeball into the orbit).

13.13 Lesions of the Plexus Lumbosacralis

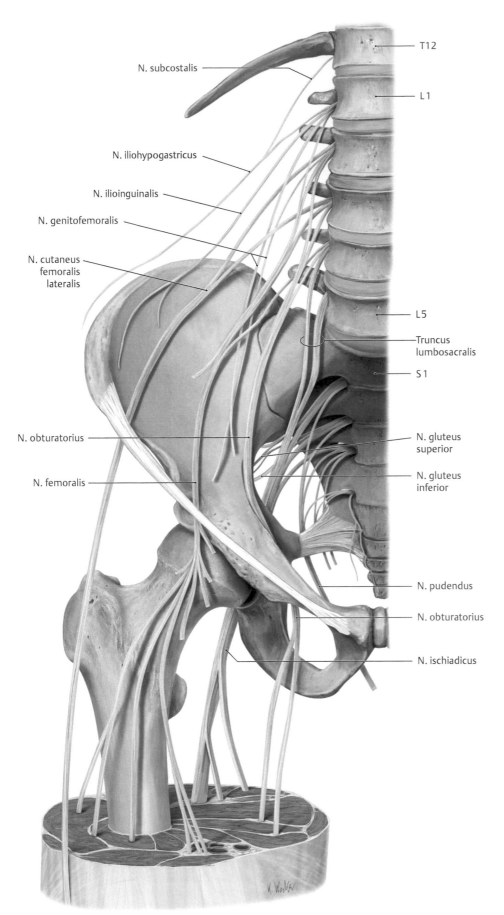

N. subcostalis

N. iliohypogastricus

N. ilioinguinalis

N. genitofemoralis

N. cutaneus femoralis lateralis

N. obturatorius

N. femoralis

T12

L1

L5

Truncus lumbosacralis

S1

N. gluteus superior

N. gluteus inferior

N. pudendus

N. obturatorius

N. ischiadicus

A Plexus lumbosacralis

Anterior view. The plexus lumbosacralis is divided into a plexus lumbalis (T12–L4) and plexus sacralis (L5–S4). The inferior fibers of L4 as well as all fibers of L5 merge to form the truncus lumbosacralis, which is the connection to the plexus sacralis. The latter runs in dorsal direction.

Note: Most nerves of the lumbar component run in ventral direction whereas the nerves from the sacral component run in dorsal direction. Since the plexus lumbosacralis lies very protected deep inside the pelvis, it is less frequently affected by lesions than the plexus brachialis which runs closer to the surface. Lesions to the plexus lumbosacralis occur in case of fractures of the pelvis ring, sacrum or hip and as a result of hip replacement.

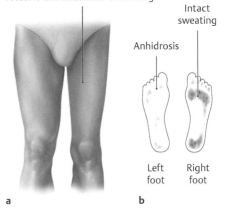

Weakness and atrophy of the hip flexors, knee extensors, and external rotators and adductors of the thigh

Intact sweating

Anhidrosis

Left foot   Right foot

a   b

B Lesion of the left plexus lumbalis (T12–L4)

The dominant feature of this condition is n. femoralis paralysis affecting the hip flexors, knee extensors, and the external rotators and adductors of the thigh (**a**). A sensory deficit is found on the anteromedial aspect of the thigh and calf. The lesion also disrupts the sympathetic fibers for the leg, which arise from the pars lumbalis medullae spinalis and pass through the plexus lumbalis. The clinical manifestations (**b**) include increased warmth of the foot (loss of sympathetic vasoconstriction) and anhidrosis on the sole of the foot (sweating is absent because of loss of sympathetic innervation to the gll. sudoriferae). When sweating is intact, the ninhydrin test is positive (footprint on a sheet of paper stains purple with 1% ninhydrin solution).

Note: Manifestations in the limbs are recognized by comparison with the unaffected side.

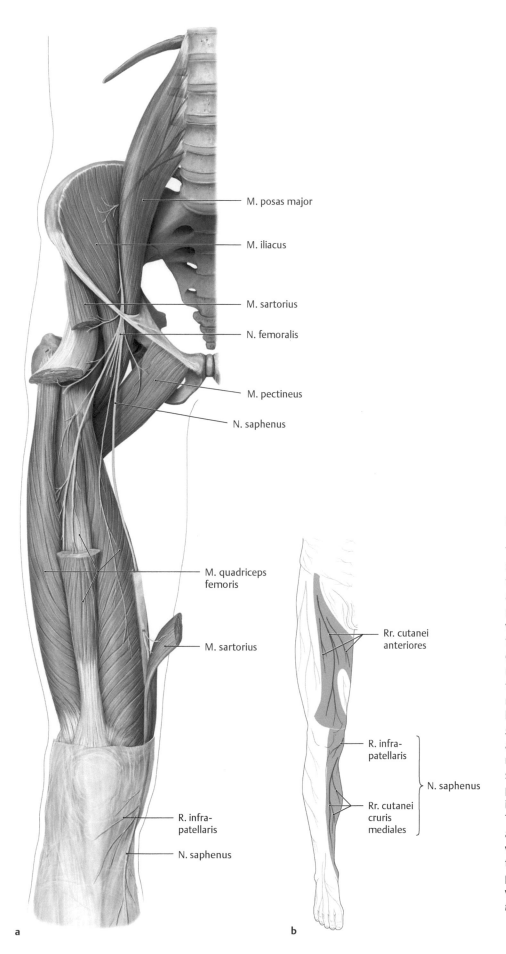

C Muscular and cutaneous distribution of the nervus femoralis
(L1– L4)
Anterior view.

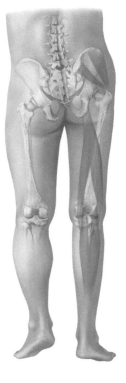

D Lesion of the right plexus sacralis
(L5 – S4)

This lesion presents clinically with *paralysis of the n. ischiadicus* and its two main branches, the nn. tibialis and fibularis communis, which are jointly affected. The results are loss of plantar flexion (n. tibialis paralysis, inability to walk on the toes) and paralysis of the foot and toe extensors (n. fibularis communis, steppage gait: the patient must raise the knee abnormally high while walking to avoid dragging the toes on the ground). Sensory disturbances are noted on the posterior surfaces of the thigh, lower leg, and foot. Because the *n. gluteus superior* is involved, the mm. glutei medius and minimus are also paralyzed. These two muscles stabilize the pelvis of the stationary side during gait. When they are paralyzed, the pelvis tilts toward the swinging leg, producing a "waddling" gait (known also as a positive Trendelenburg sign). The n. gluteus superior also innervates the m. tensor fasciae latae, which normally acts in the same manners as the two gluteal muscles. Specific categories of peripheral nerve lesions are described in the volume on *General Anatomy and Musculoskeletal System*.

13.14 Lesions of the Medulla Spinalis and Peripheral Nerves: Sensory Deficits

Overview of the next three units (after Bähr and Frotscher)
Two questions should be addressed in the diagnostic evaluation of medulla spinalis lesions:

1. What structure(s) within the *cross-section* of the medulla spinalis is (are) affected? This is determined systematically by proceeding from the periphery of the cord toward the center.
2. At what level of the medulla spinalis (in longitudinal section) is the lesion located?

In these units we will first correlate various deficit patterns (syndromes) with the structures in the cross-section of the medulla spinalis. We will then discuss the level of the lesion in the longitudinal or craniocaudal dimension. Since these syndromes present with deficits that result from damage to specific anatomical structures, they can be explained in anatomical terms. Based on the lesions and syndromes described here, the reader can test his or her ability to relate what has already been learned to the locations and effects of medulla spinalis lesions.

A Spinal ganglion syndrome illustrated for an isolated lesion of T6

As part of the radices posteriores, the ganglia sensoria nervorum spinalium are concerned with the transmission of sensory information. (Recall that the ganglia contain the cell bodies of the first sensory neurons.) When only a single ganglion sensorium nervi spinalis is affected (e.g., by a viral infection such as herpes zoster), the resulting pain and paresthesia are limited to the sensory distribution (dermatome) of the ganglion. Because the dermatomes show considerable overlap, adjacent dermatomes can assume the function of the affected dermatome. As a result, the area that shows absolute sensory loss, called the "autonomous area" of the dermatome, may be quite small.

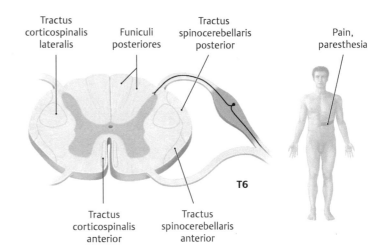

B Dorsal root syndrome illustrated for a lesion at the C4 – T6 level

When a lesion (trauma, degenerative spinal changes, tumor) affects multiple successive radices posteriores as in this example, complete sensory loss occurs in the affected dermatomes. When this sensory loss affects the afferent limb of a reflex, that reflex will be absent or diminished. If the radices posteriores (sensoriae) are irritated but not disrupted, as in the case of a herniated discus intervertebralis, severe pain may sometimes be perceived in the affected dermatome. Because pain fibers do not overlap as much as other sensory fibers, the examiner should have no difficulty in identifying the affected dermatome, and thus the corresponding medulla spinalis segment, from the location of the pain.

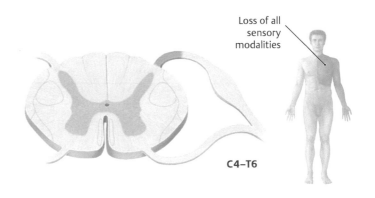

C Posterior horn syndrome illustrated for a lesion at the C5 – C8 level

This lesion, like a radix posterior lesion of the nn. spinales, is characterized by a segmental pattern of sensory disturbance. But with a *cornu posterius* lesion of the medulla spinalis, unlike a radix posterior lesion, the resulting sensory deficit is incomplete. Pain and temperature sensation are abolished in the dermatomes on the ipsilateral side because the first peripheral/afferent neuron of the tractus spinothalamicus lateralis arrives to the cornu posterius, which is within the damaged area. Position sense and vibration sense are unaffected because the fibers for these sensory modalities are both conveyed in the funiculus posterior. Bypassing the cornu posterius, these fibers pass directly via the funiculi posteriores and ascend to the nucleus gracilis or nucleus cuneatus where they synapse (see p. 404 f). A lesion of the tractus spinothalamicus anterior does not produce striking clinical signs. The deficit (loss of pain and temperature sensation with preservation of position and vibration sense) is called a *dissociated sensory loss*. Pain and temperature sensation are preserved below the lesion because the tracts in the substantia alba (tractus spinothalamicus lateralis) are undamaged. This type of dissociated sensory loss occurs in syringomyelia, a congenital or acquired condition in which threre is an expanded cavity in or near the canalis centralis of the medulla spinalis. (According to the strictest terminology, expansion of the canalis centralis itself = hydromyelia).

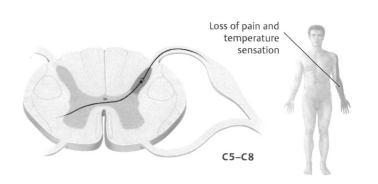

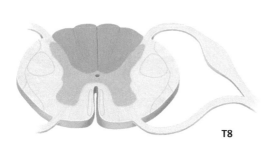

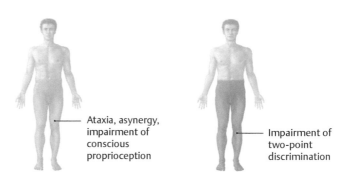

D Lesion of the funiculi posteriores at the T8 level

A lesion of the funiculi posteriores (see also p. 404 f) is characterized by a loss of

- Position sense,
- Vibration sense, and
- Two-point discrimination.

These deficits occur distal to the lesion, hence they involve the legs and lower trunk when the lesion is at the T 8 level. When the legs are affected, as in the present example, the loss of position sense (mediated by proprioception, see p. 280) leads to an unsteady gait (ataxia). When the arm is affected (not shown here), the only clinical finding is sensory impairment. The lack of feedback to the motor system also prevents the precise interaction of different muscle groups during fine movements (asynergy). Ataxia results from the fact that information on body position is essential for carrying out movements. Vision can (partly) compensate for this loss of information when the eyes are open, and so the ataxia worsens when the eyes are closed (Romberg's sign). This *sensory ataxia* differs from *cerebellar ataxia* in that the latter cannot be compensated by visual control.

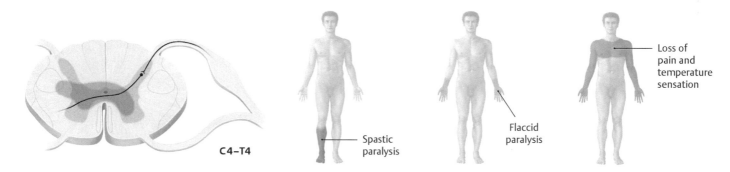

E Gray matter syndrome illustrated for a lesion at the C4 – T4 level

This syndrome results from a pathological process (e.g., a tumor) in and around the canalis centralis. All tracts that cross through the substantia grisea are damaged, i.e., the tractus spinothalamici anterior and lateralis. The result is a dissociated sensory loss (loss of pain and temperature sensation with preservation of position, vibration, and touch), in this case involving the arms and upper chest (compare with **C**). A relatively large lesion may additionally affect the cornua anteriora, which contain the alpha motor neuron, causing a flaccid paralysis in the distal portions of the upper limb. An even larger lesion may concomitantly affect the tractus pyramidalis, causing spastic paralysis of the distal muscles (here in the legs). This syndrome may result from syringomyelia (see **C**) or tumors located near the canlis centralis.

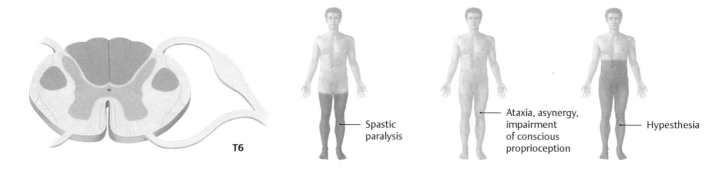

F Combined disease of the funiculi posteriores and tractus pyramidalis illustrated for a lesion at the T6 level

A *lesion of the funiculi posteriores* leads to loss of position and vibration sense. A concomitant *tractus pyramidalis lesion* additionally leads to spastic paralysis of the legs and abdominal muscles below the affected dermatome (i.e., below T6 in the example). This predominantly cervico-thoracic lesion typically occurs in funicular myelosis (vitamin B$_{12}$ deficiency), in which the funiculi posteriores are affected initially, followed by the tractus pyramidalis. This disease is characterized by degeneration of the myelin sheaths.

13.15 Lesions of the Medulla Spinalis and Peripheral Nerves: Motor Deficits

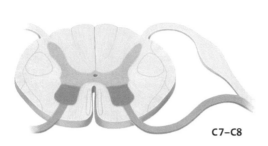

C7–C8

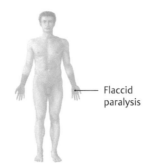

Flaccid paralysis

A Anterior horn syndrome illustrated for a lesion at the C7 – C8 level

Damage to the motor cornu anterius cells leads to ipsilateral paralysis, in this case involving the hands and forearm muscles because the lesion is at C7 – C8 and these segments innervate the muscles in this region. The paralysis is flaccid because the alpha motor neuron that supplies the muscles (lower motor neuron) has ceased to function. Because larger muscles are supplied by motor neurons from more than

one segment (see **A**, p. 398), damage to a single segment may lead only to muscular weakness (paresis) rather than complete paralysis of the affected muscle group. When the cornua lateralia are additionally involved, decreased sweating and vasomotor function will also be noted because the cornua lateralia contain the cell bodies of the sympathetic neurons that subserve these functions. This type of lesion may occur in poliomyelitis or in spinal muscular atrophy, for example. These relatively rare diseases are relentlessly progressive.

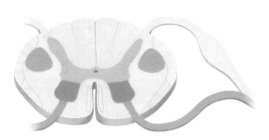

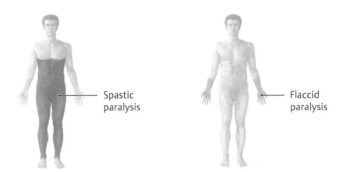

Spastic paralysis

Flaccid paralysis

B Combined lesions of the cornu anterius and tractus corticospinalis lateralis

These lesions produce a combination of flaccid and spastic paralysis. Damage to the motor cornua anteriora or lower motor neuron causes flaccid paralysis, while a lesion of the tractus corticospinalis lateralis or upper motor neuron causes spastic paralysis. The degree of injury to both types of neuron may be highly variable. In the example shown, a cornu anterius lesion at the C7 – C8 level has caused flaccid paralysis of the forearm and hand. By contrast, a lesion of the tractus corticospinalis lateralis at the T5 level would cause spastic paralysis of the abdominal and leg muscles.

Note: When the second motor neuron in the cornu anterius is already damaged (flaccid paralysis), an additional lesion of the tractus corticospinalis lateralis at the level of the same segment will not produce any noticeable effects. This lesion pattern occurs in amyotrophic lateral sclerosis, in which the first cortical motor neuron (tractus pyramidalis lesion) and second spinal motor neuron (cornu anterius lesion) both undergo progressive degeneration (etiology unclear). The end stage is marked by additional involvement of the motor n. cranialis nuclei, with swallowing and speaking difficulties (bulbar paralysis).

C Corticospinal tract syndrome

Progressive spastic spinal paralysis (Erb-Charcot disease) is characterized by a progressive degeneration of the neurons in the motor cortex with increasing failure of the corticospinal pathways (axonal degeneration of the first motor neuron). The course of the disease is marked by a progressive spastic paralysis of the limbs that begins in the legs and eventually reaches the arms.

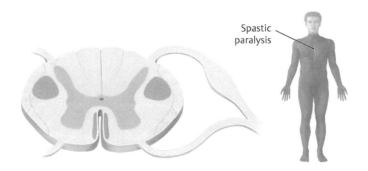

Spastic paralysis

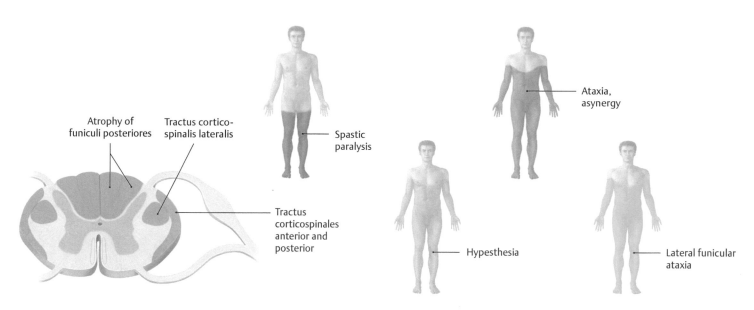

D Combined lesions of the funiculus posterior, tractus spinocerebellares, and tractus pyramidalis

This syndrome begins with destruction of the neurons in the ganglia sensoria nervorum spinalium, which transmit information on conscious position sense (loss: ataxia, asynergy), vibration sense, and two-point discrimination. This neuronal destruction leads to atrophy of the funiculi posteriores. There is little or no impairment of pain and temperature sensation, which are still transmitted to higher centers in the unaffected tractus spinothalamicus lateralis. The loss of conscious proprioception

alone is sufficient to cause sensory ataxia (lack of feedback to the motor system, see **D**, p. 471). But the lesions additionally affect the tractus spinocerebellares (unconscious proprioception), injury to which suffices to cause ataxia, and so this dual injury causes a particularly severe loss of conscious and unconscious proprioception. This is the main clinical feature of the disease. Spastic paralysis also develops as a result of tractus pyramidalis dysfunction. The prototype of this disease is hereditary Friedreich ataxia, which has several variants. The gene has been localized on chromosome 19.

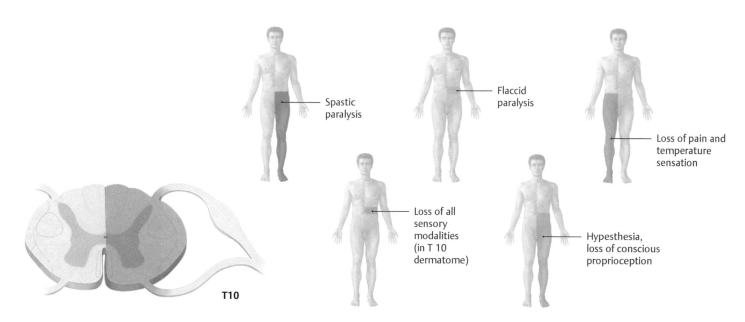

E Spinal hemisection syndrome (Brown–Séquard syndrome) illustrated for a lesion at the T 10 level on the left side

Hemisection of the medulla spinalis, though uncommon (e.g., in stab injuries), is an excellent model for testing our understanding of the function and course of the nerve tracts in the medulla spinalis. Spastic paralysis due to interruption of the tractus corticospinalis lateralis (see footnote on p. 461) occurs on the side of the lesion (and below the level of the lesion). The interruption of the funiculi posteriores (pathways for conscious proprioception) causes a loss of position and vibration sense and two-point discrimination on the side of the lesion. After spinal shock has subsided, spastic paralysis develops below the level of the lesion (here affecting the left leg). Of course, this paralysis does not produce an ataxia like that

described following interruption of the funiculi posteriores. Destruction of the alpha motor neurons in the locally damaged segment (in this case T 10) leads to ipsilateral flaccid paralysis associated with this segment. Because the axons of the tractus spinothalamicus lateralis have already crossed to the unaffected side below the lesion, pain and temperature sensation is preserved on the *ipsilateral* side below the lesion. These two types of sensation are lost on the *contralateral* side, however, because the crossed axons on the opposite side have been interrupted at the level of the lesion. If spinal root irritation occurs at the level of the lesion, radicular pain may occur because of the descending course of the radices sensoriae (and motoriae) in the segment above the lesion (see **E**, p. 463).

13.16 Lesions of the Medulla Spinalis, Assessment

A Deficits caused by complete medulla spinalis lesions at various levels

Having explored the manifestations of lesions at different sites in the cross-section of the medulla spinalis, we will now consider the effects of lesions at various levels of the cord. An example is the paralysis caused by a *complete medulla spinalis lesion*, which occurs acutely after a severe injury and is considerably more common than the incomplete lesions described earlier (see **E**, p. 473). A complete medulla spinalis lesion following acute trauma is initially manifested by *spinal shock*, the pathophysiology of which is not yet fully understood. This condition is marked by complete flaccid paralysis below the site of the lesion, with a loss of all sensory modalities from the level of the lesion downward. Loss of bladder and rectal function and impotence are also present. Because the lesion also interrupts the sympathetic fibers, sweating and thermoregulation are impaired. The substantia grisea of the medulla spinalis recovers over a period ranging from a few days to eight weeks. The spinal reflexes return, and the flaccid paralysis changes to a spastic paralysis. There is a recovery of bladder and rectal function, but only at a reflex level since voluntary control has been permanently lost. Impotence is permanent. **Lesions of the pars cervicalis medullae spinalis** above C 3 are swiftly fatal because they disrupt the efferent supply of the n. phrenicus (main root at C 4), which innervates the diaphragma and maintains abdominal respiration, while innervation to the mm. intercostales is also lost, causing a failure of thoracic respiration. A complete lesion of the lower pars cervicalis causes paralysis of all four limbs (quadriplegia), and respiration is precarious because of paralysis of the mm. intercostales. **Lesions of the upper pars thoracica medullae spinalis** (T 2 downward) spare the arms but respiration is compromised because of paralysis of the abdominal muscles. A lesion of the **lower pars thoracica medullae spinalis** (the exact site is unimportant) has little or no effect on the abdominal muscles, and respiration is not impaired. If the sympathetic nn. splanchnici are also damaged, there may be compromise of visceral motor function ranging to paralytic ileus (see p. 304).

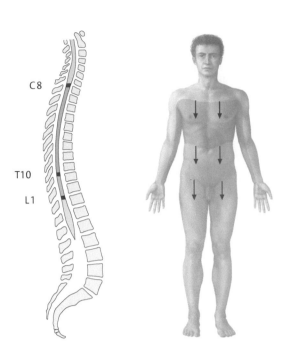

With **lesions of the pars lumbalis medullae spinalis**, a distinction is drawn between epiconus syndrome (L 4 – S 2) and conus (conus medullaris) syndrome (S 3 downward). *Epiconus syndrome* is characterized by a flaccid paralysis of the legs (only the roots are affected, causing peripheral paralysis), and reflex but not conscious emptying of the bladder and rectum is preserved. Sexual potency is lost. In *conus syndrome*, the legs are not paralyzed and only the foregoing autonomic disturbances are present. The motor deficits described here are also associated with sensory deficits (see **B**).

B Deficits associated with complete medulla spinalis lesions at various levels (after Rohkamm)

Level of lesion	Motor deficits	Sensory deficits	Autonomic deficits
C 1 – C 3 (high pars cervicalis lesion)	• Quadriplegia • Paralysis of nuchal muscles • Spasticity • Respiratory paralysis (immediate death if not artificially ventilated)	• Sensory loss from occiput or mandibular border downward • Pain in occipital region, back of neck, and shoulder region	• Reflex visceral functions (bladder, bowel) with no voluntary control • Horner syndrome
C 4 – C 5	• Quadriplegia • Diaphragmatic respiration only	• Sensory loss from clavicula or shoulder downward	• See above
C 6 – C 8 (lower pars cervicalis lesion)	• Quadriplegia • Diaphragmatic respiration • Spasticity	• Sensory loss from upper chest wall and back downward, and on the arms (sparing the shoulders)	• See above
T 1 – T 5	• Paraplegia • Decreased respiratory volume	• Sensory loss from inside of forearm, upper chest wall and back	• Reflex function of bladder and rectum • Erection without voluntary control
T 5 – T 10	• Paraplegia, spasticity	• Sensory loss from affected level in chest wall and back	• See above
T 11 – L 3	• Paraplegia	• Sensory loss from groin region or front of thigh, depending on site of lesion	• See above
L 4 – S 2 (epiconus, radices nervorum spinalium paralyzed)	• Distal paraplegia	• Sensory loss from front of thigh, dorsum of foot, sole of foot, or back of thigh, depending on site of lesion	• Flaccid paralysis of bladder and rectum • Impotence
S 3 – S 5 (conus)	• No deficit	• Sensory loss in perianal region and inside of thigh	• See above

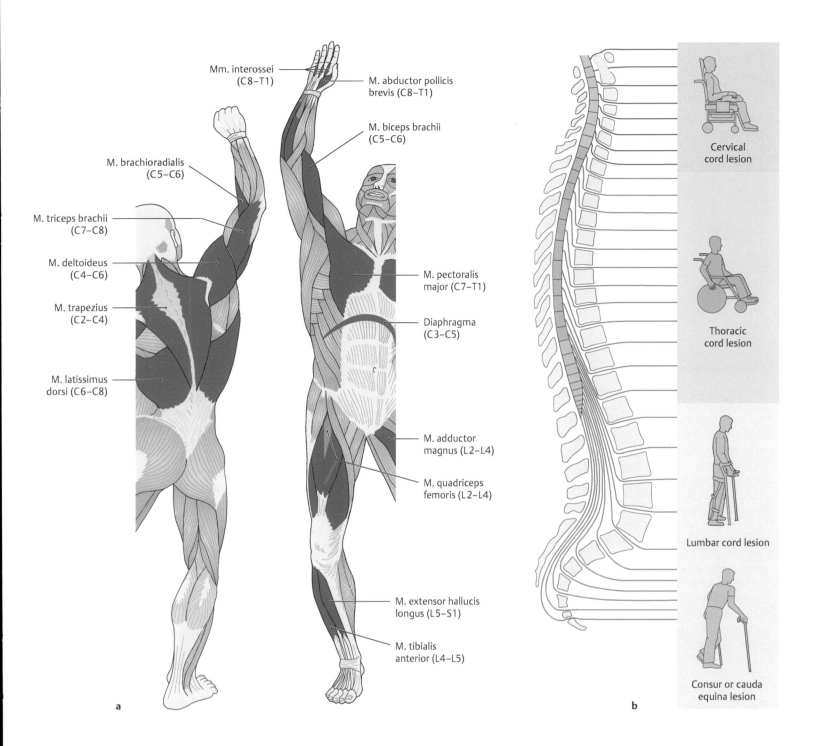

Mm. interossei (C8–T1)

M. abductor pollicis brevis (C8–T1)

M. biceps brachii (C5–C6)

M. brachioradialis (C5–C6)

M. triceps brachii (C7–C8)

M. deltoideus (C4–C6)

M. trapezius (C2–C4)

M. latissimus dorsi (C6–C8)

M. pectoralis major (C7–T1)

Diaphragma (C3–C5)

M. adductor magnus (L2–L4)

M. quadriceps femoris (L2–L4)

M. extensor hallucis longus (L5–S1)

M. tibialis anterior (L4–L5)

Cervical cord lesion

Thoracic cord lesion

Lumbar cord lesion

Consur or cauda equina lesion

a

b

C Determining the level of medulla spinalis lesions

a Muscles and the medulla spinalis segments that innervate them. Most muscles are multisegmental, that is they receive innervation from several medulla spinalis segments. Thus, for example, a lesion at the C7 level will not necessarily cause complete paralysis of the m. latissimus dorsi, because that muscle is also innervated by C6. This is

not the case with the "indicator muscles," which are supplied almost exclusively by a single segment (see **B**, p. 465). A lesion at the L3 level, for example, will cause almost complete paralysis of the m. quadriceps femoris because that muscle is innervated almost entirely by L3.

b The degree of disability varies, depending on the level of the complete cord lesion.

13.17 Visual System: Overview and Geniculate Part

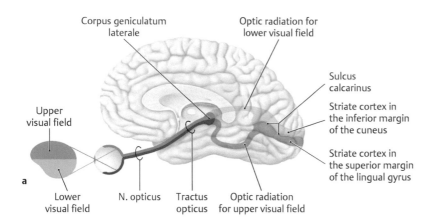

Corpus geniculatum laterale

Optic radiation for lower visual field

Sulcus calcarinus

Striate cortex in the inferior margin of the cuneus

Striate cortex in the superior margin of the lingual gyrus

Upper visual field

Lower visual field

N. opticus

Tractus opticus

Optic radiation for upper visual field

a

A Overview of the visual pathway

Left lateral view of the right cerebral hemisphere (**a**) and superior view through a transparent cerebrum (**b**).

The visual pathway begins in the retina (initial neuronal processing of visual stimuli, see **B**). The retina lies behind the pupilla. This small aperture in the eye has the effect of projecting light rays incident from above onto the lower retina and light rays incident from below onto the upper retina (**a**). The same applies to light rays incident on the left and right (**b**). Thus, the image on the retina is upside down and reversed left to right, producing a **camera obscura or pinhole image effect.**

The retina and visual field are divided into four quadrants, which are connected in a very specific manner to the four quadrants of the primary visual cortex (see **C**). The axons of the third neuronal layer in the retina form the n. opticus (second cranial nerve) of each eye. The two nn. optici leave the respective orbit through the canalis opticus. Posterior to it they come together in the chiasma opticum at the base of the diencephalon. Here the axons of the *nasal retina* cross to the contralateral side (see **b**). The fibers of the *temporal retina* continue on the ipsilateral side. This has the following effect on vision: Because the nasal halves of the retina look outward (temporal visual field, see **b**), the respective "outer half" of the visual world is conducted to the respective contralateral half of the brain whereas the "inner half" of the visual world (nasal visual field) remains in the ipsilateral half of the brain. This means that for the left half of the brain (see blue markings in **b**), it looks to the right with the temporal retina of the left eye (nerve fibers do *not cross*) and also looks to the right with the nasal retina of the right eye (fibers cross).

Note: Therefore, one half of the brain (in contrast to one eye, which sees the left and right world) only perceives the contralateral world. The *upper* and lower "worlds" are perceived as follows: Regardless of whether the fibers cross or not, information from the *upper* half of the retina (but from the lower visual field) ends in the upper visual cortex (above the sulcus calcarinus at the lower border of the cuneus), whereas information from the *lower* half of the retina ends in the *lower* visual cortex (beneath the sulcus calcarinus on the upper border of the gyrus lingualis, see **a**). The upper portions of the visual cortex thus look down and vice versa. The pathway posterior to the chiasma opticum, is no longer referred to as the n. opticus but is called the **"tractus opticus."** The vast majority of the optic nerve fibers (90%) course further in this tract to a nucleus in the thalamus, the **corpus geniculatum laterale** (the *genicular portion* of the visual pathway), where they are again connected (fourth neuron). The neurons in the corpus geniculatum laterale project the conscious visual perception onto the primary visual cortex on the occipital pole of the brain. The remaining 10% of the axons of the third neuron do not end in the corpus geniculatum laterale (*non-genicular portion* of the visual pathway, see **B**, p. 479) and do not produce a conscious visual perception. The path from the neurons in the corpus geniculatum laterale to the visual cortex (fifth neuron) is referred to as the **optic radiation**. It extends in a band over the lower and posterior horn of the ventriculus lateralis.

Note: Like the retina, the n. opticus, chiasma opticum, and tractus opticus all belong to the CNS, specifically to the diencephalon. They are invested in meninges. The n. opticus is thus not a true nerve but a diencephalic pathway that has migrated anteriorly out of the brain.

B Structure of the retina and visual cortex

a Circuitry of the retina; **b** coronal section through the lobus occipitalis.

Three layers of neurons connected in series form the retina. The first neuron is also a photoreceptor for black and white perception (rods) or color perception (cones). It is connected via bipolar cells (second neuron) with the third neuron, the ganglion cells. Its axons form the n. opticus.

Note: The photosensitive photoreceptors lie on the side of the retina facing away from the light (inversion of the retina).

A strong convergence of signal processing occurs during this connection; 125 million photoreceptor cells interact with 4 million ganglion cells. The entire primary visual cortex (striate area, area 17 after Brodmann) is subdivided into four quadrants; the longitudinal fissure divides the visual cortex into left and right halves (see **Ab**). The sulcus calcarinus (see **Aa**) in turn divides each half into an upper portion (at the cuneus) and a lower portion (at the gyrus lingualis). Within the visual cortex the fibers of the optic radiation are bundled together to form a macroscopically visible layer of substantia alba, the stria occipitalis.

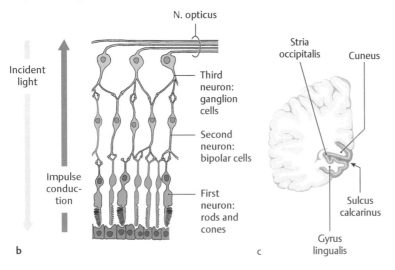

N. opticus

Incident light

Impulse conduction

Third neuron: ganglion cells

Second neuron: bipolar cells

First neuron: rods and cones

b

Stria occipitalis

Cuneus

Sulcus calcarinus

Gyrus lingualis

c

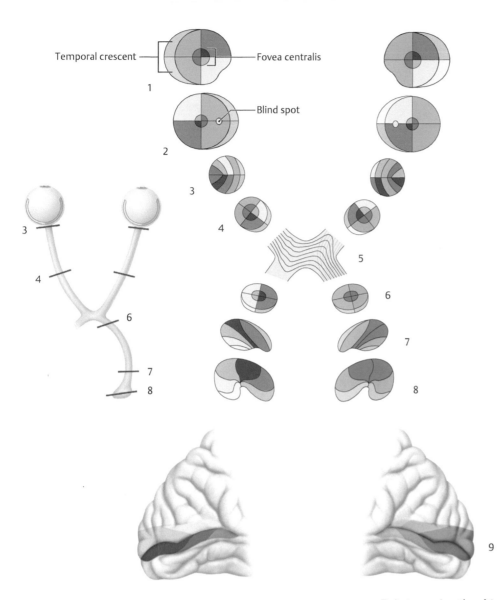

Temporal crescent —— Fovea centralis

1

Blind spot

2

3

3

4

4

5

6

6

7

7

8

8

9

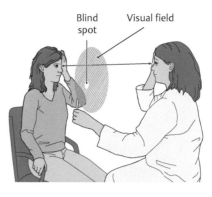

Blind spot   Visual field

D Informal visual field examination with the confrontation test

The visual field examination is an essential step in the examination of lesions of the visual pathway (see **A**, p. 478). The **confrontation test** is an *informal* test in which the examiner (with an intact visual field) and the patient sit face-to-face, cover one eye, and each fixes their gaze on the other's open eye, creating identical visual axes. The examiner then moves his or her index finger from the outer edge of the visual field toward the center until the patient signals that he or she can see the finger. With this test the examiner can make a gross assessment as to the presence and approximate location of a possible visual field defect. The *precise* location and extent of a visual field defect can be determined by **perimetry**, in which points of light replace the examiner's finger. The results of the test are entered in charts that resemble the small diagrams in **C**.

C Topographic organization of the geniculate part of the visual pathway

The fovea centralis, the point of maximum visual acuity on the retina, has a high receptor density. Accordingly, a great many axons pass centrally from its receptors, and so the fovea centralis is represented by an exceptionally large area in the visual cortex. Other, more peripheral portions of the retina contain fewer receptors and therefore fewer axons, resulting in a smaller representational area in the visual cortex.

Note: Only the left half of the complete visual field is shown. It is subdivided into four quadrants (clockwise from top left in 1): upper temporal, upper nasal, lower nasal, and lower temporal. The representation of this subdivision is continued into the visual cortex.

1 The three zones that make up a particular visual hemifield (left, in this case) are each indicated by color shading of decreasing intensity:

- The smallest and darkest zone is at the center of the fovea centralis; it corresponds to the central visual field.
- The largest zone is the macular visual field, which also contains the "blind spot" (= optic disk, see **2**).
- The "temporal crescent" represents the temporal, monocular part of the visual field.
- Note that the lower nasal quadrant of each visual field is indented by the nose (small medial depression).

2 Retina: Because the pupilla acts as a pinhole aperture (see **Aa**), the image on the retina is inverted and reversed temporal to nasal.

3, 4 In the initial part of the n. opticus, the fibers that represent the macular visual field first occupy a lateral position (**3**) and then move increasingly toward the center of the nerve (**4**).

5 In traversing the **chiasma opticum**, the nasal fibers of the n. opticus cross the midline to the opposite side.

6 At the **start of the tractus opticus**, the fibers from the corresponding halves of the retinae unite—the right halves of the retinae in the right tract, the left halves in the left tract. The impulses from the right visual field finally terminate in the left striate area. Initially the macular fibers continue to occupy a central position in the tractus opticus.

7 At the **end of the tractus opticus**, just before it enters the corpus geniculatum laterale, the fibers are collected to form a wedge.

8 In the **corpus geniculatum laterale**, the wedge shape is preserved, the macular fibers occupying almost half the wedge. These fibers synapse with the fourth neurons, which project to the posterior end of the polus occipitalis (visual cortex).

9 This figure shows that the central part of the visual field is represented by the largest area in the **visual cortex** compared with other portions of the field. This is due to the large number of axons that run to the n. opticus from the fovea centralis. This large proportion of axons is continued into the visual cortex, establishing a point-to-point (retinotopic) correlation between the fovea centralis and the visual cortex. The other parts of the visual field also show a point-to-point correlation but have fewer axons. The central lower half of the visual field is represented by a large area on the polus occipitalis above the sulcus calcarinus, while the central upper half of the visual field is represented below the sulcus. The region of central vision also occupies the largest area within the corpus geniculatum laterale (see **8**).

477

13.18 Visual System: Lesions and Nongeniculate Part

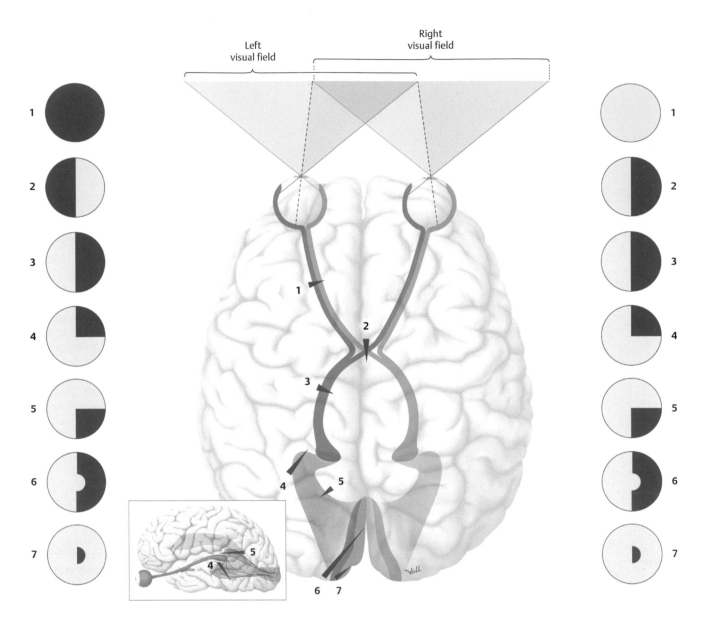

A Visual field defects (scotomata) and their location along the visual pathway

Visual field defects and lesion sites are illustrated here for the left visual pathway. Lesions of the visual pathway may result from a large number of neurological diseases. The patient perceives the lesion as a visual disturbance. Because the nature of the visual field defect often points to the location of the lesion, it is clinically important to know the patterns of defects that may be encountered. Division of the visual field into four quadrants is helpful in determining the location of a lesion. The quadrants are designated as upper and lower temporal, and upper and lower nasal (see also p. 477).

1 A unilateral n. opticus lesion produces blindness (amaurosis) in the affected eye only.
2 A lesion of the chiasma opticum causes bitemporal hemianopia (as in a horse wearing blinders) because it interrupts the fibers from the nasal portions of the retina (the only ones that cross in the chiasma opticum), which represent the temporal visual fields
3 A unilateral lesion of the tractus opticus causes contralateral homonymous hemianopia because it interrupts fibers from the temporal portions of the retina on the ipsilateral side and the nasal portions on the opposite side. Thus the right or left half of the visual field is affected in each eye.

Note: All homonymous visual field defects are caused by a retrochiasmal lesion.

4 A unilateral lesion of the radiatio optica in the anterior temporal lobe (Meyer's loop) leads to contralateral upper quadrantanopia (a "pie-in-the sky" deficit). This occurs because the affected fibers wind around the cornu inferius of the ventriculus lateralis in the lobus temporalis and are separated from the fibers that come from the lower half of the visual field (see p. 476).
5 A unilateral lesion in the medial part of the radiatio optica in the lobus parietalis leads to contralateral lower quadrantanopia. This occurs because the fibers course superior to those for the upper quadrant in Meyer's loop (see p. 476).
6 A lesion of the lobus occipitalis leads to homonymous hemianopia. Because the radiatio optica fans out widely before entering the visual cortex, lesions of the lobus occipitalis have been described that spare foveal vision. These lesions are most commonly due to intracerebral hemorrhage. The visual field defects may vary considerably because of the variable size of the hemorrhage.
7 A lesion confined to the cortical areas of the polus occipitalis, which represent the macula, is characterized by a homonymous hemianopic central scotoma.

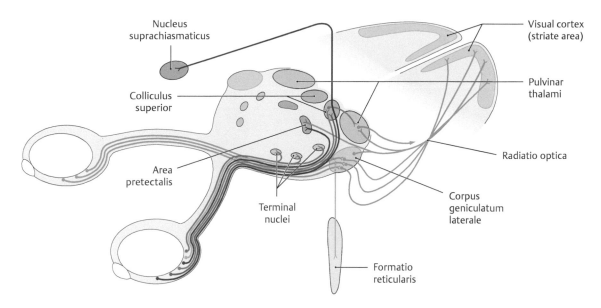

Labels (clockwise): Nucleus suprachiasmaticus; Colliculus superior; Area pretectalis; Terminal nuclei; Visual cortex (striate area); Pulvinar thalami; Radiatio optica; Corpus geniculatum laterale; Formatio reticularis

B Nongeniculate part of the visual pathway

Approximately 10% of the axons of the n. opticus do not terminate on neurons in the corpus geniculatum laterale for projection to the visual cortex. They continue along the radix medialis of the tractus opticus, forming the *nongeniculate part* of the visual pathway. The information from these fibers is not processed at a conscious level but plays an important role in the unconscious regulation of various vision-related processes and in visually mediated reflexes (e.g., the afferent limb of the pupillary light reflex). Axons from the nongeniculate part of the visual pathway terminate in the following regions:

- Axons to the colliculus superior: transmit kinetic information that is necessary for tracking moving objects by unconscious eye and head movements (retinotectal system).

- Axons to the area pretectalis: afferents for pupillary responses and accommodation reflexes (retinopretectal system). Subdivision into specific nuclei has not yet been accomplished in humans, and so the term "area" is used.
- Axons to the nucleus suprachiasmaticus of the hypothalamus: influence circadian rhythms.
- Axons to the thalamic nuclei (tractus opticus) in the tegmentum of the mesencephalon and to the nuclei vestibulares: afferent fibers for optokinetic nystagmus (jerky, physiological eye movements during the tracking of fast-moving objects). This has also been called the "accessory visual system."
- Axons to the pulvinar thalami: visual association cortex for oculomotor function (neurons are relayed in the colliculus superior).
- Axons to the nucleus reticularis parvocellularis: arousal function.

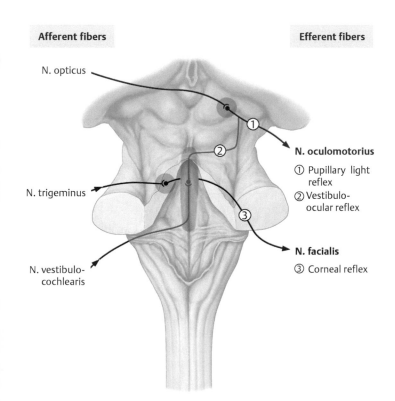

Afferent fibers | **Efferent fibers**

Labels: N. opticus; N. trigeminus; N. vestibulo-cochlearis; N. oculomotorius — ① Pupillary light reflex, ② Vestibulo-ocular reflex; N. facialis — ③ Corneal reflex

C Brainstem reflexes: Clinical importance of the nongeniculate part of the visual pathway

Brainstem reflexes are important in the examination of comatose patients. Loss of all brainstem reflexes is considered evidence of brain death. Three of these reflexes are described below:

Pupillary light reflex: The pupillary light reflex relies on the nongeniculate parts of the visual pathway (see p. 481). The afferent fibers for this reflex come from the n. opticus, which is an extension of the diencephalon (since the diencephalon is not part of the truncus encephali, "brainstem reflex" is a somewhat unfortunate term). The efferents for the pupillary reflex come from the nuclei accessorii nervi oculomotorii (CN III), which is located in the truncus encephali. Loss of the pupillary reflex may signify a lesion of the diencephalon or mesencephalon (midbrain).

Vestibulo-ocular reflex: Irrigating the meatus acusticus externa with cold water in a normal individual evokes nystagmus that beats toward the opposite side (afferent fibers are conveyed in the n. vestibulocochlearis: CN VIII, efferent fibers in the n. oculomotorius: CN III). When the vestibulo-ocular reflex is absent in a comatose patient, it is considered a poor sign because this reflex is the most reliable clinical test of truncus encephali function.

Corneal reflex: This reflex is not mediated by the visual pathway. The afferent fibers for the reflex (elicited by stimulation of the cornea, as by touching it with a sterile cotton wisp) travel in the n. trigeminus and the efferent fibers (contraction of the m. orbicularis oculi in response to corneal irritation) in the n. facialis. The relay center for the corneal reflex is located in the pontine region of the truncus encephali.

13.19 Visual System: Reflexes

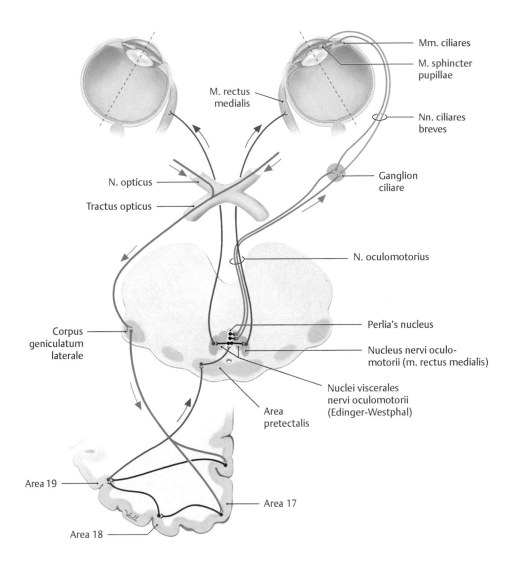

A Pathways for convergence and accommodation

When the head moves closer to an object, the visual axes of the eyes must move closer together (convergence) and *simultaneously* the lenses must adjust their focal length (accommodation). Both processes are necessary for a sharp, three-dimensional visual impression. Three subprocesses can be identified in convergence and accommodation:

1. In **convergence**, the two mm. recti mediales move the ocular axis inward to keep the image of the approaching object on the fovea centralis.
2. In **accommodation**, the curvature of the lens is increased to keep the image of the object sharply focused on the retina. The lens is flattened by contraction of the fibrae zonulares, which are attached to the m. ciliaris. When the m. ciliaris contracts during accommodation, it relaxes the tension on the fibrae zonulares, and the intrinsic pressure of the lens causes it to assume a more rounded shape.
3. The pupil is constricted by the m. sphincter pupillae to increase visual acuity.

Convergence and accommodation may be conscious (fixing the gaze on a near object) or unconscious (fixing the gaze on an approaching automobile). Most of the axons of the third neuron in the visual pathway course in the n. opticus to the corpus geniculatum laterale. There they are relayed to the fourth neuron, whose axons project to the primary visual cortex (area 17). Axons from the secondary visual area (19) finally reach the area pretectalis by way of synaptic relays and interneurons. Another relay occurs at that level, and the axons from these neurons terminate in Perlia's nucleus, which is located between the two Edinger-Westphal nuclei (nuclei viscerales nervi oculomotorii). Two functionally distinct groups of neurons are located in Perlia's nucleus:

- For accommodation, one group of neurons relays impulses to the *somatomotor* nucleus nervi oculomotorii, whose axons pass directly to the m. rectus medialis.
- The other group relays the neurons responsible for accommodation and pupillary constriction to the *visceromotor* (parasympathetic) nuclei accessorii nervi oculomotorii (parasympathetic innervation is illustrated here for one side only).

After synapsing in this nuclear region, the preganglionic parasympathetic axons pass to the ganglion ciliare, where they synapse with the postganglionic parasympathetic neurons. Again, two groups of neurons are distinguished: one passes to the m. ciliaris (accommodation) and the other to the m. sphincter pupillae (pupillary constriction). The pupillary sphincter light response is abolished in tertiary syphilis, while accommodation (m. ciliaris) and convergence are preserved. This phenomenon, called an Argyll Robertson pupil, suggests that the connections to the mm. ciliaris and sphincter pupillae are mediated by different tracts, although the anatomy of these tracts is not yet fully understood.

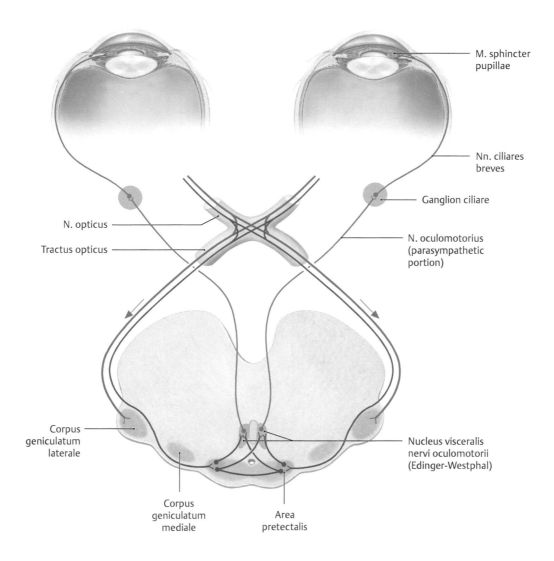

M. sphincter pupillae

Nn. ciliares breves

Ganglion ciliare

N. opticus

Tractus opticus

N. oculomotorius (parasympathetic portion)

Corpus geniculatum laterale

Nucleus visceralis nervi oculomotorii (Edinger-Westphal)

Corpus geniculatum mediale

Area pretectalis

B Regulation of pupillary size — the light reflex
The pupillary light reflex enables the eye to adapt to varying levels of brightness. When a large amount of light enters the eye, like the beam of a flashlight, the pupil constricts (to protect the photoreceptors in the retina); when the light fades, the pupil dilates. As the term "reflex" implies, this adaptation takes place without conscious input (*nongeniculate* part of the visual pathway).
Afferent limb of the light reflex: The first three neurons (first neurons: rods and cones; second neurons: bipolar cells; third neurons: ganglion cells) in the *afferent* limb of the light reflex are located in the retina. The axons from the ganglion cells form the n. opticus. The axons responsible for the light reflex (blue) pass to the area pretectalis (nongeniculate part of the visual pathway) in the radix medialis of the tractus opticus. The other axons pass to the corpus geniculatum laterale (purple). After synapsing in the nuclei pretectales, the axons from the fourth neurons pass to the parasympathetic nuclei viscerales nervi oculomotorii (nuclei accessorii nervi oculomotorii: Edinger-Westphal nuclei). Because both sides are innervated, a *consensual light response* will occur (see below).
Efferent limb of the light reflex: The neurons located in the nuclei viscerales nervi oculomotorii (preganglionic parasympathetic neurons) distribute their axons to the ganglion ciliare. There they are relayed to postganglionic parasympathetic neurons that send their axons to the m. sphincter pupillae.

The *direct* pupillary light response is distinguished from the consensual (indirect) response:
The **direct light response** is tested by covering both eyes of the conscious, cooperative patient and then uncovering one eye. After a short latency period, the pupil of the light-exposed eye will contract.
To test the **indirect light response**, the examiner places his hand on the bridge of the patient's nose, shading one eye from the beam of a flashlight while shining it into the other eye. The object is to test whether shining the light into one eye will cause the pupil of the shaded eye to contract as well (*consensual light response*).
Loss of the light response due to certain lesions: With a unilateral n. opticus lesion, shining a light into the *affected* side will induce no direct light response on the affected side. The consensual light response on the opposite side will also be lost because of impairment of the afferent limb of the light response on the affected side. Illumination of the *unaffected* side will, of course, elicit pupillary contraction on that side (direct light response). A consensual light response is also present because the afferent signals for this reflex are mediated by the unaffected side while the efferent signals are not mediated by the n. opticus. With a lesion of the parasympathetic oculomotor nucleus or ganglion ciliare, the efferent limb of the reflex is lost. In either case the patient has no direct or indirect pupillary light response on the affected side. A lesion of the radiatio optica or visual cortex (*geniculate* part of the visual pathway) does not abolish this reflex given that it will affect only the geniculate part of the visual pathway.

13.20 Visual System: Coordination of Eye Movement

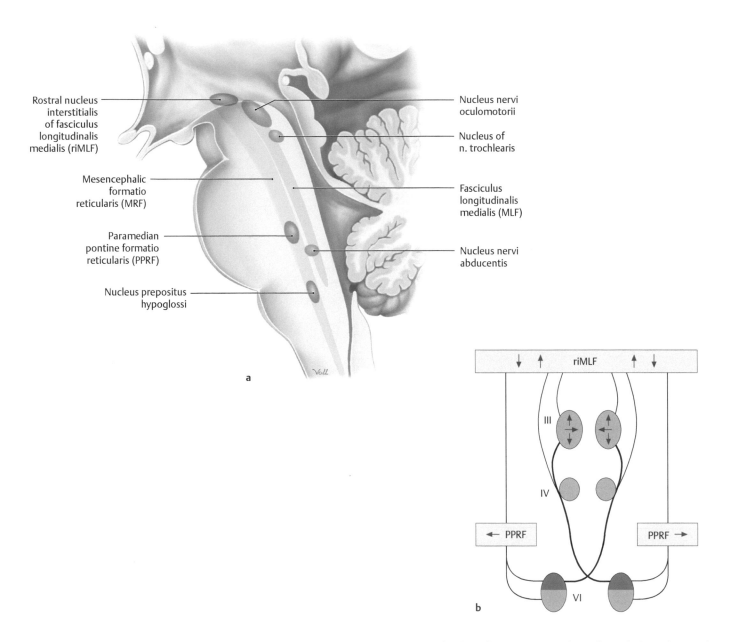

Rostral nucleus interstitialis of fasciculus longitudinalis medialis (riMLF)

Mesencephalic formatio reticularis (MRF)

Paramedian pontine formatio reticularis (PPRF)

Nucleus prepositus hypoglossi

Nucleus nervi oculomotorii

Nucleus of n. trochlearis

Fasciculus longitudinalis medialis (MLF)

Nucleus nervi abducentis

A Nuclei nervi oculomotorii and their higher connections in the truncus encephali

a Midsagittal section viewed from the left side. **b** Circuit diagram showing the supranuclear organization of eye movements.

When we shift our gaze to a new object, we swiftly move the axis of vision of our eyes toward the intended target. These rapid, precise, "ballistic" eye movements are called *saccades*. They are preprogrammed and, once initiated, cannot be altered until the end of the saccadic movement. The nuclei of all the nerves that supply the eye muscles (nuclei of nn. craniales III, IV, and VI, shaded red) are involved in carrying out these movements. They are interconnected for this purpose by the *fasciculus longitudinalis medialis* (shaded blue; see **B** for its location). Because these complex movements essentially involve all of the extraocular muscles and the nerves supplying them, the activity of the nuclei must be coordinated at a higher or *supranuclear level*. This means, for

example, that when we gaze to the right with the *right* eye, the right m. rectus lateralis (CN VI, nucleus nervi abducentis activated) must contract while the right m. rectus medialis (CN III, nucleus nervi oculomotorii inhibited) must relax. For the *left* eye, the left m. rectus lateralis (CN VI) must relax while the left m. rectus medialis (CN III) must contract. Movements of this kind that involve both eyes are called *conjugate eye movements*. These movements are coordinated by several centers (premotor nuclei, shaded purple). Horizontal gaze movements are programmed in the nuclear region of the paramedian pontine reticular formation (PPRF), while vertical gaze movements are programmed in the rostral nucleus interstitialis of the fasciculus longitudinalis medialis (riMLF). Both gaze centers establish bilateral connections with the nuclei of nn. craniales III, IV, and VI. The tonic signals for maintaining the new eye position originate from the nucleus prepositus hypoglossi (see **a**).

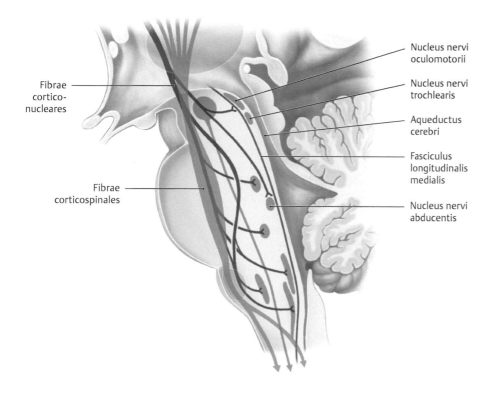

B Course of the fasciculus longitudinalis medialis in the truncus encephali

Midsagittal section viewed from the left side. The fasciculus longitudinalis medialis runs anterior to the aqueductus cerebri on both sides and continues from the mesencephalon to the pars cervicalis medullae spinalis. It transmits fibers for the coordination of conjugate eye movements. A lesion of the MLF results in internuclear ophthalmoplegia (see **C**).

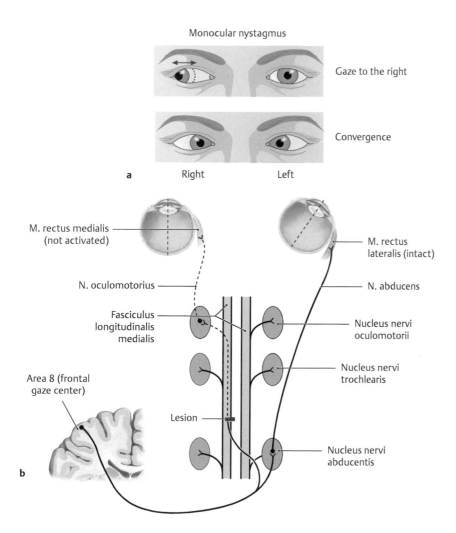

C Lesion of the fasciculus longitudinalis medialis and internuclear ophthalmoplegia

The fasciculus longitudinalis medialis interconnects the nuclei nervi oculomotorii and also connects them with the opposite side (**b**). When this "information highway" is interrupted, internuclear ophthalmoplegia develops. This type of lesion most commonly occurs between the nucleus nervi abducentis and the nucleus nervi oculomotoriis. It may be unilateral or bilateral. Typical causes are multiple sclerosis and diminished blood flow. The lesion is manifested by the loss of conjugate eye movements (**a**). With a lesion of the left fasciculus longitudinalis medialis, as shown here, the left m. rectus medialis is no longer activated during gaze to the right. The eye cannot be moved *inward* on the side of the lesion (loss of the m. rectus medialis), and the opposite eye goes into an abducting nystagmus (m. rectus lateralis is intact and innervated by the n. abducens). Reflex movements such as convergence are not impaired because there is no peripheral or nuclear lesion and this reaction is not mediated by the fasciculus longitudinalis medialis.

483

13.21 Auditory Pathway

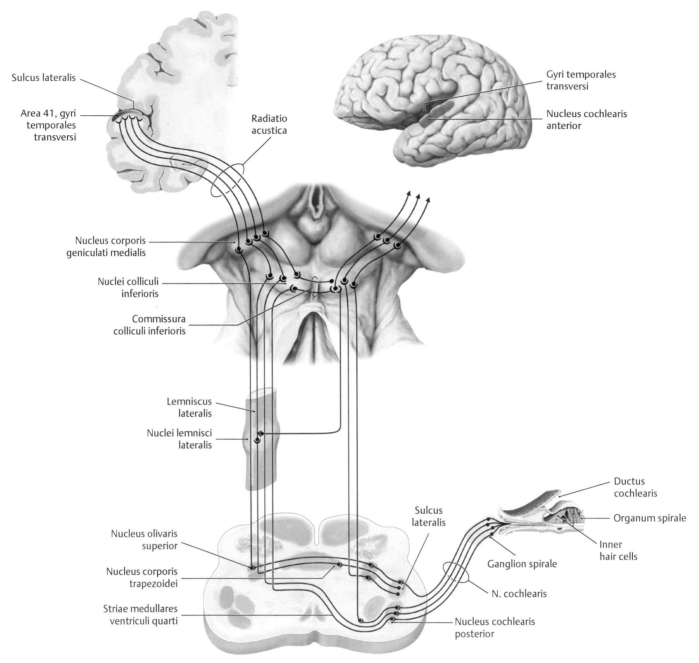

A Afferent auditory pathway of the left ear

The receptors of the auditory pathway are the inner hair cells of the organum spirale. Because they lack neural processes, they are called *secondary sensory cells*. They are located in the ductus cochlearis of the lamina basilaris and are studded with stereocilia, which are exposed to shearing forces from the membrana tectoria in response to a traveling wave. This causes bowing of the stereocilia (see p. 153). These bowing movements act as a stimulus to evoke cascades of neural signals. Dendritic processes of the bipolar neurons in the ganglion spirale pick up the stimulus. The bipolar neurons then transmit impulses via their axons, which are collected to form the n. cochlearis, to the nuclei cochleares anterior and posterior. In these nuclei the signals are relayed to the second neuron of the auditory pathway. Information from the nuclei cochleares is then transmitted via 4–6 nuclei to the primary auditory cortex, where the auditory information is consciously perceived (analogous to the visual cortex). The primary auditory cortex is located—somewhat hidden in the lateral sulcus—in the gyri temporales transversi (Heschl gyri, Brodmann area 41). The auditory pathway thus contains the following key stations:

- Inner hair cells in the organum spirale
- Ganglion spirale

- Nuclei cochleares anterior and posterior
- Nuclei corporis trapezoidei and nuclei olivares superior
- Nucleus lemnisci lateralis
- Nucleus colliculi inferioris
- Nucleus corporis geniculati lateralis
- Primary auditory cortex in the lobus temporalis (gyri temporales transversi: Heschl gyri or Brodmann area 41)

The individual parts of the cochlea are correlated with specific areas in the auditory cortex and its relay stations. This is known as the *tonotopic organization of the auditory pathway*. This organizational principle is similar to that in the visual pathway. Binaural processing of the auditory information: stereo hearing) first occurs at the level of the nuclei olivares superiores. At all further stages of the auditory pathway there are also interconnections between the right and left sides of the auditory pathway (for clarity, these are not shown here). A cochlea that has ceased to function can sometimes be replaced with a cochlear implant.

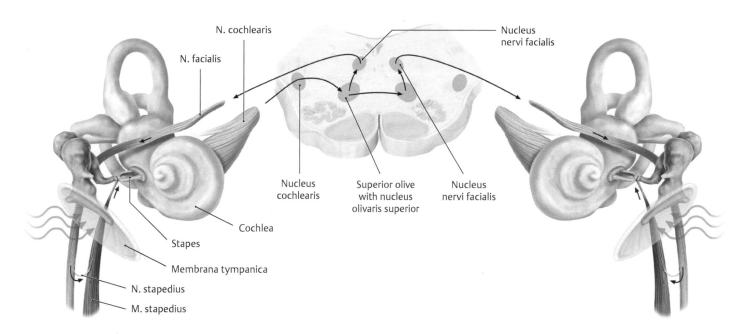

B The stapedius reflex

When the volume of an acoustic signal reaches a certain threshold, the stapedius reflex triggers a contraction of the m. stapedius. This reflex can be utilized to test hearing without the patient's cooperation ("objective" auditory testing). The test is done by introducing a sonic probe into the meatus acusticus externa and presenting a test noise to the membrana tympanica. When the noise volume reaches a certain threshold, it evokes the stapedius reflex and the membrana tympanica stiffens. The change in the resistance of the membrana tympanica is then measured and recorded. The *afferent* limb of this reflex is in the n. cochlearis. Information is conveyed to the nucleus nervi facialis on each side by way of the nuclei olivares superiores. The *efferent* limb of this reflex is formed by special visceromotor fibers of the n. facialis.

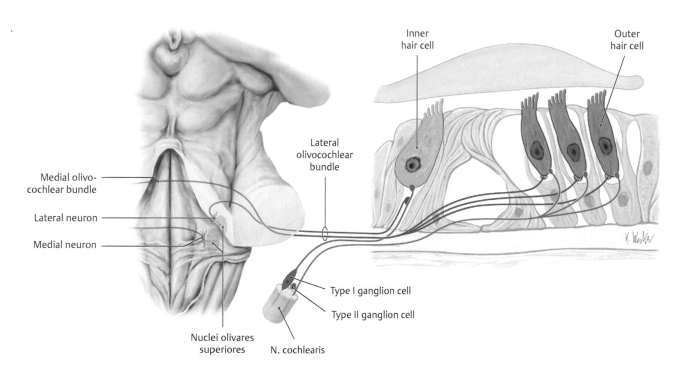

C Efferent fibers from the olive to the organum spirale

Besides the afferent fibers from the organum spirale (see **A**, shown here in blue), which form the n. vestibulocochlearis, there are also efferent fibers (red) that pass to the organum spirale in the auris interna and are concerned with the active preprocessing of sound ("cochlear amplifier") and acoustic protection. The efferent fibers arise from neurons that are located in either the nucleus olivaris superior lateralis or medialis and project from there to the cochlea (tractus olivocochlearis). The fibers of the lateral neurons pass *uncrossed* to the dendrites of the *inner* hair cells, while the fibers of the medial neurons cross to the opposite side and terminate at the base of the *outer* hair cells, whose activity they influence. When stimulated, the outer hair cells can actively amplify the traveling wave. This increases the sensitivity of the inner hair cells (the actual receptor cells). The activity of the efferents from the olive can be recorded as otoacoustic emissions (OAE). This test can be used to screen for hearing abnormalities in newborns.

13.22 **Vestibular System**

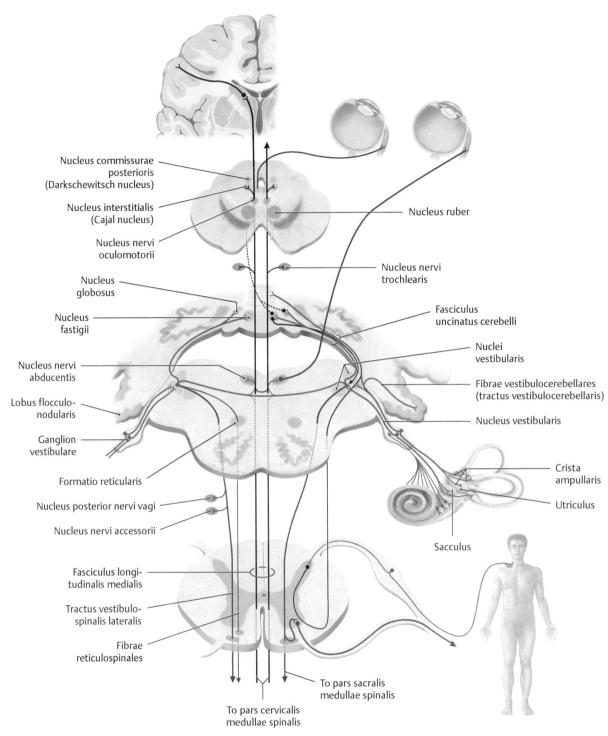

Nucleus commissurae posterioris (Darkschewitsch nucleus)

Nucleus interstitialis (Cajal nucleus)

Nucleus nervi oculomotorii

Nucleus globosus

Nucleus fastigii

Nucleus nervi abducentis

Lobus flocculo-nodularis

Ganglion vestibulare

Formatio reticularis

Nucleus posterior nervi vagi

Nucleus nervi accessorii

Fasciculus longi-tudinalis medialis

Tractus vestibulo-spinalis lateralis

Fibrae reticulospinales

Nucleus ruber

Nucleus nervi trochlearis

Fasciculus uncinatus cerebelli

Nuclei vestibularis

Fibrae vestibulocerebellares (tractus vestibulocerebellaris)

Nucleus vestibularis

Crista ampullaris

Utriculus

Sacculus

To pars sacralis medullae spinalis

To pars cervicalis medullae spinalis

A Central connections of the nervus vestibularis

Three systems are involved in the regulation of human balance:

- Vestibular system
- Proprioceptive system
- Visual system

The latter two systems have already been described. The peripheral receptors of the vestibular system are located in the labyrinthus membranaceus (see pars petrosa ossis temporalis, pp. 142, 154), which consists of the utriculus and sacculus and the ampullae of the three canales semicirculares. The maculae of the utriculus and sacculus respond to linear acceleration, while the semicircular canal organs in the cristae ampullares respond to angular (rotational) acceleration. Like the hair cells of the inner ear, the receptors of the vestibular system are secondary sensory cells. The basal portions of the secondary sensory cells are

surrounded by dendritic processes of bipolar neurons with their bodies located in the ganglion vestibulare. The axons from these neurons form the n. vestibularis and terminate in the four nuclei vestibulares (see **C**). Besides input from the vestibular apparatus, these nuclei also receive sensory input (see **B**). The nuclei vestibulares show a topographical organization (see **C**) and distribute their efferent fibers to three targets:

- Motor neurons in the medulla spinalis via the tractus vestibulospinalis lateralis. These motor neurons help to maintain upright stance, mainly by increasing the tone of extensor muscles
- Lobus flocculonodularis of the cerebellum (direct sensory input to the cerebellum) via fibrae vestibulocerebellares
- Ipsilateral and contralateral nuclei oculomotorii via the ascending part of the fasciculus longitudinalis medialis

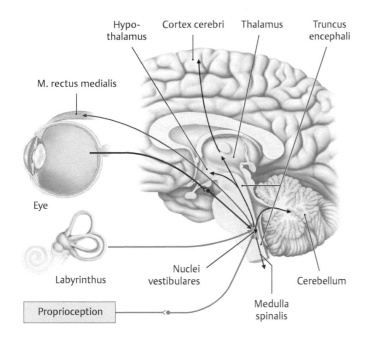

B Central role of the nuclei vestibulares in the maintenance of balance

The afferent fibers that pass to the nuclei vestibulares and the efferent fibers that emerge from them demonstrate the central role of these nuclei in maintaining balance. The nuclei vestibulares receive afferent input from the vestibular system, proprioceptive system (position sense, muscles, and joints), and visual system. They then distribute efferent fibers to nuclei that control the motor systems important for balance. These nuclei are located in the

- Medulla spinalis (motor support),
- Cerebellum (fine control of motor function), and
- Truncus encephali (nuclei nervi oculomotorii for oculomotor function).

Efferents from the nuclei vestibulares are also distributed to the following regions:

- Thalamus and cortex (spatial sense)
- Hypothalamus (autonomic regulation: vomiting in response to vertigo)

Note: Acute failure of the vestibular system is manifested by rotary vertigo.

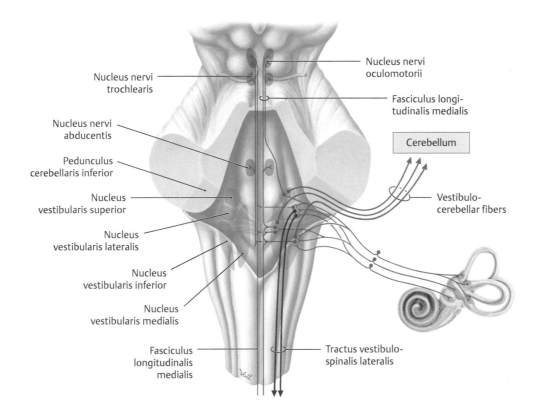

C Nuclei vestibulares: Topographic organization and central connections

Four nuclei are distinguished:

- Nucleus vestibularis superior (of Bechterew)
- Nucleus vestibularis lateralis (of Deiters)
- Nucleus vestibularis medialis (of Schwalbe)
- Nucleus vestibularis inferior (of Roller)

The vestibular system has a topographic organization:

- The afferent fibers of the macula sacculi terminate in the inferior nucleus vestibularis inferior and nucleus vestibularis lateralis.
- The afferent fibers of the macula utriculi terminate in the medial part of the nucleus vestibularis inferior, the lateral part of the nucleus vestibularis medius, and the nucleus vestibularis lateralis.

- The afferent fibers from the cristae ampullares of the canales semicirculares terminate in the nucleus vestibularis superior, the upper part of the nucleus vestibularis inferior, and the nucleus vestibularis lateralis.

The efferent fibers from the nucleus vestibularis lateralis pass to the tractus vestibulospinalis lateralis. This tract extends to the pars sacralis of the medulla spinalis, its axons terminating on motor neurons. Functionally it is concerned with keeping the body upright, chiefly by increasing the tone of the extensor muscles. The vestibulocerebellar fibers from the other three nuclei act through the cerebellum to modulate muscular tone. All four nuclei vestibulares distribute ipsilateral and contralateral axons via the fasciculus longitudinalis medialis to the three motor nuclei of the nerves to the extraocular muscles (i.e., the nuclei of the nn. abducens, trochlearis, and oculomotorius).

487

13.23 Gustatory System (Taste)

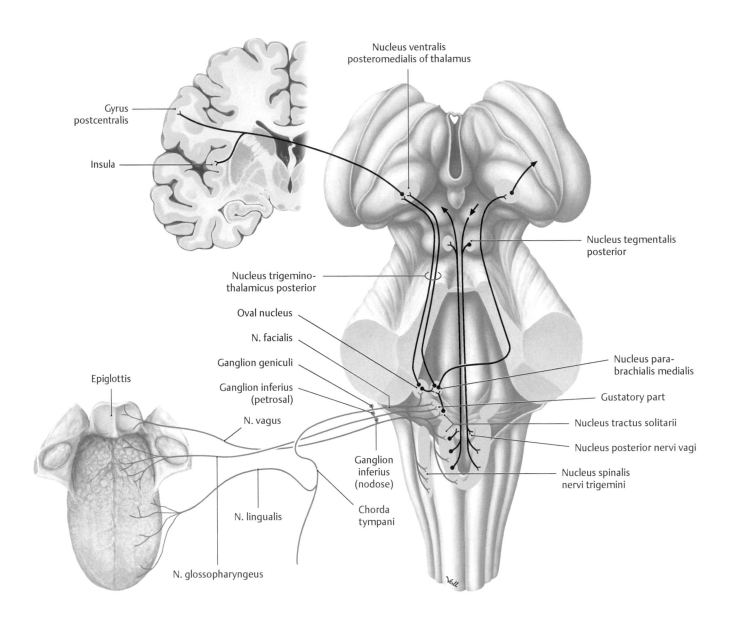

Nucleus ventralis posteromedialis of thalamus

Gyrus postcentralis

Insula

Nucleus trigemino-thalamicus posterior

Oval nucleus

N. facialis

Ganglion geniculi

Ganglion inferius (petrosal)

N. vagus

Epiglottis

N. lingualis

N. glossopharyngeus

Ganglion inferius (nodose)

Chorda tympani

Nucleus tegmentalis posterior

Nucleus para-brachialis medialis

Gustatory part

Nucleus tractus solitarii

Nucleus posterior nervi vagi

Nucleus spinalis nervi trigemini

A Gustatory pathway

The receptors for the sense of taste are the gemmae gustatoriae of the tongue (see **B**). Unlike other receptor cells, the receptor cells of the gemmae gustatoriae are specialized epithelial cells (secondary sensory cells given that they do not have an axon). When these epithelial cells are chemically stimulated, the base of the cells releases glutamate, which stimulates the peripheral processes of afferent nn. craniales. These different nn. craniales serve different areas of the tongue. It is rare, therefore, for a complete loss of taste (ageusia) to occur.

- The **anterior two-thirds** of the tongue are supplied by the n. facialis (CN VII), the afferent fibers first passing in the n. lingualis (branch of the n. trigeminus) and then in the chorda tympani to the ganglion geniculi of the n. facialis.
- The *posterior third of the tongue* and the *papillae vallatae* are supplied by the n. glossopharyngeus (CN IX).
- The *epiglottis* is supplied by the n. vagus (CN X).

Peripheral processes from pseudounipolar ganglion cells (which correspond to pseudounipolar spinal ganglion cells) terminate on the gemmae gustatoriae. The central portions of these processes convey taste information to the gustatory part of the nucleus tractus solitarii. Thus, they function as the first afferent neuron of the gustatory pathway. Their cell bodies are located in the ganglion geniculi for the n. facialis,

in the ganglion inferius (petrosal) for the n. glossopharyngeus, and in the ganglion inferius (nodose) for the n. vagus. After the first neurons synapse with the second neurons in the gustatory part of the nucleus tractus solitarii, some of the axons of the second neurons run ipsi- and contralaterally with the tractus trigeminothalamicus to the nucleus ventralis posteromedialis (VPM) of the thalamus, where they terminate on the third neurons. These neurons then project to the gyrus postcentralis and the insular cortex. However, some of the axons of the second neurons travel to an additional intermediate station in the truncus encephali, the nucleus parabrachialis medialis, which in turn projects (as third neurons) to the thalamus, which further projects (as fourth neurons) to the insular cortex and gyrus postcentralis. Collaterals from the first and second neurons of the gustatory afferent pathway are distributed to the nuclei salivatorii superior and inferior. Afferent impulses in these fibers induce the secretion of saliva during eating ("salivary reflex"). The parasympathetic preganglionic fibers exit the truncus encephali via nn. craniales VII and IX (see the descriptions of these nn. craniales for details). Besides this purely gustatory pathway, spicy foods may also stimulate trigeminal fibers (not shown), which contribute to the sensation of taste. Finally, olfaction (the sense of smell), too, is a major component of the sense of taste as it is subjectively perceived: patients who cannot smell (anosmosia) report that their food tastes abnormally bland.

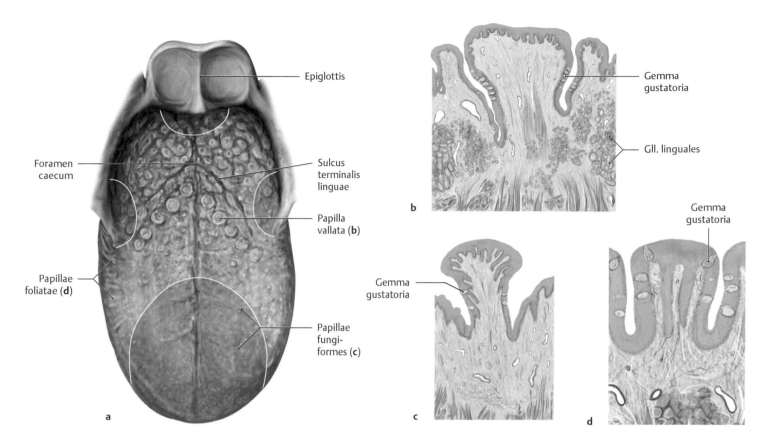

b

c   d

Epiglottis

Foramen caecum

Sulcus terminalis linguae

Papilla vallata (b)

Papillae foliatae (d)

Papillae fungiformes (c)

Gemma gustatoria

Gll. linguales

Gemma gustatoria

Gemma gustatoria

a

B Organization of the taste receptors in the tongue

The human tongue contains approximately 4600 gemmae gustatoriae in which the secondary sensory cells for taste perception are collected. They are concentrated in the white bordered areas. The gemmae gustatoriae (see **C**) are embedded in the epithelium of the lingual mucosa and are located on the surface expansions of the lingual mucosa—the papillae vallatae (principal site, **b**), the papillae fungiformes (**c**), and the papillae foliatae (**d**). Additionally, isolated gemmae gustatoriae are located in the tunica mucosa of the palatum molle and pharynx. The surrounding serous gll. linguales (Ebner glands), which are most closely associated with the papillae vallatae, constantly wash the taste buds clean to allow for new tasting. Humans can perceive five basic tastes: sweet, sour, salty, bitter, and a fifth "savory" taste, called umami, which is activated by glutamate (a taste enhancer).

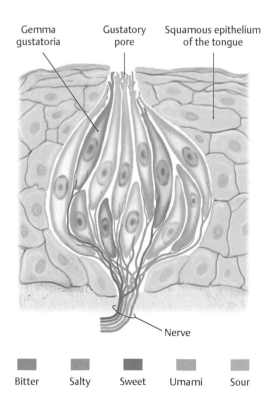

Gemma gustatoria   *Gustatory pore*   *Squamous epithelium of the tongue*

Nerve

Bitter   Salty   Sweet   Umami   Sour

C Microscopic structure of a gemma gustatoria

(after: Chandrashekar, Hoon et al.)

Nerves induce the formation of gemmae gustatoriae in the oral mucosa. Processes of neurons of the three above mentioned nn. craniales, which grow into the tunica mucosa oris from the basal side, induce the epithelium to differentiate into the depicted taste cells (modified epithelial cells). Their microvilli extend to the gustatory pore. Specialized taste receptor proteins in the cell membrane of the microvilli are responsible for taste perception (for details, see physiology textbooks). After low-molecular-weight flavored substances bind to the receptor proteins, a signal transduction is induced, which causes the release of glutamate. This in turn excites the peripheral processes of the pseudounipolar neurons with the bodies in the ganglia of the mentioned three nn. craniales. Based on their features, each receptor cell is specialized in one of the five tastes (see color coding); the entire range of the perception of taste qualities is coded within each individual gemma gustatoria. This explains why the old notion that particular areas of the tongue are sensitive to specific taste qualities is incorrect.

489

13.24 Olfactory System (Smell)

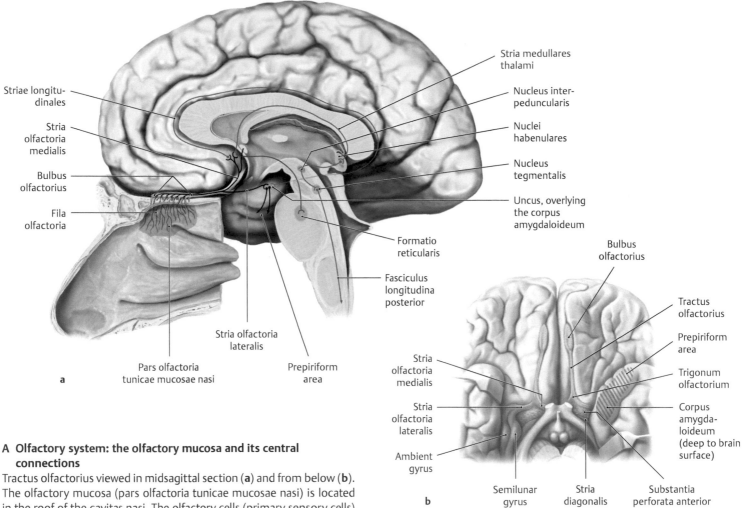

a

Striae longitudinales
Stria olfactoria medialis
Bulbus olfactorius
Fila olfactoria
Pars olfactoria tunicae mucosae nasi
Stria olfactoria lateralis
Prepiriform area

Stria medullares thalami
Nucleus interpeduncularis
Nuclei habenulares
Nucleus tegmentalis
Uncus, overlying the corpus amygdaloideum
Formatio reticularis
Fasciculus longitudina posterior

b

Stria olfactoria medialis
Stria olfactoria lateralis
Ambient gyrus
Semilunar gyrus
Stria diagonalis
Substantia perforata anterior

Bulbus olfactorius
Tractus olfactorius
Prepiriform area
Trigonum olfactorium
Corpus amygdaloideum (deep to brain surface)

A Olfactory system: the olfactory mucosa and its central connections

Tractus olfactorius viewed in midsagittal section (**a**) and from below (**b**). The olfactory mucosa (pars olfactoria tunicae mucosae nasi) is located in the roof of the cavitas nasi. The olfactory cells (primary sensory cells) are bipolar neurons. Their peripheral receptor-bearing processes are found in the epithelium of the tunica mucosa nasi, while their central processes pass to the bulbus olfactorius (see **B** for details). The bulbus olfactorius, where the second neurons of the olfactory pathway (mitral and tufted cells) are located, is considered an extension of the telencephalon. The axons of these second neurons pass centrally as the *tractus olfactorius*. In front of the substantia perforata anterior, the tractus olfactorius widens to form the trigonum olfactorium and splits into the striae olfactoriae lateralis and medialis.

- Some of the axons of the tractus olfactorius run in the **stria olfactoria lateralis** to the olfactory centers: the corpus amygdaloideum, semilunar gyrus, and ambient gyrus. The prepiriform area (Brodmann area 28) is considered to be the primary olfactory cortex in the strict sense. It contains the third neurons of the olfactory pathway.
  Note: The prepiriform area is shaded in **b**, lying at the junction of the basal side of the lobus frontalis and the medial side of the lobus temporalis.
- Other axons of the tractus olfactorius run in the **stria olfactoria medialis** to nuclei in the septal (subcallosal) area, which is part of the limbic system (see p. 492), and to the tuberculum olfactorium, a small elevation in the substantia perforata anterior.
- Yet other axons of the tractus olfactorius terminate in the **nucleus olfactorius anterior**, where the fibers that cross to the opposite side branch off and are relayed. This nucleus is located in the trigonum olfactorium, which lies between the two striae olfactoriae and in front of the substantia perforata anterior.

Note: None of these three tracts are routed through the thalamus. Thus, the olfactory system is the only sensory system that is not relayed in the thalamus before reaching the cortex. There is, however, an indirect route from the primary olfactory cortex to the neocortex passing through the thalamus and terminating in the pars basalis telencephali. The olfactory signals are further analyzed in these basal portions of the forebrain (not shown).

The olfactory system is linked to other brain areas well beyond the primary olfactory cortex, with the result that olfactory stimuli can evoke complex emotional and behavioral responses. Noxious smells may induce nausea, while appetizing smells evoke watering of the mouth. Presumably these sensations are processed by the hypothalamus, thalamus, and limbic system (see next unit) via connections established mainly by the fasciculus medialis telencephali and the striae medullares thalami. The fasciculus medialis telencephali distributes axons to the following structures:

- Hypothalamic nuclei
- Formatio reticularis
- Nuclei salivatorii
- Nucleus posterior nervi vagi

The axons that run in the striae medullares thalami terminate in the nuclei habenulares. This tract also continues to the truncus encephali, where it stimulates salivation in response to smell.

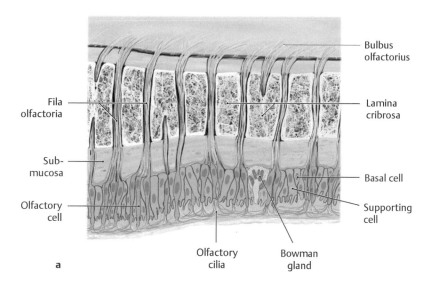

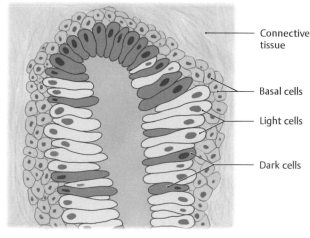

Fila olfactoria

Sub-mucosa

Olfactory cell

Bulbus olfactorius

Lamina cribrosa

Basal cell

Supporting cell

Olfactory cilia

Bowman gland

a

Connective tissue

Basal cells

Light cells

Dark cells

c

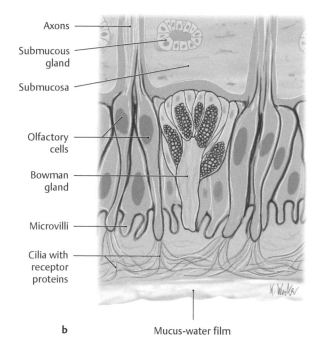

Axons

Submucous gland

Submucosa

Olfactory cells

Bowman gland

Microvilli

Cilia with receptor proteins

b

Mucus-water film

B Olfactory mucosa and vomeronasal organ (VNO, organum vomeronasale)

The **pars olfactoria tunicae mucosae nasi** occupies an area of approximately 2 cm² on the roof of each cavitas nasi, and 10⁷ primary sensory cells are concentrated in each of these areas (**a**). At the molecular level, the olfactory receptor proteins are located in the cilia of the sensory cells (**b**). Each sensory cell has only one specialized receptor protein that mediates signal transduction when an odorant molecule binds to it. Although humans are microsmatic, having a sense of smell that is feeble compared with other mammals, the olfactory receptor proteins still make up 2% of the human genome. This underscores the importance of olfaction in humans. The primary olfactory sensory cells have a life span of approximately 60 days and regenerate from the basal cells (lifelong division of neurons). The bundled central processes (axons) from hundreds of olfactory cells form fila olfactoria (**a**) that pass through the lamina cribrosa of the os ethmoidale and terminate in the *bulbus olfactorius* (see **C**), which lies above the lamina cribrosa. The organum vomeronasale (**c**) is located on both sides of the anterior septum nasi. Its central connections in humans are unknown. It responds to steroids and evokes unconscious reactions in subjects (possibly influences the choice of a mate). Mate selection in many animal species is known to be mediated by olfactory impulses that are perceived in the organum vomeronasale.

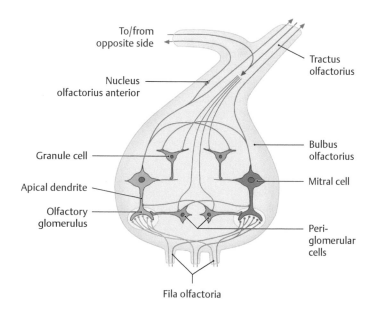

To/from opposite side

Nucleus olfactorius anterior

Granule cell

Apical dendrite

Olfactory glomerulus

Tractus olfactorius

Bulbus olfactorius

Mitral cell

Peri-glomerular cells

Fila olfactoria

C Synaptic patterns in a bulbus olfactorius

Specialized neurons in the bulbus olfactorius, called mitral cells, form apical dendrites that receive synaptic contact from the axons of thousands of primary sensory cells. The dendrite plus the synapses make up the *olfactory glomeruli*. Axons from sensory cells with the same receptor protein form glomeruli with only one or a small number of mitral cells. The basal axons of the mitral cells form the tractus olfactorius. The axons that run in the tractus olfactorius project primarily to the olfactory cortex but are also distributed to other nuclei in the CNS. The axon collaterals of the mitral cells pass to granule cells: both granule cells and periglomerular cells inhibit the activity of the mitral cells, causing less sensory information to reach higher centers. These inhibitory processes are believed to heighten olfactory contrast, which aids in the more accurate perception of smells. The tufted cells, which also project to the primary olfactory cortex, are not shown.

13.25 Limbic System

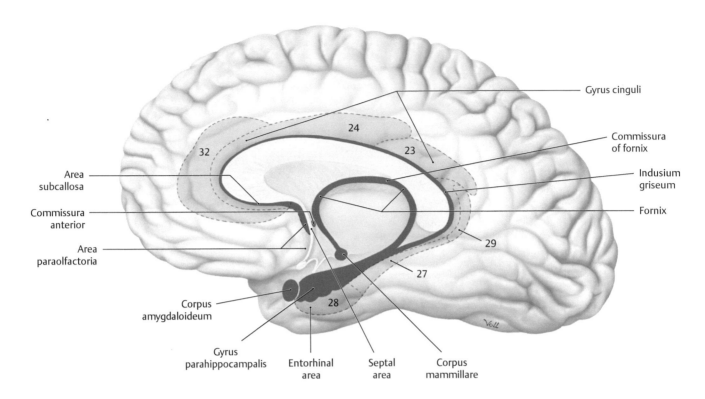

A Limbic system viewed through the partially transparent cortex
Medial view of the right hemispherium. The term "limbic system" (Latin *limbus*: "border" or "fringe") was first used by Broca in 1878, who collectively described the gyri surrounding the corpus callosum, diencephalon, and nuclei basales as the *grand lobe limbique*. The limbic system encompasses neo-, archi-, and paleocortical regions as well as subcortical nuclei. The anatomical extent of the limbic system is such that it can exchange and integrate information between the telencephalon (hemispheria cerebri), diencephalon, and mesencephalon. Viewed from the medial aspect of the hemispheria cerebri, the limbic system is seen to consist of an inner arc and an outer arc. The outer arc is formed by

- Gyrus parahippocampalis,
- Gyrus cinguli (also called the limbic gyrus),
- Area subcallosa (area paraolfactoria), and
- Indusium griseum.

The inner arc is formed by

- Hippocampal formation,
- Fornix,
- Septal area (also known simply as the septum),
- Stria diagonalis of Broca (not visible in this view), and
- Gyrus paraterminalis.

The limbic system also includes the corpora amygdaloidea and corpora mammillaria. The following nuclei are also considered part of the limbic system but are not shown: the nuclei anteriores thalami, nuclei habenulares, nucleus tegmentalis posterior, and nucleus interpeduncularis.
The limbic system is concerned with the regulation of drive and affective behavior and plays a crucial role in memory and learning. The numbers in the diagram indicate the Brodmann areas.

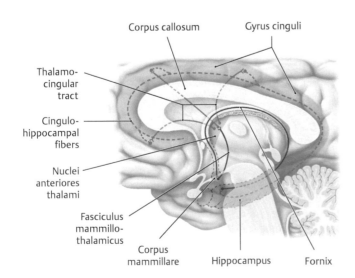

B Neuronal circuit (Papez circuit)
View of the medial surface of the right hemispherium. Several nuclei of the limbic system are interconnected by a *neuronal circuit* (see below) called the Papez circuit after the anatomist who first described it. MacLean later (1949) expanded the concept by introducing the term limbic system. The sequence below indicates the nuclei (normal print) and tracts (*italic print*) that are the successive stations of this neuronal circuit:

Hippocampus → *fornix* → corpus mammillare → *fasciculus mammillothalamicus* (Vicq d'Azyr bundle) → nuclei anteriores thalami → *tractus thalamocingularis (radiation)* → gyrus cinguli → *fibrae cingulohippocampales* → hippocampus.

This neuronal circuit interconnects ontogenically distinct parts of the limbic system. It establishes a connection between information stored in the unconscious and conscious behavior.

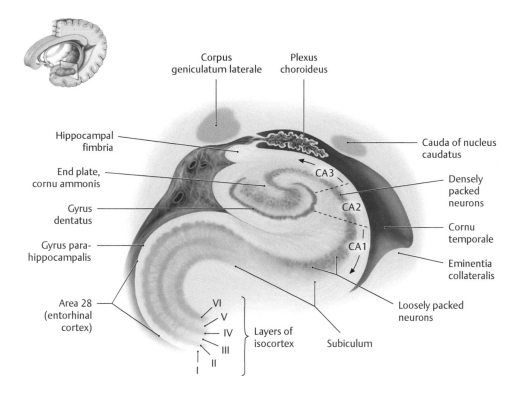

Corpus geniculatum laterale

Plexus choroideus

Hippocampal fimbria

End plate, cornu ammonis

Gyrus dentatus

Gyrus para-hippocampalis

Area 28 (entorhinal cortex)

CA3

CA2

CA1

Cauda of nucleus caudatus

Densely packed neurons

Cornu temporale

Eminentia collateralis

Loosely packed neurons

VI
V
IV
III
II
I

Layers of isocortex

Subiculum

C Cytoarchitecture of the hippocampal formation (after Bähr and Frotscher)

View from anterior left.

Note: The hippocampal formation has a three-layered allocortex instead of a six-layered isocortex (lower left in diagram). It is a phylogenetically older structure than the isocortex. At the center of the allocortex is a band of neurons that forms the neuronal layer of the hippocampus (hippocampus proprius [cornu ammonis]). The neurons in this layer are mainly pyramidal cells. Three regions, designated CA1–CA3, can be distinguished based on differences in the density of the pyramidal cells. *Region CA 1*, called also the "Sommer sector," is important in neuropathology because the death of neurons in this sector is the first morphologically detectable sign of cerebral hypoxia. Besides the hippocampus proprius, we can also identify the stratum granulare of the gyrus dentatus (dentate fascia), which consists mainly of granule cells.

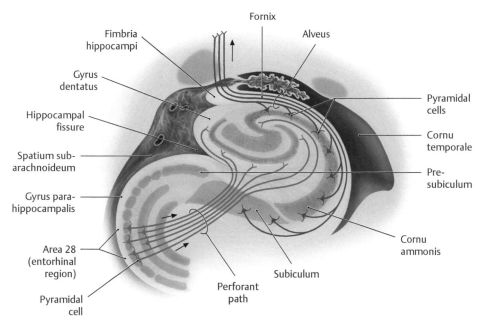

Fornix

Fimbria hippocampi

Alveus

Gyrus dentatus

Hippocampal fissure

Spatium sub-arachnoideum

Gyrus para-hippocampalis

Area 28 (entorhinal region)

Pyramidal cell

Pyramidal cells

Cornu temporale

Pre-subiculum

Cornu ammonis

Subiculum

Perforant path

D Connections of the hippocampus

Left anterior view. The most important afferent pathway to the hippocampus is the *perforant path* (blue), which extends from the entorhinal region (triangular pyramidal cells of Brodmann area 28) to the hippocampus proprius (where it ends in a synapse). The neurons that project from area 28 into the hippocampus receive afferent input from many brain regions. Thus, the entorhinal region is considered the gateway to the hippocampus. The pyramidal cells of the cornu ammonis (triangles) send their axons into the fornix, and the axons transmitted via the fornix continue to the corpus mammillare (Papez neuronal circuit) or to the nuclei septales.

E Important definitions pertaining to the limbic system

Archicortex
Phylogenetically old structures of the cortex cerebri; does not have a six-layered architecture

Hippocampus (retrocommissural)
Cornu ammonis (hippocampus proprius), gyrus dentatus (dentate fascia), subiculum (some authors consider it part of the hippocampal formation rather than the hippocampus itself)

Hippocampal formation
Hippocampus plus the entorhinal area of the gyrus parahippocampalis

Limbic system
Important coordinating system for memory and emotions. Includes the following telencephalic structures: gyrus cinguli, gyrus parahippocampalis, hippocampal formation, nuclei septales, and corpus amygdaloideum. Its diencephalic components include the nuclei anteriores thalami, corpora mammillaria, nucleus accumbens, and nuclei habenulares. Its truncus encephali components are the nuclei raphes. The fasciculus medialis telencephali and the fasciculus longitudinalis posterior contribute to the fiber tracts of the limbic system.

Periarchicortex
A broad transitional zone around the hippocampus, consisting of the gyrus cinguli, the isthmus gyri cinguli, and the gyrus parahippocampalis

493

13.26 Brain: Functional Organization

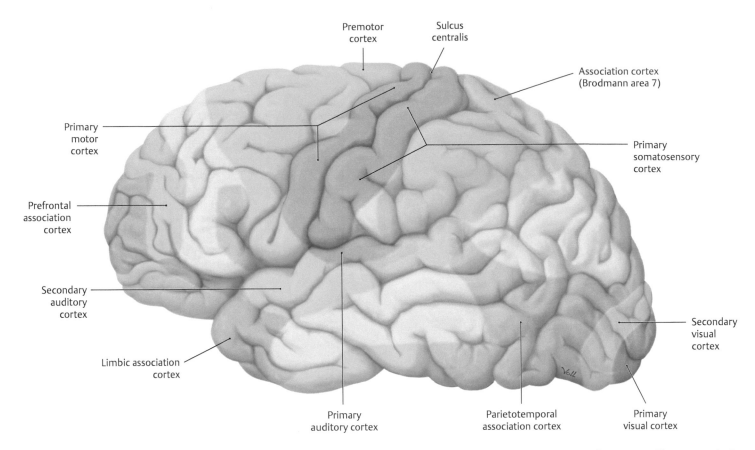

A Functional organization of the neocortex

Left lateral view. The primary sensory and motor areas are shown in red, and the areas of the association cortex are shown in different shades of green. Projection tracts begin or end, respectively, in the primary motor or sensory areas. More than 80% of the cortical surface area is association cortex, which is secondarily connected to the primary sensory or primary motor areas. The neuronal processing of differentiated behavior and intellectual performance takes place in the association cortex,

which has increased greatly in size over the course of human evolution. The functional organization pattern shown here, such as the localization of the primary motor cortex in the gyrus precentralis, can be demonstrated in living subjects with modern imaging techniques. The results of such studies are illustrated in the figures below. Interestingly, the correlations described in these studies correspond reasonably well with the cortical areas defined by Brodmann.

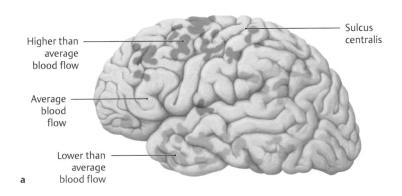

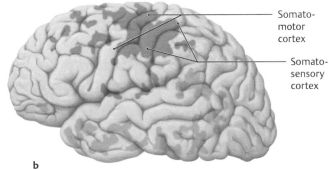

B Analysis of brain function based on studies of regional cerebral blood flow

Left lateral view of the brain. When neurons are activated they consume more glucose and oxygen, which must be delivered to them via the bloodstream. This may produce a detectable increase in regional blood flow. These brain maps illustrate the local patterns of cerebral blood flow

at rest (**a**) and during movement of the right hand (**b**). When the right hand is moved, increased blood flow is recorded in the left gyrus precentralis, which contains the motor representation of the right hand (see motor homunculus in **B** on p. 457). Simultaneous activation is noted in the sensory cortex of the postcentral region, showing that the sensory cortex is also active during motor function (feedback loop).

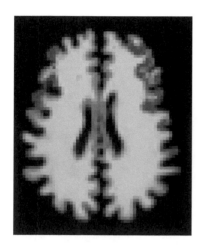

Female

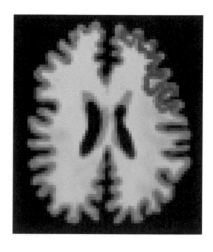

Male

C Sex differences in neuronal processing
(after Stoppe, Hentschel, and Munz)

Patterns of brain activity can also be demonstrated by functional magnetic resonance imaging (fMRI). This provides a noninvasive method for investigating the metabolic activity of the brain. Because no human brain is identical to any other, a comparison of several brains will show slight variations in the distribution of specific functions. By superimposing the results of examinations in different brains, we can produce a generalized map that shows the approximate distribution of brain functions. Compare the summation map for female brains on the left with a map for male brains on the right. Both groups of subjects were given phonological tasks based on recognizing differences in the meaning of spoken sounds. While the female subjects activated both sides of their brain when solving the tasks, the male subjects activated only the left side (the sectional images are viewed from below).

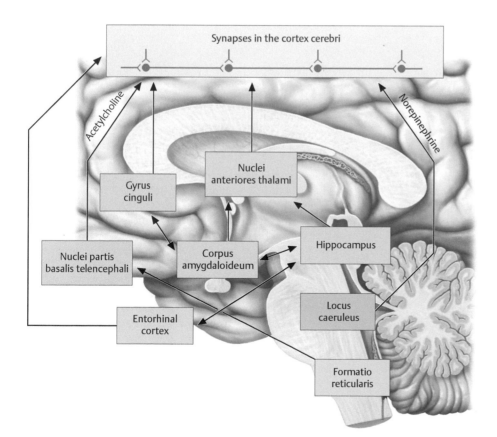

D Modulating subcortical centers
The cortex cerebri, the seat of our conscious thoughts and actions, is influenced by various subcortical centers. The parts of the limbic system that are crucial for learning and memory are indicated in light red.

13.27 Brain: Hemispheric Dominance

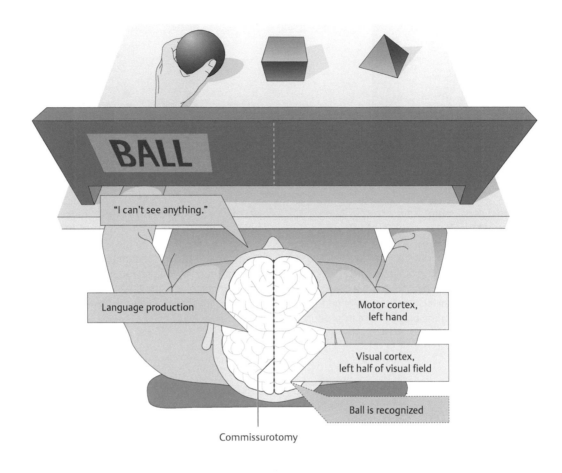

Commissurotomy

A Demonstration of hemispheric dominance for language in splitbrain patients (after Klinke, Pape, and Silbernagl)

The corpus callosum is by far the most important commissural tract, interconnecting areas of like function in both hemispheria of the encephalon. Because lesions of the corpus callosum were once considered to have no clinical effects, surgical division of the corpus callosum was commonly performed at one time in epileptic patients to keep epileptic seizures from spreading across the brain. This operation interrupts the connections in the *upper telencephalon* while leaving intact the more deeply situated *diencephalon*, which contains the tractus opticus. Patients who have undergone this operation are called "split-brain patients." They have no obvious clinical abnormalities, but special neuropsychological tests reveal deficits, the study of which has improved our understanding of brain function. In one test the patient sits in front of a screen on which words are projected. Meanwhile, the patient can grasp objects behind the screen without being able to see them. When the word "Ball" is flashed briefly on the left side of the screen, the patient perceives it in the visual cortex on the right side (the tractus opticus has not been cut). Because language production resides in the *left* hemispherium in 97% of the population, the patient cannot verbalize the projected word out loud because communication between the hemispheria has been interrupted at the level of the telencephalon (seat of speech production). But the patient is still able to feel the ball manually and pick it out from other objects. The function of the corpus callosum is to enable both hemispheres (which can function independently to a degree) to communicate with each other when the need arises. Because of the phenomenon of hemispheric dominance, the corpus callosum in humans is more elaborately developed than in other animal species. The male and female brain differs in the assignment of functional roles to the cortical areas. In the male, only one hemispherium participates in the execution of linguistic tasks whereas females activate both hemispheria (see **C**, p. 495). This fact is believed to also have an impact on the structure of the corpus callosum. According to several studies, the number of axons in the isthmus of the corpus callosum is said to be larger in the female (approximately 25% larger isthmus area), who are supposed to show better speech comprehension ability than males (one man, one word—one woman, one dictionary). However, these findings are highly controversial.

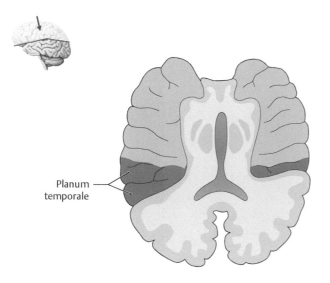

Planum
temporale

B Hemispheric asymmetry (after Klinke and Silbernagl)
Superior view of the lobus temporalis of a brain that has been taken
apart (i.e., the lobi frontales have been removed) along the lateral fissure. The *planum temporale*, located on the posterior and superior surface of the lobus temporalis, has different contours on the two sides
of the encephalon, being more pronounced on the left side than on
the right in two-thirds of individuals. The functional significance of this
asymmetry is uncertain. We cannot explain it simply by noting that
Wernicke's speech area is located in that part of the lobus temporalis,
because while temporal asymmetry is present in only 67% of the population, the speech area is located on the left side in 97%.

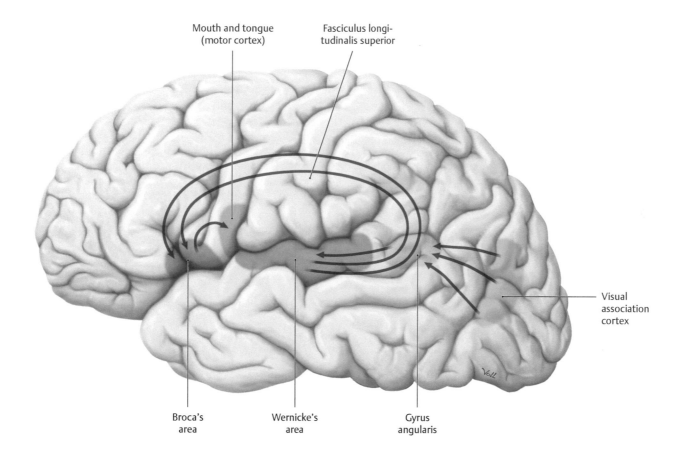

Mouth and tongue
(motor cortex)

Fasciculus longi-
tudinalis superior

Visual
association
cortex

Broca's
area

Wernicke's
area

Gyrus
angularis

C Language areas in the normally dominant left hemispherium
Lateral view. The brain contains several language areas whose loss is
associated with typical clinical symptoms. *Wernicke's area* (the posterior
part of area 22) is necessary for language comprehension, while *Broca's
area* (area 44) is concerned with language production. The two areas
are interconnected by the fasciculus longitudinalis superior (fasciculus
arcuatus). Broca's area activates the mouth and tongue region of the
motor cortex for the articulation of speech. The gyrus angularis coordinates the inputs from the visual, acoustic, and somatosensory cortices
and relays them onward to Wernicke's area.

497

13.28 Brain: Clinical Findings

The figures in this unit illustrate the correlations that have been discovered between specific brain areas and clinical findings. Studies of this kind have enabled us to link particular patterns of behavior, some abnormal, and particular clinical symptoms to specific areas in the brain.

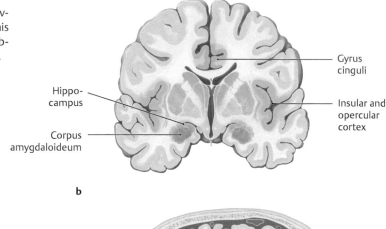

Gyrus cinguli

Hippocampus

Insular and opercular cortex

Corpus amygdaloideum

b

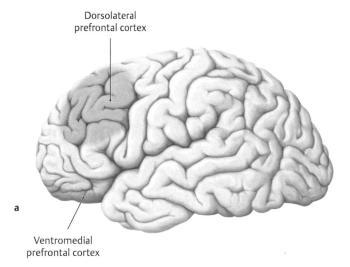

Dorsolateral prefrontal cortex

a

Ventromedial prefrontal cortex

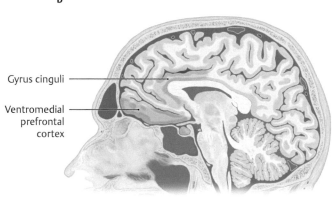

Gyrus cinguli

Ventromedial prefrontal cortex

c

A Neuroanatomy of emotions (after Braus)
a Lateral view of the left hemispherium. **b** Anterior view of a coronal section through the corpus amygdaloideum. **c** Midsagittal section of the right hemispherium, medial aspect.
Emotion is linked to specific regions of the brain. The ventromedial prefrontal cortex is connected primarily to the corpora amygdaloidea and is believed to modulate emotion, while the dorsolateral prefrontal cortex is connected primarily to the hippocampus. This is the area of the cortex in which memories are stored along with their emotional valence. Abnormalities of this network are believed to play a role in depression.

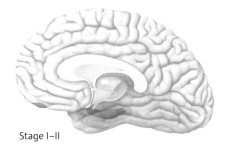

Stage I–II

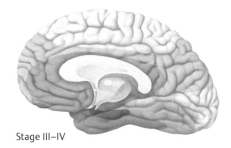

Stage III–IV

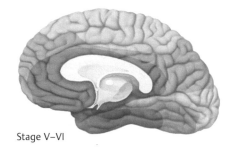

Stage V–VI

B Spread of Alzheimer's disease through the brain
(after Braak and Braak)

Medial view of the right hemispherium. Alzheimer's disease is a relentlessly progressive disease of the cortex cerebri that causes memory loss and, eventually, profound dementia. The progression of the disease can be demonstrated with special staining methods and can be divided into stages using the classification of Braak and Braak:

- Stages I–II: the appearance of the nerve cells is altered in the periphery of the entorhinal cortex (=transentorhinal region), which is considered part of the allocortex (see p. 330). These stages are still asymptomatic.

- Stages III–IV: the lesions have spread to involve the limbic system (also part of the allocortex), and initial clinical symptoms appear. These stages may be detectable by imaging studies in some cases.
- Stages V–VI: the entire isocortex is involved, and the clinical manifestations are fully developed.

Thus, the allocortex is important in brain pathophysiology as the site of origin of Alzheimer's dementia, even though it makes up only 5% of the cortex cerebri.

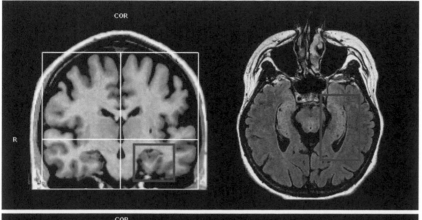

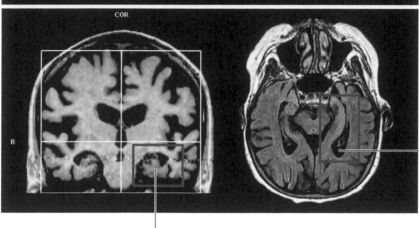

C MRI changes in the hippocampus in a patient with Alzheimer's dementia
Comparing the brain of a healthy subject (**a**) with that of a patient with Alzheimer's dementia (**b**), we notice that the latter shows atrophy of the hippocampus, a brain region that is part of the allocortex. We notice, too, that the ventriculi laterales are enlarged in the patient with Alzheimer dementia (from D. F. Braus: *Ein Blick ins Gehirn*. Thieme, Stuttgart 2004).

Enlarged ventriculus lateralis

Atrophy of the hippocampus

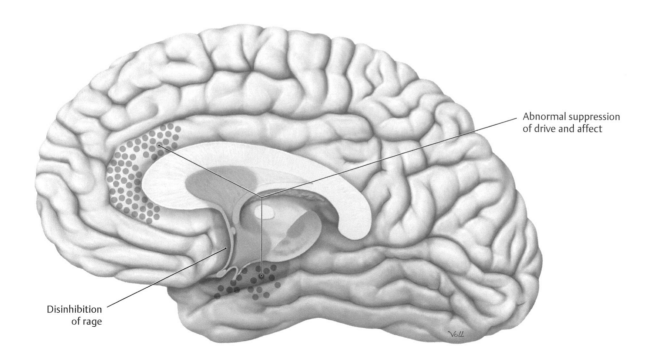

Abnormal suppression of drive and affect

Disinhibition of rage

D Lesions of certain brain areas and associated behavioral changes (after Poeck and Hartje)
Medial view of the right hemispherium. Bilateral lesions of the medial lobus temporalis and the frontal part of the gyrus cinguli (blue dots) lead to a suppression of drive and affect. This structural abnormality in the limbic system produces clinical changes that include apathy, a blank facial expression, monotone speech, and a dull, nonspontaneous mode of behavior. The condition may be caused by tumors, decreased blood flow, or trauma. On the other hand, tumors involving the septum pellucidum and hypothalamus (pink-shaded area) and certain forms of epilepsy may cause a disinhibition of anger, and the patient may respond to seemingly trivial events with attacks of "hypothalamic rage" accompanied by screaming and biting. This outburst is not directed against any particular person or object and persists for some time.

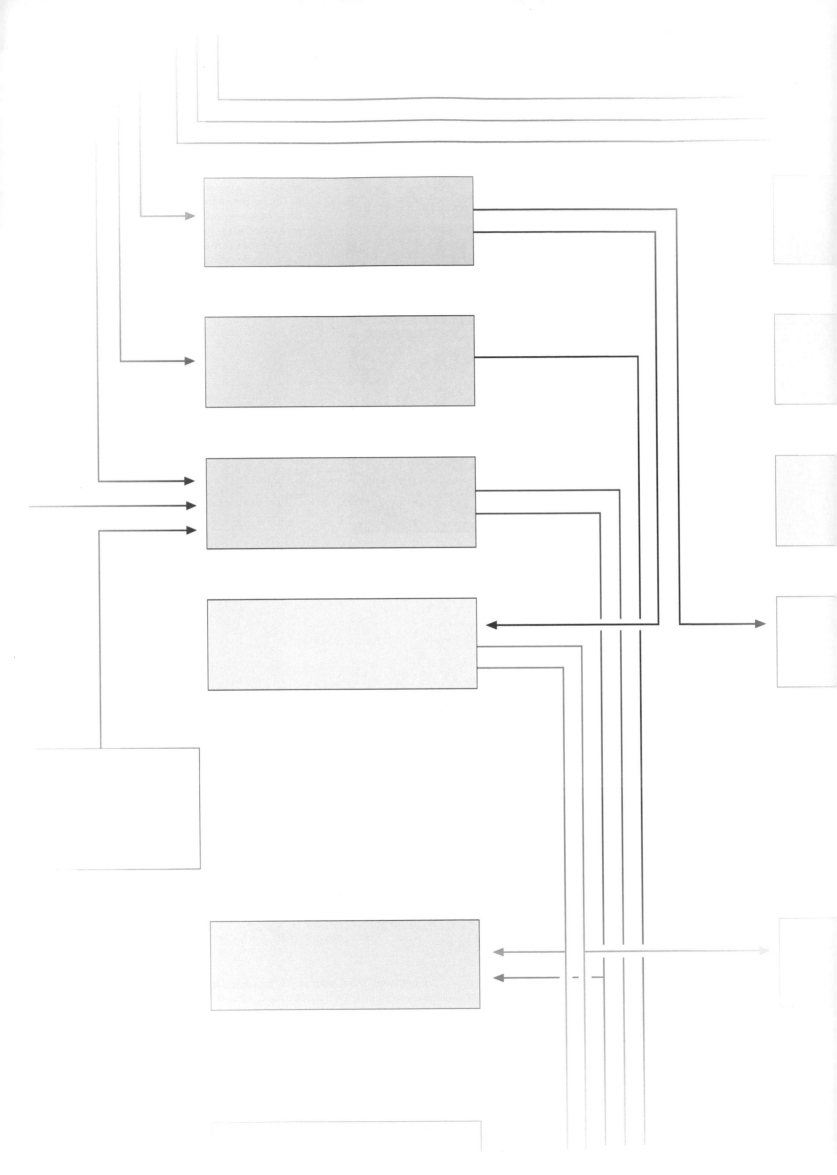

C CNS: Glossary and Synopsis

1.1 Substantia Grisea (Gray Matter)

- **Definition "gray matter"** (substantia grisea):
  collection of neuronal cell bodies (perikarya, somata)

- **Distribution:**
  - in the CNS as cortex and nucleus
  - in the PNS as ganglion (sensory or autonomic)

Substantia grisea in the CNS, morphological terms

Cortex
- *Definition:* layered arrangement of neuronal cell bodies at the outer surface of the CNS and thus visible from outside, in the majority of cases
- *Distribution:*
  - telencephalon (cortex cerebri)
  - cerebellum (cortex cerebelli)

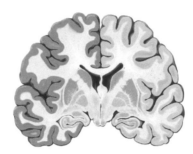

Cortex cerebri

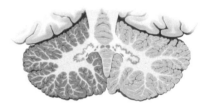

Cortex cerebelli

Nucleus:
- *Definition:* localized collection of neuronal cell bodies within the substantia alba (see p. 494f), thus visible only in sections
- *Distribution:* all parts of the CNS, in the medulla spinalis also in specific morphological arrangements:
  - as columna: term used for three-dimensional representation of the clusters of neuron cell bodies arranged in nuclei or cornu, respectively: term used for two-dimensional representation, thus a cross-section of the columna. On a cross-section, all columns of

substantia grisea give the typical butterfly shape of the medulla spinalis.
  - as formatio reticularis (reticulum = net): net-like arrangement of numerous, very small nuclei, which, based on their small size are morphologically hardly identifiable as nuclei; therefore the substantiae grisea and alba appear "mixed" in a net-like pattern. formatio reticularis also exists in the truncus encephali.

Note: Per definition, nuclei exist only in the CNS, not in the PNS!

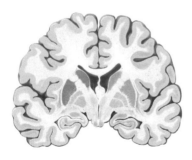

Nuclei in the telencephalon
(nuclei basales or ganglia)

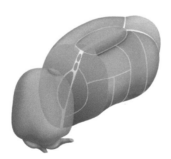

Nucleus in the diencephalon (here: thalamus as collection of nuclei = nuclear area)

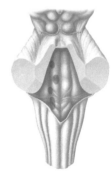

Nuclei in the truncus encephali
(here: some of the nuclei nervorum cranialium)

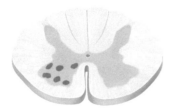

Nuclei in the medulla spinalis

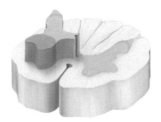

Arranged in columnae
in the medulla spinalis

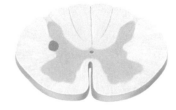

Arrangement resembling a "net"
in the medulla spinalis

Lamina:
- *Definition:* layered arrangement of neurons; microscopically or barely macroscopically visible. In the cerebellum and at the hippocampus, the layers are also referred to as stratum/strata.
- *Distribution:* cortex and nuclei (not in all nuclei!) and medulla spinalis. The laminae in the medulla spinalis are classified cytomorphologically according to Rexed, even if they don't always feature a classical layer pattern.

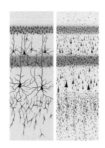

Cortex cerebri
(here: isocortex)

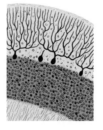

Cortex cerebelli

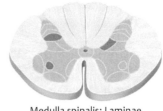

Medulla spinalis: Laminae
according to Rexed

Substantia grisea in the CNS, functional terms: nuclei of origin and terminal nuclei

- **Nucleus of origin [A]:**
  a tract originates from it (originating neuron)

- **Terminal nucleus [B]:**
  at which a fiber tract ends (terminating neuron)

- **Motor nucleus**
  is always the original nucleus, from which a motor fiber emerges.
  Note: Not every nucleus of origin is a motor nucleus!

- **Sensory nucleus**
  is always a terminal nucleus, at which a sensory tract or afferent fibers from nn. craniales or spinales end.
  Note: Not every terminal nucleus is a sensory nucleus!

Substantia grisea in the CNS, terminology aspects

Note: For historical reasons, some nuclei are not called "nucleus" but have proper names. otable examples:

- **Telencephalon**
  - Putamen
  - Globus pallidus
  - Claustrum
- **Diencephalon**
  - Thalamus
  - Zona incerta
- **Midbrain (mesencephalon)**
  - Substantia nigra
- **Truncus encephali**
  - Substantia grisea centralis

Gray matter in the PNS, morphological terms

Ganglion: cluster of neuronal cell bodies in the PNS. Based on their function (see below), ganglia are divided into

- Sensory ganglion (ganglion craniospinale sensorium, somatic nervous system) and

- Autonomic ganglion (ganglion autonomicum, autonomic nervous system).

Note: Per definition, ganglia are found only in the PNS. Thus, the term "basal ganglia" is incorrect. Accurately, they are basal nuclei, which is also expressed in the Latin term "nuclei basales."

Ganglion craniospinale sensorium:
Ganglion of the somatic nervous system, which would be

- Dorsal root ganglion (ganglion sensorium nervi spinalis), on the radix posterior of the n. spinalis in the proximity of the medulla spinalis or as
- Ganglion sensorium nervi cranialis along the course of the sensory component of a n. cranialis.

Note: Synapses are found only in autonomic ganglia, not in sensory ones.

Ganglion autonomicum:
Ganglion of the autonomic nervous system, which could be

- Ganglion sympathicum either paravertebral in the truncus sympathicus or prevertebral (only in abdomen and pelvis);
- Ganglion parasympathicum, which is close to the organs; usually very small.

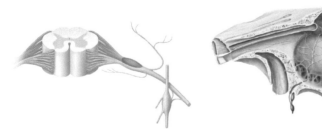

Ganglion sensorium
nervi spinalis

Ganglia sensoria of the
n. glossopharyngeus

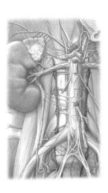

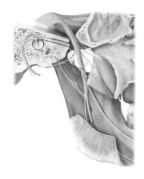

Ganglia sympathica: truncus spinalis
and prevertebral ganglia

Ganglion parasympathicum:
ganglion pterygopalatinum

1.2   Substantia Alba (White Matter)

- **Definition "white matter"** (substantia alba):
  Accumulation of bundled and myelinated neuronal processes, which appear white in the unstained cross-section specimens, because the myelin sheaths mainly consist of lipids

- **Distribution:**
  – in the telencephalon and cerebellum as subcortical substantia alba (located underneath the cortex); it appears morpholog-

ically homogeneous, yet functionally it is divided into microscopically detectable tracts,
  – in the PNS, the substantia alba consists of nerve fibers.

The distinction between the following terms is not always clearly defined and is not consistently used.

Morphological terms

Funiculus (cord)
- Cord-like strand, morphologically loose arrangement of white matter
- Example: Funiculus posterior in the medulla spinalis

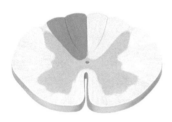

Tractus (tract):
- Group of nerve fibers with a common origin and destination
- Example: tractus spinothalamicus that runs from the medulla spinalis to the thalamus

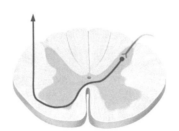

Fasciculus (bundle):
- Morphologicially clearly defined accumulation of neuronal processes; contains at least one, p.r.n. multiple tracts
- Example: Fasciculus cuneatus

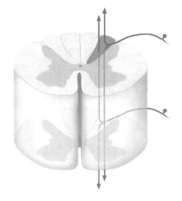

Stria (strand):
- strandlike accumulation of bundles of substantia alba
- Example: corpus striatum (part of the nuclei basales in the telecephalon): rapidly growing, diverging bundles of substantia alba mix with the substantia grisea which gives the corpus striatum its striped appearance

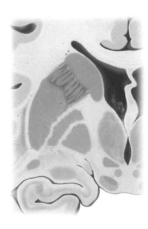

Lemniscus (ribbon):
Historically used term, specifically for four sensory tracts in the truncus encephali, which exhibit a ribbon-like course: lemnisci medialis, lateralis, spinalis and trigeminalis

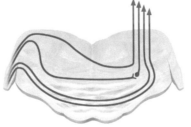

Course:
Everywhere in the CNS, particularly in the medulla spinalis and the truncus encephali, a distinction is made between the ascending (running from caudal to cranial) and descending (running from cranial to caudal) trajectory

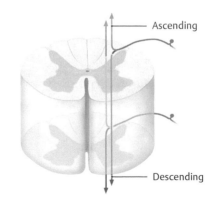

Ascending

Descending

Terminological particularities regarding tracts

Note: For historical reasons, some tracts are not termed "tract" or "fasciculus," but have proper names. Notable examples:

- **In the telencephalon:** capsula interna, externa and extrema; corpus callosum
- **Diencephalon and telencephalon:** fornix (vault)
- **Truncus encephali:** lemniscus (ribbon)

Substantia alba in the CNS, functional terms

Projection fibers (fibrae projectionis):
- Substantia alba bundles, which connect the cortex cerebri (Co = Cortex) with so-called subcortical (sc) structures
- Course: running from the cortex (corticofugal, e.g., tractus pyramidalis) or toward the cortex (corticopetal, e.g., fibrae thalamoparietales)

Note: one fibra projectionis conveys information in only one direction.

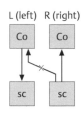

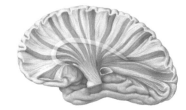

Target neuron ipsi- or contralateral to the originating neurons

Commissure (commissura):
- Tracts that connect similar structures on the left and right side of the CNS
- Example: commissura anterior (cf. p. 540)
- **Commissural fibers (fibrae commissurales):** the fibers that form a commissura

Note: Commissurae always convey information bidirectionally.

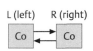

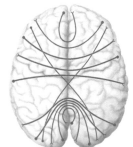

Target neuron contralateral to the originating neuron

Association fibers (fibrae associationis):
- Substantia alba bundles that connect different parts of the same hemispherium cerebri (cf. p. 530)
- Example: fasciculus longitudinalis superior

Note: An association fasciculus usually conveys information bidirectionally.

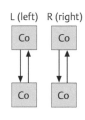

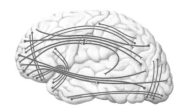

Target neuron ipsilateral to the originating neuron

Decussation (decussatio, crossing):
- Nerve fibers crossing the midline to the opposite side of the CNS
- Connecting different structures
- Example: decussatio pyramidum (crossing of the tractus pyramidales; cf. p. 541)

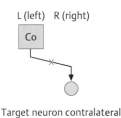

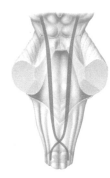

Target neuron contralateral to the originating neuron

Substantia alba in the PNS, functional terms

Afferent fibers (blue): nerve fibers bundled in one nerve, carrying impulses toward the CNS

Efferent fibers (red): nerve fibers bundled in one nerve, carrying impulses away from the CNS

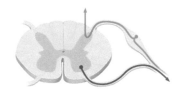

Somatic fibers: Fibers that innervate skeletal mucles and the skin

Autonomic fibers: Fibers that innervate the internal organs (not shown here)

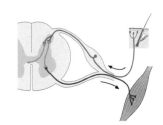

Preganglionic fibers (purple):
- Nerve fibers from the CNS to a ganglion autonomicum
- In the sympathetic nervous system as r. communicans albus to the paravertebral ganglion (ganglia sympathica) or as thoracic or lumbar n. splanchnicus to the prevertebral ganglion
- In the parasympathetic nervous sytem in the composition of certain nn. craniales or as pelvic nn. splanchnici

Postganglionic fibers (green):
- Nerve fibers from the ganglion autonomicum to the target organ
- In the sympathetic nervous system as r. communicans griseus to the n. spinalis or as autonomic plexus to the target organ

Autonomic plexus:
- Network of autonomic fibers
- Example: plexus hypogastricus inferior

Visceral plexus (plexus visceralis):
- Specific part of an autonomic plexus, directly at the organ
- Example: plexus rectalis inferior

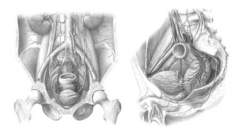

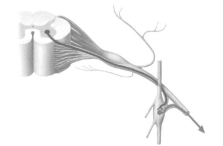

1.3 Sensory and Motor Functions; Overview of the Medulla Spinalis and Tracts in the Medulla Spinalis

A Sensory and motor functions in the CNS and PNS: General terminology

Sensory functions of the CNS and PNS	Motor functions of the CNS and PNS
Somatosensation:	**Somatomotor:**
• General somatosensation: including the following:	The Innervation of striated muscles of the trunk, limbs, neck and extraocular muscles is provided by the somatomotor component of the corresponding nn. spinales and craniales.
– *Exteroception* (external perception, or superficial sensation): transmission of impulses from the skin – *Proprioception* (self-perception, or deep sensation), transmission of impulses from muscle spindles and stretch receptors in tendons and articular capsules (via the sensory components of the nn. craniales and spinales)	
• Based on the type of sensation, exteroception is further divided into	
– *Epicritic sensation* (fine touch, vibration; two-point discrimination and pressure) and – *Protopathic sensation* (diffuse touch and pressure; temperature and pain).	
• Special somatosensation: Processing of impulses from the retina (vision) and inner ear (hearing; acceleration) via the n. opticus and n. vestibulocochlearis respectively	
Visceral sensation:	**Visceromotor** (innervation of the "internal organs"):
• General visceral sensation: Transmission of impulses from the internal organs and blood vessels (e.g., wall tension, blood pressure, oxygen saturation); via afferent autonomic fibers, (especially sympathetic fibers), mainly via the nn. splanchnici, but also via the nn. craniales IX and X;	• General visceromotor Innervation of the smooth muscles of the organs (viscera) and the blood vessels as well as glands and the heart. It is conveyed through the vegetative nervous system via parasympathetic and sympathetic nerve fibers, which partly run with nn. spinales or craniales (in case of the latter only parasympathetic) and partly independently (e.g., as nn. splanchnici).
• Special visceral sensation: Transmission of impulses from the gemmae gustatoriae (via the nn. craniales VII, IX and X) and the olfactory mucosa (via the nn., bulbi and tractus olfactorii).	• Special visceromotor Embryology concept. They supply the striate muscles innervated by the nerves of arcus pharyngei: mastication (V_3); facial expression (VII); pharynx and larynx (IX and X) as well as craniofugal muscles (XI). (From a phylogenetic perspective, it refers to somatomotor innervation of muscles that were "visceral muscles" in fish).
Note: The perikarya of the pseudounipolar neurons, which convey visceral sensation, are located in the ganglia sensoria nervorum spinalium or cranialium (e.g., n. vagus).	

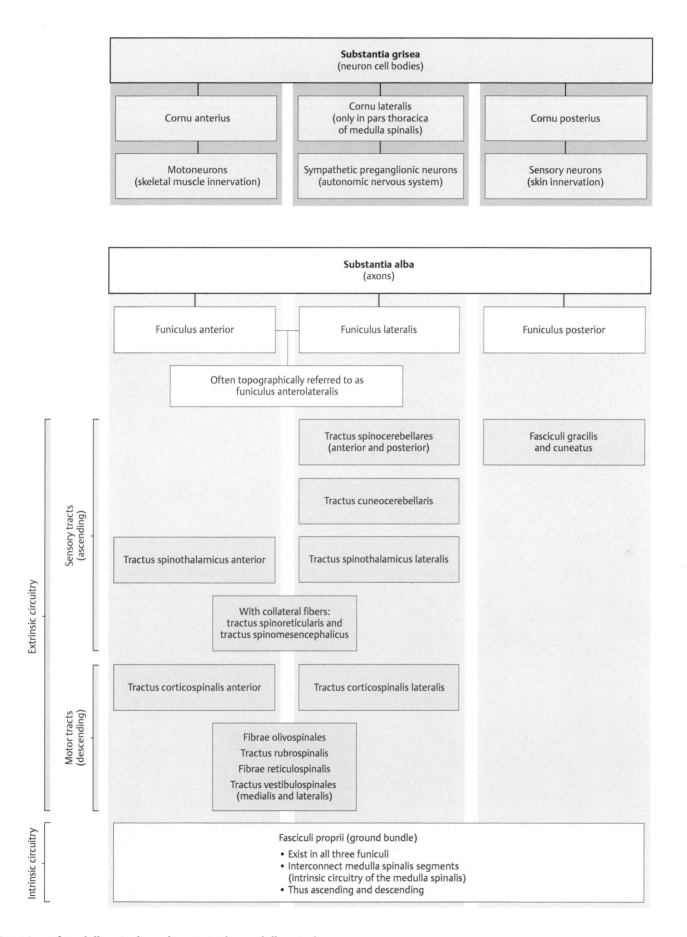

B Overview of medulla spinalis and tracts in the medulla spinalis
Note: In the truncus encephali, the tractus spinothalamici are known as
the lemniscus spinalis, while the fasciculi gracilis and cuneatus continue
with the lemniscus medialis, see p. 508 f.

2.1 Sensory Tracts of the Medulla Spinalis

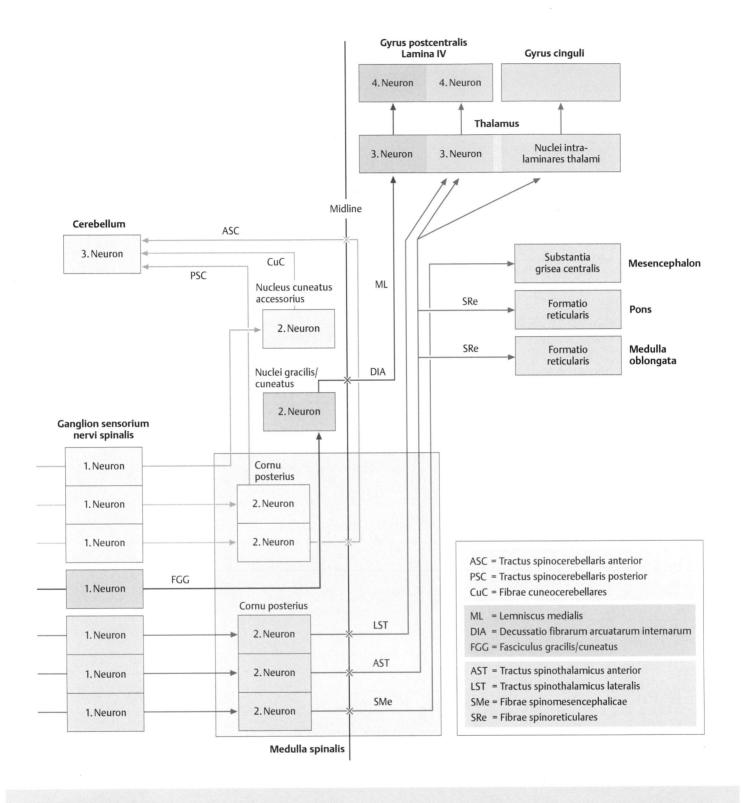

Definition and function

The sensory tracts in the medulla spinalis carry all somatosensory modalities related to the trunk, neck, and limbs to the cerebellum or to the telencephalon. Since they share very important features, they are presented together in this chapter. The clearest classification of the tracts is the one based on the type of information they transmit:

- The type of sensation that can be perceived consciously reaches the telencephalon via the thalamus (spinocortical) and is transmitted through a four-neuron chain.

- The type of sensation that is unconscious ascends to the cerebellum (spinocerebellar) without thalamic involvement and is transmitted through a three-neuron chain.

Note: Pathways to the telencephalon always cross; pathways to the cerebellum terminate on the same side with the point of origin. Even the tractus spinocerebellaris anterior eventually ends ipsilaterally, albeit crossing first.

Qualities of somatosensation

- Exteroception (conscious external sensation through the skin):
  - epicritic sensation is carried in the *fasciculi gracilis* and *cuneatus* (dorsal column)
  - protopathic sensation is carried in the tractus spinothalamici *anterior* and *lateralis*; important collaterals exist for this tract (see below).
- Proprioception (largely unconscious), the responsible tracts run to the cerebellum as

- *tractus spinocerebellares anterior* and *posterior* (responsible for the lower part of the body and lower limb) and
- *fibrae cuneocerebellares* (responsible for the upper part of the body and upper limb, see below).
- A small part of proprioception happens consciously and the input is carried by the *fasciculi gracilis* and *cuneatus* (thus fasciculi gracilis/cuneatus carry extero- and proprioceptive information).

Neural wiring and topography of tracts

4 (spinocortical) or 3 (spinocerebellar) consecutive neurons. For all tracts, the first neuron is located in the ganglion sensorium nervi spinalis. For the tracts ascending to the telencephalon, the third and sometimes the fourth neuron have the same location.

First neuron:
Pseudounipolar neuron in the ganglion sensorium nervi spinalis: Its peripheral process receives the information from a receptor (for pain transmission, the receptor is the ending of the neuronal process itself) and the axon (central process) carries it with via the radix posterior of the n. spinalis to the medulla spinalis.

Second neuron:
- *Fasciculi gracilis* and *cuneatus* consist of axons of the first neurons. They end in the ipsilateral nuclei gracilis and cuneatus respectively (in the medulla oblongata) where the bodies of the second neurons are located. After crossing the midline immediately rostral to the nuclei (at the decussatio lemnisci medialis), the axons of the second neurons form the lemniscus medialis, thus reaching the third neuron in the contralateral thalamus.
- *Tractus spinothalamici anterior* and *lateralis:* The second neurons' cell bodies are in the ispilateral cornu posterius of the medulla spinalis. The axons of the second neurons cross the midline and ascend in the contralateral tractus anterolaterales to the thalamus. In the truncus encephali, the axons of the second neurons are refferred to as the lemniscus spinalis. Axons of the second neurons can also ascend to the formatio reticularis (*fibrae spinoreticulares*) or to the mesencephalon (*fibrae spinomesencephalicae*) for the subcortical processing of painful stimuli (e.g., reacting to painful stimuli);
- *Tractus spinocerebellares anterior* and *posterior:* The cell bodies of the second neurons that form the tractus spinocerebellaris posterior are located at the base of the *ipsilateral cornu posterius* in the nucleus thoracicus posterior. These axons remain uncrossed and travel in the funiculus lateralis of the medulla spinalis to the ipsilateral truncus encephali. The cell bodies of the second neurons that form the tractus spinocerebellaris anterior are located in the middle of the ipsilateral cornu posterius. Their axons run in the funiculus lateralis either crossed (at the commissura alba anterior) or uncrossed and reach the truncus encephali. The axons of the tractus spinocerebellaris posterior travel via the pedunculus cerebellaris inferior to the ipsilateral cerebellum.
Note: Collaterals of the tractus spinocerebellaris posterior

reach to a truncus encephali nucleus ("Nucleus Z"; adjacent to nucleus gracilis), which further projects via the lemniscus medialis to the thalamus (VPL nucleus), which in turn projects to the gyrus postcentralis (ensuring conscious propriocepion of the lower part of the body, not shown here). The axons of the tractus spinocerebellaris anterior reach the mesencephalon and then the cerebellum through the pedunculus cerebellaris superior. The fibers in this tract that crossed in the medulla spinalis, cross back to their original side.
- *Fibrae cuneocerebellares:* The second neurons are located in the nucleus cuneatus accessorius, which is immediately next to the nucleus cuneatus of the medulla oblongata. The axons of the second neurons travel uncrossed through the ipsilateral pedunculus cerebellaris inferior to the cerebellum. Similar to tractus spinocerebellaris posterior, collaterals from the fibrae cuneocerebellares project to the thalamus, which in turn projects to the telencephalon (ensuring conscious proprioception for the upper body).

Third neuron:
- *Fasciculi gracilis/cuneatus* and tractus spinothalamicus *anterior/lateralis:* The body of the third neuron is located in the nucleus ventralis posterolateralis (VPL) of the thalamus. Their axons travel to the cortex cerebri (to the fourth neurons) in the radiationes thalamicae in the crus posterius of the capsula interna.
- *Only for the tractus spinothalamici:* Bodies of third neurons are also located in the nuclei intralaminares thalami, which project to the gyrus cinguli (limbic system; emotional meaning of pain).
- *Tractus spinocerebellares* and *fibrae cuneocerebellares:* The bodies of the third neurons are located in the cerebellum, either in the nuclei cerebelli (mainly the nuclei emboliformis and globosus) or as granule cells in the cortex of the spinocerebellum (in the lobus cerebelli anterior, vermis, paramedial zone) that synapse with mossy fibers.

Fourth neuron:
- *Fasciculi gracilis/cuneatus* and *tractus spinothalamici:* The body of fourth neurons are located in the lamina granularis interna (layer IV) of the gyrus postcentralis. In case of the spinothalamic pathway, bodies of fourth neurons are also located in the gyrus cinguli.
- Tracts running to the cerebellum don't have a fourth neuron.

Somatotopic organization of tracts

Fibers corresponding to the sacral spinal segments are located medial or dorsal, while those corresponding to the cervical segments are positioned lateral or ventral.

Symptoms

- Dysfunction of fasciculus gracilis leads to impaired epicritic perception (e.g., numbness of skin).
- Dysfunction of the tractus spinothalamici leads to impaired perception of pain and temperature.

- Dysfunction of tractus spinocerebellares leads to gross motor functional and gait impairment (sensory ataxia).

2.2   Motor Tracts of the Medulla Spinalis

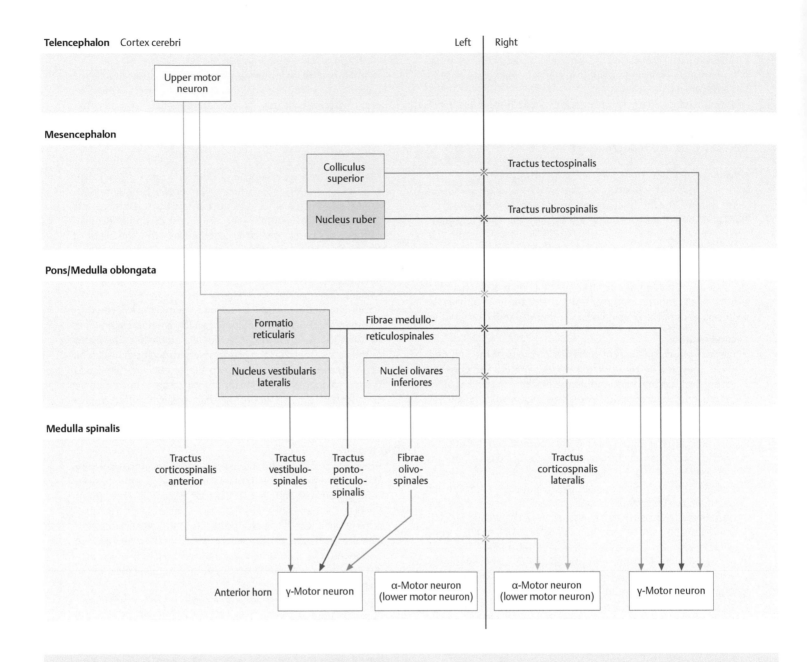

Definition and function

Motor tracts of the medulla spinalis can de divided into two groups:

- Pyramidal fibers (passing through the pyramis in the medulla oblongata)
- Extrapyramidal fibers (don't run in caudal direction in the pyramis, but in the tegmentum)

Pyramidal fibers originate in the cortex cerebri; extrapyramidal tracts originate in nuclei of the truncus encephali. A rough classification based on their functions, which is still used in the clinic, is analogous to the tracts, as one refers to pyramidal and extrapyramidal motor functions. However, physiologically, both systems work closely together.

Pyramidal fibers in the medulla spinalis (tractus corticospinales anterior and lateralis)

Definition and function:
- Major motor tract (voluntary motor function, conscious movement control of neck, trunk and limbs)
- The part of the *tractus pyramidalis*, which extends from the primary motor cortex to the medulla spinalis. Only when it reaches the medulla spinalis, is it called *tractus corticospinales*;

before entering the medulla spinalis, the fibers of this descending tract are usually referred to as *fibrae corticospinales*. Like the other fibers of the tractus pyramidalis (fibrae corticonucleares bulbi to the nuclei nervorum cranialium and fibrae corticoreticulares to the formatio reticularis), they include axons of the large pyramidal cells.

Pathway characteristics:
Somatomotor; descending; efferent.
Note: Per definition, the fibrae corticonucleares and corticoreticulares should not be referred to as part of the tractus pyramidalis, since they end above the pyramis which means they don't pass through it. On functional grounds, they are considered in the same category as the fibrae corticospinales and based on their neurons of origin, they are usually considered part of the "pyramidal fibers."

Neural wiring and topography of the tract (fibrae corticospinales): total of two neurons:

Upper motor neuron:
Large pyramidal cells in the lamina pyramidalis interna (layer V) of the gyrus precentralis (primary motor cortex); 40% of which are located in the Brodmann area 4; the remaining 60% are located in neighboring brain regions.

Course of the axons of the upper motor neurons: On their descending way from the telencephalon, to the decussatio pyramidum the *fibrae corticospinales* travel through the

• Primary motor cortex → crus posterius of the capsula interna, → pedunculi cerebri of the mesencephalon → pars basilaris pontis (basal pons) → pyramis medullae oblongatae

• At the decussatio pyramidum (thus above the medulla spinalis), 80% of fibers cross to the opposite side. From there

– The uncrossed 20% run ipsilaterally in the medulla spinalis as the tractus corticospinalis anterior; they cross in the commissura alba anterior only at the level of the spinal segment where those fibers end. This component of the tract ends at about the middle of the thoracic region.
– The crossed fibers run contralaterally in the medulla spinalis as the tractus corticospinalis lateralis (all medulla spinalis segments contain a portion of this tract).

Lower motor neuron:
α- or γ-motor neurons in the cornu anterius of the medulla spinalis, largely in the laminae A-C after Rexed, on which the axons of the tractus corticospinalis terminate. The axon terminals form excitatory synapses. Axons of the lower motor neuron end on target organs, in this case striate muscles. The neurotransmitter is acetylcholine.
Note: The tractus corticospinalis ends on the lower motor neuron. The axons of the lower motor neurons form the somatomotor fibers in the composition of the n. spinalis.

Extrapyramidal fibers in the medulla spinalis

Definition and function:
Major motor pathways (mainly for fine movement control).

Pathway characteristics:
Somatomotor; descending; efferent.
The extrapyramidal pathways originate as upper motor neurons in nuclei trunci encephali and the premotor cortex, end mostly on γ-motor neurons in the medulla spinalis (as lower motor neurons), and are usually collectively called "extrapyramidal motor" pathways. They are responsible for fine-tuning motor function and subcortical preparation of a cortically initiated movement. Topographically, they run in the funiculus anterior or lateralis.

Major extrapyramidal pathways are as follows:
• Tractus vestibulospinalis lateralis/medialis: originate in the nuclei vestibulares.

• Fibrae olivospinales: originates in the nuclei olivares inferiores.
• Tractus pontoreticulospinalis and bulboreticulospinalis: originate in the formatio reticularis nuclei of the pons and medulla oblongata respectively
• Tractus rubrospinalis: originates in the nucleus ruber.
• Tractus tectospinalis: originates in colliculus superior of the tectum mesencephali. This tract is detectable only in the pars cervicalis.

Extrapyramidal pathways largely cross (either completely or partially). Only the tractus vestibulospinalis lateralis has not been verified to cross.

Somatotopic organization of the tractus corticospinales anterior and lateralis
(not known for extrapyramidal pathways in humans)

• In the crus posterius of the capsula interna: cervical fibers rostral; sacral fibers occipital
• In the pedunculi cerebri (mesencephalon): cervical fibers medial; sacral fibers lateral

• In the medulla spinalis: cervical fibers medial; sacral fibers lateral

---

Symptoms

Dysfunction of the tractus corticospinales leads to impaired voluntary movement of the neck, trunk, and limbs. Depending on the extent of the damage, it can result in paresis (loss of crude voluntary movement) or plegia (complete paralysis) of muscles or muscle groups. Since damage of the fibrae corticospinales or tractus corticospinales as a result of the mechanism of injury (e.g., impairment of blood flow in the truncus encephali; medulla spinalis transection) usually also affects the extrapyramidal pathways

which exert an inhibitory influence on medulla spinalis excitation, the paralysis (dysfunction of the tractus corticospinalis) is accompanied by spasticity (increased muscle tone, increased reflexes).
Note: Damage to the upper motor neuron of the tractus pyramidalis leads to spastic paralysis. Damage to the lower motor neuron leads to flaccid paralysis (same as in the loss of motor fibers in a peripheral nerve).

511

2.3 Sensory Trigeminal Pathway

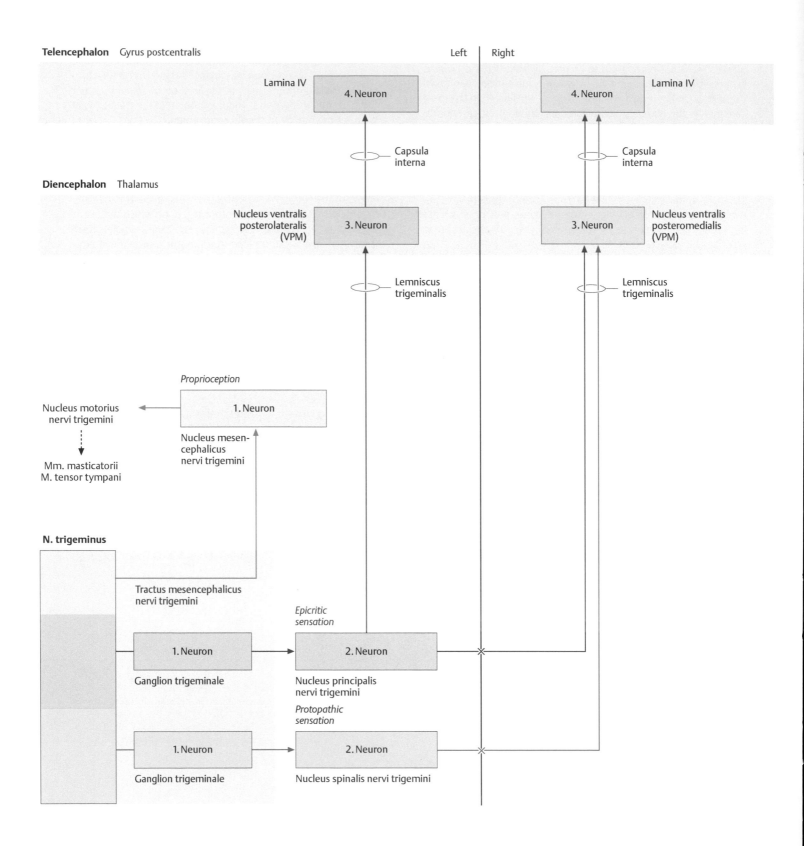

Definition and function

Major pathway of superficial sensation and (partially conscious) deep sensation.

- Superficial sensation (exteroception): information received from specific receptors on the skin surface and mucous membranes is carried to the telencephalon for conscious perception of

  - light touch, two-point discrimination and vibration (epicritic perception) as well as

  - crude touch and pressure, pain and temperature (protopathic perception). In addition to the skin surface and mucosae, pain receptors are also found in the meninges.

- Deep sensation (proprioception); information from receptors of muscles, tendons, and articular capsules located within the skull is carried to the telencephalon for conscious perception (and also unconscious perception) of increased muscle tension (proprioceptive perception).

Pathway characteristics

Somatosensory, ascending; afferent.
Note: All information concerning superficial and deep sensation from the head is transmitted via one single sensory trigeminal pathway. For the trunk and limbs, however, the respective information is conducted via two pathways: anterolateral system (protopathy, thus pain and temperatue) and posterior column (epicritic, conscious proprioception).

Neural wiring and topography of the tract

A total of 4 serially connected neurons:

- **First neuron:** Pseudounipolar cell in the ganglion trigeminale located in the fossa cranii media. It receives the stimulus via its peripheral process and carries it to the truncus encephali via the central process (that enters the pons) to the ipsilateral second neuron in the nuclei trigeminales.
  Note: The first neuron for the quality of "proprioception" is not located in the ganglion trigeminale but in nucleus mesencephalicus nervi trigemini. The nucleus mesencephalicus is per definition a ganglion trigeminale which is positioned in the CNS and consists of pseudounipolar cells.

- **Second neuron:** For the epicritic sensation nucleus principalis nervi trigemini (located in the pons); for the protopathic sensation in the nucleus spinalis nervi trigemini (located in the medulla oblongata and extending into the medulla spinalis). The axons of the second neurons ascend as part of the tractus trigeminothalamicus to the thalamus. These fibers are called the lemniscus trigeminalis and join the lemniscus medialis.

Note: The axons of the second neuron of the nucleus principalis travel both uncrossed and crossed to the thalamus; those of the nucleus spinalis travel crossed. The stimuli about epicritic sensation through the n. trigeminus reach both contraand ipsilateral gyri postcentrales.

- **Third neuron:** In the nucleus ventralis posteromedialis (VPM) of the ipsi- and contralateral thalamus. From there, the axons of the third neurons travel in the radiationes thalami in the crus posterius of the capsula interna to the fourth neuron.

- **Fourth neuron:** In the telencephalon in the lamina granularis interna (layer IV) of the gyrus postcentralis.

Note: The n. trigeminus also has a nucleus motorius that provides its motor component for the mm. masticatorii and the m. tensor tympani in the auris media. However, the cortical control of this motor nucleus is an exception which is why it is not discussed here but as part of the "control of the motor nuclei of nn. craniales," see p. 520 f.

Somotopic organization of the pathway

The fibers of the fourth neuron end in the gyrus postcentralis in the area which begins superior to the sulcus centralis and extends toward the parietal cortex to the middle of the gyrus postcentralis.

Symptoms

A dysfunction of the sensory trigeminal pathway (e.g., as a result of vascular disorders, cranial fractures or tumors) leads to impaired conscious perception of crude and light pressure, crude and light touch, pain, temperature and proprioception.
Note: Due to the (partial) crossing of the tract in the truncus encephali

- A lesion of the tract from the n. trigeminus all the way to the second neuron leads to ipsilateral loss of sensation;

- A lesion of the tract from the thalamus to the gyrus postcentralis leads to

  - contralateral disorder for the entirely contralateral projection of protopathic sensation
  - ipsi- and contralateral dysfunction in terms of epicritic sensation but usually not a complete loss due to the representation on the gyrus postcentralis on both sides

2.4 Auditory Pathway

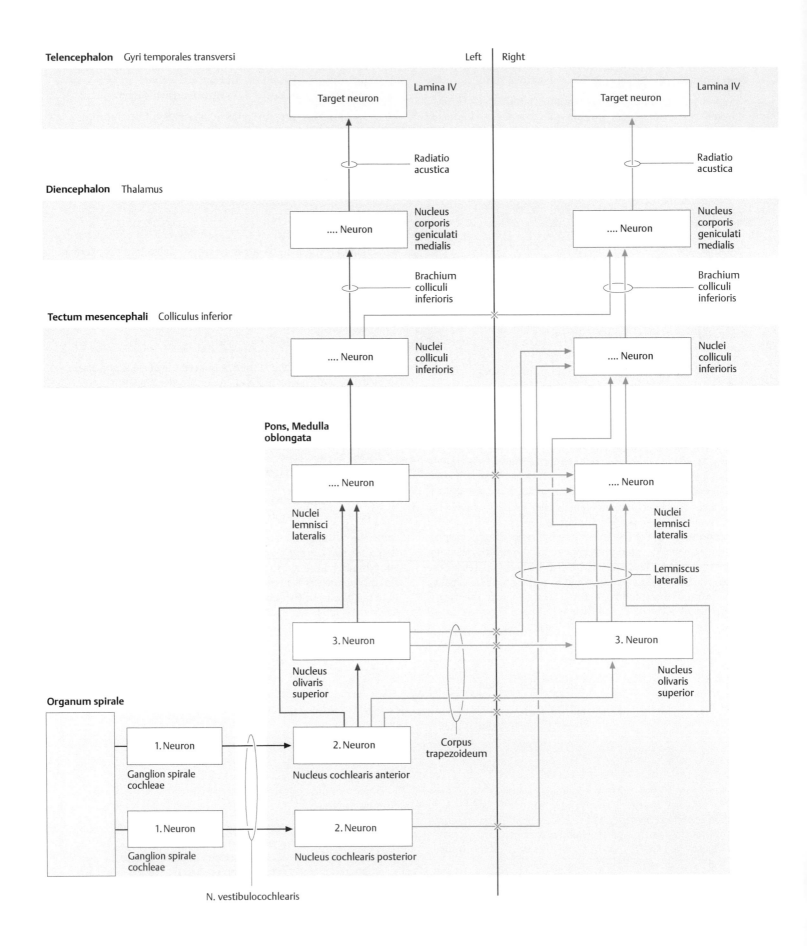

Telencephalon   Gyri temporales transversi

Left | Right

Target neuron   Lamina IV

Target neuron   Lamina IV

Radiatio
acustica

Radiatio
acustica

Diencephalon   Thalamus

.... Neuron   Nucleus
corporis
geniculati
medialis

.... Neuron   Nucleus
corporis
geniculati
medialis

Brachium
colliculi
inferioris

Brachium
colliculi
inferioris

Tectum mesencephali   Colliculus inferior

.... Neuron   Nuclei
colliculi
inferioris

.... Neuron   Nuclei
colliculi
inferioris

Pons, Medulla
oblongata

.... Neuron

.... Neuron

Nuclei
lemnisci
lateralis

Nuclei
lemnisci
lateralis

Lemniscus
lateralis

3. Neuron

3. Neuron

Nucleus
olivaris
superior

Nucleus
olivaris
superior

Organum spirale

1. Neuron

2. Neuron

Corpus
trapezoideum

Ganglion spirale
cochleae

Nucleus cochlearis anterior

1. Neuron

2. Neuron

Ganglion spirale
cochleae

Nucleus cochlearis posterior

N. vestibulocochlearis

Definition and function

Pathway for the perception of acoustic stimuli including information about the amplitude, frequency and spatial location of a sound.

Characteristics of pathway

(special) somatosensory (sensory); afferent.
Note: The information is processed by a sensory organ (organum spirale) in the cochlea (in the os temporale), which contains specialized sensory cells (hair cells). The mechanic stimulation of these cells result in impulses that are transmitted via the n. cochlearis part of the n. vestibulocochlearis (VIII).

Neural wiring and topography of the pathway

A total of at least six serially connected neurons:

- **First neuron:** Bipolar neuron in the ganglion spirale cochleae). It receives the information from the receptor cells (inner hair cell in the organum spirale). The axon travels via the n. cranialis VIII and enters the truncus encephali at the angulus pontocerebellaris.
- **Second neuron:** Is located in the ipsilateral nucleus cochlearis anterior/or posterior of the truncus encephali, in the floor of the ventriculus quartus close to the recessus lateralis. Axons of the second neurons travel crossed and uncrossed to the third neuron. All ascending fibers that leave the nuclei cochlearis are collectively called lemniscus lateralis.
- **Third neuron:** Nucleus olivaris superior (axons of the second neuron predominantly originate in the nucleus cochlearis anterior). From the nucleus olivaris superior and the nucleus cochlearis anterior, fibers travel to the opposite side. When crossing over, they can (but not necessarily have to) terminate in a small nuclear group (not shown) called nuclei corporis trapezoidei. All of these small nuclei together with the crossing fibers are collectively called the corpus trapezoideum.

Note: One characteristic of the auditory pathway is that the successive stations of this neuronal circuit are not always followed by all parts of the tract. Groups of axons can bypass individual neural relay stations shown here. Only first (in the ganglion cochleare) second (in the nuclei cochleares) and last (cortical neuron; see target neuron) are constant stations of this neuronal circuit. Thus, a strict neuron enumeration after the third neuron of this particular pathway is no longer useful.

- **Additional stations of the neuronal circuit:**
  - Nuclei of the lemniscus lateralis (receive input from both nuclei cochleares)
  - Nucleus of the colliculus inferior (in the colliculus inferior of the mesencephalon); from here, axons travel to the thalamus via the brachium colliculi inferioris.
  - Nucleus corporis geniculati medialis (in the corpus geniculatum mediale of the metathalamus). From here, axons travel as radiatio acustica to the primary auditory cortex.

- **Target neuron:** Primary auditory cortex, lamina granularis interna (layer IV) in the gyri temporales transversi (Heschl's gyri), Brodmann area 41

Note: The pattern of crossing of axons of the the second neuron and the following neurons of the pathway leads to the primary auditory cortex receiving information from both cochlear organs, which substantially contributes to the auditory spatial perception.

Somatotopic (= in this case tonotopic) organization of pathway

The tonotopic organization of the auditory cortex adapts to the structure of Heschl's gyri. In the primary auditory cortex, high frequencies are rather located near the occipital bone, and low frequencies rather frontally.

Symptoms

Unilateral damage to the auditory pathway proximal to the nuclei cochleares leads to impaired auditory spatial perception. Bilateral damage leads to deafness.

2.5 Gustatory Pathway

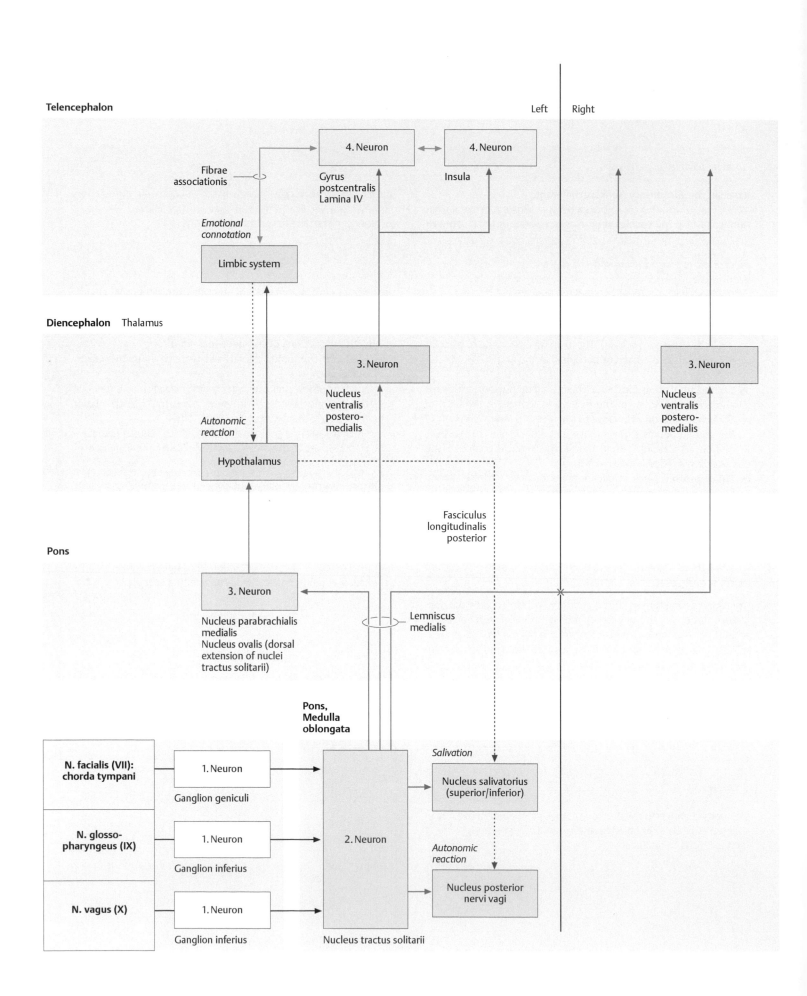

Telencephalon

Left | Right

4. Neuron — Gyrus postcentralis Lamina IV

4. Neuron — Insula

Fibrae associationis

Emotional connotation

Limbic system

Diencephalon Thalamus

3. Neuron
Nucleus ventralis postero-medialis

3. Neuron
Nucleus ventralis postero-medialis

Autonomic reaction

Hypothalamus

Fasciculus longitudinalis posterior

Pons

3. Neuron
Nucleus parabrachialis medialis
Nucleus ovalis (dorsal extension of nuclei tractus solitarii)

Lemniscus medialis

Pons, Medulla oblongata

N. facialis (VII): chorda tympani

1. Neuron
Ganglion geniculi

Salivation

Nucleus salivatorius (superior/inferior)

N. glosso-pharyngeus (IX)

1. Neuron
Ganglion inferius

2. Neuron

Autonomic reaction

N. vagus (X)

1. Neuron
Ganglion inferius

Nucleus posterior nervi vagi

Nucleus tractus solitarii

Definition and function

Pathway for the conscious taste sensation from the tongue (sensation of sweet, sour, salty, bitter, umami)

Characteristics of pathway

(special) viscerosensory (sensory); afferent.
Note: Taste information is conveyed via three nn. craniales: n. facialis (VII), n. glossopharyngeus (IX) and n. vagus (X). They all pick up signals from taste receptors on the tongue surface and carry them first to a common, centrally located nucleus, the nucleus tractus solitarii. This pathway ends in two different cortical locations: insula and gyrus postcentralis.

Neural wiring and topography of the pathway

- **First neuron:** Pseudounipolar neuron with the body in the ganglion of the corresponding n. cranialis. Its peripheral process receives the information from a taste receptor. The central process of the pseudounipolar neuron with the body in the n. cranialis ganglion ascends ipsilaterally to the truncus encephali where it synapses with the second neuron in the nucleus tractus solitarii.
  Note: The afferent fibers of the n. facialis initially run with the n. lingualis, then with the chorda tympani before joining the n. facialis in the canalis nervi facialis of the os temporale and traveling as part of the n. facialis to the truncus encephali.
- **Second neuron:** In the medulla oblongata ipsilateral in the nucleus tractus solitarii (pars gustatoria). The axons of the second neurons ascend uncrossed to the pons (where they terminate on third neurons) or bypass the nuclei pontis and directly join the ipsilateral lemniscus medialis (and apparently to a lesser degree the contralateral one) on the way to the thalamus (where the third neurons are located in this case).
- **Third neuron:**
  - in the pons: in a pontine nuclear group close to the recessus lateralis of the ventriculus quartus: nucleus parabrachialis and nucleus ovalis. From there, the pathway ascends uncrossed to the hypothalamus and further to parts of the limbic system.
  - in the thalamus: located in the nucleus ventralis posteromedialis. From there, fibers of the radiatio thalamica ascend in the crus posterius of the capsula interna.

- **Fourth neuron** in the gyrus postcentralis (lamina granularis interna [IV]) or the insular cortex.

Note: Thus, the gustatory pathway ends on two cortical regions, where apparently different type of information is processed. Collaterals of the nucleus parabrachialis and oval nucleus reach the hypothalamus (autonomic reaction) and areas of the limbic system (gustatory sensation and their emotional connotations). From the second neuron, the collaterals ascend to the nucleus salivatorius (reflex of salivation). Via the fasciculus longitudinalis posterior (PLF), the hypothalamus can control autonomic reactions by influencing the autonomic nuclei of the truncus encephali.

Somatopic organization of pathway

Not known.

Clinical correlations

A dysfunction of the gustatory pathway leads to a loss of taste sensation (ageusia). It is extremely rare, since a bilateral peripheral lesion of the nn. craniales VII, IX, and X is highly unlikely and a central lesion, in the truncus encephali for instance, would affect so many other structures that the clinical presentation would be dominated by more severe manifestations.

2.6 Olfactory Pathway

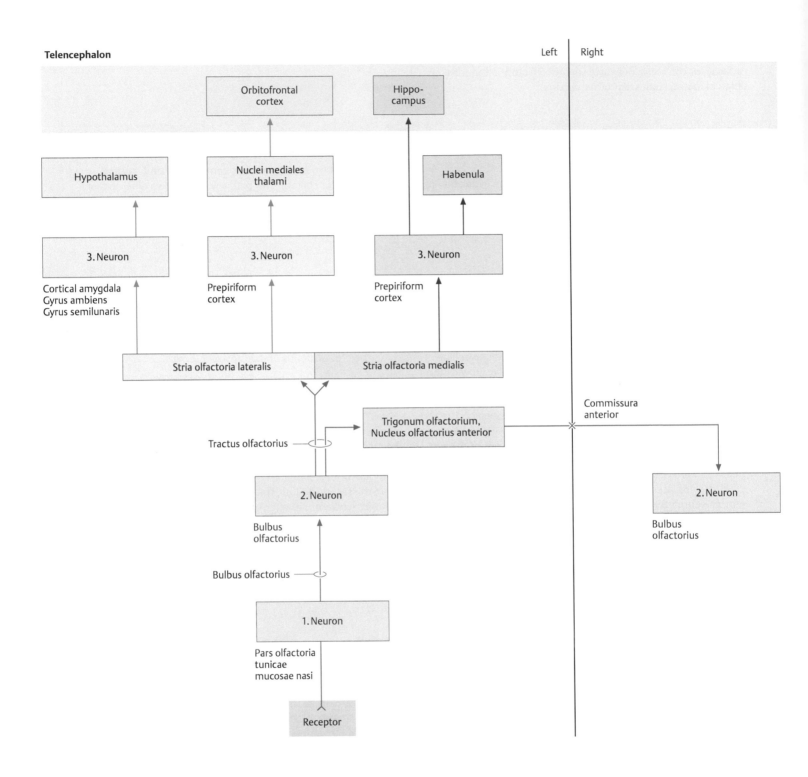

Telencephalon

Left | Right

Orbitofrontal cortex

Hippo-campus

Hypothalamus

Nuclei mediales thalami

Habenula

3. Neuron

3. Neuron

3. Neuron

Cortical amygdala
Gyrus ambiens
Gyrus semilunaris

Prepiriform cortex

Prepiriform cortex

Stria olfactoria lateralis | Stria olfactoria medialis

Commissura anterior

Tractus olfactorius

Trigonum olfactorium,
Nucleus olfactorius anterior

2. Neuron

2. Neuron

Bulbus olfactorius

Bulbus olfactorius

Bulbus olfactorius

1. Neuron

Pars olfactoria tunicae mucosae nasi

Receptor

Definition and function

Pathway of conscious sensation of the olfactory system for the perception of olfactory stimuli.

Characteristics of pathway

(special) viscerosensory (sensory); afferent.

Note: Part of the olfactory pathway is represented by the first n. cranialis (n. olfactorius). The n. olfactorius, however, is not a true cranial nerve but, per definition, an extension segment of the telencephalic cortex (in this case paleocortex), that is the CNS:

- Therefore, it is surrounded by meninges,
- it is bathed in liquor cerebrospinalis,

- the axons of the neurons contained in them are surrounded by neuroglia systematis nervosi centralis (oligodendrocytes).

The n. olfactorius on the other hand does not represent a coherent structure but consists of the sum of the numerous individual fila olfactoria. The fila olfactoria are the axons of the primary sensory cells (receptor cells) of the epithelium olfactorium. The n. olfactorius is by definition a component of the peripheral nervous system.

Neural wiring and topography of the pathway

A total of 3 serially connected neurons:

- **First neuron:** lies as receptor cell (primary sensory cell) in the roof of the cavitates nasi. The peripheral process has at its end a receptor located in the tunica mucosa nasi. The central process (part of fila olfactoria) passes thorough the lamina cribrosa of the os ethmoidale to reach the second neuron.
- **Second neuron:** in the bulbus olfactorius, located on the os ethmoidale, in the fossa cranii anterior. There are two types of second-order neurons: mitral cells and tufted cells. The axons of the second neurons travel via the tractus olfactorius that divides into a stria olfactoria medialis and lateralis.
- **Third neuron:** projects to successive neurons, and is found in three locations:

  – for the stria olfactoria lateralis: in the prepirifom area (Brodmann area 28); it conveys information via the thalamus (nuclei mediales thalami) to the orbitofrontal cortex or neurons in the cortex surrounding the corpus amygdaloideum (semilunar and ambient gyri); further to the hypothalamus;

  – for the stria olfactoria medialis: nuclei in the area subcallosa (with nuclei septales) convey information to the habenula and hippocampus. Both connections remain ipsilateral;
  – for crossed fibers: nucleus olfactorius anterior (in the trigonum olfactorium) conveys information from the bulbus olfactorius.

Note: The second neuron in the the stria olfactoria lateralis reaches cortical areas without thalamic participation. The olfactory pathway is thus, according to present knowledge, the only afferent pathway that can reach telencephalic neurons without passing through the thalamus. The extensive projection of the stria olfactoria to neurons of the limbic system (mainly the cortex surrounding the corpus amygdaloideum) explains the strong emotional connotations of olfactory impressions. The projection to the hypothalamus is responsible for autonomic reactions (e.g., nausea, p.r.n. vomiting) related to unpleasant olfactory sensations.

Somatopic organization of pathway

Not known.

Clinical correlations

Olfactory pathway dysfunction leads to anosmia. It can result from damages to both bulbi olfactorii or both tractus olfactorii in the case of basal skull fracture.

2.7 Control of Motor Nuclei of Nervi Craniales

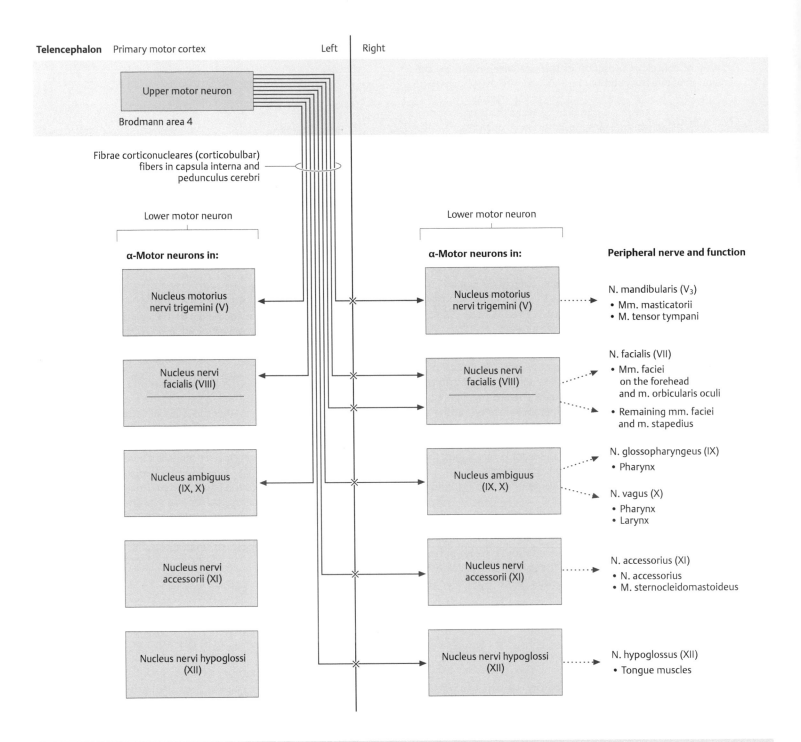

Organization of the motor nuclei of nervi craniales

Based on their function, they are divided into two groups:

- Nuclei for the motor function of eye muscles (III, IV, and VI) and
- Nuclei for the other motor functions controlled by n. craniales (Vmotor; VII, IX, X, XI, and XII).

Usually, the cortical control is mediated via a common pathway, the fibrae corticonucleares or corticobulbar tract (fibers). This pathway, however, differentiates into two parts: one for the eye muscles, one for the other motor functions. Control of eye movement is mediated through one section of the tract via multiple centers in the truncus encephali before the eye muscle nuclei are reached, via the fasciculus longitudinalis medialis (see "control of motor functions of eye muscles," p. 522 f). Only the control of the other n. cranialis motor nuclei is explained here, those that are reached directly by the second part of the fibrae corticonucleares. This is analogous to the fibrae corticospinales that project to motor neurons in the medulla spinalis.

Definition and function of the fibrae corticonucleares for the control of the motor nuclei of nervi craniales

- Major pathway for voluntary motor function: conscious movement control of mm. masticatorii, mm. faciei, mm. linguae, other muscles attached to the skull, as well as subconscious motor control of pharyngeal and laryngeal muscles
- The part of the tractus pyramidalis between the primary motor cortex and the motor nuclei in the truncus encephali. Similar to the other fibers of the tractus pyramidalis (i.e., fibrae corticospinales to the medulla spinalis and fibrae corticoreticulares to the formatio reticularis), these fibers are axons of the large pyramidal neurons.

Characteristics of pathway

Somatomotor; descending; efferent

Neural wiring and topography of the pathway

Total of two serially connected neurons:

- **Upper motor neuron:** large pyramidal cells in the lamina pyramidalis interna (layer V) of the gyrus precentralis (primary motor cortex); they are located in the Brodmann area 4. Most other neurons origimate in neighboring cortical regions. On their descending way from the telencepahlon to the truncus encephali, the axons of the upper motor neurons pass through the following structures:

Primary motor cortex → genu capsulae internae → pedunculus cerebri (mesencephalon) → tegmentum pontis

Decussation of the upper motor neuron axons: partial crossing (largely in the pons), thus resulting in crossed and uncrossed projections from the motor cortex to the lower motor neurons

Axons of the upper motor neurons terminate only contralaterally on
- Portion of the nucleus nervi facialis that controls the facial expression of the lower face,
- Nucleus nervi accessorii,
- Nucleus nervi hypoglossi.

Axons of the upper motor neurons terminate both contra- and ipsilaterally axons on the
- Nucleus motorius nervi trigemini,
- Nucleus nervi facialis that controls the superior part of the face (muscles of the forehead and m. orbicularis oculi),
- Nucleus ambiguus (innervation of pharynx and larynx).

- **Lower motor neurons:** α-motor neurons in the
  - Nucleus motorius nervi trigemini (mm. masticatorii and m. tensor tympani),
  - Nucleus nervi facialis (mm. faciei),
  - Nucleus ambiguus that projects via the nn. glossopharyngeus and vagus (pharynx and larynx),
  - Nucleus nervi accessorii (trapezius and sternocleidomastoideus), and
  - Nucleus nervi hypoglossi (most muscles of the tongue).

The axons of the fibrae corticonucleares end as excitatory synapses on these nuclei. The axons of the lower motor neurons terminate in the target organ, in this case the muscles; therefore they represent the motor component of the respective n. cranialis. The neurotransmitter is acetylcholine.

Note: The fibrae corticonucleares end on the lower motor neurons. The axons of the lower motor neurons forms the motor component of the respective n. cranialis.

Somatopic organization of the pathway

- Capsula interna: in the genu, rostral to the fibrae corticospinales that run in the posterior limb
- Mesencephalon: in the pedunculi cerebri; medial to the fibrae corticospinales.

Clinical correlations

Dysfunction of the fibrae corticonucleares leads to impaired voluntary movement related to chewing (n. trigeminus), facial expression (n. facialis), turning the head and shrugging the shoulder (n. accessorius) and movements of the tongue (n. hypoglossus).

Note: Dysfunction of the upper motor neurons leads to a central type of palsy and dysfunction of the lower motor neurons to a peripheral palsy (similar to a lesion to the motor fibers in the n. cranialis).

Since only one part of the nucleus nervi facialis is innervated ipsi- and contralaterally, a distinction can be made between a nuclear or infranuclear lesion palsy (lower motor neuron or peripheral nerve is affected) vs. a supranuclear lesion palsy (upper motor neuron is affected):

- In case of a palsy due to a peripheral nerve lesion, all fibers are affected (including those that control forehead muscles and the m. orbicularis oculi).
- In case of a supranuclear palsy, the forehead muscles and part of the m. orbicularis oculi are not paralyzed because the lower motor neurons controlling these muscles are influenced by fibers arriving from the ipsilateral motor cortex as well.

2.8   Ocular Motor Control

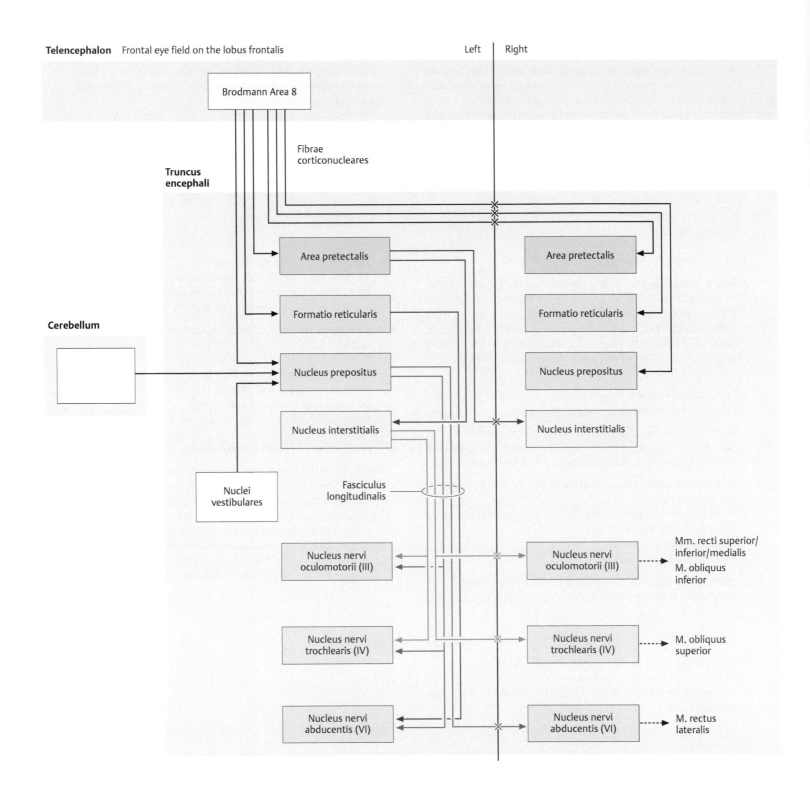

Definition and function

The control of eye movements is extremely complex. In order to guarantee an unambiguous visual impression, images fall on corresponding areas of the retina. This requires that both eyes move in a coordinated way. If that doesn't happen and light rays don't fall on the corresponding retinal points, double vision results. The ocular motor control is mainly a reflexive response mediated by subcortical centers (see "projections of the retina," p. 526 f). Voluntary eye movements are possible. However, they are not initiated by the gyrus precentralis (somatomotor function) but are controlled by a specialized command center in the lobus frontalis (as opposed to the gyrus precentralis), called the frontal eye field (part of Brodmann area 8). Unlike the gyrus precentralis, the frontal eye field doesn't send its efferents directly to α-motor neurons in nuclei of the nn. craniales but they reach control centers in the truncus encephali (mesencephalon and pons), which further project to the motor nuclei responsible for eye movements.

Characteristics of pathway

Somatomotor; descending; efferent.

Neural wiring and topography of pathway

The originating neurons are located in the frontal eye field (in this case, neurons are usually not numbered, thus the term "originating neuron"). Their axons travel along with axons of neurons of the gyrus precentralis in the capsula interna as fibrae corticonucleares. The neurons from area 8 project ipsi- and contralaterally to neurons in the area pretectalis (at the diencephalic-mesencephalic junction) and to the formatio reticularis and nucleus prepositus. Neurons from the area pretectalis project bilaterally to the nucleus interstitialis. The nuclei prepositus and interstitialis further project to the motor nuclei of nn. craniales III, IV and VI as listed below.

- Nucleus prepositus projects ipsilaterally to all nuclei and contralaterally to the nucleus of n. cranialis VI.

- The nucleus interstitialis projects ipsi- and contralaterally to the nuclei of nn. craniales III and IV,
- Neurons of the formatio reticularis in the truncus encephali project ipsilaterally to the nucleus of n. cranialis VI.

The connections between the cerebellum and the nuclei vestibulares, especially the nucleus prepositus, coordinate the movements that maintain balance with the help of eye movements (e.g., vestibular nystagmus—involuntary eye movement during head turning, for example, when driving a car).
In the truncus encephali, the fasciculus longitudinalis medialis contains fibers responsible for interconnecting the nuclei responsible for eye muscles with the command centers and with the vestibular system (see also "Truncus Encephali Pathways," p. 524 f).

Clinical correlations

- Only dysfunction of a single motor nucleus that controls eye muscles leads to dysfunction of a single muscle or muscle group in one eye.
- Dysfunction of command centers (e.g., in case of vascular lesions in the truncus encephali or lesions in the area surrounding the frontal eye field) are always associated with complex eye movement dysfunctions affecting both eyes.

2.9 Truncus Encephali Pathways

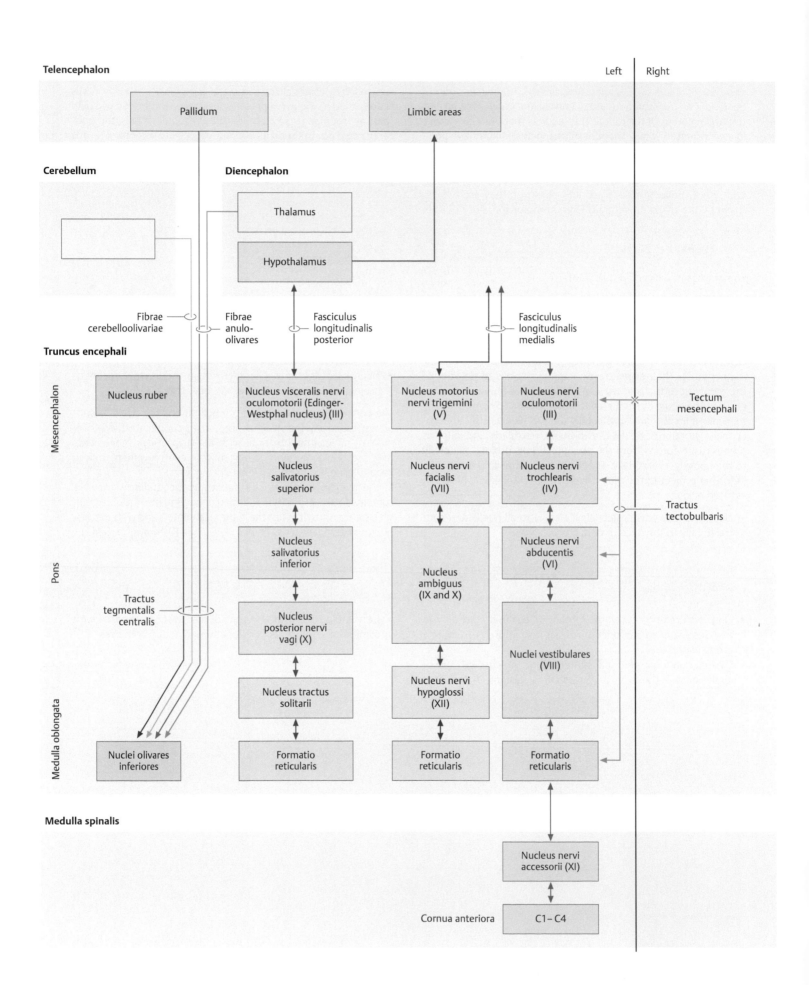

Telencephalon

Left | Right

Pallidum

Limbic areas

Cerebellum

Diencephalon

Thalamus

Hypothalamus

Fibrae cerebelloolivariae

Fibrae anulo-olivares

Fasciculus longitudinalis posterior

Fasciculus longitudinalis medialis

Truncus encephali

Mesencephalon

Nucleus ruber

Nucleus visceralis nervi oculomotorii (Edinger-Westphal nucleus) (III)

Nucleus motorius nervi trigemini (V)

Nucleus nervi oculomotorii (III)

Tectum mesencephali

Nucleus salivatorius superior

Nucleus nervi facialis (VII)

Nucleus nervi trochlearis (IV)

Tractus tectobulbaris

Pons

Tractus tegmentalis centralis

Nucleus salivatorius inferior

Nucleus nervi abducentis (VI)

Nucleus ambiguus (IX and X)

Nucleus posterior nervi vagi (X)

Nuclei vestibulares (VIII)

Medulla oblongata

Nuclei olivares inferiores

Nucleus tractus solitarii

Nucleus nervi hypoglossi (XII)

Formatio reticularis

Formatio reticularis

Formatio reticularis

Medulla spinalis

Nucleus nervi accessorii (XI)

Cornua anteriora

C1– C4

Essentially, truncus encephali pathways can be divided into two groups:

- Longitudinal pathways that exclusively or mainly pass through the truncus encephali
- Pathways that interconnect nuclei of the truncus encephali

The four major truncus encephali interconnections are explained below.

Longitudinal pathways (not shown here)

Either descending, thus mainly somatomotor or visceromotor, or ascending, thus mainly sensory:

- Descending pathways
  - **Tractus pyramidalis** (with its different parts, see p. 510 f)
  - **Tractus corticopontinus** as part of the corticopontocerebellar pathway (see p. 510 f);
- Ascending pathways: the four lemnisci:
  - **Lemniscus medialis** (continuation of the pathway includes the posterior column, see p. 508)

- **Lemniscus spinalis** (continuation of the sensory anterolateral system, see p. 508)
- **Lemniscus trigeminalis** (continuation of trigeminal pathway) (see p. 512 f)
- **Lemniscus lateralis** (part of the auditory pathway) (see p. 514 f)

Interconnecting pathways

- **Tractus tegmentalis centralis:** Descending pathway, most important pathway of the extrapyramidal system in the truncus encephali. Formed by several pathways: fibers originate from the telencephalon (pallidum), diencephalon (thalamus), cerebellum and—from the truncus encephali itself—the nucleus ruber. These individual pathways combine to form the tractus tegmentalis centralis that ends in the nuclei olivares inferiores. The nuclei olivares inferiores are therefore a central relay nucleus of the extra-pyramidal motor system.
- **Fasciculus longitudinalis posterior:** This pathway contains both ascending and descending fibers and interconnects various parts of the autonomic nervous system. The hypothalamus as the main autonomic control center interconnects with parasympathetic nuclei and the nucleus gustatorius (nucleus tractus solitarii). At the same time, there are collaterals reaching the motor nuclei of nn. craniales involved in chewing, swallowing, sucking, and gagging. The reflex motor activities related to these functions are carried on via the motor nuclei

of nn. craniales V, VII, nucleus ambiguus (for the nn. craniales IX and X), and XII. The pathway crosses at multiple levels (not shown here).
- **Fasciculus longitudinalis medialis:** This functionally mixed pathway—which also contains both ascending and descending fibers—interconnects motor nuclei of the systems that control the movements of the eyes (III, IV, VI) and head (XI, cornu anterius C1–C4) with nuclei vestibulares (balance) for smooth pursuit eye movements but also motor nuclei of nn. craniales involved in the voluntary motor control of chewing, swallowing, sucking. The motor nuclei of nn. craniales are thus interconnected via both fasciculi. The pathway crosses at multiple levels (not shown here).
- **Tractus tectobulbaris:** Crossed pathway that originates in the colliculus superior (in the tectum mesencephali) and projects to the motor nuclei responsible for eye movements and the formatio reticularis for reflex oculomotor activity.

525

2.10 Retinal Projections

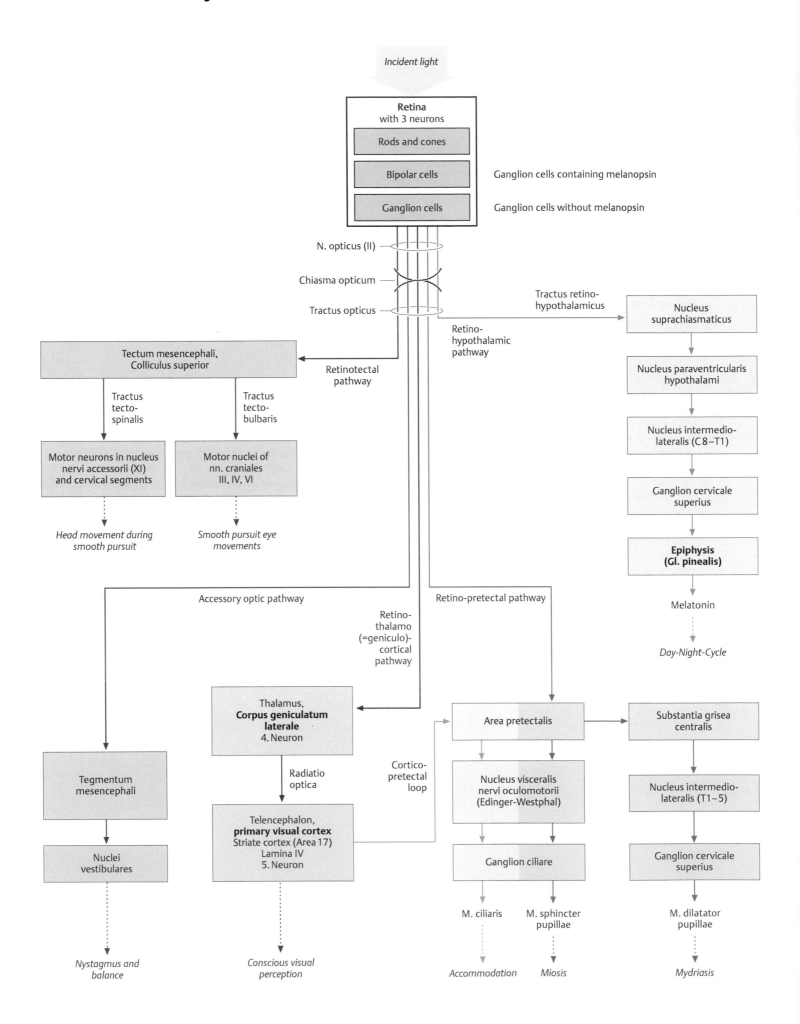

The visual system is responsible for processing visual stimuli. This includes not only the conscious perception of visual impressions but encompasses five different functions with the retina (a diencephalic derivative) as the common starting point.

Visual pathway

Mediates conscious perception and processing of visual impression (color, shape, size, position, movement, etc. of an object).

- Morphologically, largest part of the visual system.
- Passes through the thalamus (fourth neuron in the corpus geniculatum laterale; first to third neurons in the retina) and from the thalamus to the primary visual cortex, where it ends above and below the sulcus calcarinus in the striate cortex of cuneus and gyrus lingualis.
- From the primary visual cortex, association pathways run to the secondary and tertiary visual cortical areas for further processing of complex visual information (not shown here).

Retinopretectal pathway

- Control of the visceral motor innervation mediates the pupillary light reflex for which smooth muscles are responsible.
- Extends to the area pretectalis, a nuclear region rostral to the colliculi superiores of the mesencephalon, which topographically is part of the diencephalon (epithalamus).
- The area pretectalis projects to the parasympathetic nucleus visceralis nervi oculomotorii (Edinger-Westphal nucleus) in the mesencephalon and via the substantia grisea centralis of the truncus encephali (periaqueductal gray) to sympathetic neurons in the medulla spinalis (C8–T1). The Edinger-Westphal nucleus mediates pupil constriction (miosis) and lens accomodation and the sympathetic neurons are responsbile for contraction of m. dilatator pupillae (mydriasis).
- The area pretectalis, plays, therefore, a key functional role in two neuronal circuits: one without the participation of the thalamus and visual cortex (retinopretectal pathway) and one involving the participation of the visual cortex (corticopretectal loop). In the first case, the information is related to the amount of light that enters the eye, which causes the pupil to dilate or constrict. Since the cerebral visual cortex is not involved, this response can also be triggered in an unconscious patient. In the second case, information about image sharpness is transmitted which causes the lens to adjust to shift focus between near and far objects (and thus leads to focusing of the image). This requires a perception of the actual sharpness by the visual cortex, which means that only fully conscious people can respond adequately.

Retinotectal system

- Responsible for reflex tracking eye movements and accommodation.
- Passes through the colliculi superiores of the tectum mesencephali and the tractus tectospinalis and tectobulbaris to motor neurons that innervate various striate muscles, involved in head or eye movements. This way, the head and eyes automatically "follow" the moving object so that the image always falls on the site of the sharpest vision in both eyes.

Accessory optic system

Transmits visual information via the mesencephalon to the vestibular system (to analyze head motion). This way, balance and eye movements are coordinated (e.g., reflex head turning to compensate for eye movement). The accessory optic system thus supports (accessory) the retinotectal system.

Retino-hypothalamic system

Influences the circadian rhythm (e.g., day/night cycle) by measuring the daily light levels. Information relayed to the hypothalamus passes through several relay stations to reach the epiphysis (melatonin production and release).

Note: Axons from the nasal retina cross in the chiasma opticum (approx. 48% of all fibers). Thus, for all above mentioned systems, axons from both eyes enter the respective relay stations, meaning bilateral processing of information. For a general overview, the diagram indicates only the junction of the chiasma opticum, between the n. opticus and tractus opticus. The crossed fibers are not displayed.

2.11 Autonomic and Sensory Ganglia of the Head

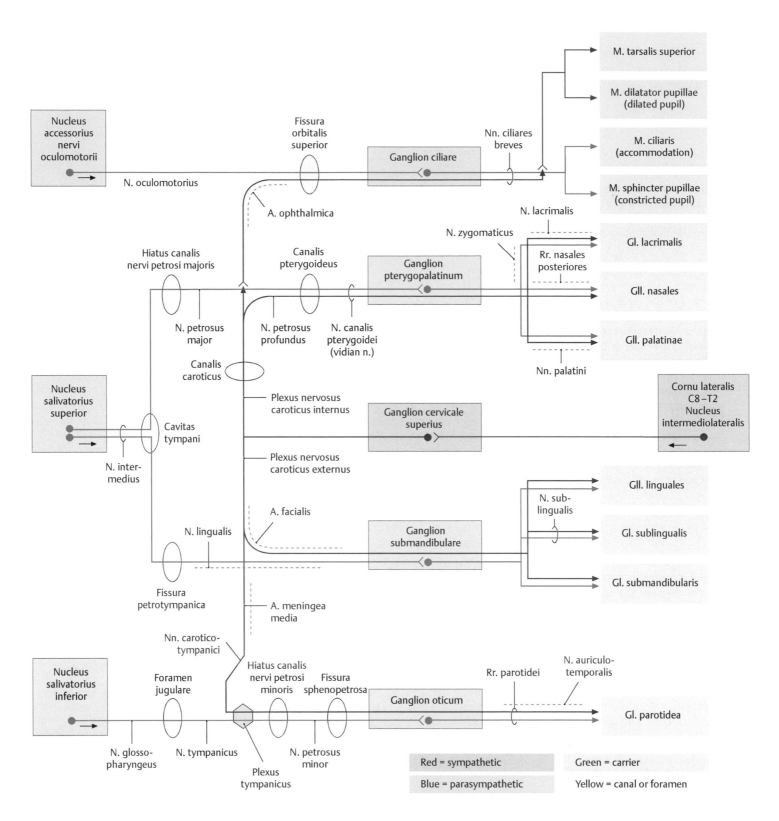

Red = sympathetic

Blue = parasympathetic

Green = carrier

Yellow = canal or foramen

A Autonomic ganglia of the head

Autonomic and sensory ganglia of the head can be easily confused. This is why both types are depicted here along with the direction in which the ganglia relay impulses (see arrows).

The autonomic ganglia of the head are always parasympathetic. Inside the ganglia, fibers of preganglionic neurons from the brainstem terminate at the perikaryon of the postganglionic neurons, which project their axons to the target organs. On their way to the target, the very thin and thus mechanically very sensitive fibers use other structures by traveling along them, including blood vessels or other nerves running to the same region as the autonomic fibers although they serve different functions. This is initially confusing which is why the autonomic fibers are represented here in blue (parasympathetic) or red (sympathetic) and the "main fibers" which have nothing to do with the autonomic fibers are represented in green. All structures mentioned here exit the skull through specific openings (canals and foraminae) which are represented in yellow.

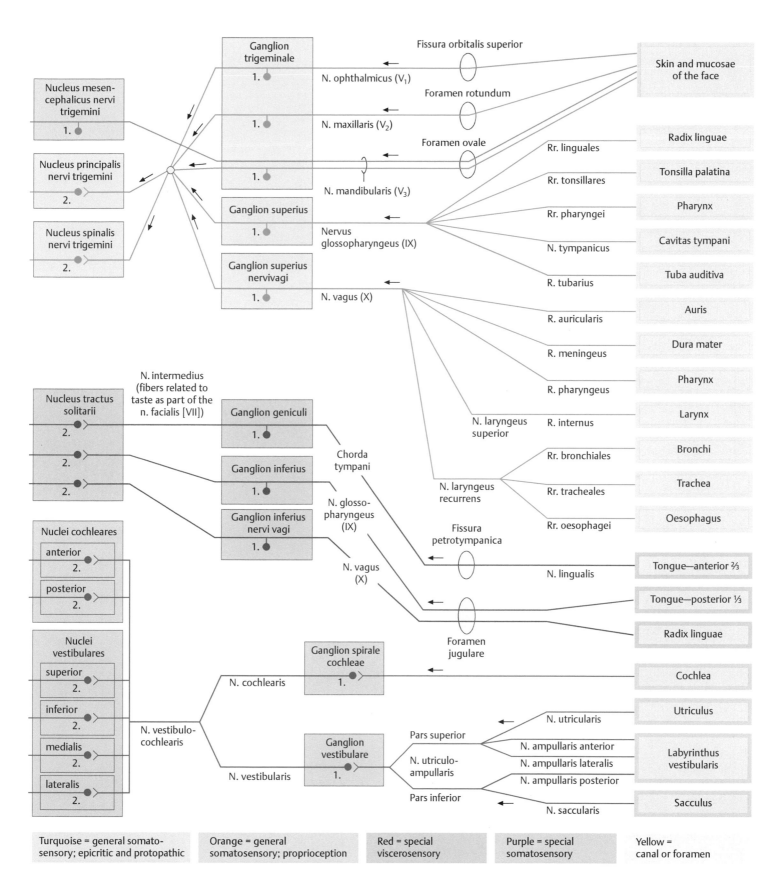

Turquoise = general somato-sensory; epicritic and protopathic

Orange = general somatosensory; proprioception

Red = special viscerosensory

Purple = special somatosensory

Yellow = canal or foramen

B Sensory ganglia of the head

Unlike the autonomic ganglia, the sensory ganglia contain no synapses. The sensory ganglia contain the bodies of the pseudounipolar or bipolar (in case of the n. vestibulocochlearis) neurons (primary afferent neurons). Their peripheral processes bring impulses from a receptor, their central process synapse in the CNS. As an example, the n. glossopharyngeus carries taste information from the posterior third of the tongue, the fibers pass through the ganglion inferius and end in the nucleus tractus solitarii in the CNS. This specific information is viscerosensory (here represented in red). The n. glossopharyngeus also carries information from the pharynx, in this case general somatosensory information. Its fibers pass through the ganglion superius and end in the nucleus spinalis nervi trigemini, which conveys protopathic information from several nn. craniales (thus not only the n. trigeminus for which it is named). Temperature and pain sensation of the pharynx (e.g., very hot beverage) can thus be detected by the n. glossopharyngeus. The n. vagus also conducts (via the ganglion superius (jugular) of the n. vagus) protopathic information (mainly pain) from the larynx to the nucleus spinalis nervi trigemini (e.g., pain caused by laryngitis).

2.12 **Motor System Connectivity**

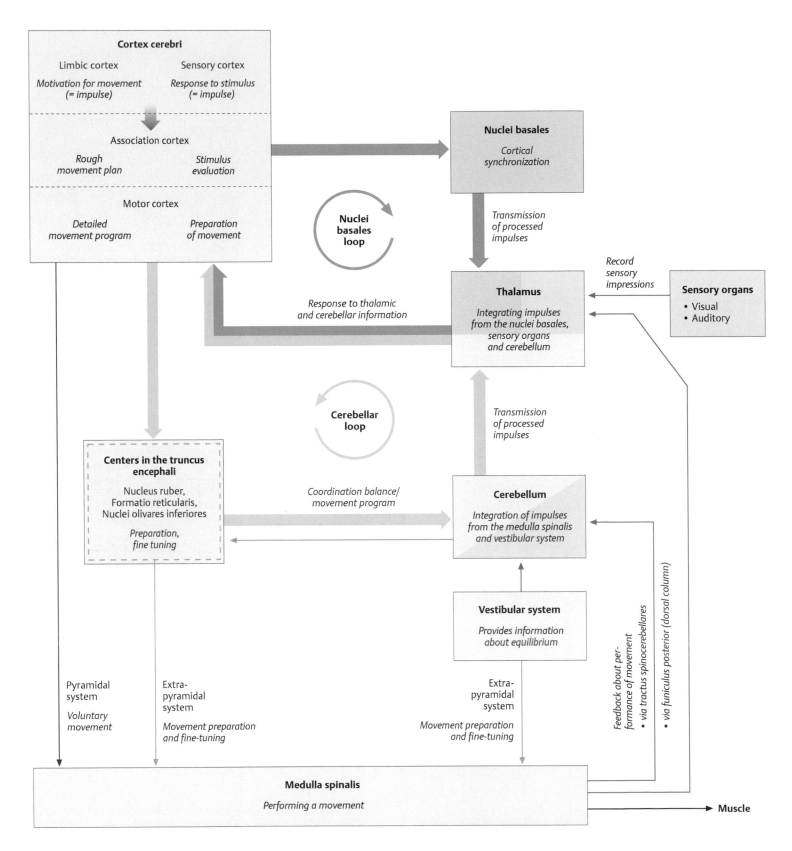

An overview of the functions of neurons, pathways and their interaction is depicted on the left, while the individual pathways, their structures, and nuclei are shown on the right.

Note: The cortex cerebri is the starting and ending point for two loops, the nuclei-basales loop and the cerebellar loop. The thalamus participates in both loops ("motor thalamus"). It picks up signals from the nuclei basales and the cerebellum and relays the integrated impulse pattern to the motor cortex. At the same time, the thalamus receives input from the sensory organs ("sensory thalamus"). If these signals are relevant for movement, the thalamus feeds them into the impulse pattern as above. Thus, the thalamus is the major integration center for both loops as well as for sensory input.

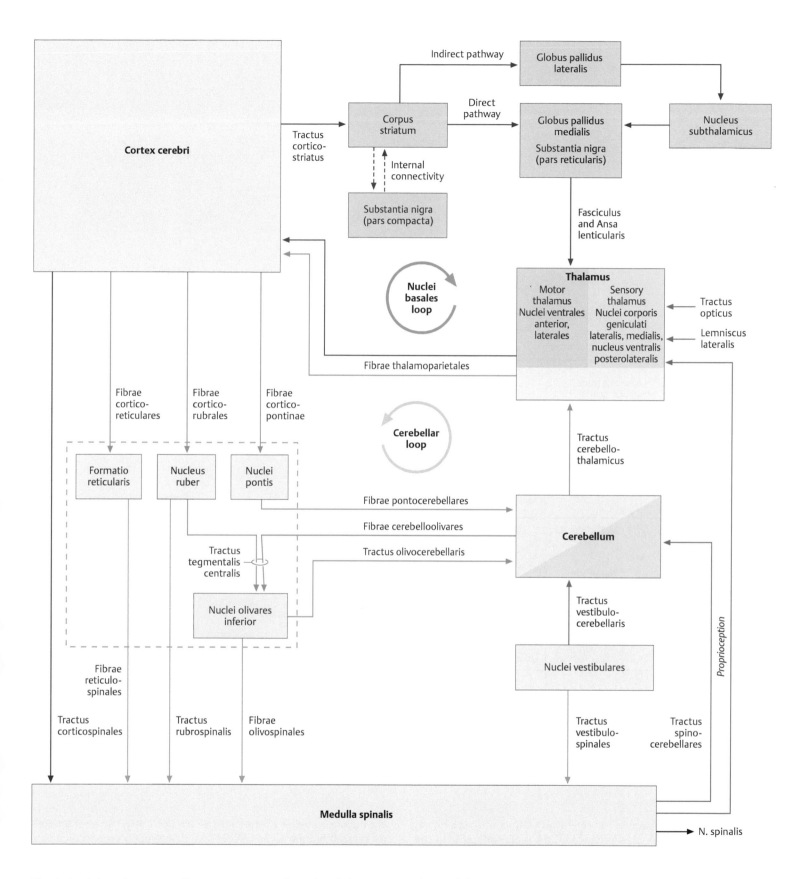

The thalamic impulses eventually generate a "complete" detailed movement program. It is relayed to centers in truncus encephali (nucleus ruber, formatio reticularis, nuclei olivares inferiores) for fine tuning. The nuclei olivares inferiores represent a particularly significant connection of the cerebellar loop toward the medulla spinalis. The movement is ultimately initiated by impulses from the motor cortex (mostly gyrus precentralis), which reach the medulla spinalis via the tractus pyramidalis (here tractus corticospinales) (for voluntary movement).

The medulla spinalis itself executes the movement and sends the impulse via the nn. spinales to the corresponding muscles. Information about the execution of movement is sent via tractus spinocerebellares from the medulla spinalis to the cerebellum, which uses this information for constantly making postural adjustments in order to maintain balance. The cerebellum does not have direct efferent connections to the medulla spinalis but can indirectly influence the medulla spinalis via the nuclei olivares inferiores.

2.13 Cerebellar Connectivity

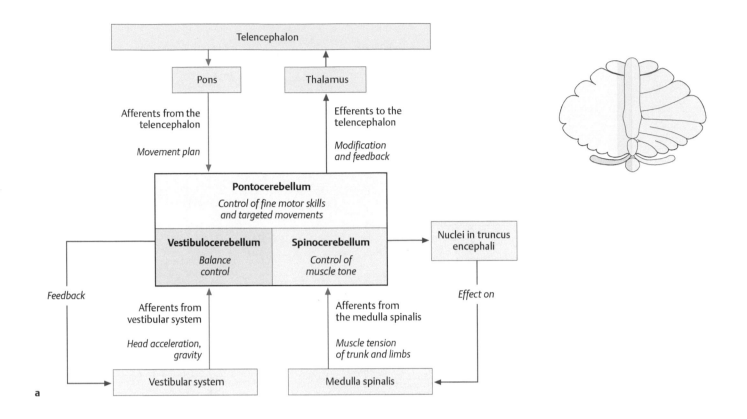

a

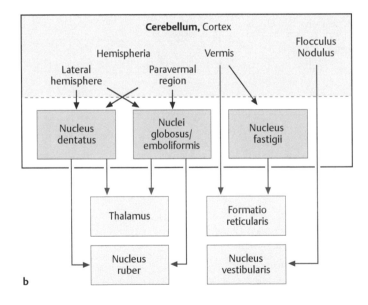

b

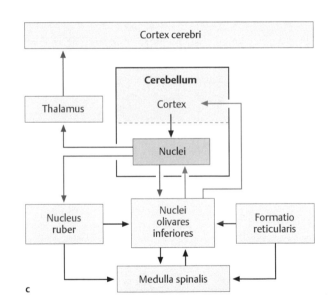

c

The functional organization of the cerebellum into ponto-, spino- and vestibulocerebellum (**a**) takes into account the **major afferents to the cerebellum:**

- From the telencephalon (via pons) for fine motor skills as part of planning of movements
- From the medulla spinalis for the regulation of muscle tone
- From the vestibular system for the control of head position and acceleration

Cerebellar efferent loops exist directly with the vestibular system and indirectly via the thalamus to the telencephalon and via nuclei of the truncus encephali to the medulla spinalis.

The **major cerebellar efferents** (**b**) usually don't originate from the cortex cerebelli but the nuclei cerebelli, which are largely assigned one particular cortical area. These nuclei project to the thalamus or to nuclei in the medulla spinalis. The nuclei olivares inferiores of the truncus encephali play a significant role (**c**): They project both to the cerebellum and to the medulla spinalis and receives afferents from both regions. Additionally, the oliva receives afferents from other brainstem nuclei (nucleus ruber and formatio reticularis). The oliva thus integrates cerebellar and spinal impulses. The purpose of this complex wiring is to allow the cerebellum—indirectly via the nuclei of the truncus encephali—to influence the medulla spinalis's motor activity in order to maintain balance and to control fine and precise motor skills.

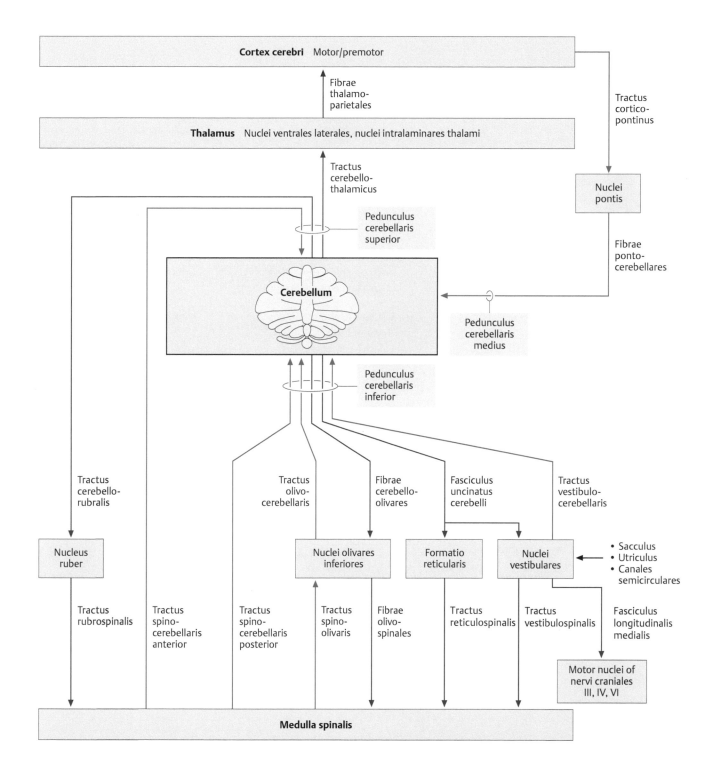

Cerebellar pathways

All pathways running to and from the cerebellum pass through one of the pedunculi cerebellares. The pedunculus cerebellaris medius contains only afferents. All afferents end in the cortex with collaterals ending in nuclei cerebelli (not shown here). Histologically, the tractus olivocerebellaris is the only one that provides climbing fibers (they directly end on the Purkinje cells in the cortex). All other afferents end as mossy fibers on the granule cells in the cortex cerebelli. The cerebellar efferents largely originate from the nuclei (see left side, **b**) and run either

to the thalamus (feedback loop to the telencephalon (see left side, **a**) or to nuclei in the truncus encephali, which in turn project to the medulla spinalis via extrapyramidal tracts and thus control motor functions (cf. "Tractus Pyramidalis" and "Truncus Encephali Pathways"). The projection from the nuclei vestibulares to the nuclei that control eye movements help with compensatory eye movements during head movement.

Note: A direct projection of the cerebellum to the medulla spinalis has not been so far proven in humans.

2.14 Functional Cortical Areas

A Functional cortical areas

Functional lobes	Specialization	Localization	Symptoms in case of damage
Lobus frontalis	Personality	① Gyri orbitales	Abulia; impaired decision-making ability and absence of goal-oriented behavior; Witzelsucht (compulsive wisecracking) ("frontal lobe syndrome")
	Somatomotor function (primary motor cortex)	② Gyrus precentralis	Contralateral paralysis; damage dependent on the localization of lesion on the cortex ("motor homunculus")
	Motor center for speech (Broca)	③ Gyrus frontalis inferior (pars opercularis; pars triangularis) lateralization (dominant hemisphere mostly left)	Motor aphasia/Broca aphasia: inability to formulate more or less complex sentences
	Olfactory cortex	④ Substantia perforata anterior, gyrus ambiens, gyrus semilunaris	Anosmia
Lobus parietalis	Somotosensation (primary somatosensory cortex)	⑤ Gyrus postcentralis	Loss of tactile and temperature sensation and/or pain localization
	Abstract (non-pictorial) thinking, reading	⑥ Gyrus angularis and gyri supramarginales Lateralization (dominant hemisphere)	Abstract thinking, reading, inability to perform mathematical calculations
Lobus occipitalis	Visual cortex (primary visual cortex)	⑦ Above and below the sulcus calcarinus, cuneus and gyrus lingualis	Loss of half of the visual field (homonymous hemianopsia) on the opposite side or defect in one quadrant of the contralateral visual field (quadrantanopsia)
Lobus temporalis	Auditory cortex (primary auditory cortex)	⑧ Gyri temporales transversi (Heschl)	Only in case of bilateral damage: impaired auditory perception
	Sensory speech center (Wernicke)	⑨ Gyrus temporalis superior	Sensory aphasia/Wernicke aphasia: inability to comprehend sentences
Lobus limbicus	Learning, memory, emotional reponse	⑩ Hippocampal formation	Only in case of bilateral damage Impaired explicit memory
Insula	Gustatory cortex	⑪ Gyri insulae	p.r.n. ageusia

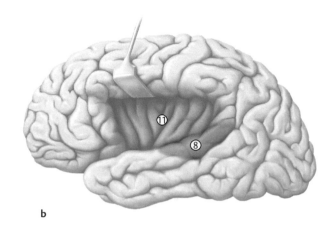

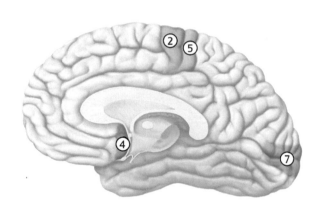

a

b

B Left hemispherium
a Lateral view; **b** Lateral view, sulcus lateralis widely open by retractors

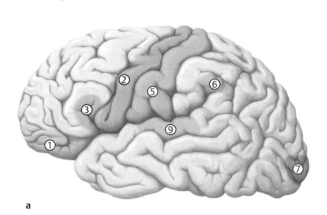

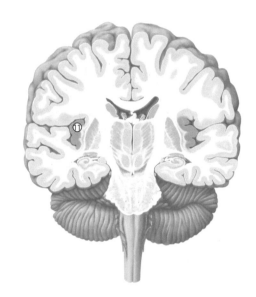

C Right hemispherium
Medial view.

D Frontal section of the telencephalon
Anterior view.

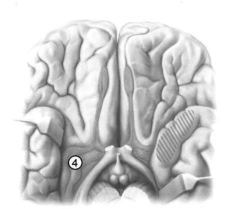

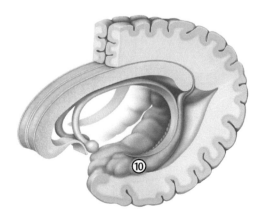

E Rostral part of the hemispheria cerebri
Basal view.

F Left hippocampal formation
Left anterior-superior view.

2.15 Association and Projection Pathways

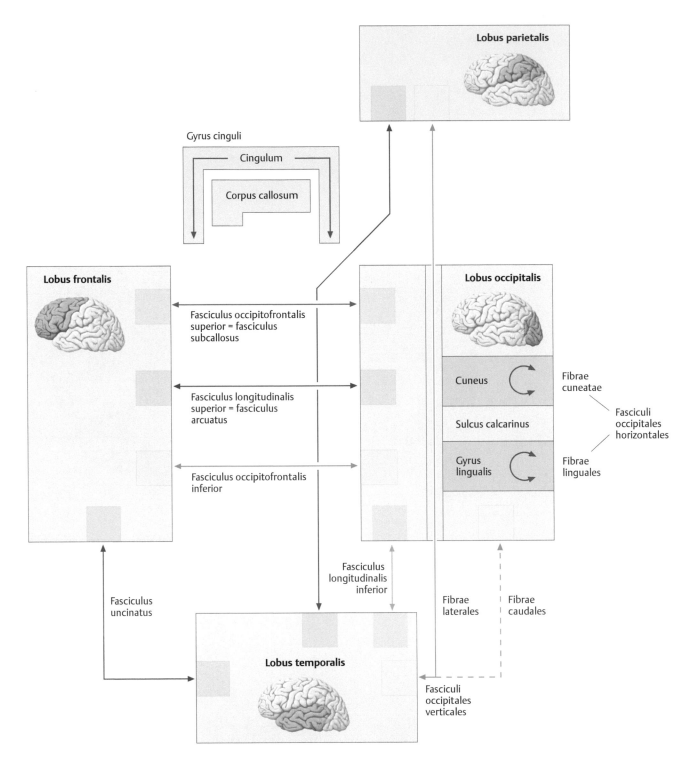

A Association pathways (association fibers in the telencephalon)
Association pathways connect different cortical regions, in order to, for instance, combine visual and acoustic information. Although such functional connections exist in all parts of the CNS, the term "association pathway" only refers to tracts of the telencephalon. There, association pathways connect different cortical areas of the same hemispherium (they never cross). There are three distinct type of association fibers:

- Fibrae arcuatae cerebri (not shown here) connect adjcent gyri.
- Fibrae associationis breves connect areas within one lobe (represented here are only the fibrae occipitales horizontales that connect lateral and medial parts of the lobus occipitalis).

- Fibrae associationis longae connect cortical areas of different lobes. These tracts are always individually named.

Note: The fibers of the fasciculi occipitales verticales connect lateral lobi temporalis and parietalis and cross the lobus occipitalis.

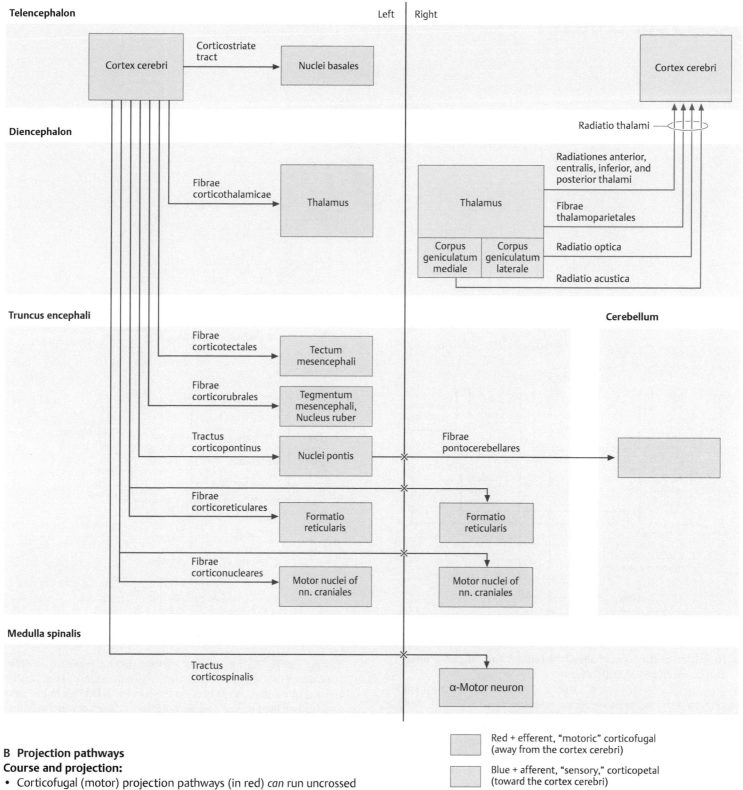

B Projection pathways

Course and projection:

- Corticofugal (motor) projection pathways (in red) *can* run uncrossed yet mostly cross. Motor impulses from the cortex cerebri thus travel to contralateral subcortical centers and influence motor activity of the contralateral side of the body.

- Corticopetal (sensory) projection pathways (in blue) never cross. Thus, they reach the cortex cerebri only from the ipsilateral thalamus. Yet, the thalamus itself, is reached by pathways of subordinate centers, most of which are located contralaterally. Subsequently, sensory impulses to the cortex cerebri originate mainly from the contralateral side of the body.

Exceptions to this basic principle:

- Motor function: cortical projections to individual motor nuclei of nn. craniales (see p. 520 f and 522 f)
- Somatosensation: innervation of the head via the n. trigeminus (see p. 512)

Red + efferent, "motoric" corticofugal (away from the cortex cerebri)

Blue + afferent, "sensory," corticopetal (toward the cortex cerebri)

- Special senses: olfactory pathway, gustatory pathway, auditory pathway, visual pathway (see respective wiring diagram)

The following **major pathways** are distinguished:

- In the telencephalon: to the basal ganglia (nuclei basales), particularly to the corpus striatum (corticofugal: corticostriate tract), not shown here, see "Motor System Connections," p. 530 f
- In the diencephalon: to and from the thalamus (corticofugal: fibrae corticothalamicae; corticopetal: radiationes thalami)
- To the truncus encephali: (e.g., tractus corticopontinus, fibrae corticonucleares, fibrae corticorubrales, fibrae corticoreticulares)
- In the medulla spinalis: tractus corticospinalis

537

2.16 Nuclei Olivares Superior and Inferior as well as the Four Lemnisci

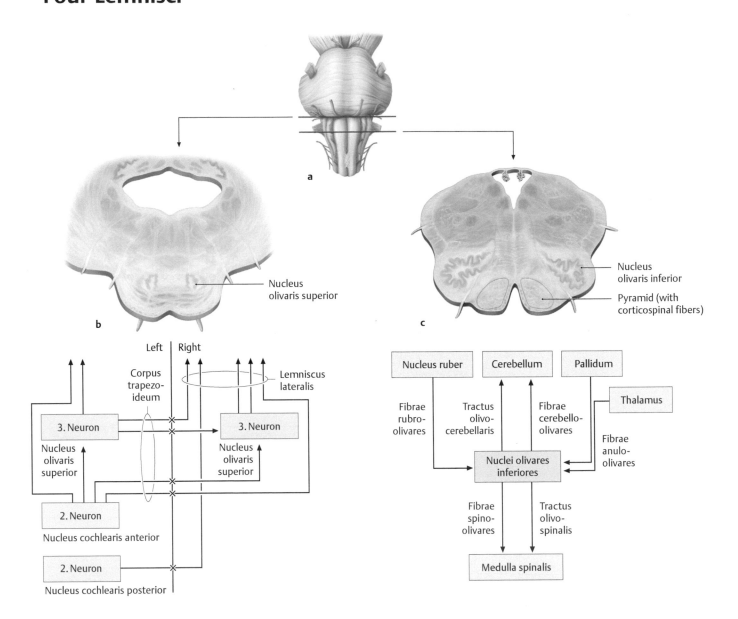

A Definition of the terms "olive," "inferior," and "superior olive" and connections of both olives

a Truncus encephali, ventral view; **b** Cross-section of the medulla oblongata near the pons—superior view; **c** Cross-section of medulla oblongata—inferior view.

- **Oliva:** The oliva is a distinct olive-shaped protrusion, located on the ventral aspect of the medulla oblongata. It lies lateral to the pyramis. The term "oliva" is thus a descriptive macroscopic term.
- **Superior olive** (*Nucleus olivaris superior*): The superior olive is significantly smaller than the inferior olive; it alone would not be identifiable as a protrusion. It is located inside the medulla oblongata, mediodorsal and largely cranial to the inferior olive and is thus clearly visible on cross-sections directly caudal to the pons (**b**). The superior olive continues into the most inferior parts of the pons. Due to the partial overlap of the inferior and superior olive, both nuclear complexes are sometimes visible on same cross-sections. Similar terms are used for the superior and inferior olive, which are adjacent topographically. Functionally, however they are not conected and have to be strictly separated.
- **Connections of the superior olive:** The nucleus olivaris superior is a major nucleus with role in the localization of sound and connections involved in the stapedius reflex (a protective reflex for the sense of

hearing, see p. 485). It receives afferents from the nucleus cochlearis anterior (both ipsi- and contralateral); both nuclei olivares superiores are connected and project via the lemniscus lateralis to ipsi- and contralateral hierarchically upper nuclei of the auditory pathway. For more details see p. 484 f and 514.

- **Inferior olive** (*complexus olivaris inferior; nuclei olivares inferiores*) (**c**): The inferior olive is located in the medualla oblongata. It consists of several nuclei; this is why it is also often referred to as "complexus olivaris inferior." Due to its size, the complexus olivaris inferior gives the protrusion called the "oliva" on the ventral aspect of the truncus encephali. Not all nuclei of the complex are visible to the naked eye.

Connections of the inferior olive: The inferior olive is involved in the coordination of motor activities and thus extensively connected to other neural regions concerned with motor functions:

- Tractus olivocerebellaris and fibrae cerebelloolivares: connections with the cerebellum
- Tractus olivospinalis: pathway to the the cornu anterius of the medulla spinalis
- Fibrae spinoolivares: pathway originating in the medulla spinalis
- Fibrae anuloolivares: pathway from the nuclei basales and diencephalon (for more details see p. 514 and 537–539)

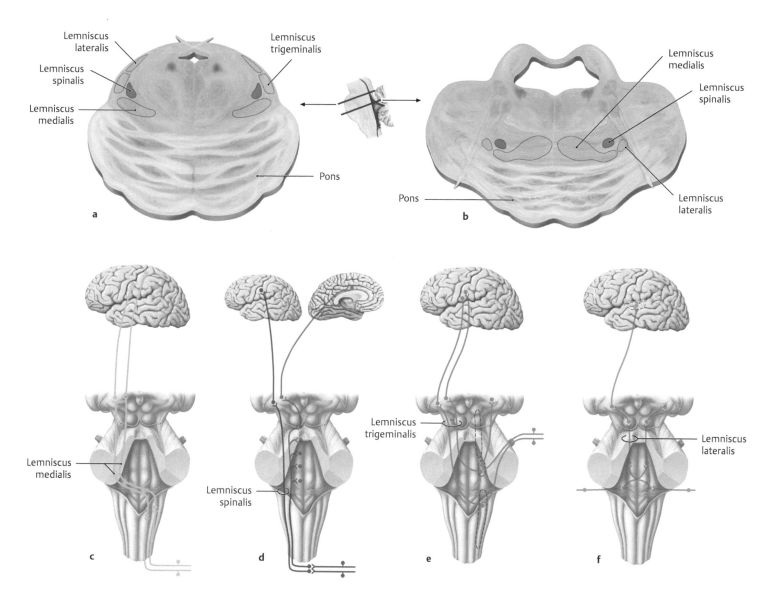

B The four lemnisci in the truncus encephali

a and **b** Cross-section of the pons—superior and medial view respectively; **c-f** Schematic representation of the four lemnisci

The term lemniscus (ribbon) refers to the ribbon-like course of a total of four specific afferent (ascending) pathways in the truncus encephali. A lemniscus is not a "new" pathway but rather the name of a portion of a pathway. The specific names of the individual lemnisci are based on

- their location relative to each other in the truncus encephali (lemnisci medialis and lateralis),
- their origin in the medulla spinalis (lemniscus spinalis), or
- their origin in a nucleus of a n. cranialis (lemniscus trigeminalis).

The terms are historically related; they are not based on any classification. **a** and **b** display on two cross-section samples the respective location of the four lemnisci. A lemniscus contains axons of the second neuron which is located in the CNS. It starts with the course of the second axon in the truncus encephali and ends at the entry into the thalamic nucleus (diencephalon). Some fibers in all lemnisci are uncrossed. Details follow:

- *Lemniscus medialis* (**c**): Continuation of the fasciculus gracilis or cuneatus. Second neurons (with the bodies in nucleus gracilis or cuneatus) are already in the truncus encephali. The entire lemniscus is formed by fibers that crossed in the decussatio lemnisci medialis and ends in the contralateral nucleus ventralis posterolateralis of the thalamus. It conveys epicritic sensation from the trunk, limbs, and back of the head.

- *Lemniscus spinalis* (**d**): Continuation of the tractus spinothalamici anterior and lateralis. The bodies of the second neurons are located in the cornu posterius of the medulla spinalis and all of them decussate while still in the medulla spinalis; therefore the lemniscus spinalis

itself does not cross. It ends in the nucleus ventralis posterolateralis of the thalamus. The lemniscus spinalis runs very close to the lemniscus medialis in some parts of the truncus encephali; therefore an "individual" course is rarely described. It relays the protopathic sensation from trunk, limbs, and back of the head.
Note: Unlike the other three terms, "lemniscus spinalis" is not frequently used; occasionally it is used as a synonym for the tractus spinothalamicus lateralis.

- *Lemniscus trigeminalis* (tractus trigeminothalamicus; **e**): originates in the trigeminal nuclei. The second neurons (with the bodies in the nucleus principalis or nucleus spinalis nervi trigemini) cross only partially and end in the contra- and ipsilateral nuclei ventrales posteriomediales of the thalamus. It conveys the epicritic and protopathic sensation from the head (not including the back of the head). Distinctive feature: it divides into a tractus trigeminothalamicus anterior (uncrossed fibers) and posterior (crossed fibers). Due to a particular role of the nucleus mesencephalicus nervi trigemini, which is discussed in a different chapter, this illustration depicts only a part of the trigeminal pathways.

- *Lemniscus lateralis* (**f**): Auditory pathway. Second neurons (with the bodies in the nucleus cochlearis anterior) in the truncus encephali; some cross and some remain ipsilateral; therefore they end in the contra- and ipsilateral corpora geniculata medialia (medial geniculate bodies) of the thalamus. It conveys information from the organs of hearing. Distinctive feature: the lemniscus contains "its own nuclei" (nuclei lemnisci lateralis), which serve as relay stations for the auditory pathway. It terminates in the nuclei colliculi inferioris of the mesencephalon.

2.17 Left to Right Connections in the CNS: Commissures and Decussations

A Commissures

Note: Commissures connect specific areas on the left side of the CNS with the analogous areas on the right side of the CNS and vice versa. For instance, they connect specific areas of the left and right visual cortex.

Per definition, commissural projections are contralateral. The term commissure is generally used for the entire pathway. The site at which this pathway crossed the midline does not have a name. For further details see the term "decussation."

Name of pathway	Location/course	Structures connected by the pathway
Telencephalic commissures		
Corpus callosum • Forceps frontalis (lobus frontalis) • Forceps occipitalis (lobi parietalis and occipitalis)	Roof and anterior wall of the ventriculi laterales	Hemispheria cerebri with the exception of the lobi temporales; the lobi temporales are connected via the pars posterior of the commissura anterior
Commissura anterior with a pars anterior and posterior	Adjacent to the lamina terminalis (anterior wall of the ventriculus tertius)	• Pars anterior: Nuclei olfactorii • Pars posterior: Gyri temporales mediales and inferiores
Commissura fornicis (Hippocampal commissure)	Border between telencephalon/ diencephalon, crus of fornix	Left and right hippocampus via the fimbria of the fornix
Commissura habenularis	Epithalamus, parietal to the recessus pinealis	Connection between left and right nuclei habenulares
Diencephalic commissures (Diencephalon)		
Commissura posterior (Commissura epithalamica)	Between the recessus pinealis and aqueductus cerebri	Connection between left and right epithalamus
Commissures of the truncus encephali (Medulla oblongata, Pons, Mesencephalon)		
Commissurae supraopticae ventralis and dorsalis	Parts of it pass through the diencephalon superior to the chiasma opticum	Connection between the left and right pons and mesencephalon: the commissure thus passes through the diencephalon but connects parts of the truncus encephali.
Commissura colliculi superioris	Tectum mesencephali	Colliculi superiores
Commissura colliculi inferioris	Tectum mesencephali	Colliculi inferiores
Commissura cochlearis pontis	Tegmentum pontis (corpus trapezoideum)	Nucleus cochlearis anterior
Commissura cerebelli	Cerebellum; medulla; close to nucleus fastigii	Hemispheria cerebelli
Pathways of the medulla spinalis		
Commissurae albae anterior/posterior	In each case between the cornua anterius and posterius	Connection between symmetrical halves of the medulla spinalis; part of the fasciculi proprii (propriospinal fibers)
Commissurae griseae anterior/posterior	Anterior and posterior to the canalis centralis	Layer of substantia grisea; not a real functional commissure.

B Decussations

Note: The term "decussationes" refers to the crossover of tracts, not to analogous sites on the opposite side but to topographically different regions. For instance, the tractus pyramidalis runs from one hemispherium cerebri to contralateral half of the medulla spinalis. For these tracts (which are called tractus, fasciculi, funiculi, or fibrae), the site at which the tract crosses over—meaning it crosses the midline—lies in the median plane of the CNS, somewhere along the course of the the tract. This is in contrast to the commissures, for which the crossover point is located in the middle between left and right analogous structures. As a result, the crossover point of each crossing is individually named (cf. the term "commissure").

Name of decussation	Location	Name of the crossed pathway(s)	Structures connected by the pathway(s)
Decussatio tegmentalis anterior	Tegmentum mesencephali at the level of the colliculi superiores	Fibers of the tractus rubrospinales	Nucleus ruber in the mesencephalon with γ-motor neurons in the cornu anterius of the medulla spinalis
Decussatio tegmentalis posterior	Tegmentum mesencephali at the level of the colliculi superiores	Fibers of the tractus tectospinalis and tectobulbaris	Connects the colliculus superior with γ-motor neurons in the cornu anterius of the medulla spinalis
Decussatio pedunculorum cerebellarium superiorum	Tegmentum mesencephali at the level of the colliculi inferiores	Pedunculi cerebellares superiores (for more details see the information in right column)	• Tractus spinocerebellaris anterior: connects medulla spinalis with cortex cerebelli and nuclei cerebelli • Tractus dentothalamicus: from the nucleus dentatus of the cerebellum to the thalamus • Tractus cerebellorubralis: from the nuclei cerebelli to the nucleus ruber in the mesencephalon
Decussatio fibrarum nervorum trochlearium	Tectum mesencephali in the substantia alba	Crossing of the axons of the nn. trochleares; This is the only crossing of a peripheral nerve.	The n. trochlearis crosses at this level in order to innervate the opposite m. obliquus superior
Decussatio lemnisci medialis (sensory decussation)	Medulla oblongata, at the level of the oliva	Crossing of the axons originating in the nuclei gracilis/ cuneatus (part of fibrae arcuatae internae)	Connect the nuclei gracilis and cuneatus nuclei with the nucleus ventralis posterolateralis of the thalamus
Decussatio pyramidum	Medulla oblongata; ventral aspect, level of pyramides	About 80% of the tractus pyramidalis cross here	Connect the gyrus precentralis and other areas of the cortex cerebri with α motor neurons in the cornu anterius of the medulla spinalis

Note: With the exception of the n. trochlearis (the only crossing of a peripheral nerve), all the above mentioned decussations refer to crossings of pathways in the central nervous system.

2.18 Diencephalic Nuclei and Thalamic Nuclear Regions

A Diencephalic nuclei

Part of diencephalon	Nuclear region	Function
Epithalamus	• Nuclei habenulares (in the habenula) • Gl. pinealis (epiphysis)	• Circadian rhythm and melatonin production • Relay station for vegetative processing of olfactory impulses
Thalamus	• Nuclei anteriores thalami • Nuclei mediales thalami • Nuclei intralaminares and mediani thalami • Nuclei reticulares • Nuclei ventrales posterolaterales • Nucleus ventralis posteromedialis • Nucleus ventralis anterior • Pulvinar thalami • Nuclei corporis geniculati medialis • Nucleus corporis geniculati lateralis	• Limbic system • Emotional stability • Cerebellar connection • Interthalamic connection • Epicritic, protopathic, and proprioceptive information from trunk and limbs • Epicritic, protopathic, and proprioceptive information from the face • Cerebellar information • Functional relation to the association cortex • Relay station on the auditory pathway • Relay station on the visual pathway
Hypothalamus	• Nucleus infundibularis • Corpus mammillare (with nuclei mammillares medialis and lateralis) • Nucleus paraventricularis hypothalami • Nucleus supraopticus • Nucleus suprachiasmaticus	• Releasing and inhibiting hormones that act on the hypophysis • Limbic system • Oxytocin • Antidiuretic hormone • Circadian rhythm
Subthalamus	• Nucleus subthalamicus • Zona incerta	• (extrapyramidal) motor control

B Thalamic nuclear regions

Nuclear region	Afferent from	Efferent to	Function
Nuclei anteriores thalami	Nuclei mammillares medialis and lateralis of the corpus mammillare via the fasciculus mammillothalamicus	• Gyrus cinguli • Gyrus parahippocampalis	• Limbic system • Part of the Papez circuit
Nuclei mediales thalami	• Corpus amygdaloideum • Olfactory cortex	Frontal cortical areas	Affective function
Nuclei mediani thalami	• Telencephalon: gyrus cinguli • Diencephalon: hypothalamus • Truncus encephali: formatio reticularis	Gyrus cingulus; hippocampus; corpus amygdaloideum	Wakefulness; alertness
Nuclei ventrales thalami • Nucleus ventralis anterior/ nucleus ventrales laterales • Nucleus ventralis posterolateralis • Nucleus ventralis posteromedialis	• Globus pallidus; substantia nigra; nuclei cerebelli • Lemniscus medialis; tractus spinothalamicus • Lemniscus trigeminalis	• Motor cortical areas • Gyrus postcentralis • Gyrus postcentralis	• Motor functions • Sensation from limbs and trunk • Sensation from head/face
Nuclei dorsales thalami • Pulvinar thalami • Nuclei intralaminares thalami • Nucleus reticularis thalami	• Lemniscus trigeminalis; colliculus superior • Large parts of the cortex, truncus encephali; medulla spinalis • Cortex and other thalamic nuclei	• Association cortex • Cortex; nuclei basales • Thalamic nuclei	• Control of eye movement • Motor system; alertness (ARAS) • Interthalamic connection (largely inhibition)

2.19 Nuclei of Nervi Craniales and Autonomic Nuclei

A Nuclei of the nervi craniales

Name of nucleus	Location	Course including nerve	Target organs
Somatic motor nuclei (general somatic efferent); the axons of these nerves end directly on target organs			
Nucleus nervi oculomotorii	Mesencephalon, at the level of the colliculus superior	N. oculomotorius (III)	Mm. obliquus inferior, rectus medialis, recti superior and inferior, levator palpebrae superioris
Nucleus nervi trochlearis	Mesencephalon, at the level of the colliculus inferior	N. trochlearis (IV)	M. obliquus superior
Nucleus nervi abducentis	Midpons floor of the ventriculus quartus	N. abducens (VI)	M. rectus lateralis
Nucleus nervi accessorii	Pars cervicalis medullae spinalis (extending to C6 segment)	Accessory n. (radix spinalis) (XI)	Mm. trapezius and sternocleidomastoideus
Nucleus nervi hypoglossi	Medulla oblongata, floor of the ventriculus quartus	N. hypoglossus (XII)	Muscles of the tongue
Visceral motor nuclei (special visceral efferent or branchiomotor) (embryological term; control of skeletal muscles derived from arcus pharyngei); the axons in these nerves end directly on target organs			
Nucleus motorius nervi trigemini	Midpons	N. mandibularis (V$_3$)	Mm. masticatorii, tensor tympani, tensor veli palatini, digastricus (venter anterior), and mylohyoideus
Nucleus nervi facialis	Caudal pons	N. facialis (VII)	Mm. faciei and stapedius
Nucleus ambiguus	Medulla oblongata	• N. glossopharyngeus (IX) • N. vagus (X) • N. accessorius, radix cranialis (XI)	• Pharyngeal muscles • Pharyngeal and laryngeal muscles • Laryngeal muscles, fibers ran back in the n. vagus
Visceral efferent nuclei (general visceral motor) (control of smooth muscles of the internal organs, glands, and eyes) Nucleus accessorius nervi oculomotorii; nuclei salivatorii superior and inferior; Nucleus posterior nervi vagi, see **B**			
Somatic sensory nuclei (general somatic afferent); with the exception of the nucleus mesencephalicus nervi trigemini, all these nuclei contain bodies of second order neurons of afferent pathways, while the bodies of first neurons of the pathways are located in the respective ganglia sensoria of cranial nerves.			
Nucleus principalis nervi trigemini	Pons, rostral part	All three branches of the n. trigeminus First neuron in the ganglion trigeminale	Skin and mucosae: Epicritic sensation
Nucleus spinalis nervi trigemini	Pars cervicalis medullae spinalis, extending to segment C6	All three branches of the n. trigeminus; First neuron in the ganglion trigeminale	Skin and mucosae: Protopatic sensation
Nucleus mesencephalicus nervi trigemini	Tegmentum mesencephali	N. mandibularis First neuron in the nucleus mesencephalicus nervi trigemini	Mm. masticatorii, Mandibular joint: Proprioception
Nuclei vestibulares medialis, lateralis, superior, and inferior	From pons to medulla oblongata	N. vestibularis (VIII); first neuron in the ganglion vestibulare	Cristae ampullares in the canales semicirculares; Macula in the utriculi and sacculi; Balance
Nuclei cochleares anterior/posterior	Pontomedullary junction at the recessus lateralis of the ventriculus quartus	N. cochlearis (VIII); first neuron in the ganglion spirale cochleae	Organum spirale in the cochlea Hearing
Visceral sensory nuclei (general and special visceral afferent); these nuclei contain second neurons of an afferent pathway, while the first neurons are located in the ganglion sensorium nervi cranialis			
Nucleus tractus solitarii • Superior part • Inferior part	Medulla oblongata	• Special visceral afferent: N. VII; IX and X; first neuron in the ganglin geniculi and the ganglia inferiora of IX and X respectively • General visceral afferent: N. IX and X; first neuron in the ganglia superiora of IX and X	• Tongue papillae; taste • Lungs and bifurcatio carotidis; glomus caroticum; pulmonary stretch receptors

B Autonomic nuclei

Nuclear region	Preganglionic neuron (central), location and course of axons	Postganglionic neuron (peripheral), location of the ganglion and course of axons	Territory of distribution
Parasympathetic nuclei			
Nuclei accessorii nervi oculomotorii (Erdinger-Westphal nucleus)	Tegmentum mesencephali; travels with CN III	Orbita, ganglion ciliare, then travels via the nn. ciliares breves	M. sphincter pupillae M. ciliaris
Nucleus salivatorius superior	Tegmentum pontis; travels initially with the n. intermedius (part of CN VII, then with chorda tympani	Ganglion submandibulare Rr. glandulares to the gll. salivariae	Gll. sublingualis and submandibularis
	Or as n. petrosus major	Ganglion pterygopalatinum; rr. orbitales, n. nasopalatinus, nn. palatini major and minores	Gl. lacrimalis gll. nasales and palate
Nucleus salivatorius inferior	Tegmentum pontis; travels initially with CN IX then as n. tympanicus and n. petrosus minor	Ganglion oticum; travels with the n. auriculotemporalis	Gl. parotidea
Nucleus posterior nervi vagi	Pons/Medulla oblongata; travel with CN X	Ganglia close to the target organs, from there as plexus	Organs from the neck to the abdomen, intestinum crassum proximal to the flexura coli sinistra
Nuclei parasympathici sacrales	Medulla spinalis, intermediolateral region, S2-4; nn. splanchnici pelvici	Ganglia close to the organs in the plexus hypogastricus inferior	Urogenital system, intestinum crassum distal to the flexura coli sinistra
Sympathetic nuclei			
Nuclei intermediolateralis and intermediomedialis	Medulla spinalis, cornu laterale, C8-L2		
	As r. communicans albus to the ganglia trunci sympathici in the C8-L2 segments	All ganglia trunci sympathici: R. communicans griseus	Trunk and limbs: blood vessels, sweat glands
		T1–4 ganglia trunci sympathici as plexus cardiacus or cardiac nerves	Thoracic organs
	From the ganglia trunci sympathici (without synapsing here) T5–12: Nn. splanchnici major and minor; L1–4: Nn. splanchnici lumbales	Prevertebral ganglia: Ganglia coeliaca: ganglion mesentericum superius; ganglion mesentericum inferius (plexus with various names)	Abdominal organs to the flexura coli sinistra
	S1-4: Nn. splanchnici sacrales	Plexus hypogastricus inferior	Abdominal organs distal to the flexura coli sinistra and urogenital system

2.20 Neurovascular Structures of the Nose

A Arteries and nerves of the nose

The arterial supply to the nose and the sensory innervation of the tunica mucosa nasi follow common principles: There are **two areas of supply** in the cavitas nasi:

- the medial *septum nasi* (see a and c, left view) and
- the lateral *nasal wall* (see **b** and **d**, right view of the left lateral nasal wall).

Neurovascular structures enter the respective areas of supply via **two approaches:**
- *superiorly* (from the orbita) and
- *posteriorly* (from the fossa pterygopalatina through the foramen sphenopalatinum).

Note: In the interest of clarity this depiction of the openings through which the neurovascular structures pass is neither drawn to scale nor is it topographically precise.

Arterial supply: The arteries of the cavitas nasi arise from two flow tracts: the a. carotis interna (green) and the a. carotis externa (orange).

- The *a. carotis interna* enters the cavitas cranii through the canalis caroticus and gives off the a. ophthalmica. This artery passes through the canalis opticus into the orbit and there gives off the aa. ethmoidales anterior et posterior, which enter the cavitas nasi through the foramina ethmoidalia anterius et posterius. There they split into rr. septales posteriores and lateral nasal wall. The a. ophthalmica thus supplies the nose *superiorly*.
- The *a. carotis externa* gives off the a. maxillaris whose branch—the a. sphenopalatina—enters the cavitas nasi through the foramen sphenopalatinum and also gives off rr. septales posteriores and lateral nasal wall. The a. sphenopalatina artery supplies the nose *posteriorly*. This systematic separation of areas of supply is indicated by the dashed line.

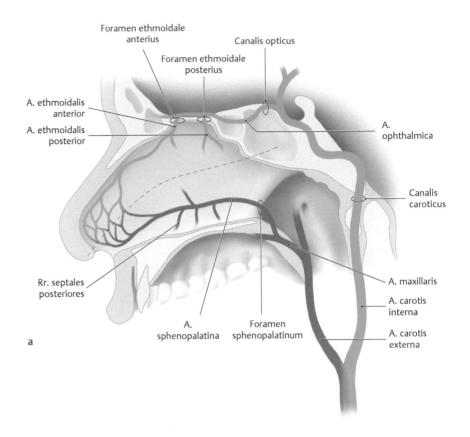

a

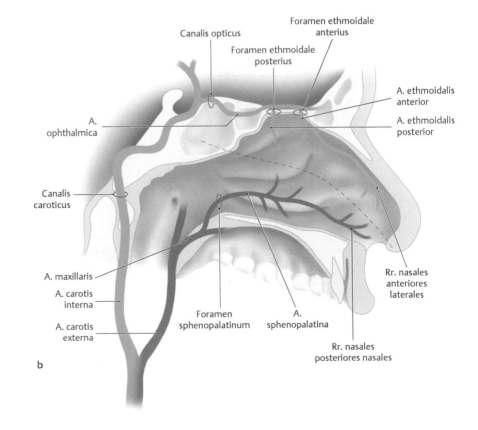

b

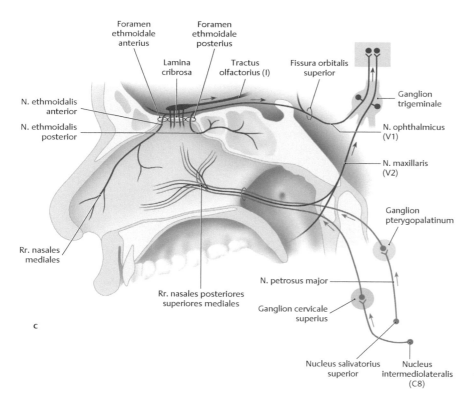

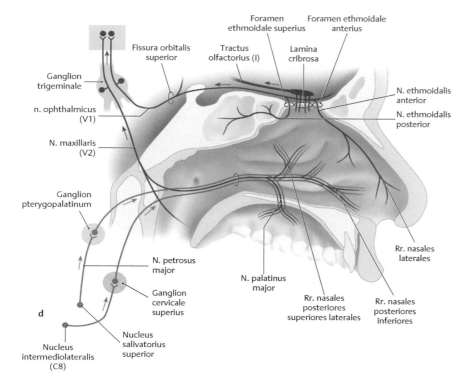

Sensory innervation:

- The nn. ethmoidales anterior et posterior pass through the foramina ethmoidalia anterius et posterius to the n. ophthalmicus (V1), which passes through the fissura orbitalis superior to the ganglion trigeminale. The n. ophthalmicus supplies the septal and lateral regions of the nose from *above*.
- Fine rr. nasales posteriores (rr. superiores medialis et lateralis) supply the septum nasi and lateral nasal wall posteriorly, exit the nose through the foramen sphenopalatinum, and extend to the n. maxillaris (V2). The n. maxillaris supplies the nose *posteriorly*.

Note: The innervation for *smell* is provided *only superiorly* by the n. olfactorius (I), which passes through the os ethmoidale in the lamina cribrosa and reaches the olfactory region in the superior cavitas nasi. The *autonomic innervation* of the nose is *only posterior*, whereby parasympathetic fibers from the ganglion pterygopalatinum (green) and the ganglion cervicale superius (brown) enter the cavitas nasi posteriorly and separate in the lateral and septal wall to innervate the nasal glands.

Overview:

- Superior arterial supply and sensory innervation of the septum nasi and lateral nasal wall: a. ophthalmica et n. ophthalmicus.
- Posterior arterial supply and sensory innervation of the septum nasi and lateral nasal wall: a. sphenopalatina et n. maxillaris.

2.21   Vessels of the Orbita

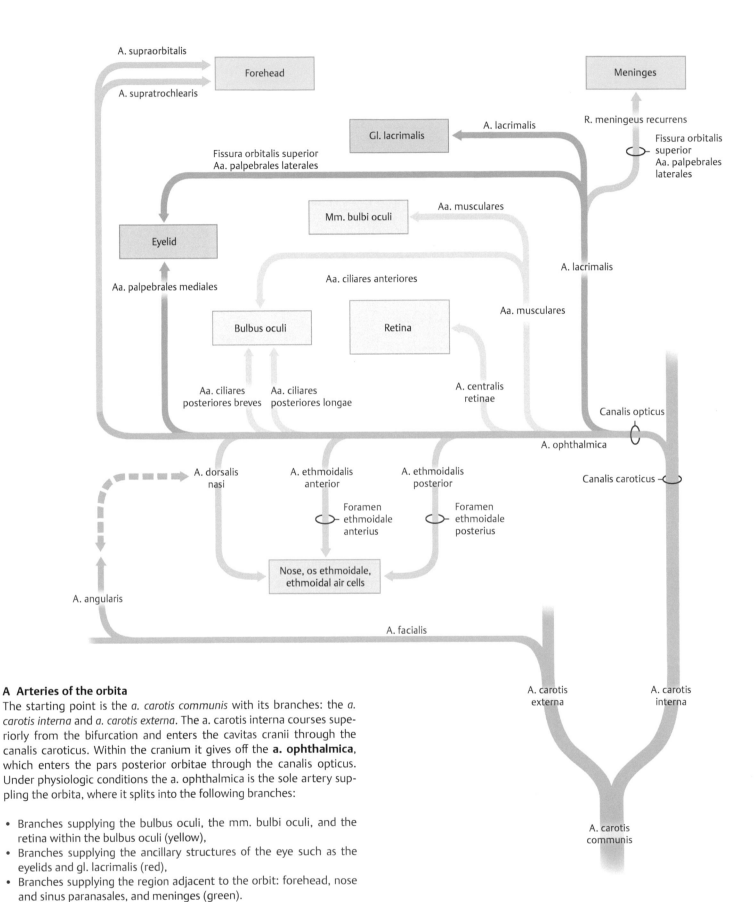

A Arteries of the orbita

The starting point is the *a. carotis communis* with its branches: the *a. carotis interna* and *a. carotis externa*. The a. carotis interna courses superiorly from the bifurcation and enters the cavitas cranii through the canalis caroticus. Within the cranium it gives off the **a. ophthalmica**, which enters the pars posterior orbitae through the canalis opticus. Under physiologic conditions the a. ophthalmica is the sole artery supplying the orbita, where it splits into the following branches:

- Branches supplying the bulbus oculi, the mm. bulbi oculi, and the retina within the bulbus oculi (yellow),
- Branches supplying the ancillary structures of the eye such as the eyelids and gl. lacrimalis (red),
- Branches supplying the region adjacent to the orbit: forehead, nose and sinus paranasales, and meninges (green).

The *a. carotis externa* only contributes to supplying the orbita under pathologic conditions when arterial supply via the a. ophthalmica is compromised. In such cases the *anastomosis* (see blue dashed line) between the *a. angularis* (courses to the angle of the eye) and the *a. dorsalis nasi* (branch of the a. ophthalmica) partially compensates the loss of arterial supply. The a. angularis enters the pars anterior orbitae.

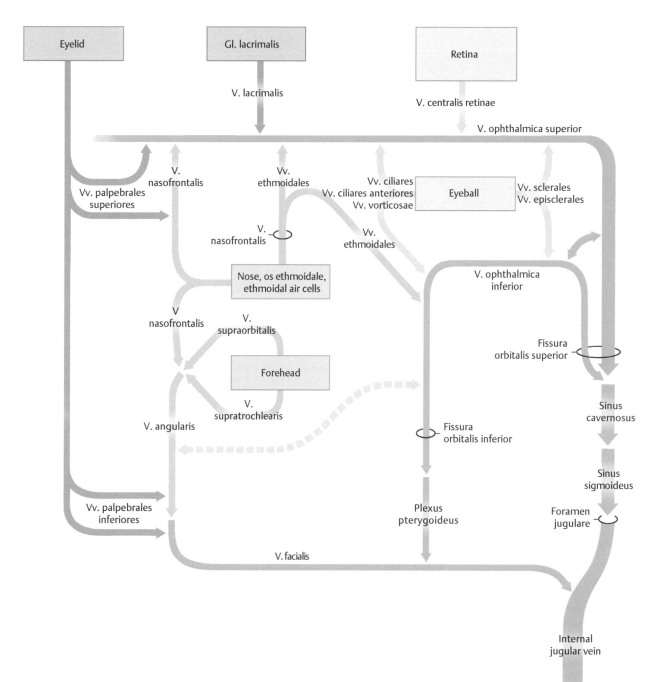

A Veins of the orbita

In contrast to its supply *via a single artery*, the orbit is drained by *two veins*. They drain the blood via different pathways that eventually converge at the v. jugularis interna. The two veins are as follows:

- **v. ophthalmica superior:** conducts the blood via the *fissura orbitalis superior* into the sinus cavernosus and *into the cranium*,
- **v. ophthalmica inferior:** similarly to the v. ophthalmica superior, it conducts the blood via the *fissura orbitalis inferior out of the cranium* and into the plexus pterygoideus to the base of the skull.

Venous drainage occurs via a network of vessels in contrast to the arterial supply, which resembles a one-way street. However, here too there are three major drainage areas with a corresponding system of branch veins:

- branches draining blood from the bulbus oculi and the retina within the bulbus oculi (yellow),
- branches draining blood from the region adjacent to the orbita: forehead, nose, and sinus paranasales (green), and
- branches draining blood from the ancillary structures of the eye such as the eyelids and gll. lacrimales (red).

The two vv. ophthalmicae are physiologically interconnected by an extensive anastomosis (see continuous blue line). There is also an anastomosis between the v. angularis and the v. ophthalmica inferior as well as a connection between the v. angularis and the v. ophthalmica superior via the v. nasofrontalis. Both of these anastomotic systems are clinically significant. The low-pressure flow of blood through the valveless veins of the cranium can easily reverse direction. This means that there is a risk that, in infections in the nasal and facial region, blood from the area drained by the v. angularis (especially skin in the nasal region) can flow in retrograde fashion to the v. ophthalmica, thus spreading germs into the orbita and further into the sinus system.

2.22 Nerves of the Orbita

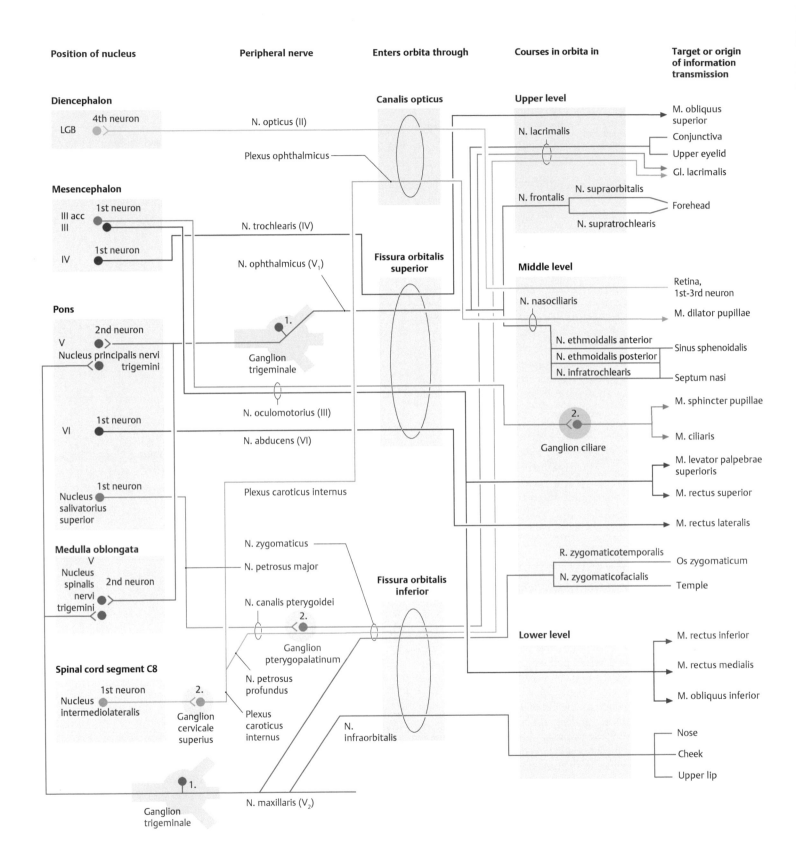

Position of nucleus

Diencephalon

LGB · 4th neuron — N. opticus (II)

Mesencephalon

III acc · 1st neuron
III

IV · 1st neuron — N. trochlearis (IV)

N. ophthalmicus (V₁)

Pons

V · 2nd neuron
Nucleus principalis nervi trigemini

Ganglion trigeminale 1.

N. oculomotorius (III)

VI · 1st neuron — N. abducens (VI)

Nucleus salivatorius superior · 1st neuron

Plexus caroticus internus

Medulla oblongata
V
Nucleus spinalis nervi trigemini · 2nd neuron

N. zygomaticus
N. petrosus major
N. canalis pterygoidei
2.
Ganglion pterygopalatinum
N. petrosus profundus

Spinal cord segment C8

Nucleus intermediolateralis · 1st neuron
2.
Ganglion cervicale superius
Plexus caroticus internus
N. infraorbitalis

Ganglion trigeminale 1.
N. maxillaris (V₂)

Peripheral nerve

Plexus ophthalmicus

Enters orbita through

Canalis opticus

Fissura orbitalis superior

Fissura orbitalis inferior

Courses in orbita in

Upper level

N. lacrimalis

N. frontalis · N. supraorbitalis
N. supratrochlearis

Middle level

N. nasociliaris

N. ethmoidalis anterior
N. ethmoidalis posterior
N. infratrochlearis

Ganglion ciliare 2.

Lower level

R. zygomaticotemporalis
N. zygomaticofacialis

Target or origin of information transmission

M. obliquus superior
Conjunctiva
Upper eyelid
Gl. lacrimalis

Forehead

Retina, 1st-3rd neuron
M. dilator pupillae

Sinus sphenoidalis

Septum nasi

M. sphincter pupillae
M. ciliaris

M. levator palpebrae superioris
M. rectus superior

M. rectus lateralis

Os zygomaticum

Temple

M. rectus inferior
M. rectus medialis
M. obliquus inferior

Nose
Cheek
Upper lip

A Nerves of the orbita

The courses of nerves within the orbit are very complex. Achieving a comprehensive understanding of them requires an appreciation of their distinctive systematic, functional, and topographic features. This text is intended to help you orient yourself using the illustration much in the manner of a road map. This scheme divides the road map into five "information columns."

Topographical aspects

The orbita as a space (information column 4, "Courses in orbit in"): The orbita can be divided into three levels. Each *level* is schematically represented by a gray box. You will find important information for the topographical demarcation of the levels on p. 174. All neurovascular structures of the orbita, and therefore many nerves, course in one of the three levels. The middle l evel is by far the largest. It contains the bulbus oculi as its salient landmark (see A, p. 174).

Access to the orbita (information column 3, "Enters orbit through"): The orbita is accessed posteriorly—from the left in the illustration—through *three openings, the canalis opticus and the fissurae orbitales superior et inferior* (see the ellipses in the gray boxes).

Note: The orbita and the cavitas cranii communicate only through the canalis opticus and the *fissura* orbitalis superior. These two openings lie *superior* to the level of the skull base and give the orbita an *intracranial connection to the internal skull base.*

In contrast, the *fissura* orbitalis inferior lies *inferior* to the level of the skull base; it gives the orbita *extracranial access to the external skull base.* All neurovascular structures that enter or leave the orbita posteriorly must therefore pass through one of these three openings. To understand the course of the neurovascular structure, it is important to recognize that structures entering the orbita through the fissura orbitalis inferior can continue into the upper level; it is entirely possible to change levels. The orbital openings are shown in greater detail in Fig. **B**, p. 36.

Functional aspects

The relay stations (information column 1, "Position of nucleus"): The nerves of the orbita transmit motor and sensory information. This information is processed in the CNS in the diencephalon, the three segments of the truncus encephali (*mesencephalon, pons,* and *medulla oblongata*), and the medulla spinalis. In these segments of the CNS there are two **types of nuclei:**

- motor nuclei which send information, nuclei of origin, and
- sensory nuclei which receive information, terminal nuclei.

The **nuclei of origin** transmit information to the muscles and glands and are either *somato*motor nuclei (dark red, for the motor nuclei of cranial nerves **III, IV,** and **VI**) or *visceral* motor nuclei. Visceral motor nuclei belong to the parasympathetic system (pale red for **III acc,** accessory nucleus of the n. oculomotorius and nucleus salivatorius superior) or to the sympathetic system (orange for the nucleus intermediolateralis in spinal segment C8). The flow of information is conducted from left to right.

The **terminal nuclei** receive information in the visual system (*lateral geniculate body [LGB]*) from the retina or surface sensations from the skin, mucosa, or surface of the eye via two of the three rr. nervi trigemini (*nucleus principalis nervi trigemini and nucleus spinalis nervi trigemini* for epicritic and protopathic sensation). Sensory nuclei are shown in blue. The flow of information is conducted from right to left.

The effector organ (information column 5, "Target or origin of information transmission"): The source of the sensory information and target of the motor information are the "effector organs," which are shown on the far right.

Systematic aspects

Designation of the neurovascular structures (information column 2, "Peripheral nerve"): The information is transmitted via nerves named according to topographical, functional, or phenomenological criteria. They are shown in column 2. Sensory nerves include sensory ganglia along the course of the nerve (blue). Where information is conducted from right to left, these ganglia contain the first neuron of a neuron chain without synaptic connections. Autonomic ganglia are embedded for transmission of visceral motor information (gray circles). Where information is conducted from left to right, these ganglia contain the second neuron of a neuron chain (with synaptic relay).

You would like to

- learn the motor area of a somatomotor or visceral motor nucleus? Begin with information column 1 and follow the nerve to the right all the way to column 5. Note the gray ganglia in applicable cases;
- learn the nucleus for a sensory source area? Begin with information column 5 and follow the course of the nerve to the left all the way to column 1. Note the blue ganglia in applicable cases. The nerve may possibly split into branches within the orbita.
- Columns 2–4, which you will pass through as you follow the course of the nerve, inform you about the levels, openings, and names of the nerves.

2.23 Larynx

Arteries

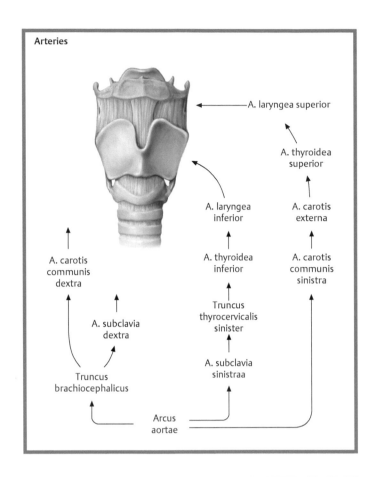

A. laryngea superior

A. thyroidea superior

A. laryngea inferior

A. carotis externa

A. carotis communis dextra

A. thyroidea inferior

A. carotis communis sinistra

A. subclavia dextra

Truncus thyrocervicalis sinister

Truncus brachiocephalicus

A. subclavia sinistraa

Arcus aortae

Veins

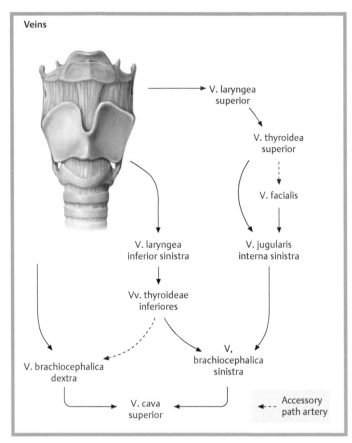

V. laryngea superior

V. thyroidea superior

V. facialis

V. laryngea inferior sinistra

V. jugularis interna sinistra

Vv. thyroideae inferiores

V. brachiocephalica dextra

V, brachiocephalica sinistra

V. cava superior

Accessory path artery

Lymph nodes

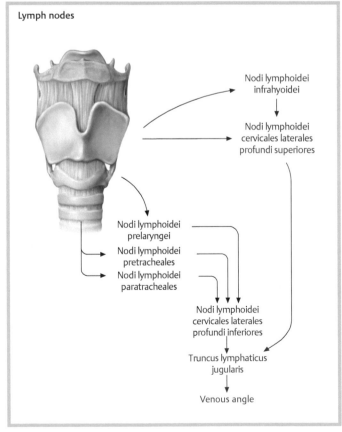

Nodi lymphoidei infrahyoidei

Nodi lymphoidei cervicales laterales profundi superiores

Nodi lymphoidei prelaryngei

Nodi lymphoidei pretracheales

Nodi lymphoidei paratracheales

Nodi lymphoidei cervicales laterales profundi inferiores

Truncus lymphaticus jugularis

Venous angle

Innervation

Sympathetic	Somatomotor	Parasympathetic
Truncus sympathicus	Nucleus ambiguus	Nucleus posterior nervi vagi
Plexus caroticus		N. vagus
Plexus laryngeus		

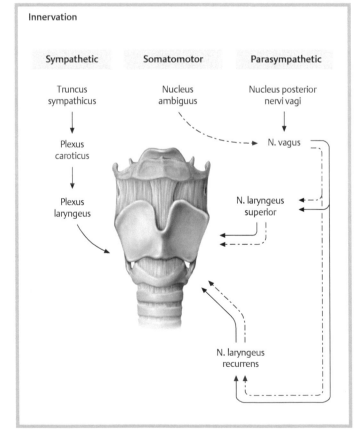

N. laryngeus superior

N. laryngeus recurrens

2.24 Gl. Thyroidea

Arteries

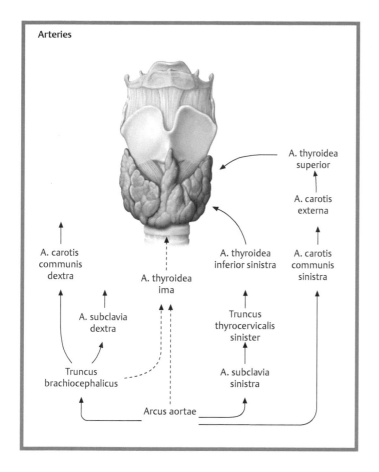

Veins

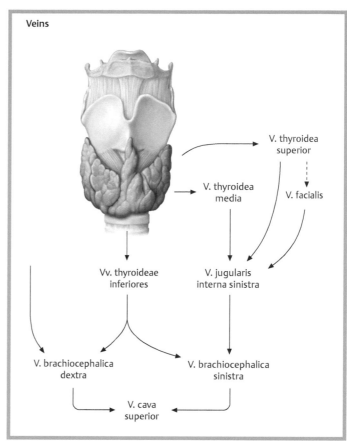

Lymph nodes

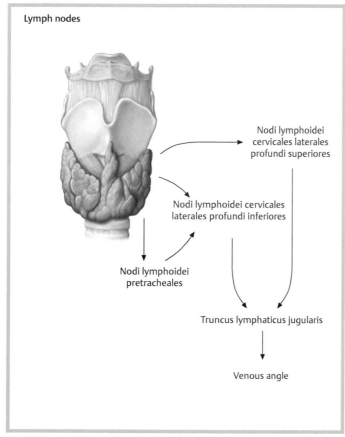

Innervation

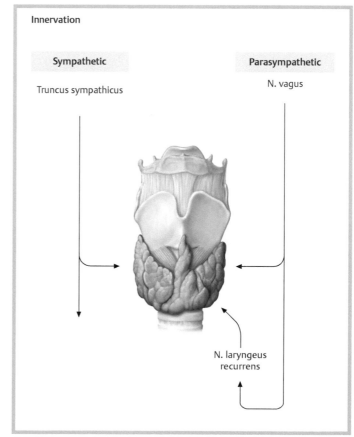

553

2.25 Pharynx*

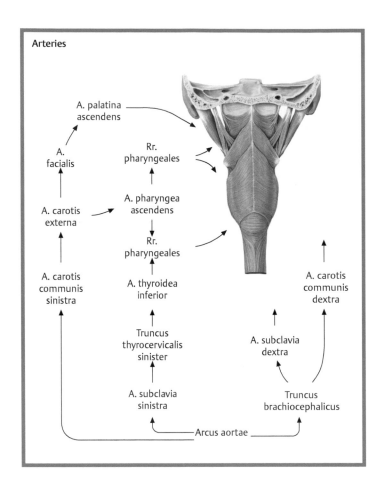

Arteries

- A. palatina ascendens
- A. facialis
- Rr. pharyngeales
- A. carotis externa
- A. pharyngea ascendens
- Rr. pharyngeales
- A. carotis communis sinistra
- A. thyroidea inferior
- A. carotis communis dextra
- Truncus thyrocervicalis sinister
- A. subclavia dextra
- A. subclavia sinistra
- Truncus brachiocephalicus
- Arcus aortae

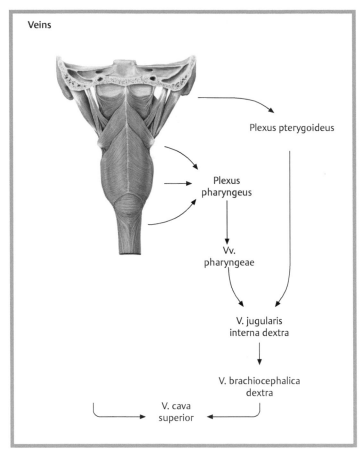

Veins

- Plexus pterygoideus
- Plexus pharyngeus
- Vv. pharyngeae
- V. jugularis interna dextra
- V. brachiocephalica dextra
- V. cava superior

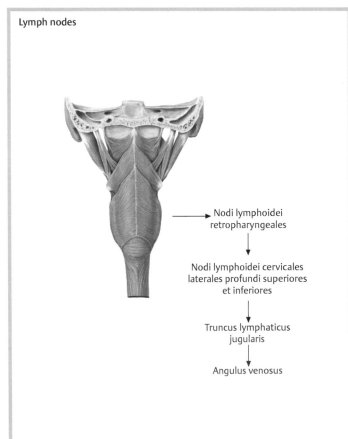

Lymph nodes

- Nodi lymphoidei retropharyngeales
- Nodi lymphoidei cervicales laterales profundi superiores et inferiores
- Truncus lymphaticus jugularis
- Angulus venosus

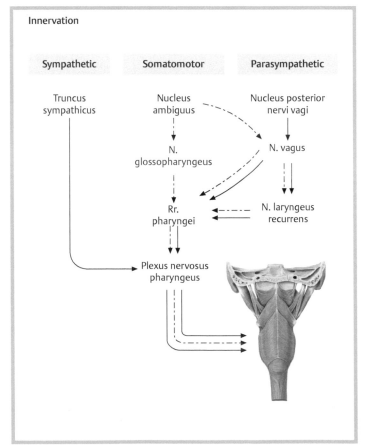

Innervation

Sympathetic	Somatomotor	Parasympathetic
Truncus sympathicus	Nucleus ambiguus	Nucleus posterior nervi vagi
	N. glossopharyngeus	N. vagus
	Rr. pharyngei	N. laryngeus recurrens
	Plexus nervosus pharyngeus	

*Posterior view

Appendix

References

Abboud B. Anatomie topographique et vascularisation artérielle de parathyroides. Presse Med 1996; 25: 1156–61

Anschütz F. Die körperliche Untersuchung. 3. Aufl. Heidelberg: Springer; 1978

Barr ML, Kiernan JA. The Human Nervous System. 5th ed. Philadelphia: JB Lippincott; 1988

Bähr M, Frotscher M. Neurologisch-topische Diagnostik. 10. Aufl. Stuttgart: Thieme; 2014

Bear MF, Connors BW, Paradiso MA. Neuroscience. Exploring the Brain. 2. Aufl. Baltimore: Williams u. Wilkins; 2000

Becker W, Naumann HH, Pfaltz CR. Hals-Nasen-Ohren-Heilkunde. 2. Aufl. Stuttgart: Thieme; 1983

Becker W, Naumann HH, Pfaltz CR. Ear, Nose and Throat Diseases. 2. Aufl. Stuttgart: Thieme; 1994

Berghaus A, Rettinger G, Böhme G. Hals-Nasen-Ohren-Heilkunde. Duale Reihe. Stuttgart: Thieme; 1996

Blum HE, Müller-Wieland D (Hrsg.). Klinische Pathophysiologie. 10. Aufl. Stuttgart: Thieme; 2018

Bossy JG, Ferratier R. Studies of the spinal cord of Galago senegalensis, compared to that in man. J Comp Neurol 1968 Mar; 132(3): 485–98. PubMed PMID: 5657526

Braak H, Braak E. Neuroanatomie. In: Beyreuther K, Einhäupl KM, Förstl H, Kurz A, Hrsg. Demenzen. Stuttgart: Thieme; 2002: 118–129

Braus DF. EinBlick ins Gehirn. 3. Aufl. Stuttgart: Thieme; 2014

Calabria G, Rolando M. Strutture e funzioni del film lacrimale. Genua: Proceedings of the 6th Symposium of the Italian Ophthalmological Society (S.O.I.); 1984: 9–35

Camper P. De Hominis Varietate (1792). Deutsche Fassung von S. Th. Sömmering (nach Kobes LWR. Quellenstudie zu Petrus Camper und der nach ihm benannten Schädelebene). Dtsch Zahnärztl Z; 1983: 38: 268–270

Carlsson GE, Haraldson T, Mohl ND. The dentition. In Mohl ND, Zarb GH, Carlsson GE, Rugh JD. A Textbook of Occlusion. Chicago: Quintessence Books; 1988

Chandrashekar J, Hoon MA, Ryba NJ, Zuker CS. The receptors and cells for mammalian taste. Nature 2006; 444: 288–294

Da Costa S, van der Zwaag W, Marques JP, Frackowiak RS, Clarke S, Saenz M. Human primary auditory cortex follows the shape of Heschl's gyrus. J Neurosci. 2011 Oct 5; 31(40): 14067–75. PubMed PMID: 21976491.

Dauber W. Bild-Lexikon der Anatomie. 10. Aufl. Stuttgart: Thieme; 2008

Faller A, Schüke M. Der Köper des Menschen. 17. Aufl. Stuttgart: Thieme; 2016

Frick H, Leonhardt H, Starck D. Allgemeine und spezielle Anatomie. Taschenlehrbuch der gesamten Anatomie. Bd. 1 und 2. 4. Aufl. Stuttgart: Thieme; 1992

Fritsch H, Künel W. Taschenatlas der Anatomie. Bd. 2. 11. Aufl. Stuttgart: Thieme; 2013

Füß H S, Middecke M. Anamnese und klinische Untersuchung. 6. Aufl. Stuttgart: Thieme; 2018

Gehlen W, Delank HW. Neurologie. 12. Aufl. Stuttgart: Thieme; 2010

Harvey R. et al. The Olfactory Strip and Its Presvervation in Endoscopic Pituitary Surgery Maintains Smell and Sinonasal Function. In: Neurolog. Surg. B 2015; 76(06): 464-470

Hegglin J. Chirurgische Untersuchung. Stuttgart: Thieme; 1976 Hempelmann G, Krier C, Schulte am Esch J, Hrsg. Gesamtreihe ains. 4 Bäde. Stuttgart: Thieme; 2001

Herrick J C. Brains of Rats and Men. Chicago: University of Chicago Press; 1926

Holodny et al. Diffusion tensor tractography of the motor white matter tracts in man–Current controversies and future directions. Ann N Y Acad Sci 2005; 1064: 88–7

Ingvar D H. Functional landscapes of the dominant hemisphere. Brain Res 1976; 107: 181–97

Jäig W. Visceral afferent neurones: Neuroanatomy and functions, organ regulations and sensations. In: Vaitl D, Schandry R, eds. From the heart to the brain. Frankfurt am Main: Peter Lang; 1995: 5–4

Kahle W, Frotscher M. Taschenatlas der Anatomie. Bd. 3. 11. Aufl. Stuttgart: Thieme; 2013

Kell Ch A, von Kriegstein K, Rösler A, Kleinschmidt A, Laufs H. The Sensory Cortical Representation of the Human Penis: Revisiting Somatotopy in the Male Homunculus. J Neurosci Jun 2005; 25: 5984–987

Kim et al. Corticospinal tract location in internal capsule of human brain: diffusion tensor tractography and functional MRI study. Neuroreport 2008; Vol 19, No 8

Kunze K. Lehrbuch der Neurologie. Stuttgart: Thieme; 1992

Kuwert T, Grüwald F, Haberkorn U, Krause T. Nuklearmedizin. 4. Aufl. Stuttgart: Thieme; 2008

Lang, G. Augenheilkunde. 5. Aufl. Stuttgart: Thieme; 2014

Lehmann KM, Hellwig E, Wenz H-J. Zahnäztliche Propäeutik. 13. Aufl. Kön: Deutscher Zahnäzte Verlag; 2015

Lippert H, Pabst R. Arterial Variations in Man. Müchen: Bergman; 1985

Lorke D. Schmerzrelevante Neuroanatomie. In: Beck H, Martin E,

Motsch J, Schulte am Esch J, Hrsg. ains. Bd. 4. Schmerztherapie. Stuttgart: Thieme; 2001: 13–8

Masuhr K F, Neumann M. Neurologie. Duale Reihe. 7. Aufl. Stuttgart: Thieme; 2013

Maurer J. Neuroootologie. Stuttgart: Thieme; 1999

Meyer W. Die Zahn-Mund-und Kiefer-Heilkunde. Bd. 1. München: Urban & Schwarzenberg; 1958

Mülreiter F. Anatomie des menschlichen Gebisses. Leipzig: Felix; 1912

Müler-Vahl H, Mumenthaler M, Stör M. Läionen peripherer Nerven und radikuläe Syndrome. 10. Aufl. Stuttgart: Thieme; 2014

Nieuwenhuys R, Voogd J, van Huijzen Chr. Das Zentralnervensystem des Menschen. 2. Aufl. Berlin: Springer; 1991

Pape HC, Kurtz A, Silbernagl S. Physiologie. 8. Aufl. Stuttgart: Thieme; 2018

Platzer W. Atlas der topografischen Anatomie. Stuttgart: Thieme; 1982

Poeck K, Hartje W. Stöungen von Antrieb und Affektivitä. In: Hartje W, Poeck K, Hrsg. Klinische Neuropsychologie. 5. Aufl. Stuttgart: Thieme; 2002: 412–22

Poisel S, Golth D. Zur Variabilitä der großn Arterien im Trigonum caroticum. Wiener medizinische Wochenschrift 1974; 124: 229–32

Probst R, Grevers G, Iro H. Hals-Nasen-Ohren-Heilkunde. 3. Aufl. Stuttgart: Thieme; 2008

Rauber/Kopsch. Anatomie des Menschen. Bd. 1–4. Stuttgart: Thieme; Bd. 1, 2. Aufl.; 1997, Bd. 2 und 3; 1987, Bd. 4; 1988

Robbins KT, Medina JE, Wolfe GT, Levine PA, Sessions RB, Pruet CW. Standardizing neck dissection terminology. Official report of the Academy's Committee for Head and Neck Surgery and Oncology. Arch Otolaryngol Head Neck Surg 1991 Jun;117(6): 601-5. PubMed PMID: 2036180

Rohkamm R. Taschenatlas Neurologie. 4. Aufl. Stuttgart: Thieme; 2017

Romer A S, Parson TS. Vergleichende Anatomie der Wirbeltiere. 5. Aufl. Hamburg und Berlin: Paul Parey; 1983

Sachsenweger M. Augenheilkunde. 2. Aufl. Stuttgart: Thieme; 2003

Sadler T W. Medizinische Embryologie. 12. Aufl. Stuttgart: Thieme; 2014

Scheibel M E, Scheibel A B. Activity cycles in neurons of the reticular formation. Recent Adv Biol Psychiatry. 1965; 8: 283–93

Schmidt F. Zur Innervation der Articulatio temporomandibularis. Gegenbaurs morphol Jb 1967; 110: 554–573

Schroeder H E. Orale Strukturbiologie. 3. Aufl. Stuttgart: Thieme; 1987

Schumacher G H: Funktionelle Anatomie des orofazialen Systems. Heidelberg: Hüthig; 1985

Schumacher G H, Aumüller G. Topographische Anatomie des Menschen. 6. Aufl. Stuttgart: G. Fischer; 1994

Schumacher GH, Schmidt H. Anatomie und Biochemie der Zähne. Stuttgart: G. Fischer; 1976

Siegenthaler W. Klinische Pathophysiologie. 8. Aufl. Stuttgart: Thieme; 2000

Stammberger H, Hawke M. Essentials of functional endoscopic sinus surgery. 2. Aufl. St. Louis: Mosby; 1993

Steiniger B, Schwarzbach H, Stachniss, V. Mikroskopische Anatomie der Zähne und des Parodonts. Stuttgart: Thieme; 2010

Stoppe G, Hentschel F, Munz DL. Bildgebende Verfahren in der Psychiatrie. Stuttgart: Thieme; 2000

Strup JR, Türp JC, Witkowski S, Hürzeler MB, Kern M. Curriculum Prothetik (Band I). 2. Aufl. Berlin Quintessenz 1999

Tillmann B. Farbatlas der Anatomie Zahnmedizin-Humanmedizin. Stuttgart: Thieme; 1997

Töndury G. Angewandte und topographische Anatomie. 5. Aufl. Stuttgart: Thieme; 1981

Vahlensieck M, Reiser M. MRT des Bewegungsapparates. 4. Aufl. Stuttgart: Thieme; 2014

Van Aken H, Wulf H (Hrsg.). Lokalanästhesie, Regionalanästhesie, Regionale Schmerztherapie. begr. von HCh Niesel. 3. Aufl. Stuttgart: Thieme; 2010

von Lanz T, Wachsmuth W. Praktische Anatomie. Bd. 1/1B Kopf. Gehirnund Augenschädel. Berlin: Springer; 2004

von Lanz T, Wachsmuth W. In: von Loeweneck u Feifel, Hrsg. Praktische Anatomie. Bd. 2, 6. Teil. Berlin: Springer; 1993

von Lanz T, Wachsmuth W. Praktische Anatomie. Bd. 1/2. Hals, Berlin: Springer; 1955

von Spee Graf F. Die Verschiebungsbahn des Unterkiefers am Schädel. Arch Anat Entwicklungsgesch. 1890; 285–294

Warshawsky H. The teeth. In Weiss L. Cell and Tissue Biology – a textbook of histology. 6. Aufl. München: Urban & Schwarzenberg; 1988

Wolpert L, Beddington R, Brockes J, Jessel T, Lawrence P, Meyerowitz E. Entwicklungsbiologie. Weinheim: Spektrum Verlag; 1999

Subject Index